W9-BSA-244

VASCULAR DIAGNOSIS

VASCULAR DIAGNOSIS

M. Ashraf Mansour, MD, RVT, FACS

Associate Professor of Surgery
Program Director, Vascular Surgery
Michigan State University
Grand Rapids Medical Education and Research Center
Grand Rapids, Michigan

Nicos Labropoulos, PhD, DIC, RVT

Associate Professor of Surgery
Director, Vascular Laboratory
Loyola University Chicago
Stritch School of Medicine
Maywood, Illinois

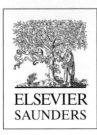

ELSEVIER
SAUNDERS

ELSEVIER
SAUNDERS

An Imprint of Elsevier

The Curtis Center
170 S Independence Mall W 300E
Philadelphia, Pennsylvania 19106

VASCULAR DIAGNOSIS   ISBN: 0-721-69426-8

Copyright © 2005, Elsevier Inc. All rights reserved.

No part of this publication may be reproduced or transmitted in any form or by any means, electronic or mechanical, including photocopying, recording, or any information storage and retrieval system, without permission in writing from the publisher. Permissions may be sought directly from Elsevier's Health Sciences Rights Department in Philadelphia, PA, USA: phone: (+1) 215 238 7869, fax: (+1) 215 238 2239, e-mail: healthpermissions@elsevier.com. You may also complete your request on-line via the Elsevier homepage (http://www.elsevier.com), by selecting 'Customer Support' and then 'Obtaining Permissions.'

NOTICE

Vascular Surgery is an ever-changing field. Standard safety precautions must be followed, but as new research and clinical experience broaden our knowledge, changes in treatment and drug therapy may become necessary or appropriate. Readers are advised to check the most current product information provided by the manufacturer of each drug to be administered to verify the recommended dose, the method and duration of administration, and contraindications. It is the responsibility of the licensed prescriber, relying on experience and knowledge of the patient, to determine dosages and the best treatment for each individual patient. Neither the publisher nor the authors assume any liability for any injury and/or damage to persons or property arising from this publication.

Previous edition copyrighted 1994.

Library of Congress Cataloging-in-Publication Data

Vascular diagnosis/[edited by] M. Ashraf Mansour, Nicos Labropoulos. – 1st ed.
     p.; cm.
    Includes bibliographical references and index.
    ISBN 0-7216-9426-8
     1. Blood-vessels—Diseases—Diagnosis.   2. Blood-vessels—Surgery.   I. Mansour, M.
  Ashraf.   II. Labropoulos, Nicos.
    [DNLM: 1. Vascular Diseases—diagnosis.   2. Diagnostic Imaging—methods.
   3. Diagnostic Techniques, Cardiovascular. WG 500 V33121 2004]
    RC691.5.V365 2004
    616.1′3–dc22   2004042977

Acquisitions Editor: Hilarie Surrena
Developmental Editor: Donna L. Morrissey
Project Manager: Mary Stermel

Printed in China

Last digit is the print number: 9 8 7 6 5 4 3 2 1

Dedication

Vascular Diagnosis is dedicated to our parents and families who supported us.

Contributors

Ali F. AbuRahma, MD
Professor of Surgery and Chief of Vascular Surgery,
Department of Surgery, Robert C. Byrd Health Sciences Center
of West Virginia University; Medical Director, Vascular Laboratory,
Charleston Area Medical Center; Charleston, West Virginia

Samuel S. Ahn, MD
Clinical Professor of Surgery, University of California, Los Angeles,
Los Angeles, California

Enrico Ascher, MD
Chief, Vascular Surgery, Division of Vascular Surgery,
Maimonides Medical Center, Brooklyn, New York

J. Dennis Baker, MD
Professor, Department of Surgery, David Geffen School of Medicine
at UCLA; Chief, Vascular Surgery Section, Department of Surgery,
VA Medical Center; Los Angeles, California

William H. Baker, MD, FACS
Professor Emeritus, Surgery, Stritch School of Medicine,
Loyola University of Chicago, Maywood, Illinois

Hisham Bassiouny, MD
Professor, Vascular Surgery, and Director, Vascular Laboratory,
Department of Surgery, University of Chicago, Chicago, Illinois

Kirk W. Beach, PhD, MD
Research Professor, Department of Surgery,
University of Washington, Seattle, Washington

Phillip J. Bendick, PhD
Director, Peripheral Vascular Diagnostic Center;
Director of Surgical Research, William Beaumont Hospital;
Royal Oak, Michigan

Marshall E. Benjamin, MD
Associate Professor of Surgery, University of Maryland School
of Medicine, Baltimore, Maryland; Chief of Surgery,
North Arundel Hospital, Glen Burnie, Maryland

George Berdejo, BA, RVT
Technical Director, Vascular Laboratories, Montefiore Hospital;
Weiler Hospital; and Albert Einstein College of Medicine,
New York, New York

Luke P. Brewster, MD
Resident, General Surgery, Loyola University Medical Center,
Maywood, Illinois

Marc Cairols, MD, FRCS (London), PhD
Professor of Surgery, University of Barcelona;
Chief, Department of Vascular Surgery,
Hospital Universitari de Bellvitge; Catalonia, Spain

Sandra C. Carr, MD
Assistant Professor, Department of Surgery, Univer-
sity of Wisconsin School of Medicine, Madison,
Wisconsin

John J. Castronuovo, Jr., MD
Clinical Professor of Surgery, University of Medicine and Dentistry,
New Jersey Medical School, Newark, New Jersey; Chairman,
Division of Vascular Surgery and Director of Noninvasive
Vascular Laboratory, Morristown Memorial Hospital, Morristown,
New Jersey

Joaquim J. Cerveira, MD
Assistant Professor of Surgery, Department of Surgery,
UMDNJ–New Jersey Medical School, Newark, New Jersey

Benjamin B. Chang, MD
Assistant Professor, Department of Surgery,
Albany Medical School; Attending Vascular Surgeon,
Department of Surgery–Vascular Surgery,
Albany Medical Center Hospital;
Albany, New York

Vasana Cheanvechai, MD
Assistant Professor of Surgery, University of Maryland School of
Medicine, Baltimore, Maryland

Jeremy Collins, BS
Department of Radiology, Feinberg School of Medicine,
Northwestern University, Chicago, Illinois

Robert F. Cuff, MD
Clinical Instructor, Department of Surgery,
Michigan State University, East Lansing, Michigan

Ronald L. Dalman, MD
Associate Professor of Surgery, Department of Surgery,
Division of Vascular Surgery, Stanford University School
of Medicine, Stanford, California; Chief, Vascular Surgery,
Surgical Service, Veterans Affairs Palo Alto Health Care System,
Palo Alto, California

R. Clement Darling III, MD
Professor, Department of Surgery, Albany Medical College;
Chief, Division of Vascular Surgery, Albany
Medical Center Hospital;
Albany, New York

Diana Eastridge, MS, RN/CNP
Nurse Practitioner, Division of Vascular Surgery,
Northwestern Memorial Hospital, Chicago, Illinois

Victor Erzurum, MD
The Cleveland Clinic, Beachwood Family Health and Surgery Center,
Beachwood, Ohio

Julie Ann Freischlag, MD
William Stewart Halsted Professor, Chair, Department of Surgery,
and Surgeon in Chief, Johns Hopkins Medical Institutions,
Baltimore, Maryland

George Geroulakos, MD, FRCS, DIC, PhD
Senior Lecturer in Vascular Surgery, Imperial College of Science
Technology and Medicine; Consultant Vascular Surgeon,
Charing Cross and Ealing Hospital; London, United Kingdom

Peter Gloviczki, MD
Professor of Surgery, Mayo Clinic College of Medicine; Chair,
Division of Vascular Surgery and Director, Gonda Vascular Center,
Mayo Clinic; Rochester, Minnesota

Maura Griffin, MSc, DIC, PhD
Chief Vascular Ultrasonographer, The Vascular Noninvasive
Screening and Diagnostic Centre, London, United Kingdom

Thomas M. Grist, MD
Professor, Department of Radiology, University of Wisconsin School
of Medicine, Madison, Wisconsin

Jennifer K. Grogan, MD
Research Fellow, Department of Surgery, University of Chicago,
Chicago, Illinois

Brian G. Halloran, MD
Adjunct Clinical Assistant Professor of Surgery, University of Michigan;
Attending Vascular Surgeon, St. Joseph Mercy Hospital; Ann Arbor,
Michigan

John Preston Harris, MD, FRACS, FRCS, FACS, DDU
Professor of Vascular Surgery, University of Sydney; Head,
Division of Surgery and Director, Vascular Laboratory,
Royal Prince Alfred Hospital; Sydney, Australia

Jennifer Heller, MD
Assistant Professor of Surgery, Johns Hopkins School of Medicine;
Assistant Professor of Surgery, Johns Hopkins Bayview Medical
Center; Baltimore, Maryland

Anil Hingorani, MD
Vascular Surgeon, Division of Vascular Surgery,
Maimonides Medical Center, Brooklyn, New York

Kim J. Hodgson , MD
Professor and Chair, Division of Vascular Surgery,
Southern Illinois University School of Medicine, Springfield, Illinois

Douglas B. Hood, MD
Assistant Professor of Surgery and Radiology,
University of Southern California, Keck School of Medicine,
Los Angeles, California

Bonnie Johnson, RDMS, RVT, FSVU
Director, Vascular Laboratory Services, Division of Vascular Surgery,
Stanford University Medical Center, Stanford, California

Stavros K. Kakkos, MD, MSc
Department of Vascular Surgery, Faculty of Medicine,
Imperial College, London, United Kingdom

Steven S. Kang, MD
Vascular Surgeon, Miami Cardiac and Vascular Institute,
Baptist Health South Florida, Miami, Florida

Kenneth K. Kao
Department of Surgery, UCLA, Los Angeles, California

John K. Karwowski, MD
Vascular Surgery Fellow, Department of Surgery,
Division of Vascular Surgery, Stanford University School of Medicine,
Stanford, California

Sandra L. Katanick, RN, RVT, FSVU, CAE
Executive Director, Intersocietal Accreditation Commission,
Columbia, Maryland

Jenifer Kidd, RVT, DMU, AMS
Emeritus Director, Camperdown Vascular Laboratory, Sydney,
Australia

Mark J. W. Koelemaij, MD, PhD
Vascular Surgery Fellow and Clinical Epidemiologist,
Academic Medical Center, University of Amsterdam, Amsterdam,
The Netherlands

George E. Kopchok, BS
Department of Surgery, Harbor-UCLA Medical Center, Torrance,
California

Paul B. Kreienberg, MD
Assistant Professor, Department of Surgery, Albany Medical College;
Attending Vascular Surgeon, Department of Surgery–Vascular Surgery,
Albany Medical Center Hospital; Albany, New York

Efthyvoulos Kyriakou
Department of Computational Intelligence, The Cyprus Institute of
Neurology and Genetics, Nicosia, Cyprus

Nicos Labropoulos, PhD, DIC, RVT
Associate Professor of Surgery, Director, Vascular Laboratory,
Loyola University Chicago, Stritch School of Medicine,
Maywood, Illinois

Brajesh K. Lal, MD
Assistant Professor, Surgery–Division of Vascular Surgery,
UMDNJ–New Jersey Medical School, Newark, New Jersey

Everett Y. Lam, MD
Resident, Division of Vascular Surgery, Oregon Health & Sciences
University, Portland, Oregon

Jason T. Lee, MD
Vascular Surgery Fellow, Division of Vascular Surgery,
Stanford University Medical Center, Stanford, California

Dink A. Legemate, MD, PhD
Professor of Vascular Surgery and Clinical Epidemiologist,
Academic Medical Center, University of Amsterdam, Amsterdam,
The Netherlands

Luis R. Leon, Jr., MD, RVT
Peripheral Vascular Surgery Fellow, Loyola University Medical Center,
Maywood, Illinois

Fred N. Littooy, MD
Professor of Surgery, Loyola University Medical Center,
Loyola University School of Medicine, Maywood, Illinois

Joann Lohr, MD
Director, John J. Cranley Vascular Laboratory,
Good Samaritan Hospital, Cincinnati, Ohio

Thanila A. Macedo, MD
Instructor in Radiology, Mayo Clinic College of Medicine;
Senior Associate Consultant, Mayo Clinic, Rochester, Minnesota

M. Ashraf Mansour, MD, RVT, FACS
Associate Professor of Surgery, Program Director, Vascular Surgery,
Michigan State University, Grand Rapids Medical Education and
Research Center, Grand Rapids, Michigan

Natalia Markevich, MD, RVT
Division of Vascular Surgery, Maimonides Medical Center,
Brooklyn, New York

Jon S. Matsumura, MD
Associate Professor of Surgery, Northwestern University Feinberg
School of Medicine; Active Staff, Northwestern Memorial Hospital;
Active Staff and Chief of Vascular Surgery, Chicago VA Healthcare
System Westside; Chicago, Illinois

James May, MD, MS, FRACS, FACS
Bosch Professor of Surgery, University of Sydney; Vascular Surgeon,
Royal Prince Alfred Hospital; Sydney, Australia

Manish Mehta, MD, MPH
Assistant Professor, Department of Surgery, Albany Medical College;
Attending Vascular Surgeon, Department of Surgery–Vascular Surgery,
Albany Medical Center Hospital; Albany, New York

Mark H. Meissner, MD
Associate Professor, Vascular Surgery, and Acting Instructor,
Interventional Radiology, University of Washington School of
Medicine, Seattle, Washington

Joseph L. Mills, Sr., MD
Professor of Surgery, University of Arizona Health Sciences Center;
Chief, Division of Vascular and Endovascular Surgery and Director,
Noninvasive Vascular Laboratory, University Physicians, Inc;
Tucson, Arizona

Gregory L. Moneta, MD
Professor of Surgery and Chief, Vascular Surgery,
Oregon Health & Science University, Portland, Oregon

Samuel R. Money, MD
Clinical Associate Professor of Surgery, Tulane University School
of Medicine; Head, Section of Vascular Surgery,
Ochsner Clinic Foundation; New Orleans, Louisiana

Mark D. Morasch, MD
Assistant Professor of Surgery, Division of Vascular Surgery,
Feinberg School of Medicine, Northwestern University; Attending
Surgeon, Northwestern Memorial Hospital; Chicago, Illinois

Terry Needham, RVT, FSVT
Director, Heart and Vascular Department, Erlanger Health System,
Chattanooga, Tennessee

Stephen C. Nicholls, MD
Associate Professor, Department of Surgery, Division of
Vascular Surgery, University of Washington School of Medicine;
Chief of Vascular Surgery, Harborview Medical Center; Seattle,
Washington

Andrew Nicolaides, MD, FRCS
Emeritus Professor of Vascular Surgery, Imperial College;
Honorary Consultant Surgeon, Ealing Hospital; London,
United Kingdom; Specialist Scientist, Department of Biological
Sciences, University of Cyprus, Nicosia, Cyprus

Paul J. Nordness, MD
Fellow, Section of Vascular Surgery, Ochsner Clinic Foundation,
New Orleans, Louisiana

Gustavo S. Oderich, MD
Vascular Surgery Fellow, Mayo Clinic College of Medicine,
Rochester, Minnesota

Kathleen J. Ozsvath, MD
Assistant Professor, Department of Surgery–Vascular Surgery,
Albany Medical College; Attending Vascular Surgeon,
Department of Surgery, Albany Medical Center Hospital;
Albany, New York

Jean M. Panneton, MD
Associate Professor of Surgery, Mayo Medical School;
Consultant, Director of Clinical Research, Mayo Clinic
and Mayo Foundation; Rochester, Minnesota

Peter J. Pappas, MD
Chief, Section of Vascular Surgery at University Hospital,
Department of Surgery, Division of Vascular Surgery,
UMDNJ–New Jersey Medical School, Newark, New Jersey

Sheela T. Patel, MD
Senior Fellow, Vascular Surgery and Endovascular Surgery,
University of Arizona Health Sciences Center, Tucson, Arizona

Philip S. K. Paty, MD
Associate Professor, Department of Surgery, Albany Medical College;
Attending Vascular Surgeon, Department of Surgery–Vascular Surgery,
Albany Medical Center Hospital; Albany, New York

William H. Pearce, MD
Violet R. and Charles A. Baldwin Professor of Vascular Surgery,
Department of Surgery, Northwestern University,
Feinberg School of Medicine; Chief, Division of Vascular Surgery,
Department of Surgery, Northwestern Memorial Hospital;
Chicago, Illinois

Brian G. Peterson, MD
General Surgery Resident, Department of Surgery, McGaw
Medical Center, Northwestern University, Chicago, Illinois

Michael A. Ricci, MD
Roger H. Allbee Professor of Surgery, Division of Vascular Surgery,
University of Vermont College of Medicine, Burlington, Vermont

Sean P. Roddy, MD
Assistant Professor, Department of Surgery, Albany Medical College;
Attending Vascular Surgeon, Department of Surgery–Vascular Surgery,
Albany Medical Center Hospital; Albany, New York

Heron E. Rodriguez, MD
Assistant Professor of Surgery and Radiology,
Loyola University Stritch School of Medicine; Attending Surgeon,
Loyola University Medical Center; Maywood, Illinois

Robert B. Rutherford, MD, FACS, FRCS(G)
Emeritus Professor of Surgery, University of Colorado School
of Medicine, Denver, Colorado

Sergio X. Salles-Cunha, PhD, RVT, FSVU
Technical Director, The Vascular Institute of New York,
Maimonides Medical Center, Brooklyn, New York

Russell H. Samson, MD, FACS, RVT
President, Mote Vascular Foundation, Inc., Sarasota, Florida

Gretchen Schwarze, MD
Clinical Associate, Department of Surgery, University of Chicago,
Chicago, Illinois

Dhiraj M. Shah, MD
Professor of Surgery, Department of Surgery, Albany Medical College;
Director, Institute for Vascular Health and Disease, Albany Medical
Center Hospital; Albany, New York

Maureen K. Sheehan, MD
Vascular Surgery Fellow, University of Pittsburgh Medical Center,
Pittsburgh, Pennsylvania

Gail P. Size, RVT, RVS, RCVT, FSVU
President, Inside Ultrasound, Inc., Pearce, Arizona

Timothy M. Sullivan, MD
Senior Associate Consultant, Divisions of Vascular Surgery and
Interventional Radiology, Mayo Clinic; Associate Professor of Surgery,
Mayo Medical School; Vascular Surgeon, Saint Marys Hospital,
Mayo Medical Center; Rochester, Minnesota

Algirdas Edvardas Tamosiunas, MD, PhD, RVT, RDMS
Associate Research Professor, Clinic of Gastroenterology and
Abdominal Surgery, Faculty of Medicine, Vilnius University;
Director, Vascular Laboratory, Vilnius University Hospital
Santariskiu Klinikos; Vilnius, Lithuania

Apostolos K. Tassiopoulos, MD
Clinical Assistant Professor, Department of Cardiovascular Surgery,
Rush Medical College; Senior Attending, Department of Surgery,
Division of Vascular Surgery, The John H. Stroger Jr. Hospital of
Cook County; Chicago, Illinois

William D. Turnipseed, MD
Preceptor, Volunteer Staff, Surgery, University of Wisconsin School
of Medicine, Madison, Wisconsin

Frank Veith, MD
Professor of Surgery, Montefiore Hospital of the Albert Einstein
College of Medicine; Vice Chairman, Department of Surgery and
William von Liebig Chair of Vascular Surgery, Montefiore Hospital;
New York, New York

Reese A. Wain, MD
Attending Surgeon, Vascular Surgery, Winthrop University Hospital,
Mineola, New York; Attending Surgeon, Stony Brook University,
Stony Brook, New York

Fred A. Weaver, MD
Professor and Chief, Division of Vascular Surgery,
University of Southern California, Keck School of Medicine,
Los Angeles, California

Franklin W. West, BSN, RN, RVT, RVS, CCP
Director of Professional Services, Pacific Vascular Inc.,
Bothell, Washington

Geoffrey H. White, MD, FRACS
Associate Professor of Surgery, University of Sydney; Head,
Department of Vascular Surgery, Royal Prince Alfred Hospital;
Sydney, Australia

Rodney White, MD
Professor of Surgery, UCLA School of Medicine, Los Angeles,
California; Chief, Vascular Surgery and Associate Chair,
Department of Surgery, Harbor–UCLA Medical Center, Torrance,
California

James S. T. Yao, MD, PhD
Magerstadt Professor of Surgery, Division of Vascular Surgery,
Feinberg School of Medicine, Northwestern University;
Attending Surgeon, Division of Vascular Surgery,
Northwestern Memorial Hospital; Attending Surgeon,
Division of Vascular Surgery, Department of Veterans Affairs
Hospital; Chicago, Illinois

R. Eugene Zierler, MD
Professor of Surgery, Department of Surgery,
University of Washington; Medical Director,
Vascular Diagnostic Service, University of Washington Medical
Center; Seattle, Washington

Robert M. Zwolak, MD, PhD
Professor of Surgery, Dartmouth Medical School;
Attending Vascular Surgeon and Medical Director,
Noninvasive Vascular Laboratory,
Dartmouth Hitchcock Medical Center; Lebanon, New Hampshire

Preface

Disorders of arteries and veins are prevalent in our society. The selection of appropriate tests supplements careful physical examination and completes the clinical evaluation of patients with vascular disease. *Vascular Diagnosis* is about the detection and management of vascular disease. The field is rapidly expanding, and technological innovations are occurring with regularity. Refinements in imaging equipment and software are being introduced at a steady pace, making it difficult to stay current. At the same time, vascular laboratories have proliferated nationwide to fill the needs of patients and physicians. Demand for experienced vascular technologists has increased. Meanwhile, concerns about the quality of work in some of these diagnostic centers have led some to demand stricter supervision by regulatory bodies. It is estimated that there are more than 10,000 vascular laboratories in North America; however, only one fifth have received certification by the Intersocietal Commission for the Accreditation of Vascular Laboratories. This book is intended to provide a comprehensive overview of the diagnosis of vascular disease and a source of information on establishing and maintaining an accredited vascular laboratory.

The last edition of *Vascular Diagnosis* was edited by the late Eugene Bernstein, MD, and published by Mosby in 1993. Dr. Bernstein conceived the idea of publishing a book dedicated to the noninvasive diagnosis of vascular disease in conjunction with a postgraduate course that assembled experts from around the world. The course and the book were very successful, and the latter was considered by many to be the standard in the field. In the last decade, many changes and innovations have occurred in the diagnosis and treatment of vascular disease. Endovascular repair of aortic aneurysms is now a commonly performed operation. Carotid stenting will soon be approved as an accepted modality to treat carotid stenosis. Endovenous procedures with laser or radiofrequency are gaining widespread acceptance. As devices become smaller, minimally invasive techniques are facilitated. Patients and practitioners are constantly demanding less invasive techniques and shorter hospital stays. It is now commonplace to have patients discharged on the following day after endovascular abdominal aortic aneurysm repair or a carotid intervention. In that last edition, Dr. Bernstein stated: "Rapid and profound strides have been made since the first edition of this book...." Indeed, much has changed in this last decade.

Physicians from multiple backgrounds and specialties are now involved in the diagnosis of vascular disease. The concept of the "vascular center"—embracing specialists from different training paradigms to treat patients with vascular disease—is promulgated as the right model for the present and future. As public awareness of vascular disease increases, a growing number of patients are seeking to be screened and educated about their atherosclerotic risk factors and cardiovascular disease. The vascular laboratory is playing a central role in this revolution by providing fast and precise answers to frequent questions. The earlier version of the vascular laboratory relied on physiologic methods of blood flow measurement such as blood pressure and waveforms. Currently, there is more emphasis on imaging blood vessels and observing blood flow with ultrasound machines or with computed tomographic angiography and magnetic resonance angiography. By necessity, some of the tools we use every day are located outside the vascular laboratory; nevertheless, their inclusion in the discussion of vascular diagnosis is germane.

Vascular Diagnosis is organized into three major parts with over 50 chapters. Tables are used liberally, and we placed an emphasis on providing images, black and white as well as color, for illustration. The first part covers some fundamental issues related to the vascular laboratory and principles of vascular diagnosis. The second part has five sections concerned with imaging the various regions of the body. The third part contains a collection of miscellaneous topics such as coding and reimbursement and database maintenance.

M. Ashraf Mansour, MD

Nicos Labropoulos, PhD

Acknowledgments

The completion of this book would not have been possible without the help and advice of some of our colleagues and mentors, as well as many individuals who have contributed time and effort to see this project through.

Robert Rutherford, MD, David Sumner, MD, and William Baker, MD, offered suggestions and encouragement. Others have contributed chapters or made suggestions to make the book more user friendly. Many individuals at Elsevier, including Donna L. Morrissey, Joe Rusko, and Hilarie Surrena, helped in assembling the work and meeting our deadlines.

Contents

Part One

General Aspects

Chapter 1

Current Role of Vascular Diagnosis

JAMES S.T. YAO

Introduction

Disease of arteries and veins is common. The spectrum of disease includes peripheral arterial occlusive disease of arteries of the upper or lower extremity, aneurysm of the aorta or peripheral arteries, carotid stenosis predisposing to stroke, venous thromboembolism, chronic venous insufficiency, and varicose veins. This variety of disease processes signifies the magnitude of the knowledge base required by vascular surgeons to provide optimal care for these patients.

In recent years it has become apparent that peripheral arterial disease (PAD) is a manifestation of systemic atherosclerosis and that its association with strokes and myocardial infarction is common. Although the prevalence of PAD in Europe and North America is estimated at approximately 27 million people, PAD remains largely an underdiagnosed and undertreated disease.[1] Prevention of death from rupture of aortic aneurysm is best achieved by early detection with a screening program. Likewise, early detection of asymptomatic, hemodynamically significant carotid stenosis followed by carotid endarterectomy prevents fatal stroke. The current role of vascular diagnosis therefore must not be confined to diagnosis of symptomatic patients but must be extended to early detection. This chapter reviews the current noninvasive and imaging techniques available for diagnosis and early detection of vascular disease.

The Vascular Laboratory and Noninvasive Tests

Although a careful physical examination (e.g., palpation of pulse and auscultation to detect a bruit) is helpful to establish the diagnosis of PAD, there remains a need for simple tests to aid the clinical examination. It would be even more helpful if the test also served as an objective and physiologic test for documentation and validation of the diagnosis and treatment. The evolution of the vascular laboratory in the last three decades has brought hemodynamic information to the practice of vascular surgery.

Early instrumentation in the studying of peripheral circulation includes the use of the oscillometer or plethysmograph. Several pioneering surgeons (e.g., Robert

Linton, Fiorindo Simeone, Norman Freeman, and Edward Edwards) used these instruments to measure peripheral bloodflow in patients with peripheral arterial disease. Most early studies concentrated on digital pulse amplitude and skin flow, especially in relation to sympathetic control. The first laboratory specially designated for the study of human peripheral circulation was established by Linton and Simeone at Massachusetts General Hospital (MGH) in 1946.[2] Other laboratories that existed in the 1950s and 1960s include the office vascular laboratory of John Cranley at Good Samaritan Hospital in Cincinnati and the "blood flow laboratory" established by Prof. W.T. Irvine at St. Mary's Hospital in London, England. The laboratory used mainly strain-gauge plethysmography to measure muscle and skin flow in patients and to test the effect of various vasodilating agents.[3] All of these laboratories, however, are considered not to be clinical vascular laboratories but sites to perform studies on humans.

The era of noninvasive tests and the development of the vascular laboratory began with the introduction of better and more easy-to-use instrumentation including various types of plethysmographs, a pulse volume recorder, and the Doppler ultrasound (continuous-wave or pulsed). With Doppler ultrasound, ankle systolic pressure and its response to exercise can be recorded readily. The simplicity of the technique has made the Doppler ankle systolic pressure measurement a standard objective test not only for diagnosis but also to grade the degree of ischemia. Ankle brachial index (ABI), as suggested by Winsor in 1950, has also proved to be a sensitive marker for detection of PAD and is currently the most powerful prognostic indicator in PAD.[4] Many epidemiologic studies use ankle systolic pressure index instead of pulse examination. Interest in systolic pressure measurement also extended to segmental (thigh and calf) and digital (finger and toe) pressure for additional information. Penile pressure as a reflection of pelvic hemodynamics has been found to be of value to evaluate sexual function in aortoiliac disease and the effect of the disease after reconstructive surgery. Later, the use of directional Doppler to record analog flow velocity waveform from peripheral arteries was added to the examination. This technique brought flow velocity waveform, something traditionally only seen in physiology textbooks, to clinical use.

In the 1970s, vascular laboratory and noninvasive tests became the focus of many vascular surgeons. In 1971, using the pulse volume recorder, R. Clement Darling and Jeff Raines reopened the vascular laboratory at MGH for clinical use. Soon after, other centers such as Northwestern University Medical School in Chicago (J. Bergan and J. Yao), Good Samaritan Hospital in Cincinnati (J. Cranley), VA Hospital, University of Washington in Seattle (D.E. Strandness), Scripps Clinic in San Diego (E. Bernstein), University of Colorado in Denver (R. Rutherford and R. Kempczinski), and St. John's

Hospital in St. Louis (F. Hershey) also established hospital-based, fee-for-service vascular laboratories.[3,5,6]

In 1972, the Inter-Society Commission for Heart Disease Resources of the American Heart Association recognized the need to standardize the laboratory, and a committee was formed to study medical instrumentation in peripheral vascular disease.[7] The committee recommended that the establishment of a clinical laboratory in hospitals was desirable to provide studies vital to preoperative, intraoperative, and postoperative management of patients undergoing arterial reconstructive surgery and to provide service to patients suffering from venous thromboembolism. This important document provides the blueprint for many hospitals in the United States to establish a fee-for-service vascular laboratory.

The development of the vascular laboratory could not have been done without the help of technologists. In 1977, the Society of Vascular Technology was chartered during a symposium on noninvasive diagnostic techniques in vascular disease organized by Eugene Bernstein in San Diego. Since then, vascular surgeons working side-by-side with technologists have fully developed the vascular laboratory into what it is today. In earlier years, most techniques used were indirect tests (e.g., supraorbital Doppler or oculoplethysmograph for carotid stenosis, or impedance plethysmograph or phleborheograph for venous thrombosis).

The introduction of duplex scan in 1979 by D.E. Strandness and David Phillips changed the scene of noninvasive tests. The combination of real-time imaging and a pulse Doppler provided direct interrogation of flow velocity at selected areas within the artery and a B-mode image of the vessel. High-resolution B-mode image and spectral analysis then became a standard test to detect and to determine the degree of stenosis. Subsequent addition of a color-coded scanner has further expanded the use of duplex technology to instantaneously display direction of bloodflow. At present, duplex scan is the initial examination for patients suspected to have carotid artery stenosis, and the velocity criterion is helpful to grade the degree of stenosis. Duplex technology has now extended to examination of mesenteric circulation, the parenchymal flow of the renal arteries and the kidneys, the aortoiliac artery, and the femoropopliteal segment. Duplex ultrasound has also found its way to the operating room to provide surgeons with an instant assessment of the technical integrity of the reconstruction. Duplex technology also offers a surveillance program to monitor patency of an infrainguinal bypass or hemodialysis graft and to detect recurrent stenosis following carotid endarterectomy. Venous mapping by duplex adds a new dimension to the planning of bypass procedures. It is now also possible to assess the middle cerebral artery bloodflow and to detect emboli using the transcranial Doppler. For venous examination, duplex scan has almost completely replaced venography as the diagnostic test. For the first time we are now able to detect femoral venous valve competency and to quantitate venous reflux objectively in patients with chronic venous insufficiency. As a result of better direct ultrasound technology, indirect tests have vanished from the vascular laboratory.

Because of the dominant role of duplex ultrasound technology, the Society of Vascular Technology has changed its name to Society of Vascular Ultrasound. The Society has been active in quality control issues including a certifying examination for technologists, an accreditation process for vascular laboratories, educational courses for interpretation of various tests, and reimbursement issues.

At present, a vascular laboratory is an integral part of fee-for-service diagnostic service in any hospital providing care to patients suffering from vascular disease. It is estimated that close to 10,000 vascular laboratories exist in the United States, and of these, only 2400 are accredited.[6] Recognizing the importance of the vascular laboratory, noninvasive vascular testing is now designated (along with open surgery, endovascular surgery, medical management, and critical care) as one of the five components of training requirements and credentials for hospital privileges in vascular surgery.[8]

Images of Arteries and Veins

Acquisition of images of arteries or veins remains an important step in vascular diagnosis. In general, this can be achieved by arteriography, venography, high-resolution B-mode ultrasound, computed tomography (CT), or magnetic resonance image (MRI). Each technique has its appropriate indication and offers unique diagnostic information.

Arteriography and Venography

These two diagnostic tests have been the gold standard for a long time. Barney Brooks of Vanderbilt University performed the first arteriogram.[9] It was an arteriogram of a patient with femoral artery occlusion. Later, Reynaldo Dos Santos and colleagues of Portugal reported the use of translumbar aortogram to visualize the aorta and iliac arteries.[10] Since then, most arteriograms are done with direct puncture. The major breakthrough was in 1953, when Sven-Ivar Seldinger introduced the selective femoral retrograde catheter technique.[11] This technique, coupled with refinement of radiographic equipment and the development of better guidewires and catheters, has extended the examination to intracranial arteries, the mesenteric circulation, the renal arteries and branches, the arch of the aorta, the innominate artery, the subclavian artery and its branches, and the aorta and its peripheral branches.

Perhaps the most significant information obtained with arteriogram is the observation by M. DeBakey and colleagues.[12] He recognized that the atherosclerotic change of arteries is often segmental in nature and occurs either in the aortoiliac or femoropopliteal level. It is the recognition of segmental occlusion that led to the concept of bypass graft, thus beginning the era of reconstructive arterial surgery. At present, arteriography plays an important role in the planning of a bypass procedure. Similar to arteriography, ascending venography was a standard diagnostic test for deep-vein thrombosis until the introduction of the duplex scan. Venography, however, remains an important diagnostic tool to evaluate deep and superficial veins in patients with chronic venous insufficiency.

High-Resolution Ultrasound

After World War II, sonar made its way to medical use. Ultrasonography was first applied in obstetrics to measure the size of the fetal head by Ian Donald and T.G. Brown in 1961.[13] Subsequently, the technique was extended to the examination of solid organs. In vascular surgery, ultrasonography was first applied to image aortic aneurysms. Gradually the resolution of images improved, and the current high-resolution ultrasound provides excellent images of small arteries and their luminal characteristics. Calcification, atherosclerotic debris, thrombus, and intima-media thickness are additional information obtainable with high-resolution ultrasound. Many investigators also have found the determination of intima-media thickness to be a powerful tool for epidemiology study of atherosclerosis, especially to assess the effect of various forms of medical management. Echolucency determined by gray scale ultrasound has been reported by several investigators to detect embolic-prone carotid plaque. No doubt, better technique for tissue characterization of an atherosclerotic plaque will add further diagnostic information in the future. Other than transcutaneous use, intravascular or transesophageal ultrasound offers important diagnostic information. The intravascular ultrasound probe offers accurate assessment of atherosclerotic plaque and its relationship to the cross-section area of the artery. Transesophageal ultrasonography provides direct examination of the aortic arch. With this technique, the source of atheroembolization from a mobile plaque of the aortic arch can be determined accurately.

Computed Tomography

One of the major advances in acquisition of an image of the arteries is computed tomography, introduced by Godfrey Newbold Hounsfield, an English electrical engineer, and Allan MacLeod Cormack.[14] They shared the 1979 Nobel Prize in medicine and physiology. Unlike arteriography, the CT scan provides cross-sectional images of the aorta and its major branches. Moreover, it also yields information on the surrounding structure of the aorta. The technique certainly revolutionized the diagnosis of many intra-abdominal organs. CT scan can better define aortic pathology such as aortic dissection, aneurysm, and intraluminal thrombus. The CT scan is of particular use as an accurate means to determine the exact size of an aortic aneurysm, to find unexpected pathology such as retroaortic vena cava or horseshoe kidney, and for incidental identification of renal tumor. The CT also helps to determine whether the aneurysm is inflammatory in nature or is in the form of contained rupture. In the 1990s, a new generation of CT scan (e.g., spiral and helical CT) was introduced. These scans provide not only faster time for image acquisition but also three-dimensional reconstruction of images. These new CT scanners offer better examination of aortic aneurysm and the thoracic outlet. They also are helpful in the diagnosis of pulmonary embolism. With CT, we now know that small aneurysms (i.e., less than 5.5 cm) seldom rupture, and that it is perfectly safe to use CT to monitor the size of the aneurysm. In the era of endovascular repair of aortic aneurysm, the CT is essential in the selection of patients for endovascular graft and to determine the proper device as well as to detect endoleaks following endograft placement.

Magnetic Resonance Technique

In addition to CT scan, another major development in imaging technique is magnetic resonance imaging (MRI) or magnetic resonance arteriography (MRA). Edward Mills Purcell first introduced the technique in the early 1950s.[15] At first, the technique was known as nuclear magnetic resonance; later it was changed to magnetic resonance imaging. This technique, like the CT scan, is able to detect aortic aneurysm. MRI, however, is superior to CT because of the ability to yield detailed examination of soft tissue and venous structure. The technique is most useful to evaluate patients with congenital atrioventricular malformation because of the ability of MRI to depict venous structure in both longitudinal and cross-sectional views. More importantly, the MRI demonstrates the surrounding muscular structure clearly, and the extent of the malformation can be determined accurately. In recent years there has been significant advancement in the understanding of embolic symptoms as a result of plaque rupture. MRI, as demonstrated recently, may be able to determine the type of plaque that is most likely to cause embolization, which would be of great clinical use.

Another great use of MR technology for vascular surgeons is MRA. Refinement of this technology, especially with the use of gadolinium to enhance the image, has led to the gradual replacement of the invasive catheter arteriography. At present, many centers use MRA and duplex scan as the preoperative diagnostic plan for carotid endarterectomy or stent placement. Similarly, MRA has replaced catheter arteriogram for patients who are candidates for aortic or femoral bypass procedures.

Conclusions

Since the early days of vascular surgery in the 1950s there have been great advancements in diagnostic techniques for vascular disease. The vascular laboratory, CT scan, high-resolution ultrasound, and MRI or MRA, each with different indications, are now available to establish the diagnosis and to plan the treatment of vascular disease. Many of these tests are well suited as screening tests for early detection of vascular disease. These tests, when used with proper indications and in an ethical manner, will improve the care of patients with vascular disease.

REFERENCES

1. Halperin JL, Fuster V: Meeting the challenge of peripheral arterial disease. Arch Intern Med 163:877–878, 2003.
2. Cranley JJ, Lohr JM: Evolution of the vascular laboratory. J Vasc Technol 25:185–193, 2001.
3. Yao JST: Technology and vascular surgery: Reflections of the past three decades. J Vasc Technol 22:183–186, 1998.
4. Winsor T: Influence of arterial disease on the systolic blood pressure gradients of the extremity. Am J Med Sci 220:117–126, 1950.
5. Kempczinski RF: Noninvasive vascular diagnosis. J Vasc Ultrasound 27:13–15, 2003.
6. Bandyk DF: Being a professional of vascular ultrasound. J Vasc Ultrasound 27:153–156, 2003.
7. Inter-Society Commission for Heart Disease Resources: Optimal resources for vascular surgery. Circulation 46:A305–A324, 1972.
8. Moore WS, Clagett GP, Veith FJ, et al: Guidelines for hospital privileges in vascular surgery: An update by an ad hoc committee of the American Association for Vascular Surgery and the Society for Vascular Surgery. J Vasc Surg 36:1276–1282, 2002.
9. Brooks B: Intra-arterial injection of sodium iodide. JAMA 82:1016–1019, 1924.
10. Dos Santos R, Lamas A, Pereirgi CJ: L'artériographie des membres de l'aorte et ses branches abdominales. Bull Soc Nat Chir 55:587, 1929.
11. Seldinger SI: Catheter replacement of the needle in percutaneous arteriography: A new technique. Acta Radiol 39(5):368–376, 1953.
12. Yao JST, Pearce WH: Dedication–Michael E. DeBakey, M.D. In Yao JST, Pearce WH (eds): Arterial Surgery: Management of Challenging Problems. Stamford, CT: Appleton & Lange, 1996.
13. Donald I, Brown TG: Demonstration of tissue interfaces within the body by ultrasonic echo sounding. Br J Radiol 34:539–546, 1961.
14. Shampo MA, Kyle RA: Godfrey Hounsfield: Developer of computed tomographic scanning. Mayo Clin Proc 71:990, 1996.
15. Shampo MA, Kyle RA: Edward M. Purcell: Nobel Prize for magnetic resonance imaging. Mayo Clin Proc 72:585, 1997.

Chapter 2

Hemodynamic Principles as Applied to Diagnostic Testing

LUIS R. LEON JR. • NICOS LABROPOULOS
• M. ASHRAF MANSOUR

Introduction

The vascular laboratory was developed to aid the clinician in reaching a diagnosis and in formulating a therapeutic plan for patients with peripheral arterial occlusive and venous disease. Early on, many experts recognized that physical examination alone was inadequate. Many studies have shown that palpation of pulses is sometimes inaccurate, even with trained and experienced observers. Similarly, recognition of deep venous thrombosis in the calf by physical examination alone is as good as a coin toss (i.e., a 50% chance of being wrong).

In the 1950s and 1960s, efforts at devising objective tests to diagnose arterial and venous disease focused on physiologic testing. For arterial disease, it was recognized that a pressure drop in an adjacent arterial segment denoted the presence of a significant arterial narrowing. Winsor, in 1950, used pneumoplethysmography to record sequential blood pressures in a limb to make this observation. Subsequently, with the development of continuous-wave Doppler, photoplethysmography, and strain gauge, physiologic testing was on its way to becoming the core of vascular disease diagnosis. The 1980s ushered a revolution in vascular diagnosis after the refinement of ultrasound technology. With color-flow scanning it became possible to image the vessel, artery, or vein, and to observe the behavior of bloodflow within that vessel. Bloodflow velocity measurement provided an accurate method to measure an arterial stenosis. This varied according to the vascular bed, with 85% to 90% accuracy for celiac stenosis and 95% accuracy for carotid disease.

This chapter provides the reader with an understanding of the basic hemodynamic principles used on a daily basis in the vascular laboratory.

Hemodynamic Concepts

Systemic and pulmonary flows depend on the maintenance of adequate force within the circulation to drive blood throughout; flow distribution depends on regional differences in vascular resistance. The latter is mediated by diameter changes in the precapillary arterioles. The entire process is governed by the basic rules of fluid hemodynamics. In the following text, the most important hemodynamic factors that determine bloodflow are analyzed separately because of marked differences that depend on the different anatomic vascular areas.

Wall Mechanics

The properties of vessel walls are largely dependent on the tissues that form them. Water forms about 70% by weight and fat about 1.5%. In dried, fat-free specimens, collagen and elastin together make 50% to 65% of the wall weight, and the amount of muscle is largely unknown, even though values around 25% have been quoted.[1] Mechanically speaking, the muscular tissue is the active part, whereas endothelium, elastin, connective tissue, and collagen are passive in their roles. However, their proportions in wall composition affect the wall distensibility. Elasticity is the inherent property of a material to regain its original figure or dimensions after the removal of an altering force. Stress (S) is the magnitude of the force that causes strain on a physical material. The intensity of stress is given in units of force divided by units of area. Stress can be resolved into three orthogonal components, and several qualifying terms can be derived: (1) tensile stress tends to elongate a material, and compressive stress does the reverse; (2) shearing stress acts in a plane parallel to that of the material in question; and (3) strain (e) refers to the degree of deformation of a physical material under the effect of a force (i.e., the ratio of change for a given dimension to its original value in the nonstressed state). As in the case of stress, strain can be also divided into three orthogonal parts: (1) coefficient of elasticity, also known as elastic modulus, is defined by the ratio of applied stress to the change in shape of an elastic material; it describes the elastic properties characteristics of a given material.

$$E = S/e \text{ (Formula 1)}$$

These principles were described assuming rectangular coordinates. To be applied to vessels, cylindrical coordinates need to be used. In a very-thin-walled blood vessel, stress is given by the (2) transmural pressure, which is governed by the Laplace's law:

$$T = P_1/r \text{ (Formula 2)}$$

where T is the wall tension or the circumferentially directed force per unit length (dyne/cm), P_1 is the transmural pressure (intravascular minus extravascular pressure), and r is the vessel radius. But Laplace's law should only be applied the very-thin-walled structures indeed, such as soap bubbles. (3) Circumferential stress is given by:

$$S_{\theta\theta} = Pr/h \text{ (Formula 3)}$$

where h is wall thickness. Later on, more appropriate and complicated formulations were developed for thick-walled vessels, and they could be applied for determinations of elastic modulus in vitro and in vivo.

Arteries can be conceptualized as viscoelastic cylinders; this means that they are not perfect elastic bodies. The latter identifies materials that can deform and recover their unstressed shape immediately after application and removal of stress. Viscoelastic materials need a certain time to achieve deformation and to regain their original shape. Blood, if thought of as a fluid suspension of elastic cells, shares viscoelastic properties. Static elastic modulus (Estat) refers to the stress/strain ratio measured in a vessel that suffered an abrupt increase of the transmural pressure: the vessel diameter had to increase gradually to a new value. The ratio has to be calculated when the vessel reaches a relative steady state (i.e., after a period when no further strain can be obtained). But that value does not give information about the viscous characteristics of the vessel wall. Complex viscoelastic modulus (Ec) yields information about the viscoelastic properties of a vessel: It is obtained using sinusoidal, as opposed to linear, stresses. The peaks of stress and strain are identical in perfectly elastic substances and different in viscoelastic materials. Therefore the lag time between those peaks is a reflection of the viscoelasticity of a material.

Wall Elasticity and Wave Velocity

A relation between the pulse wave speed in the arteries and wall elasticity has been recognized. First, it was reported in a nonviscous system and represented by the Moens-Korteweg equation; later it was reported in viscous models. All the derived formulas in some form or another contain simplified assumptions. However, even though no exact data can be obtained, a large amount of knowledge with regard to the pulse wave transmission in vivo has been obtained, focusing on vascular disease through a new approach: measurements of wave propagation.

Pulse Wave Velocity

In each heart cycle, a pulse wave travels from the heart down along the arterial wall to move the bloodstream forward. Pulse wave velocity is an estimate of the transmission speed with which the arterial pulse wave propagates down the arterial tree. Data from the literature suggest that its measurement at the aortic level is an important marker for changes in vascular stiffness caused by age. It is considered to be the best available method to noninvasively assess aortic stiffness.

Pulse wave velocity is calculated by dividing the distance traveled between ultrasound transducers by the time of travel of the pulse wave. Simultaneous recordings of the arterial flow waves from the right common carotid artery and the right femoral artery are obtained using continuous-wave Doppler flow probes. The more rigid the arterial wall, the faster the wave travels.[2] When the wave hits a major branching point it is reflected back to its origin site.[3] This normally occurs after closure of the aortic valve, which amplifies the diastolic pressure and facilitates bloodflow to the coronary arteries. However, in old arteries, the increased velocity of the initial wave,

and that of the subsequent reflected one from the arterial system periphery to the aortic root, further increase systolic rather than diastolic pressure in the central arteries.[4] This is responsible for the late systolic pressure peak observed in the central pressure waves of older but not younger subjects. It also decreases the contribution of the reflected wave to the filling of the coronary arteries. Age-related changes can have major clinical consequences in coronary bloodflow and can add to an increase in the systolic blood pressure.[4]

Clinical Applications of Hemodynamic Principles in Arteries

The mechanical properties of the vessel wall have been used in clinical practice. Both increased carotid artery wall stiffness and pulse pressure have been associated with higher rates of cardiovascular mortality, including stroke.[5] Recent clinical reviews have shown that a number of novel therapeutic interventions target the walls of large arteries. Such therapy may be preferentially directed to patients with documented elevations of pulse pressure or vessel stiffness. Nitrates, for example, have a selective action in lowering pulse pressure levels through changes in wave reflections.[6] Other drugs can decrease the arterial wall stiffness through alterations in the wall composition.[6] Lower sodium intake and increased exercise are associated with improved aortic compliance.[7–9] Angiotensin-converting enzyme inhibitors have a favorable effect on vessel walls.[7] Low-dose diuretics effectively reduce vessel stiffness and pulse pressure in elderly patients.[7] In contrast, beta blockers have been shown to increase vessel stiffness and the reflected wave magnitude. Calcium channel blockers yielded mixed results.[7] Aortic pulse wave velocity, along with age and time on dialysis before inclusion in clinical trials, are also strong predictors of cardiovascular mortality in patients with end-stage renal disease (ESRD).[10] Aortic stiffness measurements are also predictors of cardiovascular mortality in patients with ESRD and after kidney transplant.[11]

Cardiac Dynamics

The cardiac cycle has two phases: (1) diastole or ventricular filling, which results in a doubled blood volume in the ventricle (from 40 to 50 mL, to 100 to 120 mL at completion in resting conditions); and (2) systole or ventricular emptying. The first phase takes about two thirds of the cycle duration.

Diastole encompasses five phases. The first one, or protodiastole, is very brief and represents the fall of ventricular pressure immediately after the end of ventricular systole, producing the closure of the aortic valve. Isometric relaxation follows, being characterized by continuous muscle relaxation without changing the intraventricular volume. That results in the fall of the intraventricular pressure until it is exceeded by the pressure in the atria, causing the opening of the mitral valve. The next phase is of rapid filling, where blood falls rapidly into the ventricle, filling about 60% to 70% of this space. Further but much slower filling occurs during the next phase or diastasis, which is responsible for 10% to 20% of ventricular filling. The last phase is known as atrial systole; it increases ventricular filling again and takes responsibility for an additional 20% to 30% of blood volume.

Systole has three phases. Isometric contraction relates to an early period of ventricular contraction that increases the pressure but not to levels high enough to open the aortic valve. The intraventricular volume during this phase does not change. When the pressures do reach those levels (i.e., above aortic pressure), the valve opens and allows blood ejection, and the cycle enters in its maximal ejection phase. The ventricular pressure continues to rise as the blood is being rapidly ejected, up to a peak point where most of the blood has left the ventricle. After that peak point, there is a rapid decrease in blood ejection and the aortic pressure falls as the flow of blood out of the distal end of the arterial system begins to exceed the blood inflow from the ventricle. This is called reduced ejection and finishes the cycle; it is followed by the beginning of ventricular muscle relaxation with an associated fall in the intraventricular pressure.

Cardiac Cycle in Relation to Arterial Waveform

The phases of the heart cycle described above, together with the wall properties of the arteries and the peripheral resistance, determine the shape of the ultrasound waveform in these vessels. By coupling the M-mode picture and the waveform of an artery with the electrocardiogram (ECG), the relationship between the cardiac and arterial phases can be depicted (Fig. 2-1). During the R wave, ventricular contraction (cardiac systole) occurs and leads to vessel expansion (vessel diastole). At this moment, the highest velocity in the vessel is recorded (peak systolic velocity). Vessel diastole and peak systolic velocity occur a few milliseconds after cardiac systole because it takes some time for the pulse wave to travel to the site of the measurement. Therefore the larger the distance from the heart, the larger the delay. Immediately after, the beginning of cardiac diastole occurs, during which the vessel diameter starts to decrease (vessel systole) and the bloodflow decelerates rapidly. In arteries where the resistance is high (e.g., external carotid, popliteal, and superior mesenteric during fasting),

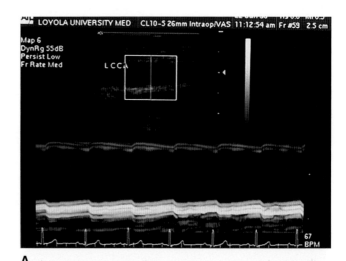

A

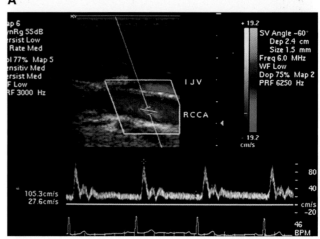

B

Figure 2-1. Arterial luminal phases and waveform in relation to cardiac cycle. **A,** *The different phases in the vessel cycle are seen in the common carotid artery by M-mode imaging coupled with electrocardiogram. A few ms after ventricular contraction (R wave), vessel diastole occurs during which the maximum diameter is achieved. In cardiac diastole the diameter of the vessel is progressively reduced (vessel systole) until it reaches its minimum just before the next cycle begins.* **B,** *The arterial systolic velocity reaches its peak during vessel diastole. The diastolic velocity occurs during vessel systole.*

the flow for a few milliseconds reverses its direction. In arteries with low resistance (e.g., internal carotid, renal, and superior mesenteric after a meal), flow reversal does not occur. The flow reversal is abolished in conditions where the resistance drops (e.g., exercise, ischemia, and inflammation). During the filling of the ventricles (after isometric relaxation), the vessel has its smallest diameter (end-diastolic velocity). Blood moves forward again as the reflective wave hits the proximal resistance of the next incoming wave and reverses direction. This phase reflects the peripheral resistance beyond the measurement as the blood travels with its own momentum (i.e., kinetic energy left during ventricular relaxation).

Cardiac Cycle in Relation to the Venous Pressure Waves

Cardiac filling pressure values are often needed in a variety of clinical situations. Typically, central venous pressure (CVP) is used to get information as to the status of the right heart. For the left heart, the pulmonary wedge pressure is commonly used. Additional information can be obtained examining the different pressure waves developed in the atria and central veins throughout the cardiac cycle (Fig. 2-2).[12]

Arterial Hemodynamics

Health care providers refer patients with arterial insufficiency to the vascular laboratory to answer the questions: Is there any evidence of arterial narrowing or obstruction? And if so, can the degree of narrowing (i.e., percent stenosis) be objectively quantified? To answer this question, a variety of direct and indirect tests are available.

In the case of occlusive arterial disease, most disease processes cause a narrowing of the arterial lumen. This is observed with atherosclerosis as well as with other arteriopathies. In the early stages of gradual arterial narrowing, most patients are asymptomatic. As the degree of stenosis increases (e.g., in patients with claudication),

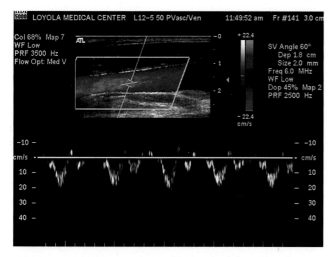

Figure 2-2. Venous waves in the internal jugular vein. During quiet breathing the respiration has little effect on the venous waveform, but it is strongly affected by the cardiac cycle. An antegrade wave is seen right after ventricular contraction. This is followed by a retrograde wave caused by atrial overfilling. Next the opening of the tricuspid valve produces an antegrade wave. Finally, a retrograde wave occurs during atrial contraction.

symptoms begin to appear.[13] In the classic description of claudication, the patient can walk for a few minutes without any symptoms of calf pain. As the metabolic demands of the calf muscle increase, the arterial narrowing prevents an adequate supply of nutrients from reaching the muscle and exercise-induced calf pain ensues. This phenomenon of arterial insufficiency causing symptoms is observed in other vascular beds as well (e.g., the coronary circulation when patients develop angina as they exert the heart muscle).

Fluid Energy

The cardiac muscle generates the pressure, or potential energy, to mobilize blood. A pressure or energy wave is created that moves throughout the vessels. The cardiac output determines the amount of blood entering the system, and the peripheral resistance determines the amount of blood that leaves it. A fraction of the generated energy is also spent in arterial distention. This causes a reservoir phenomenon that stores some of the blood and energy that were delivered to the system; it promotes the flow of blood into the tissues in diastole.

More precisely, fluid motion requires an energy differential between two points. That energy in a system is the sum of its potential and kinetic components as well as the gravitational energy. Hydrostatic pressure is a function of:

$$P = -\rho gh \text{ (Formula 4)}$$

where P is hydrostatic pressure, ρ is the density of blood, g is the force of gravity, and h is the height of the column of blood.

The formula that correlates all factors is:

$$E = P + \rho gh + 1/2\rho v^2 \text{ (Formula 5)}$$

where E is the total fluid energy, $+\rho gh$ is the gravitational energy, and $1/2\rho v^2$ is the kinetic energy. Gravitational and hydrostatic energy values are obtained using the same calculation, but they have opposite signs. The former describes the ability to do work because of its elevation. They often, but not always, cancel each other out.

Viscosity

Blood viscosity plays a major role in the loss of energy in the peripheral circulation. Blood viscosity is defined as the extent of internal friction between contiguous layers of fluid, or "lack of slipperiness," as described by Isaac Newton. He described the first equation that governs fluid viscosity: if two layers of fluid move at different velocities (v) and slide past each other, several values are derived. A is the area where both layers contact; dx refers to their individual thickness; and S is the amount of force per area unit (F/A) needed to move the fluid laminae by virtue of the friction between them. S is also termed *stress*. It is proportional to the velocity gradient, dv/dx, as is shown in the following equation:

$$S = F/A = \eta\, dv/dx \text{ (Formula 6)}$$

where η represents fluid viscosity, implying that viscosity is inherent to the fluid in question and the velocity gradient is a function of the applied stress. Viscosity is measured in poises, which equals 1 dyn sec/cm,[2] and it is affected by environmental factors such as variation in temperature. Blood has a viscosity that ranges from 0.03 to 0.04 poises at 37 °C.[1]

Inertia

Inertia is a characteristic property of pulsatile as opposed to steady flows. In the former, inertial forces are added to the unvarying kinetic energy of the latter. Energy losses caused by inertia (ΔE) are dependent of a constant K, blood specific gravity (ρ), and the square of blood velocity (v) as follows:

$$\Delta E = K\, 1/2\rho v^2 \text{ (Formula 7)}$$

Therefore inertial energy losses result from accelerations and decelerations of pulsatile flow and when blood goes from a large to a small vessel (and vice versa). Velocity is a vector quantity; therefore changes in flow direction at curves, junctions, and branches signify accelerations.

Turbulence

Also known as nonlaminar flow, turbulence arises from the random motion of parts of the fluid in axial and radial directions simultaneously, forming eddy currents and vortices. It causes an abrupt change in pressure gradient-flow relationships when flow is increased above a critical threshold. It is also an important source of fluid energy loss.

The Reynolds number (Re) is a dimensionless value that refers to the point at which flow transforms from laminar into turbulent and it is proportional to the ratio of internal forces acting over the fluid to the viscous forces:

$$Re = \rho v d/\eta = v d/\nu \text{ (Formula 8)}$$

where ν is the kinematic viscosity ($\nu = \eta/\rho$). The threshold where turbulence occurs is 2000. There is a transitional zone (2000 to 4000 Re) where the laminar flow is converted to turbulence. Above this zone true, turbulent flow occurs. Most vessels in the periphery are below that number, and therefore in normal circumstances turbulence should not occur except for brief exceptions (e.g., the ascending aorta during the peak systolic ejection period).[13]

Steady Flow

The basic principles of hemodynamics are based on simplifying bloodflow (i.e., considering it steady and through a rigid cylinder); this starting point to the knowledge of fluid flow principles has been built on over the course of the years. Flow and pressure are factors that are most commonly described in hemodynamics. J.L.M. Poiseuille first described the relation between steady flow and pressure in a cylinder. He established that in a rigid tube flow has a parabolic or laminar shape, and showed that the volume flow (Q) and the pressure drop ($P_1 - P_2$) along a tube of a given length (L) and inner diameter (D = 2r) were related as follows:

$$Q = (P_1 - P_2)\pi\, r^4/8\eta L \text{ (Formula 9)}$$

Therefore as a derivation of that equation, in a cylinder, resistance is expressed as:

$$R = 8\eta L/\pi\, r^4 \text{ (Formula 10)}$$

This concept can be applied to the pulmonary or circulatory system as a whole. In the latter, P_1 is the ascending aortic pressure, P_2 is the central venous (or right atrial) pressure, and Q is the left ventricular output. The average value over repeated complete cardiac cycles must be used. The flow that arises from the pulsatile effect of the heart muscle can be seen as steady flow with superimposed pulsations. Flow is directly proportional to a pressure gradient and vessel size; it is inversely proportional to blood viscosity and vessel length, which are elements of resistance. It is important to note that small changes in the radius result in very large flow changes because of the fact that the radius measurement is raised to the fourth power.

Pulsatile Flow

Pulsatile flow depicts changes in the driving pressure conditions and the vascular bed response to them. As opposed to steady flow, in which pressure and flow remain constant, these factors vary continuously over time in pulsatile flow. Associated changing velocity profiles occur throughout the cardiac cycle. The different parts of the arterial cycle in relation to the cardiac function have previously been described.

Pulsatile flow is important for adequate organ function, probably through the effects on the microcirculation via a mechanism that is not fully understood. Experimental work has revealed that the function of certain organs decreases under steady blood perfusion.[14]

Resistance

The measurement of the extent to which a system of conduits opposes flow is called resistance; it is defined as the relationship of mean pressure gradient to mean pressure flow, as follows:

$$S = (P_1 - P_2) / Q \text{ (Formula 11)}$$

Resistance expresses the energy dissipation per flow unit within a given system; its values are often given in dyne sec/cm.[5] The peripheral resistance unit (1 PRU = 1 mmHg per milimeter per minute = 8×10^4 dyne sec/cm[5]) is most commonly used.

Local and remote neurohormonal mediators of smooth muscle activity perform the moment-to-moment control of the vasculature; however, resistance is also influenced by the geometry of the vessel, by wall distensibility, and by transmural pressure. The smooth muscle cell layers in the arterial wall are progressively attenuated from 3 in the 100- to 150-μm arteries to 2 in intermediate branches and to 1 at the arteriolar level. Simultaneously, the elastic layer suffers fenestration and fragmentation until it completely disappears in the 20- to 25-μm arterioles. This changes the vessel compliance and the wall thickness/lumen ratio. Because of a significant decrease in the vessel inner lumenal circumference in relation to its outer perimeter, inner wall layers bear higher levels of strain caused by intravascular pressure. This may contribute to patterns of structural adaptation of large and small arteries in response to pressure stress.

Other commonly used terms in vascular hemodynamics are *impedance* and *conductance*. *Impedance* is the term used to describe the resistance to pulsatile flow offered by a peripheral vascular bed. Impedance shows how the resistance changes in time; it is a more realistic term than the *resistance*, which is applied to ideal situations only.[15] *Conductance* is the reciprocal of the resistance for the entire array of vessels from arteries, capillaries, and veins.

Stenosis and Critical Stenosis

The bloodstream changes direction as the flow narrows at a stenotic segment (contraction), and it enlarges (expansion) as it exits the stenosis. Bloodflow velocity increases through the stenotic vessel because velocity and area are inversely related. Inertial energy losses occur at the beginning and at the end of a stenotic segment. This is caused by the resulting turbulence, eddies, and vortices produced by the change in bloodflow direction. Inertial loss is proportional to the square of the velocity. Viscous energy losses also occur within the stenotic segment but are of less magnitude when compared with inertial losses. From the Poiseuille equation, the vessel radius has a greater effect on viscous energy losses than does vessel length.

The stenosis shape also influences energy losses. Gradual tapering geometry is associated with fewer losses than is irregular geometry; converging vessels stabilize laminar flow, whereas diverting vessels have a less stable flow pattern. Irregular stenoses are associated with high turbulence, producing vibrations of the vessel wall that in turn produce audible sounds known as bruits. After a significant stenosis, poststenotic dilatation occurs. Its development has been attributed to the following factors: turbulent flow leading to fatigue of the elastin fibers and collagen breakdown distal to stenotic lesions; conversion of high kinetic to high potential energy; and continuous change from high to low pressure. Subsequently, when some dilatation occurs, the decrease in the velocity near the wall will increase the lateral pressure, leading to further dilatation.[16] The sudden expansion of bloodstream, and the kinetic energy dissipation caused by the associated turbulence, can cause large energy losses at the exit site of the stenosis. That loss can be expressed by the following:

$$\Delta P = K \, 1/2\rho v^2 \, (r/r_s)^2 - 1^2 \text{ (Formula 12)}$$

where r is the radius of the normal vessel and r_s is the radius of the stenotic segment.

There is a stenotic threshold below which the reduction in flow or pressure is; this is known as critical stenosis. According to Formula 7, the energy losses across a stenotic vessel are inversely proportional to the fourth power of the radius at that site.

Mathematic and biologic models in the experimental and clinical setting have investigated mechanical and physiologic consequences linked to critical arterial stenosis. Critical stenosis has been shown to occur when the vessel diameter has been reduced by about 50%, or when the cross-sectional area is reduced by 75%. Other investigators, by using invasive techniques and correlating trans-stenotic pressure differential versus stenotic measurements, found the critical level to be 60% in diameter and 80% in area (Fig. 2-3).[16] The effects of proximal or distal stenosis on the arterial waveform are illustrated in Figure 2-4.

Several findings were derived from observations that applied only to unbranched vessels. Stenoses in series affecting a single conduit are a common occurrence. The length of the stenosis affects energy losses from viscosity, but according to Poiseuille's equation, the effect of length is less significant than is the effect of the lesion diameter. An important observation to consider is that the energy

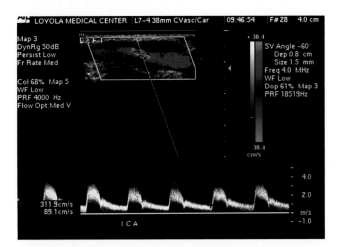

Figure 2-3. Hemodynamically significant stenosis in the internal carotid artery. This stenosis is defined as such when the pressure or flow is reduced distal to it. In general, most people accept this cutoff at a 50% diameter reduction. However, experimental work has shown that this is closer to 60% diameter stenosis. In this figure the diameter stenosis is greater than 60% but less than 80%. This is indicated by the elevated peak systolic velocity (PSV): 312 cm/sec and end-diastolic velocity (EDV): 89 cm/sec and the PSV ratio of internal carotid artery (ICA) to common carotid artery (CCA), which was 312/81 = 3.8.

loss caused by two stenoses of equal diameter is not the same as that of a single stenosis of a length that equals the sum of the lengths of the shorter lesions.[13] This is caused by entrance and exit effects for each short stenosis, as opposed to the same effects for only a single segment. That would explain several clinical observations. Multiple, subcritical arterial stenoses have been shown to have the potential for significant hemodynamic consequences. Diminished pressure and flow at the poststenotic site were correlated with the experimental serial application of subcritical stenoses in a cumulative, nonlinear fashion.[17] Stenoses of unequal diameter positioned in series get most of the hemodynamic effect from the one with smaller diameter, regardless of the order in which they are placed. Removal of the most severe, therefore, might result in significant hemodynamic benefit.[13]

Blood velocity affects energy losses as well. Because velocity depends on the distal vascular bed resistance, the latter also affects critical stenosis.

The flow characteristics need to be specified for this concept to be valid. Nonsignificant stenoses at resting flow rates may become critical when the flow is increase (e.g., during exercise). This shows the importance of clinical angiographic correlation of apparently benign lesions that may be hemodynamically significant when the patient exercises. That constitutes the basis for physiologic testing through blood pressure assessment to clinically categorize stenoses.

The preferred test to assess the circulation is the exercise or treadmill test. It produces physiologic stress that resembles the patient's ischemic symptoms. After obtaining Doppler pressure values at rest, the patient is asked to walk on a treadmill at a speed of 1.5 mph and at less than 10% elevation for about 5 minutes or until limiting symptoms occur. Duration of walking, speed, onset, location, and progression of symptoms are all recorded. Ankle-brachial indexes are calculated immediately after exertion. In normal subjects, the value should be higher than pre-exercise levels. If the value decreases, pressures are obtained every 2 minutes until pre-exercise values are reached. Single-level disease is associated with a recovery time between 2 and 6 minutes; multilevel disease with a recovery time of 6 to 12 minutes.

Alternative techniques have been developed for stressing the peripheral circulation in cases where the examined subject is unable to exercise. Postocclusive or reactive hyperemia is performed by inflating bilateral thigh cuffs to pressure levels above the systolic value and maintaining the pressure for about 5 minutes. This technique produces transient ischemia and consequent vasodilatation distal to the cuffs, which in normal subjects may produce a drop in the ankle-brachial index of 17% to 34%. In patients with disease at a single level, a less than 50% drop in the ankle pressure is seen, whereas multiple level disease is associated with a greater than 50% drop. Drug-induced hyperemia, simulating exercise, is another method based on pharmacologic arteriolar vasodilatation. This effect is readily seen with intravenous adenosine-like drugs such as dipyridamole, which are strong arteriolar dilators that lack any effect on larger arteries. It is a drug widely used in myocardial perfusion studies in humans based on that principle; it is also used in patients with peripheral arterial atherosclerotic disease during angiography.

Pressure Flow Relationships

Along a streamline of bloodflow, the total fluid energy is constant, and velocity and pressure are inversely related according to the Bernoulli principle. With or without arterial disease, the vessel geometry produces pressure gradients that, in turn, create areas of flow separation with areas of stagnation.

Clinicians are used to measuring blood pressure and not bloodflow. Bloodflow varies depending on the clinical situation. In healthy extremities, the heart produces a pressure pulse, later modified by the inherent properties of the arterial wall and by changes in the distal vascular bed resistance. As the pulse progresses distally there is a reduction in the vessel wall compliance and a reflection caused by the peripheral resistance, resulting in amplification of the peak systolic pressure. That translates into a higher pressure at the ankle level than in the upper arm. The ankle-arm pressure ratio is then defined, being normally 1.11 ± 0.18.

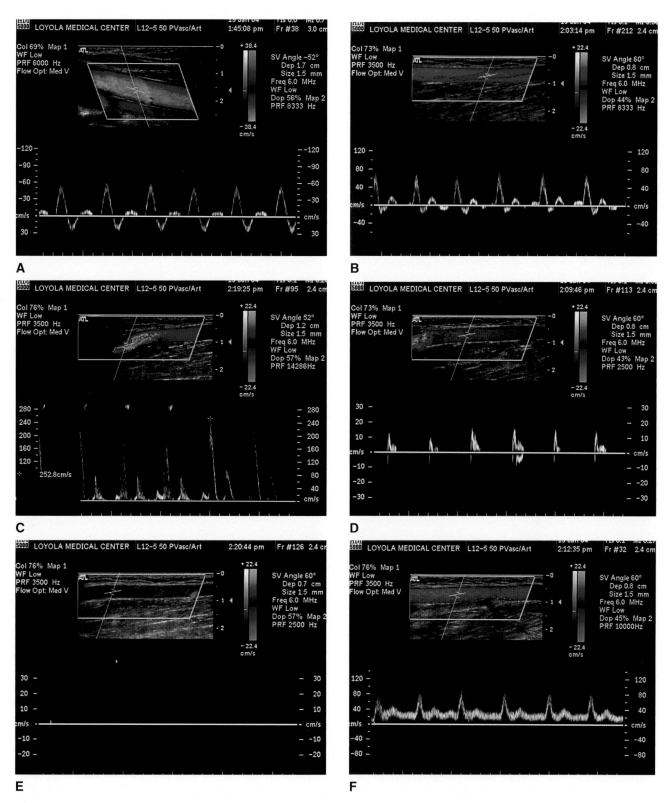

Figure 2-4. *Hemodynamic effects of stenosis, occlusion, and inflammation on the arterial waveform.* **A,** *In peripheral arteries the waveform is triphasic, as seen in the SFA of a young, healthy volunteer.* **B,** *In the upper extremities the arteries have usually more than three phases, as shown in this normal brachial artery.* **C,** *Increased peak systolic velocity in a normal brachial artery after digital compression that produced greater than 50% stenosis (peak systolic velocity ratio 253/70: 3.6).* **D,** *Low amplitude flow velocities distal to near-total occlusion of the brachial artery with digital compression.* **E,** *No flow is seen after complete occlusion.* **F,** *Absence of flow reversal, increased peak systolic and end- diastolic velocities with prolonged forward flow caused by decreased vascular resistance as seen in reactive hyperemia.*

Continued

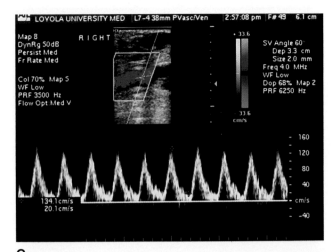

G

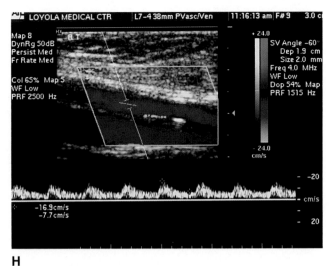

H

Figure 2-4, cont'd. **G**, *High flow in a normal common femoral artery secondary to inflammation in a patient with severe cellulitis. Areas with inflammation have significant vasodilation and therefore lower resistance.* **H**, *Low amplitude flow distal to a chronic superficial femoral artery stenosis (**I**).*

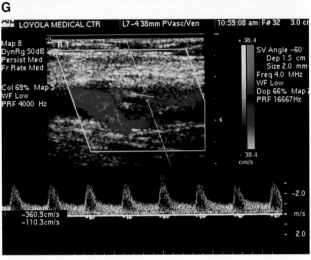

I

The mean and diastolic pressures progressively decrease at the same time. The fall in the mean value between the heart and ankle is less than 10 mmHg. Exercise in normal limbs is not associated with major changes in ankle systolic pressures, which return to resting levels within 1 to 5 minutes after exercise cessation.

In atherosclerotic limbs there is an increase in segmental vascular resistance. After exertion, metabolic products accumulate, and in normal flow conditions they are removed from the circulation. The ability to increase flow in diseased extremities is limited, and pain in exertion is assumed to be caused by those products. A dramatic fall in the ankle systolic blood pressure also occurs. Its extent and duration are proportional to the severity of the stenosis. The recovery time to resting levels can take up to 30 minutes. The hyperemia that follows exercise lasts longer, and the peak calf bloodflow decreases and recovery is delayed.

As atherosclerosis progresses, the compensatory effects of a diminished peripheral vascular resistance eventually disappear and resting flow falls below normal, producing ischemic rest pain.

Aneurysms

Important hemodynamic concepts have been derived from ideal models of arterial aneurysms. Considering them as perfect cylinders, the tangential stress applied over the aneurysmal wall (τ) is given by the product of the transmural pressure (P) times the inside arterial radius (r_1) divided by the thickness of its wall (δ). The larger the aneurysm and the higher the systemic pressure, the higher are the chances for aneurysmal rupture. Laminar thrombus formation, a layering of the inner wall of the aneurysm, forms in an attempt to keep the arterial lumen as close to normal as possible. That thickens the wall and, in theory, could be protective against rupture; this has not been shown conclusively:

$$\tau = Pr_1/\delta \text{ (Formula 13)}$$

But aneurysms are not perfect cylinders; they are asymmetric, which causes increased wall stress (Fig. 2-5). That, combined with the weakening of the aneurysm wall produced by atherosclerosis and endogenous enzymes, increases the chances of vessel rupture.

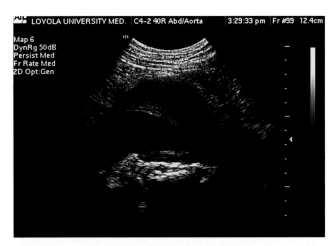

Figure 2-5. *Abdominal aortic aneurysm (AAA) with a large amount of thrombus lining the inner aneurysmal wall and asymmetric contours. These arise as a consequence of abnormal arterial wall contents of elastin and collagen. Their etiology is not known, but metalloproteinase activity, genetic predisposition, immunoreactive proteins, certain infectious diseases, and atherosclerosis have been related. Inflammation with media thinning and loss of elastin are commonly seen in surgical specimens. AAAs enlarge in an asymmetric fashion at a rate of about 0.2 to 0.8 mm/y and eventually break. The sites of rupture often correlate with areas of high arterial wall stress.*

Age

Arterial wall remodeling, along with its hemodynamic consequences, occurs with increasing age, even without atherosclerotic risk factors. Wall stiffness increases in a nonpathological process that begins in the third decade of life. This is thought to be caused by the relative decrease in elastin and fraying of the elastic layer, as well as by an increase in collagen content. The increase in the arterial stiffness has been correlated with higher rates of early atherosclerosis; it is also the most important cause of increasing systolic and pulse pressure, and for decreasing diastolic pressure with aging.

The viscoelastic properties of the carotid arteries were analyzed by Labropoulos and colleagues.[19] Analysis of the intima-media thickness in these vessels showed that 0.88 mm was the critical value at which the arterial segments became significantly stiffer compared with patients with values below that level (p < 0.01) and with controls (p < 0.001), as determined by the measurement of arterial elastic modulus.

Hypertension

Hypertension, by definition, is a hemodynamic disorder that affects about one quarter of the population. Hypertension is much more prevalent in the old, and the risk of cardiovascular morbidity increases with age. As in the case of aging, a loss of arterial distensibility was correlated with hypertension. This was first noted in a study by Freis, who analyzed the externally recorded arterial pulse wave at the carotid and brachial arteries for calculations of vessels compliance.[20]

Treatment of hypertension reduces this risk considerably; however, it should not only target arterial blood pressure but also other hemodynamic parameters and structural changes of the cardiovascular system. Excluding beta blockers, all other antihypertensives, including the vasodilating beta blockers, do not decrease cardiac output while lowering the systemic impedance. In the future, the capability to recognize preclinical arterial injury will improve cardiovascular risk stratification and act as a better guide in assessing the value of therapeutic methods than monitoring blood pressure alone.

Alternative methods to assess response to therapy are also developed. Regression of ECG evidence of left ventricular hypertrophy (LVH) has been verified with antihypertensive therapy since the Veterans' Administration trial. In this study and others, abnormal ECG changes in the treated patients developed only in one fourth of the occurrence in the control group. Furthermore, in patients who presented with ECG changes before randomization, they corrected 2.5 times more often in the treated group than in the control.[21]

Venous Hemodynamics

Venous structures have significant differences in their wall composition: these are mainly caused by the presence of valves; by a much lesser wall thickness; and by the lack of elastic tissue, with marked preponderance of muscle fiber in the media layer. Larger veins have adventitial tissue as a major component of their walls, and venules have no media layer and no smooth muscle. Because of their wall properties and size, they are called capacitance vessels, and at any given time they contain about two thirds of the total blood in the body.

Hydrostatic Pressure

Hydrostatic pressure is given by the weight of the blood columns extending from the heart to the level where the pressure is being measured (Formula 1). In supine patients, hydrostatic pressure is negligible; it becomes considerable in the standing position because of the passage of blood to the lower extremity veins of about 0.5 L. A marked increase in the transmural venous pressure at the feet occurs because gravity forces fluid out of the capillaries and into the tissues. This phenomenon occurs without a significant change in the pressure differential across foot capillaries. The calf pump is the most important factor in preventing interstitial fluid accumulation, returning it to the circulation. Other factors also aid in edema prevention in the erect position but to a lesser degree. Distal vasomotor changes occur in the lower extremity arteriolar system (the venoarterial reflex) by dependency (the elective lowering of the leg of a subject lying horizontally). The venoarterial reflex causes a mean decrease in the amplitude of plethysmographic recordings as compared with the values obtained in the horizontal position. By limiting the arterial inflow, the increased venous blood volume that results from an elevated hydrostatic pressure is limited.

Unlike arteries, veins are very compliant, being able to expand as the intraluminal pressure rises and to collapse as it decreases (i.e., when the pressure of neighboring tissues exceeds the intraluminal pressure). Vein diameter is often three to four times that of the accompanying artery, and consequently they can carry much more blood without increasing their pressure. Therefore, the transmural pressure determines venous shapes. In normal conditions they have a flattened shape, which offers a large amount of flow resistance. Very small changes in intraluminal pressure can cause vein expansion and a change of shape; but once expanded, much greater pressure changes are needed to expand it further because of the reduced wall compliance at that point. The most common consequences of abnormal venous function include varicosities and the post-thrombotic syndrome; these will be detailed in Chapters 41, 42, and 43.

Effects of Calf Pump, Cardiac Activity, and Breathing

In the resting state, veins function as reservoirs for blood. During activity, the effect of calf muscle contraction results in vein squeezing and blood ejected toward the heart. The venous pressure and pooling is decreased, and the venous return is diminished as is the cardiac output. Vein valves are bicuspid structures essential to proper function; their role is to ensure antegrade flow, from the superficial to the deep system and from there to the heart, thereby preventing reflux. Consequently, they are more heavily distributed where the effect of gravity is the largest. After muscle relaxation, a very low-pressure state is created in the deep veins; this results in bloodflow from the superficial to the deep system via perforators, pushed by the pressure gradient created. This phenomenon reduces peripheral venous pressure.

Contraction of the right heart elevates the central venous pressure, causing a brief period of flow reversal. During ventricular contraction the atrium relaxes, increasing the venous flow and decreasing the venous pressure.

During diastole, the flow decreases until the pressure gradient opens the tricuspid valve; this causes another brief period of increased flow that gradually drops to 0. Cardiac-induced pulsations are not normally perceived in the lower limb veins because of the obscuring effect of breathing activity producing significant fluctuations of bloodflow. They can be clinically seen in the jugular veins or with the aid of ultrasound in the upper extremity veins of subjects at rest. In cases of congestive heart failure or of venous valve insufficiency, the increase in central venous pressure overcomes the respiratory effect in the lower limb veins and pulsatile venous structures can become prominent (Fig. 2-6). Vein pulsatility can also be seen in arteriovenous fistulas. This pulsatility is strongest at the site of the fistula and gradually dissipates at more proximal levels.

The work of breathing also affects flow. Inspiration causes an increase in the intra-abdominal pressure while decreasing intrathoracic pressure. This reduces the gradient between the pressure in the lower extremity veins and the pressure of those in the abdomen, in turn reducing the blood return. Expiration produces the opposite effect, halting flow from the upper limbs. The Valsalva maneuver differs substantially, increasing both intrathoracic and intra-abdominal pressures (Fig. 2-7). The deep breath initially causes cessation of the spontaneous venous signal at the common femoral vein level. Augmentation of the signal is a normal response after releasing the strain. If the contrary occurs, it suggests flow reversal caused by incompetent valves. The Valsalva maneuver is contraindicated in patients with coronary heart disease, acute myocardial infarction, or hypovolemia because of the decrease in the blood return to the heart. The effects of other maneuvers on the vein flow velocity are shown in Figure 2-8.

Effect of Exercise

Venous disease becomes apparent with activation of the calf muscle pump because of its effect on venous pressure, flow rate, and direction. With activity, the venous pressure falls to very low levels and only returns to pre-exertion levels after several seconds.[22] In normal subjects, the pressure remains at constantly low levels throughout the exercise period. The calf blood volume eventually rises because of an increase in the arterial blood volume. These effects depend on a completely normal valve system; they keep the venous system empty with calf contraction and nearly empty with relaxation, ensuring normal venous return and protecting the extremity. Venous pressure testing and plethysmographic techniques have been used to measure these physiologic changes. The details and indications for testing methods will be discussed in Chapters 41, 42, and 43.

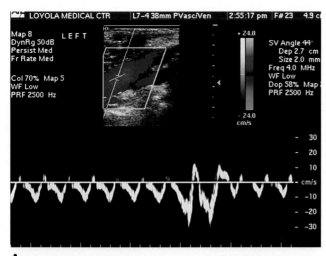

A

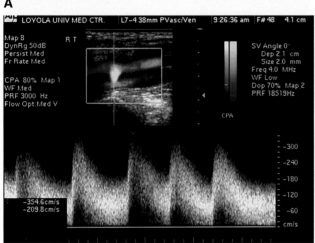

B

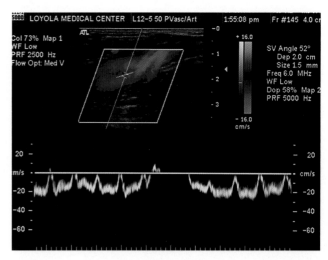

Figure 2-7. *The Valsalva maneuver is performed by forceful exhalation of air while keeping the mouth and nose closed. It usually lasts for about 20 seconds and often achieves increments of intrathoracic pressure up to 40 mmHg. Its first phase (strain beginning) causes a brief rise in the mean arterial blood pressure (MABP) because of the transmission of the high intrathoracic pressure to the arterial tree. The increased pressure is also transmitted to the femoral vein, leading to flow cessation, as shown in this figure. In phase IIa the atrial filling pressure drops, causing a decrease in the MABP. Phase IIb is associated with augmented sympathetic activation, increasing the peripheral vascular resistance and leading to a slight increase in MABP and pulse. In phase III (strain release) the MABP suddenly falls because of the release of the intrathoracic pressure. Phase IV is characterized by an "overshoot" in MABP because of a persistent increased sympathetic tone and systemic vascular resistance. Then arterial baroreceptors are stimulated, causing reflex bradycardia; this causes both MABP and pulse to return to baseline levels.*

Figure 2-6. *Pulsatile venous segments are generally ascribed to arteriovenous fistula; however, they can be associated with congestive heart failure or tricuspid valvular regurgitation.* **A,** *The popliteal vein Doppler examination of a 58-year-old male patient with severe right-sided heart failure awaiting cardiac transplantation. The right ventricle cannot meet the demands of the blood volume returning to it. The resulting congestion of the systemic venous system and decreased output to the lungs causes venous distention, hepatomegaly, splenomegaly, and peripheral edema. The increased venous pressure causes the transmission of the normal physiologic, rhythmic, pulsatile motion of the arteries from a moving myocardium into venous conduits. This phenomenon can clinically translate into pulsatile varicose veins on lower extremity examination.* **B,** *Arteriovenous fistula between the common femoral artery and vein after cardiac catheterization. Both the peak systolic and end diastolic velocities are very high because the resistance is very low.*

Edema

Edema occurs in the extremities when the rate of filtration is higher than the rate of absorption. In cases of venous obstruction or reflux, the resulted augmentation in the capillary pressure leads to edema formation. This increases the flow of fluid through the microcirculation into the interstitium and prevents normal fluid reabsorption. Eventually, normal cellular functions are distorted and skin discoloration and ulceration may occur.

Vein Stenosis

Unlike the work done in the arterial area, venous stenosis has not been the subject of intensive noninvasive research. There are few data published on the use of transcutaneous ultrasound for this purpose. A few reports describe the use of intravascular ultrasound, but otherwise, venous pressure measurements have been confined to the use of trans-stenotic recordings or venography. In the authors' experience (unpublished data), a veno-venous ratio above 2.5 has been found to correlate with more than 50% venous stenosis (Fig. 2-9). Duplex ultrasonography is able to identify the presence of stenoses in venous segments in the clinical arena. Such cases include the diagnosis of subclavian stenosis, caused by

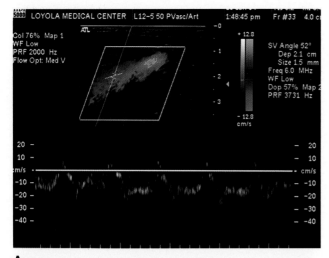

A

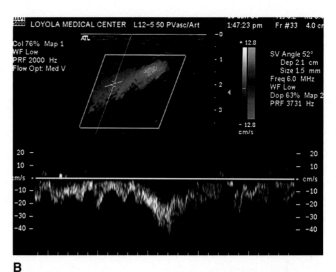

B

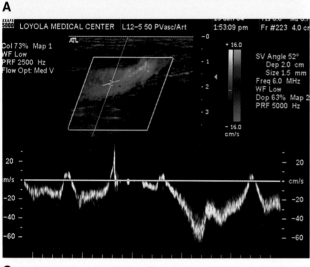

C

*Figure 2-8. The flow velocity in the veins is affected by cardiac activity, respiration, and compression. **A,** Normal waveform in a common femoral vein during quiet breathing. The changes seen in this condition are mainly caused by atrial activity (see Fig. 2-2). **B,** Distal compression augments the flow. This maneuver is used to test proximal obstruction (i.e., iliofemoral veins) and reflux (reversed flow after the release of the compression). Significant flow augmentation is seen during calf muscle contraction. This is the main mechanism by which the flow returns to the heart. **C,** Abdominal compression reduces the diameter of the pelvic veins and therefore increases the venous outflow resistance. This leads to flow reversal and interruption in the common femoral vein.*

thoracic outlet syndrome or after dialysis catheter placement; iliac vein compression in May-Thurner syndrome; extrinsic compression from different masses (e.g., tumors, aneurysms, hematomas, or cysts); and IVC stenosis after liver transplant.

Clinical Applications of Hemodynamic Principles in Veins

Like in their arterial counterpart, hemodynamic parameters have been used in clinical research in veins. Ciardullo and colleagues[23] studied the association between sex hormones and varicose veins. Vein distensibility was assessed through the use of plethysmography; it was found to increase with higher levels of endogenous steroids, suggesting a role for these compounds in the pathogenesis of venous disease. Investigation of the cause of varicose veins in high-risk groups revealed a decreased vein wall elasticity compared with normal extremities, and the role of venous valves in the origin of varicosi-

ties appeared to be secondary to those hemodynamic wall changes.[24]

The hemodynamic effect of several therapeutic interventions has been also addressed. Leon and colleagues[25] analyzed the elastic modulus of vessels affected by superficial or deep venous disease, before and after 1 month of therapy with elastic stockings. A marked increase in elasticity was found after the use of stockings, and this was found to be in a negative linear relationship with duration of the disease. The same group evaluated elastic stockings in patients with grade 2 venous disease, analyzing the effects on venous reflux and the ejecting capacity of the calf pump. The beneficial effect of elastic stockings on venous hemodynamic parameters was present mainly when the stockings are worn; it completely disappeared within a day after removal.[26] Some medications proved to have a positive effect over the hemodynamic characteristics of venous conduits through the effect in the venous elastic modulus. In patients with abnormal vein elasticity but without varicose veins, Daflon 500 mg improved the venous tone, which was evident by a significant increase in the venous elasticity.[27]

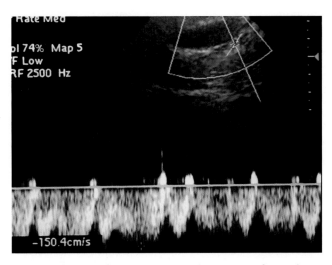

Figure 2-9. *Significant stenosis in the common femoral vein in a patient with ipsilateral lower extremity swelling. The vein is compressed by a hematoma after cardiac catheterization. The poststenotic vein velocity is 150 cm/sec and the velocity ratio across the stenosis was 7.9 (150/19). Although data for detecting significant vein stenosis in peripheral veins have not been validated, in the authors' experience, such a stenosis is present when the velocity ration across the stenosis is greater than 2.5.*

Conclusions

Circulation can be summarized as the effect of forces generated by the cardiac muscle over the bloodstream and its motion throughout blood vessels. It is governed by several principles that are ultimately based on basic hemodynamic concepts described in this chapter. It should be of interest to all who are involved in cardiovascular research, as well as health care providers taking care of patients with vascular disorders. An understanding of these principles represents the foundation for a rational diagnostic methodology and therapy of vascular disease.

REFERENCES

1. Milnor WR: Properties of the Vascular Wall. In Milnor WR (ed): Hemodynamics, 2nd ed. Baltimore: Williams & Wilkins, 1989.
2. Kelly R, Hayward C, Avolio A, et al: Noninvasive determination of age-related changes in the human arterial pulse. Circulation 80:1652–1659, 1989.
3. http://ucsfagrc.org/supplements/cardiovascular/1.14_pulse_wave_velocity.html
4. Nichols WW, Nicolini FA, Pepine CJ: Determinants of isolated systolic hypertension in the elderly. J Hypertens (Suppl 10):S73–S77, 1992.
5. Laurent S, Katsahian S, Fassot C, et al: Aortic stiffness is an independent predictor of fatal stroke in essential hypertension. Stroke 34:1203–1206, 2003.
6. Safar ME, Blacher J, Mourad JJ, et al: Stiffness of carotid artery wall material and blood pressure in humans: Application to antihypertensive therapy and stroke prevention. Stroke 31:782–790, 2000.
7. Domanski MJ, Davis BR, Pfeffer MA, et al: Isolated systolic hypertension, prognostic information provided by pulse pressure. Hypertension 34:375–380, 1999.
8. Safar ME, Asmar R, Benetos A, et al: Sodium, large arteries, and diuretic compounds in hypertension. Am J Med Sci 307:S3–S8, 1994.
9. Parnell MM, Holst DP, Kaye DM: Exercise training increases arterial compliance in patients with congestive heart failure. Clin Sci 102:1–7, 2002.
10. Blacher J, Safar ME, Guerin AP, et al: Aortic pulse wave velocity index and mortality in end-stage renal disease. Kidney Int 63:1852–1860, 2003.
11. Blacher J, Safar ME, Pannier B, et al: Prognostic significance of arterial stiffness measurements in end-stage renal disease patients. Curr Opin Nephrol Hypertens 11:629–634, 2002.
12. Abu-Yousef MM: Normal and respiratory variations of the hepatic and portal venous duplex Doppler waveforms with simultaneous electrocardiographic correlation. J Ultrasound Med 11:263–268, 1992.
13. Sumner DS: Essential Hemodynamic Principles. In Rutherford RB (ed): Vascular Surgery, 5th ed. Philadelphia: WB Saunders, 2000.
14. Nakamura K, Koga Y, Sekiya R, et al: The effects of pulsatile and nonpulsatile cardiopulmonary bypass on renal bloodflow and function. Jpn J Surg 19:334–345, 1989.
15. Nichols WW, O'Rourke MF: Vascular Impedance. In Nichols WW, O'Rourke MF (eds): McDonald's Blood Flow in Arteries: Theoretical, Experimental, and Clinical Principles, 4th ed. New York: Oxford University Press, 1998.
16. Chirossel P, Barbe R, Clermont A, et al: The concept of critical arterial stenosis: Value of a model of measures obtained by an angiographic method and the Doppler technique before and after transluminal angioplasty of the iliac arteries. J Mal Vasc 13:89–94, 1988.
17. Flanigan DP, Tullis JP, Streeter VL, et al: Multiple subcritical arterial stenoses: Effect on poststenotic pressure and flow. Ann Surg 186:663–668, 1977.
18. Yao JST: Hemodynamic studies in peripheral arterial disease. Br J Surg 57:761–766, 1970.
19. Labropoulos N, Mansour MA, Kang SS, et al: Viscoelastic properties of normal and atherosclerotic carotid arteries. Eur J Vasc Endovasc Surg 19:221–225, 2000.
20. Freis ED: Studies in hemodynamics and hypertension. Hypertension 38:1–5, 2001.
21. Freis ED: Electrocardiographic changes in the course of antihypertensive treatment. Am J Med 75:111–115, 1983.
22. Pollack AA, Wood EH: Venous pressure in the saphenous vein at the ankle in man during exercise and changes in posture. J Appl Physiol 1:649–662, 1949.
23. Ciardullo AV, Panico S, Bellati C, et al: High endogenous estradiol is associated with increased venous distensibility and clinical evidence of varicose veins in menopausal women. J Vasc Surg 32:544–549, 2000.
24. Clarke GH, Vasdekis SN, Hobbs JT, et al: Venous wall function in the pathogenesis of varicose veins. Surgery 111:402–408, 1992.
25. Leon M, Volteas N, Labropoulos N, et al: The effect of elastic stockings on the elasticity of varicose veins. Int Angiol 12:173–177, 1993.
26. Labropoulos N, Leon M, Volteas N, et al: Acute and long-term effect of elastic stockings in patients with varicose veins. Int Angiol 13:119–123, 1994.
27. Ibegbuna V, Nicolaides AN, Sowade O, et al: Venous elasticity after treatment with Daflon 500 mg. Angiology 48:45–49, 1997.

Chapter 3

Qualifications and Competence of Vascular Laboratory Personnel

MICHAEL A. RICCI

Introduction

With the increased scrutiny surrounding medical errors, credentialing, and competence,[1-3] clear-cut definitions for the qualifications of personnel working in the vascular diagnostic laboratory (VDL) have assumed added importance. In addition, many states and private insurers will now reimburse for noninvasive vascular testing only if it is performed by qualified personnel, even though the definitions of qualifications may vary.[4] Because a variety of specialists with diverse backgrounds and training have become involved in vascular diagnosis in recent years, the standardization of qualifications for both technologists and physicians has become a quality of care issue in the VDL.[4-6] Although the Intersocietal

Commission for the Accreditation of Vascular Laboratories (ICAVL) has established standards for vascular laboratories and technologists, physician standards are still lacking.[7] This chapter will review the existing standards and recommendations for training and qualifications for technologists, physicians, and physician directors of the VDL, and conclude with recommendations for assessing clinical competence of these individuals.

Technologist Qualifications

Definition and Scope of Practice

The vascular laboratory technologist is a specialist among a diverse group of diagnostic ultrasound professionals.[8,9] These technologists are qualified by professional credentialing and academic and clinical experience to provide diagnostic patient care services using ultrasound and related technologies. According to the scope of practice outlined by their professional societies, diagnostic ultrasound professionals perform the following:

- Patient assessments
- Acquire and analyze data using ultrasound and related diagnostic technologies

- Provide a summary of findings to the physician to aid in patient diagnosis and management
- Use independent judgment and systematic problem-solving methods to produce high-quality diagnostic information and optimize patient care[8,9]

"The Scope of Practice" of the diagnostic ultrasound professional, as reported by two journals, developed each of these practice areas in considerable depth.[8,9] For instance, patient assessment includes verifying patient identification and that the requested procedure is appropriate for the patient's history and complaints. The technologist is expected to take a history and review the patient's medical record in addition to assessing the patient's ability to tolerate the procedure and determining if any contraindications to the procedure exist.[8,9] These skills distinguish the vascular laboratory technologist from a technician who performs an examination by rote. Obtaining this highly specialized set of skills requires adequate training and clinical experience.

Education and Training

In December 2000, the Society for Vascular Ultrasound (SVU) proposed academic standards for undergraduate education in vascular technology.[10] The proposal closely aligned with the scope of practice.[9] Educational programs should be designed to offer graduates the required knowledge to perform the four basic aspects of their practice as outlined above. The proposal recommended that the Commission on Accreditation of Allied Health Education Programs (CAAHEP) accredit all undergraduate programs.[10] The proposal stated that undergraduate programs must contain didactic learning sessions and hands-on clinical experience in a clinical vascular laboratory for a period of 12 months of each, with a minimum of 1680 clinical hours.[10] Suggested curriculum in vascular technology, additional coursework, and standards for laboratories offering externships are all outlined.[10] This document gives technical or physician directors of laboratories a standard by which they can judge applicants who have attended such programs, even before applicants obtain the Registered Vascular Technologist (RVT) credential.

The Registered Vascular Technologist

The ICAVL has recommended that all technologists in the VDL should obtain the RVT certification from the American Registry of Diagnostic Medical Sonographers (ARDMS). As a minimum, the technical director should have this credential. To obtain the RVT certificate, an individual must pass an ARDMS-administered examination consisting of two parts: (1) vascular physical principles and instrumentation and (2) clinical vascular technology. Though passing this examination and obtaining the RVT credential is only one feature that might indicate a technologist's qualifications (i.e., it has

no applied practical test component), it is an accepted standard for many states, insurers, and the ICAVL. Completing the examination developed by practicing vascular technologists at least guarantees a minimum level of knowledge and, at present, represents the only available standard.[11]

The ARDMS has defined several pathways whereby an individual can qualify to take the examination.[12] One common mechanism is for individuals who have a 2-year degree in an allied health field or a 4-year bachelor's degree (in any field) to take additional coursework specific to vascular technology (12 credit hours) and to work in a VDL for 12 months (full-time clinical vascular ultrasound) to qualify for the examination. Historically, this has probably been the most common mechanism but, more recently, completion of a formal program in vascular technology has become more commonplace. These programs qualify an individual to take the certification examination without further clinical experience. The RVT examination may also be taken if the person is a high school graduate, takes 12 credit hours of additional coursework, and works for 48 months in a vascular lab (or 24 months in a VDL and 24 months in another allied health area). Finally, someone with a 2-year degree in a nonmedical area can also qualify for the examination with additional coursework and 24 months working in clinical vascular ultrasound.

Physician Qualifications

The vascular laboratory originated in the vascular surgery community. The first vascular laboratory is attributed to Dr. Robert Linton at the Massachusetts General hospital in Boston in 1946.[4] The list of physicians that followed in the ensuing decades reads like a who's who in vascular surgery: Cranley, Strandness, Hobbs, Fronek, Sumner, Darling, Rutherford, Kempczinski, Nicolaides, Yao, and so on.[4] Yet today, a variety of other specialists also participate in the VDL including radiologists, neurologists, neurosurgeons, cardiologists, and vascular internists.[7] How then do we ensure some level of consistency because no one specialty necessarily has all the requisite skills and knowledge?[5,7] The components listed in Table 3-1 show that specialty training, even in vascular surgery, probably does not provide a thorough knowledge. In fact, no specialty will possess all the requisite skills without some additional exposure, training, education, and experience.[5,7]

One key requirement for any physician working in the VDL is clinical knowledge and experience with the pathology, pathophysiology, symptoms, signs, and differential diagnosis of vascular diseases. It follows that an understanding of these diseases will allow a better understanding of the appropriate diagnostic testing, its sensitivity to detect disease, and the pitfalls associated with the diagnostic technique.[7] Although not every physician interpreting studies must have all the knowledge listed in Table 3-1, focused areas may be designated for certain specialties (e.g., transcranial Doppler and carotid duplex testing for neurologists and neurosurgeons).[13]

Training Background

Though the training will vary according to specialties, Abbott defined three levels of competence for the vascular surgery fellow that may be appropriate for any specialty: (1) interpretation of studies, (2) understanding how tests are performed, and (3) technologic competence in performing the tests.[14] He states that the first level is easily obtainable within the vascular surgery training period of 1 year, though it is unlikely for the other levels. In that instance, additional time is necessary, which he suggests could be 2 half days per week for the second level and 2 full days each week for the third.[14]

TABLE 3-1. Educational Components of Training in Vascular Laboratories

Ultrasound and Doppler physics

Plethysmographic principles

Hemodynamic principles

Instrumentation

Extremity arterial disease

- Continuous-wave Doppler
- Segmental limb pressures and plethysmography
- Duplex ultrasound scanning
- Provocative testing (e.g., reactive hyperemia, exercise)

Cerebrovascular disease

- Duplex ultrasound Scanning
- Transcranial Doppler (TCD)
- Oculopneumoplethysmography (OPG)

Visceral diseases

- Renal arterial duplex ultrasound
- Mesenteric artery duplex ultrasound
- Organ transplant duplex ultrasound
- Portal venous duplex ultrasound

Venous disease (acute and chronic)

- Duplex ultrasound scanning
- Photoplethysmography
- Air plethysmography

Erectile dysfunction

Ophthalmic ultrasound

From Ricci MA, Rutherford RB: Qualifications of the physician in the vascular diagnostic laboratory. In AbuRhama A, Bergan J (eds): Noninvasive Vascular Diagnosis. London: Springer-Verlag, 2000.

The Association of Program Directors in Vascular Surgery has produced a comprehensive training curriculum that includes a section on vascular diagnosis.[15] The aspects pertinent to noninvasive diagnosis are listed in Table 3-2. Obviously, considerable overlap is seen between the general components in Table 3-1 and the outline for trainees in Table 3-2.

The American Academy of Neurology also put forth guidelines in 1996 that covered all aspects of neuro-imaging, including "neurosonology" for both residency training as well as physicians who have completed training.[16] If the neurologist's training program had verifiable training in the area of interest, no additional training is needed for privileges to interpret noninvasive neurologic studies. However, training must have included appropriate physics, biologic effects and instrumentation, anatomy, pathology, pathophysiology, technique, indications, interpretation, and quality assurance. Additionally, practical experience in performance and/or interpretation of 100 studies under qualified supervision is required.[16] This level of training would likely provide level 1 and level 2 competence, as suggested by Abbott,[14] and achieves some of the criteria for level 3. In addition to didactic continuing medical education (CME) to obtain the basic fund of knowledge listed above, 40 hours of specific neurosonology training with interpretation of 100 studies is recommended.[16]

TABLE 3-2. Curriculum Outline in Noninvasive Diagnosis for Vascular Surgery Trainees

To be familiar with commonly used noninvasive instruments and modalities such as Doppler ultrasound, duplex and color-flow scanning, B-mode imaging, plethysmography (air, mercury, and impedance), magnetic resonance imaging (MRI), magnetic resonance angiography (MRA), and computerized x-ray tomography (CT), and to understand the basic principles involved in their design and operation.

To be familiar with noninvasive pressure measurements (including ankle/brachial indices, segmental pressures, digital pressures), arterial and venous velocity tracings, Doppler frequency spectral analysis, segmental and digital plethysmography, transcutaneous oxygen tension measurements ($TcPO_2$), venous outflow plethysmography, calf venous air-plethysmography (Nicolaides method) and to understand the hemodynamic principles underlying exercise testing (treadmill walking and claudication times, postexercise ankle pressure) and reactive hyperemia.

To understand the physiologic basis of these tests and their limitations, know when to order noninvasive tests, which to select, and how to interpret the results.

To perform simple noninvasive assessments (e.g., Doppler venous and arterial surveys and measurement of Ankle Brachial Index and be able to interpret duplex scans, MRIs, MRAs, and CT scans.

From Sumner DS, Blebea J: 16. Diagnostic techniques. apdvs.vascularweb.org./APDVS_Contribution_Pages/Archive/Old_Curriculum/463.html, accessed March 12, 2004.

Similarly, the American College of Cardiology has made recommendations for training in vascular medicine that includes the vascular laboratory.[6] This group suggests trainees should spend at least 3 months in the VDL. They suggest hands-on experience performing and interpreting all vascular laboratory tests, including physiologic and ultrasound tests. Whether this time is sufficient to achieve the third level of competence suggested by Abbott[14] seems unlikely based on the number of hours involved in 3 months (compared to 2 full days per week for 1 year[14]). Hands-on performance of the tests is stressed and that, at least, will go toward achieving competence at that level. Level 2, however, is easily obtained in the time suggested by the American College of Cardiology.

Necessary Skills

Rutherford has described the skills needed for the physician interpreting noninvasive vascular studies.[5] He states first and foremost that the physician must have a thorough understanding of vascular diseases and the clinical manifestations, prognosis, and treatment options of diseases of the arteries, veins, and lymphatics. The individual must understand the principles of vascular testing including hemodynamics, physiology, and ultrasound and Doppler physics. The physician must have an understanding of the appropriate indications for each test to avoid abuses or unnecessary tests, including experimental indications.[17] In order to have this understanding, the physician must have a fundamental knowledge of the equipment used for tests, the false-positive, false-negative, and accuracy rates of each test. The individual, therefore, must know the limitations of each test. Finally, the physician interpreting diagnostic tests should have the ability to perform the tests.[5,7] Though it is not expected that the interpreting physician have the same working knowledge as the technologist performing many studies each day, he or she should ideally have enough practical experience to help troubleshoot problems or even assist the technologist perform a difficult test. There is no substitute for the operating surgeon. For example, a technologist who is having trouble with a study needs to be shown where the surgeon did the anastomosis or the course of the graft using the ultrasound transducer, rather than describing it or pointing with a finger. In addition, increased use of intraoperative ultrasound almost mandates that the surgeon be able to perform and interpret the findings in the operating room.[18]

This latter requirement is perhaps more controversial, or is at least not universally recommended. The ability to perform and interpret noninvasive VDL studies has been recommended by Rutherford,[5] the American Academy of Neurology,[16] and the American College of Cardiology,[6] as well as the American College of Radiology.[19] The SVU[20] has recommended minimum standards for physicians interpreting VDL studies that are very similar to Rutherford's recommendations[5] in every aspect except the requirement for the ability to perform testing. However, the majority of recommendations from various medical specialty societies favor the idea that interpreting physicians obtain experience in the performance of vascular noninvasive studies.

The SVU has also recommended "suggested experience levels"[20] for physicians working in the VDL. For experienced physicians, over 3 years, the minimum number of examinations would include 300 carotid duplex studies, 300 transcranial Doppler studies, 300 peripheral arterial physiologic studies, 300 arterial duplex studies, 225 visceral vascular tests, and 300 venous duplex studies. For those recently completing residency training, required numbers during training are considerably less. For those without formal training, reduced numbers over a 2-year period are suggested as a minimum.[20] These numbers certainly represent a busy VDL and, in some cases, will be difficult to obtain in smaller hospitals or practices.

The American College of Radiology has also put forth standards for physicians interpreting ultrasound examinations.[19] These recommendations require experience in examination performance and include the requirement for a thorough knowledge of ultrasound principles, physics, anatomy, physiology, pathophysiology, indications, and limitations of tests (but hemodynamics is not mentioned). Additional requirements include: (1) certification in radiology and the performance of 300 ultrasound examinations in 36 months; (2) completion of an accredited residency program with the performance of 500 examinations within 36 months; or (3) certification in a nonradiology specialty with 200 hours of CME and 500 cases relative to the specialty in 36 months.[19] In fact, these recommendations are extremely limiting such that only radiologists could practically fulfill their requirements. In addition, the requirements do not address noninvasive physiologic testing other than ultrasound imaging, further limiting their usefulness outside of a department of radiology or radiology training program.

Although the background and experience may vary for physicians interpreting vascular noninvasive studies, general agreement exists regarding the cognitive skills necessary to work in this environment. Though the amount of time (or number of tests) recommended to obtain the skills varies with specialty organizations, all agree that a thorough understanding of vascular diseases and the principles of testing is necessary. Whether the interpreting physician should also have the skills needed to perform the examination is the opinion expressed by most of the references and societies cited. Ultimately, it remains for the individual institution or department to develop minimum standards for physicians interpreting in the vascular laboratory. These should set a high standard but allow for inclusion of multiple specialties. Whether absolute numbers are added to these minimum standards (e.g., as in the SVU recommendations[20] or like those developed at the University of Vermont[7,13]) must be addressed by each institution.

The Physician Registered Vascular Technologist

Obtaining an RVT certification by the physician working in the VDL has been encouraged,[7,11,14,20] although this does not guarantee their qualifications and training are adequate, nor does it ensure their competence. The RVT examination prerequisites, however, satisfy the recommendations of most of the specialty societies. The examination tests physics, ultrasound and Doppler principles, hemodynamics, and a clinical knowledge of vascular diseases. Actual performance of examinations is also a prerequisite. No equivalent or even similar credential exists for physicians and, therefore, some have chosen to take the RVT examination. In spite of this, the overall number remains small: of 10,575 active RVT registrants, only 342 are physicians.[21]

Physician Directors

The physician director of the laboratory is in a unique position of having general oversight of the operation and performance of the laboratory, technologists, physicians, and equipment. Typically, this is the most experienced physician, but it should always be someone who is an active participant in the clinical care of patients.[5] Clinical experience is necessary for the medical director to solve controversies or to provide less experienced clinicians with advice. Additionally, as a minimum, this individual must possess the complete breath of knowledge and skills described above.[5,7,22] Kempczinski favors obtaining an RVT for the VDL director even though it is not an accreditation requirement.[4]

Rutherford[22] described the ideal characteristics of the VDL director as being able to:

- Understand the instrumentation (and troubleshoot)
- Perform noninvasive tests
- Instruct others in the performance of tests
- Possess a thorough knowledge of clinical vascular disease
- Understand the meaning of test results, including accuracy and limitations, and interpret them in light of the clinical setting
- Engage in other activities (e.g., supervision, teaching, and consulting)
- Have no conflict of interest

For the ideal VDL director, one must add several additional qualities. The director should have the ability to be an effective administrator and supervisor because he or she must manage personnel, schedules, and human resources issues in addition to assessing the competence of both technologists and physician interpreters. The VDL director should be able to build a business plan and strategies with a sound budgeting approach.[4] This individual must be an expert in constantly evolving coding and compliance issues to ensure the laboratory is fairly compensated while adhering to laws and regulations. Directors are ultimately responsible for all procedural protocols and standardized interpretation criteria as well as accreditation applications. Finally, he or she needs to be a diplomat when dealing with physicians who demand inappropriate tests or when managing different specialties within the laboratory. This is a job full of significant responsibilities, and the selection of a VDL director should be a thoughtful and careful process.[7]

Competence

Defining competence is likely the most difficult component to be considered. Although one may specify minimum qualifications, recommended numbers of tests, and certifying examinations before allowing an individual to work in the VDL, none of these items ensures that someone is truly competent at the task. In fact, there is no universally accepted definition of competence with regard to medical practice.[3] The Accreditation Council for Graduate Medical Education (ACGME) has tried, however, by defining the following six areas of competence[23]:

- Patient care that is compassionate, appropriate, and effective for the treatment of health problems and the promotion of health

- Medical knowledge about established and evolving biomedical, clinical, and cognate (e.g., epidemiologic and social-behavioral) sciences and the application of this knowledge to patient care

- Practice-based learning and improvement that involves investigation and evaluation of their own patient care, appraisal and assimilation of scientific evidence, and improvements in patient care

- Interpersonal and communication skills that result in effective information exchange and teaming with patients, their families, and other health professionals

- Professionalism, as manifested through a commitment to carrying out professional responsibilities, adherence to ethical principles, and sensitivity to a diverse patient population

- Systems-based practice, as manifested by actions that demonstrate an awareness of and responsiveness to the larger context and system of health care and the ability to effectively call on system resources to provide care that is of optimal value

This definition has gained widespread acceptance in the assessment of resident trainees[3] and can be applied by the VDL director when assessing the competency of personnel in the vascular laboratory. Ultimately, this assessment is related to a quality improvement process that links data collection to outcomes to provide feedback to technologists and physicians that, together with the medical literature, improves and updates practice patterns and results.[24]

The technology professional societies have also produced a scope of practice document that serves as a model for defining most aspects of technologist competence.[8,9] The basic clinical practice standards were listed above and are detailed in the scope of practice.[8,9] This is an excellent means to judge technologist performance. The practice standard also includes other aspects that a competent technologist could master including clear, precise, accurate, timely documentation with appropriate diagnostic images, quality assurance planning, maintaining a safe and functional workplace, self-assessment, collaborative skills, ethical practices, and continuing education.[8,9] It has also been suggested that participation in professional societies may be considered a component of competence assessment.

Assessing Competence

The components of competence listed by the ACGME[23] can be adapted for application to technologists and physicians working in the VDL. The ACGME has provided a framework for assessing competence as well.[23] To begin, objectives must be set up by which competency can be measured. For technologists, the scope of practice document largely meets this need.[9] In this way, determination of competency goes beyond merely counting numbers (though quality assessment and accuracy are still vitally important) and can provide a true assessment, ultimately leading to quality improvements.[24] For the assessment of resident physicians, the ACGME has produced a "toolbox" that has a description of assessment methods and references.[23] This is not specific and can easily be applied to physician interpreters in the vascular laboratory.

Continuing Education

One area of universal agreement for both physician and technologist societies is the need for continuing education as an absolute requirement.[5,8,9,11,13,16,19,20] To maintain competency, a working knowledge of new developments in the medical literature is essential and a key component of process improvement.[24] It is generally accepted that the CME should be in the area of vascular diagnosis, though it is important to include general education about the clinical, pathologic, and hemodynamic processes that one sees in the VDL to meet the knowledge requirements described above. It is a requirement that technologists and physicians receive CME for ICAVL accreditation. To maintain RVT certification by the ARDMS, 30 hours of CME every 3 years is a minimum requirement. The SVU has adapted this requirement in its recommendations as well.[20] The American Academy of Neurology[16] suggests 25 hours of neuroimaging CME every 5 years, whereas at the other end of the spectrum, the American College of Radiology[19] suggests 60 hours of Category 1 credits every 3 years. Though each institution and VDL should address this requirement, it does not seem unreasonable to ask for the minimum of 30 hours every 3 years as suggested by the SVU and ARDMS.

REFERENCES

1. Institute of Medicine Committee on Quality of Health Care in America (Kohn LT, Corrigan JM, Donaldson MS, eds): To Err is Human: Building a Safer Health System. Washington, DC: National Academy Press, 2000.
2. Nahrwold DL: The competence movement: A report on the activities of the American Board of Medical Specialties. Bull Am Coll Surg 85:14–18, 2000.
3. Epstein RM, Hundert EM: Defining and assessing professional competence. JAMA 287:243–244, 2002.
4. Kempczinski R: Challenging times for the vascular laboratory. Sem Vasc Surg 7:212–216, 1994.
5. Rutherford RB: Physicians in the vascular diagnostic laboratory: Educational background, prerequisite skills, credentialing, and continuing medical education. Sem Vasc Surg 7:217–222, 1994.
6. Spittell JA Jr, Creager MA, Dorros G, et al: Recommendations for training in vascular medicine. J Am Coll Cardiol 22:626–628, 1993.
7. Ricci MA, Rutherford RB: Qualifications of the Physician in the Vascular Diagnostic Laboratory. In AbuRhama A, Bergan J (eds): Noninvasive Vascular Diagnosis. London: Springer-Verlag, 2000.
8. Sonography Coalition: Scope of practice of the diagnostic ultrasound professional. J Diag Med Sono 16:206–211, 2001.
9. Sonography Coalition: Scope of practice of the diagnostic ultrasound professional. J Vasc Tech 16:206–211, 2001.
10. Society for Vascular Ultrasound: Standards for undergraduate educational programs in vascular technology. www.svunet.org/about/positions/standard.education.htm, accessed March 12, 2004.
11. Jones AM: Training and certification of the vascular technologist. Sem Vasc Surg 7:228–233, 1994.
12. Examination prerequisite chart, www.ardms.org/applicants/prechart.html, accessed March 12, 2004.
13. Shackford SR, Ricci MA, Hebert JC: Education and credentialing. Prob Gen Surg 14:126–132, 1997.
14. Abbott WM: Training vascular surgical residents in the noninvasive vascular laboratory. Sem Vasc Surg 7:223–227, 1994.
15. Sumner DS, Blebea J: Diagnostic techniques. www.vascularweb.org/APDVSdoc/463.
16. Gomez C, Kinkel P, Masdeu J, et al: Guidelines for credentialing in neuroimaging; Report from the task force on updating guidelines for credentialing in neuroimaging. www.asnweb.org/practice/niguidelines.htm, accessed March 12, 2004.

17. Strandness DE Jr: Indications for and frequency of noninvasive testing. Sem Vasc Surg 7:245–250, 1994.
18. Ricci MA: The changing role of duplex scan in the management of carotid bifurcation disease and endarterectomy. Sem Vasc Surg 11:3–11, 1998.
19. Grant EG, Barr LL, Gooding GAW, et al: ACR standard for performing and interpreting diagnostic ultrasound examinations. 1992; revised 2000, www.acr.org/dyna/?doc = departments/stand_accred/ standards/standards.html, accessed March 12, 2004.
20. Johnson B, Moneta G, Oliver M: Suggested minimum qualifications for physicians interpreting noninvasive vascular diagnostic studies. www.svunet.org/about/positions/standard.physicianquals.htm, accessed March 12, 2004.
21. Personal communication, American Registry of Diagnostic Medical Sonographers, September 11, 2002.
22. Rutherford RB: Qualifications of the physician in charge of the vascular diagnostic laboratory. J Vasc Surg 8:732–735, 1988.
23. Accreditation Council for Graduate Medical Education Outcome Project, www.acgme.org/outcome, accessed March 12, 2004.
24. Ricci MA, Beardall RW: Documentation of competency: Maintaining an outcomes database. Sem Vasc Surg 15:191–197, 2002.

Chapter 4

Quality Assurance and Certification of the Vascular Laboratory

SANDRA L. KATANICK • GAIL P. SIZE

Introduction

Establishing and following standard protocols and ensuring staff certification are of paramount importance in ensuring that the vascular testing center has the basic tools for quality patient testing and care.[1] The first non-invasive vascular laboratory appeared in the early 1970s as a small department or testing area, usually located within the university setting and often employing only one or two nurses or technicians. As the role of noninvasive vascular testing began to grow and develop beyond pressure measurements, continuous-wave Doppler, and plethysmographic devices, so did the role and number of nurses and technicians. Today's vascular testing center offers a myriad of testing services from the conventional ankle brachial pressures to interoperative duplex, and the technician of yesterday is now a registered vascular technologist (RVT).

History of Vascular Technology

The profession of vascular technology evolved in response to a need for a simple method of diagnosing or following the progression of vascular disease in symptomatic or asymptomatic patients. At the time, laboratory personnel were trained either by self-study, by observation of patient testing at another laboratory, or by attending a manufacturer's seminar. Many supplemented their initial training by attending educational seminars. As responsibilities increased, the vascular technician evolved into the vascular technologist. The technologist was not only responsible for performing more sophisticated testing but also became responsible for evaluating the findings, recommending alternative testing, and producing a preliminary report. The qualifications to perform vascular diagnostic studies were very subjective and were usually measured by the technologist's experience. In 1979 the Society of Vascular Ultrasound (SVU), then known as the Society of Noninvasive Vascular Technology (SNIVT), began to investigate the possibility of national certification.[2] The American Registry of Diagnostic Medical Sonographers (ARDMS) administered the first vascular technology examination in 1983. Even though the RVT credential assured the employer and public that the technologist had demonstrated a minimum level of knowledge, it did not ensure that the technologist was proficient in all areas of testing, nor that quality testing was being performed.

With the ever-increasing amount of required knowledge and the level at which the vascular technologist must perform, certification is now considered the standard of practice in ultrasound. Certification brings credibility and professional legitimacy to the ultrasound professional.[3] There are currently three recognized credentialing organizations: the ARDMS, which awards the RVT; Cardiovascular Credentialing International (CCI), which awards the registered vascular specialist (RVS); and the American Registry of Radiologic Technologists, which awards the RT(VS). Which credential is favored is likely to depend on the practice setting and background; the SVU endorses the RVT as the official credential.

As more and more vascular technologists became registered, there was concern that the registry did not ensure the RVT was proficient in all areas of testing, or that the studies were accurate. In addition, as ultrasound systems became more refined, many studies (e.g., venous and carotid duplex) became a gold standard upon which treatment was based; therefore, the question of the accuracy and reliability of noninvasive vascular testing needed to be addressed. With increasing levels of noninvasive vascular testing, there was an increasing need for creation and standardization of laboratory guidelines. The Intersocietal Commission for the Accreditation of Vascular Laboratories (ICAVL) was formed in part to address the issues of standardization of techniques and reporting and quality assurance, and to recognize those laboratories that consistently produced quality noninvasive vascular examinations in a reliable fashion.

Scope of Practice

The success of any vascular testing center depends on the quality and expertise of its entire staff, on the testing center's internally generated specific testing protocols, and on its operational policies. Each testing center should begin by defining the technologist's scope of practice. This can easily be adopted from the SVU's position paper entitled *Scope of Practice for the Diagnostic Ultrasound Professional*. This position paper is endorsed by the Society of Medical Sonography, American Institute of Ultrasound Medicine, American Society of Echocardiography, Canadian Society of Diagnostic Medical Sonographers, and the Society of Vascular Sonography; its contents can be applied to all ultrasound professionals, not just the vascular technologist. This document defines in detail the roles, performance, and behavior expected of the diagnostic ultrasound professional. The scope of practice states that: "The diagnostic ultrasound professional is an individual qualified by professional credentialing and academic and clinical experience to provide diagnostic patient care services using ultrasound and related diagnostic procedures."[3]

Ultrasound professionals are required to perform patient assessments, acquire and analyze data obtained using ultrasound and related diagnostic technologies, provide a summary of findings to the physician to aid in patient diagnosis and management, and use independent judgement and systematic problem solving methods to produce high-quality diagnostic information and optimize patient care.[5] There is no one mechanism to ensure technical competence; however, acquiring national board certification is the current standard of practice in ultrasound. The established national certification perquisites are an aid in ensuring that specific didactic instruction and clinical experience are at an acceptable level. Having board certification; following standard protocols; and developing a system of peer review, quality assurance, quality control, and testing validation will ensure the competence of the technologist and the vascular testing center.

Standardized Protocols

Every testing center must establish and provide comprehensive procedure protocols. This is extremely important to ensure standardized quality testing, and it is mandated in the Scope of Practice. This document states that the ultrasound professional is responsible for "analysis and determination of a procedure plan for conduction of the diagnostic examination," and that the procedure plan must fall within the established protocol.[1] Why are standard protocols important and how is follow-up performed to ensure test quality? A procedure protocol is a written document describing the specific elements for performing a testing procedure; it should reflect the testing center's actual testing procedure in a step-by-step description that includes, at a minimum, the ICAVL standards for techniques and components of each noninvasive vascular test performed. Consistent quality testing and patient care can only be provided through the use of standardized protocols to produce high-quality examinations, performed by credentialed personnel in accredited laboratories.

Practice Patterns and Membership Opinion Regarding the Value of Credentialing and Accreditation

Members of the Society of Diagnostic Medical Sonography and the SVU recently conducted a practice survey to evaluate member opinions about the credentialing and accreditation process, and to assess current practice patterns in the performance of carotid duplex studies. The randomized survey was sent to varying practice settings including vascular surgery, radiology, cardiology, and sonography in the states of Indiana and Kentucky. Based on the findings, 4782 or 12% of carotid duplex examinations performed annually were repeat studies necessitated by the initial study being inadequate; 57% of those initial studies had significant discrepancies "often" or "very often." Noncredentialed personnel nearly always performed the inadequate initial examinations in nonaccredited facilities. The most common reason for repeat carotid duplex studies were inadequate diagnostic criteria (40%), incompetent technical staff (40%), incomplete interpretation by the physician (39%), and failure to adhere to a diagnostic standard (30%). Other reasons included poor instrumentation or technique; and insufficient waveform/gray scale data. When asked if the carotid duplex results alone were used to determine eligibility for carotid surgery, 60% of members responded that their practices "often" or "very often" determined patient management based solely on carotid duplex results. When asked if they believed that credentialing and or accreditation improves appropriateness of vascular sonography services, 91% agreed, 6% disagreed, and 3% abstained; overall, 98% of those surveyed support crediting and accreditation.[6,7]

History of the ICAVL

In 1989, an informal meeting of leaders in the field of noninvasive testing proposed studying the possibility of establishing a voluntary accreditation process. This initial group included vascular surgeons, radiologists, and technologists. The discussion group concluded that there was no suitable existing accreditation option and that they needed to study the feasibility of creating a new accrediting organization.[4]

Support and financial sponsorship were sought from a variety of professional societies whose members were involved in noninvasive vascular testing. One of the initial goals was to have a broad base of support across different specialty lines; another was to have an independent entity that was not specifically allied with any one specialty or society. From the very beginning, the emphasis was on an intersocietal approach. The American Academy of Neurology (AAN), the American College of Radiology (ACR), the American Institute of Ultrasound in Medicine (AIUM), the International Society for Cardiovascular Surgery (North American Chapter) (ISCVS), the Society for Vascular Surgery (SVS), the Society for Vascular Medicine and Biology (SVMB), the Society of Diagnostic Medical Sonographers (SDMS), and the Society of Vascular Technology (SVT) all committed to sponsor the initial efforts, and a work group was formed with two representatives from each society.

The ICAVL is truly an illustration of the concept of intersocietal effort, and in 1993 four additional sponsoring organizations were added: the American College of Cardiology; the American Society of Neuroimaging, combined with the American Academy of Neurology; the Joint Section on Cerebrovascular Surgery/American Association of Neurological Surgeons/Congress of Neurological Surgeons; and the Society of Cardiovascular and Interventional Radiology. In 2000, the Society of Radiologists in Ultrasound joined the ICAVL. In 1996 the American College of Radiology withdrew from the board of directors.

The initial meetings were dedicated to defining the scope of vascular laboratory accreditation and the minimum guidelines necessary for the assurance of quality. The overall objective was "To ensure high-quality patient care by providing a mechanism that recognizes laboratories providing quality vascular diagnostic techniques through a process of voluntary accreditation." This goal was to be achieved by establishing an accreditation process, issuing certificates of accreditation, and maintaining a registry of accredited laboratories. An important principle that was established early was that the accreditation should be as inclusive as possible, something that could be achieved by even the smallest laboratory that was doing quality work: It would not be limited to academics only. Another important principle adopted was that accreditation would not require any one specific medical specialty training but would evaluate the particular education and experience of all of the doctors and the technologists in each laboratory.

The ICAVL was incorporated in 1990 for the purpose of providing a peer review evaluation of laboratories and facilities providing noninvasive vascular testing in North America. The process itself is one of peer review performed by trained reviewers, and it places significant emphasis on the judgment of the quality of the work that a laboratory produces.

Because there previously has been no mechanism in place to recognize the quality and appropriateness of testing, certification and accreditation have been viewed as a benefit not only for the laboratories, departments, and facilities providing the testing but also to patients and payers who previously had no way of determining the quality of the study they were receiving or paying for. The awareness of the significance of accreditation, both within and beyond the medical community, has elevated the numbers of laboratories seeking accreditation to unprecedented rates. The major implication for the noninvasive vascular diagnostic laboratory that is not yet accredited will likely be denial of reimbursement. In addition, because of the increased public awareness of the importance of accreditation, patient avoidance of the nonaccredited laboratory may also be a reality.

In 2000, the ICAVL published its first electronic application. This application allows all answers to be entered into a database that allows for retrieval of accurate statistics regarding the national practice of noninvasive vascular testing (Fig. 4-1). One of the more interesting statistics to follow has been the change in specialty of the medical director and medical staff over the past 10 years (Fig. 4-2). The electronic application also eliminates the need for laboratories to re-enter previously submitted information when completing their reaccreditation applications. The newest version allows laboratories to even embed their attachments such as protocols and diagnostic criteria, thereby keeping all laboratory operational materials in one place.

As an accreditation organization, the ICAVL is expected to maintain a program that balances the changing needs of both the vascular ultrasound community and the general public. Therefore, the *Essentials and Standards* are reviewed and revised by the board of directors as necessary every 2 years to maintain that balance. They also are evaluated with respect to recently published scientific literature to be certain that they reflect current practice and are scientifically accurate. The application for accreditation is also revised as necessary to provide the best mechanism to objectively evaluate the laboratory operation and its compliance with the current *Essentials and Standards*. In 1999 the ICAVL added a random site

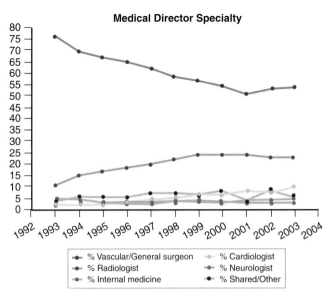

Figure 4-2. *The specialty of the medical director from 1992 through 2003.*

visit process to its program. Each quarter two applicant laboratories are randomly selected to undergo an on-site visit at the expense of the ICAVL. This allows the ICAVL to evaluate the accuracy of the written application and the efficacy of judging a laboratory solely on a written application; it also forms the basis of an internal quality assurance mechanism. To date, these random site visits have validated the accuracy of the program and support the continued evaluation and accreditation of laboratories based solely on the written application.

Essentials and Standards

The ICAVL *Essentials and Standards* form the basis for the entire accreditation program. They are intended to provide the infrastructure for laboratory organization that ensures standardization of procedures from laboratory to laboratory and person to person. The following summary of the standards was published in 2003. The standards are published in their entirety on the ICAVL Web site at www.icavl.org.

Part I: Organization

- Section 1—Supervision and Personnel
- Section 2—Support Services
- Section 3—Physical Facilities
- Section 4—Examination Interpretation, Reports, and Records
- Section 5—Miscellaneous
- Section 6—Quality Assurance and Quality Control

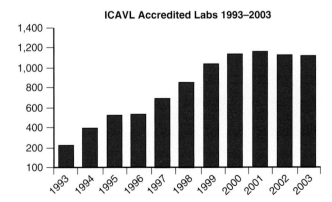

Figure 4-1. *The number of accredited labs from 1993 through 2003.*

Section 1 outlines the requirements for all physicians interpreting noninvasive vascular studies; it contains three pathways for meeting appropriate experience and training, all a combination of formal or informal training, number of years of experience, and number of examinations interpreted.

There are also multiple pathways for all technologists/sonographers to be considered appropriately experienced and trained; these range from holding an appropriate credential (e.g., RVT from the American Registry of Diagnostic Medical Sonographers; RVS from Cardiovascular Credentialing International; or RT(VS) by the American Registry of Radiologic Technologists) to on-the-job training combined with education and/or volume of studies performed.

All medical and technical staff working in the laboratory must acquire at least 15 hours of continuing medical education (CME) related to vascular testing every 3 years. All CME must be accredited (AMA Category I, SDMS, SVU), and physicians must have at least 10 hours that are AMA Category I.

In Section 4 there are specific standards addressing reporting and dealing with everything from report components to report timeliness. Specifically, all final reports must have the data reviewed by the interpreting physician, be completed within 2 working days, and have reporting standardized in content for the entire laboratory. All reports must contain at a minimum the date of the examination, the clinical indications leading to the performance of the examination, an adequate description of the test performed, an overview of the results of the examination (including pertinent positive and negative findings), the reasons for any limited examinations, a summary of the test findings, comparison with previous related studies (where available), and a physician signature and/or electronic verification.

Each one of the *Essentials and Standards* for the five testing areas (extracranial cerebrovascular, intracranial cerebrovascular, peripheral arterial, peripheral venous, and visceral vascular) is constructed in the same fashion. They each contain six sections that address that specific area of testing.

Part II – Vascular Laboratory Operations

- Section 1—Instrumentation
- Section 2—Indications
- Section 3—Techniques and Components of Examination Performance
- Section 4—Diagnostic Criteria
- Section 5—Procedure Volumes
- Section 6—Quality Assurance

Of significant importance in all testing areas is the section outlining the techniques and components of examination performance. There are specific guidelines for the number of views and Doppler samples for each vascular examination. Although the standards do not specify the exact diagnostic criteria that must be used for each examination, they do require that all examinations adhere to the criteria that the laboratory has validated for use.

Quality assurance requirements are clearly outlined for each testing section, with minimum numbers of correlations required for all areas except venous testing. Generally, a laboratory is required to correlate at least 30 vessels per area of testing every 3 years to continue to validate the laboratory's accuracy over time. Although there is no threshold defined for overall accuracy, if a laboratory finds that its accuracy is low (e.g., less than 80%), they should be able to document that a quality improvement plan has been put in place.

Benefits of Accreditation

There is no denying that applying for accreditation is a lengthy and somewhat laborious process. It requires that all staff are appropriately experienced and trained and that the training is documented, the physical facilities are adequate, the record-keeping and final reporting processes are appropriate, and that there are step-by-step written protocols for all testing procedures performed in the laboratory. It also mandates that there are validated diagnostic criteria for each test performed, and that a valid quality assurance program routinely correlates the noninvasive vascular laboratory results to another testing modality. Even though this may be time consuming, once everything is in place the laboratory will function at its peak performance and quality will be ensured. When all of the documentation has been completed, the laboratory submits, as part of the application, actual case studies performed by current staff members using current equipment. The case studies are carefully analyzed for compliance with the standards regarding performance and interpretation; this represents the most important aspect of the application process.

Once accreditation is granted, the ICAVL offers a press release program to accredited laboratories in order to help advertise their accomplishment. A camera-ready logo is also provided for use on reports, laboratory stationery, and other printed materials used in the laboratory. The laboratory is also listed on the ICAVL Web site for the duration of its accreditation

Impact of Accreditation

The ICAVL is dedicated to promoting high-quality noninvasive vascular diagnostic testing in the delivery of health care by providing a peer review process of laboratory accreditation. This mission is realized every time an application is reviewed and a laboratory is granted accreditation based on the quality of its work. Completing the accreditation application enables laboratory personnel to do a self-evaluation of their work. They often identify and correct problems during the document completion phase (e.g., revising protocols and reviewing and validating their diagnostic criteria), ultimately improving the diagnostic accuracy of the testing performed.

In addition to improving the quality of the testing, there have been other indirectly related benefits of the ICAVL accreditation program. These include an increase in the number of credentialed technologists and sonographers, increased job security for the technical staff in laboratories, and increased support staff in the operation of some laboratories. Because of the required continuing education requirements for all staff members in the laboratory, there has been an increase in the number of relevant noninvasive vascular educational programs, and an increase in attendance at these meetings. By increasing the educational level of the field in general, ultimately the quality of care the patient receives is improved by providing the basis for a more accurate diagnosis.

Conclusions

History has shown that the highest quality noninvasive vascular examinations are performed by credentialed diagnostic ultrasound professionals in accredited facilities. If either of these are absent, the quality can be improved by using as models the *Standards for Assurance of Minimum Entry Level Competence for the Diagnostic Ultrasound Professional* and *Scope of Practice of the Diagnostic Ultrasound Profession*, and by mandating national certification within a specific time frame established when hiring new staff. These efforts, coupled with strict adherence to established protocols, participation in peer review, and quality assurance programs that include testing validation, will help ensure that the patient is receiving quality care while the laboratory proceeds toward accreditation.

REFERENCES

1. Burnham C, Nix ML: Establishing Technical Competence in the Vascular Laboratory. In Bernstein E (ed): Vascular Diagnosis, 4th ed. St Louis: Mosby, 1993.
2. Jones AM: Education and Certification of the Vascular Technologist. In Bernstein E (ed): Vascular Diagnosis, 4th ed. St Louis: Mosby, 1993.
3. Sonography Coalition: Scope of Practice for the Diagnostic Ultrasound Professional, Pp. 1-4, 2000.
4. Baker JD: Accreditation of Noninvasive Vascular Laboratories. In AbuRahma AD, Bergan JJ (eds): Noninvasive Vascular Diagnosis. New York: Springer, 2000.
5. Standards for assurance of minimum entry level competence for the diagnostic ultrasound professional. JDMS, 17:301–311, 2001.
6. Jones A, West F, Benge C: A case study of the value of Society for Vascular Ultrasound Membership participation in defining local medical review policy: Results of an Indiana and Kentucky practice survey. J Vasc 27(4):223–226, 2003.
7. Boswell S, Jones A, Benge C: Practice patterns and membership opinion about the value of credentialing and accreditation: Results of a membership survey. JDMS 19(6):387–390, 2003.

Chapter 5

What Are We Measuring in the Vascular Patient?

MARK J.W. KOELEMAIJ • DINK A. LEGEMATE

Introduction

In a systematic review of the physical examination of patients suspected of peripheral arterial occlusive disease (PAOD), McGee and Boyko found low predictive value for abnormal pulses, unilateral coolness, prolonged venous filling time, and femoral bruits to diagnose PAOD.[1] Other signs (e.g., capillary refill, skin atrophy or discolorations, and absence of hair) were of no help in establishing a diagnosis. It is not only the lower extremity that is difficult to assess by physical examination alone; only 43% of patients in whom palpation suggested the presence of an abdominal aortic aneurysm larger than 3.0 cm actually had this condition.[2] In patients with a carotid artery stenosis greater than 50%, a carotid bruit is found 4.4 times more often than in those without a stenosis.[3]

These examples illustrate the limitations of diagnostic accuracy of physical examination in patients with vascular disease, and that additional testing is often necessary to establish a definitive diagnosis. This chapter addresses issues related to the assessment of the clinical value of diagnostic tests in vascular patients.

Diagnostic Accuracy

The aim of additional diagnostic testing is to increase the probability of identifying a disease in patients who may benefit from an intervention; and to increase the probability of ruling out disease in patients, thereby reducing the chance of doing harm by unnecessary interventions. The clinical value of a diagnostic test is determined by its diagnostic accuracy and reproducibility, and by the availability of an effective treatment for the disease.

Reference Standard

In the development phase, new diagnostic tests are usually compared to a "gold standard" test to determine their value to discriminate between the presence and absence of disease. The term *gold standard test* implies that a test provides absolute certainty on the true disease status of the patient. Because this is virtually never the case, it is more appropriate to use the term *reference standard*. When tests are evaluated against a reference standard, the diagnostic performance, by definition, can at best approximate the reference standard but never perform better. The limitations of a reference standard can be illustrated by the use of angiography for the evaluation of lower extremity arterial disease. Although conventional angiography served as reference standard for a long time, it became apparent that intra-arterial digital subtraction angiography (iaDSA) has an even better diagnostic accuracy.[4] In addition, recent studies comparing magnetic resonance angiography (MRA) and iaDSA found that MRA detected more patent crural arteries than does iaDSA.[5]

Sensitivity and Specificity

The ability of a test to discriminate between the presence and absence of disease (diagnostic accuracy) can be expressed in terms of sensitivity and specificity. The sensitivity of a test (true-positive rate) is the proportion of patients with a positive test result and the presence of disease as determined by the reference test (Table 5-1). The specificity, or true-negative rate, is the proportion of patients with a negative test result and the absence of disease. The sensitivity and specificity can be calculated from the 2×2 contingency table (see Table 5-1).

It is important to realize that the sensitivity and specificity of a test are dynamic entities. In the first place, the sensitivity and specificity may vary within different subgroups. This can be illustrated by exercise testing in cardiology patients. It was found that exercise testing in women has a lower diagnostic accuracy to detect significant coronary artery stenosis than it does in men.[6]

A similar problem arises when the tested population does not include a broad enough spectrum of disease. It is not difficult, for instance, for duplex scanning (DS) to discriminate between totally occluded arteries and those with minimal stenosis. Should a population comprise only patients with a borderline stenosis (i.e., peak systolic velocity [PSV] ratios between 2.0 and 2.5), the sensitivity and specificity will decrease markedly because it is likely that patients will be misclassified.[7] Likewise, DS of the tibial arteries may perform well in patients with claudication,[8] whereas it may perform less well in patients with critical limb ischemia.[9]

Predictive Value

Predictive values of a test can be derived from Table 5-1. The positive predictive value (PPV) of a test is the proportion of diseased patients with a positive test result to all patients with a positive test result. Similarly, the negative predictive value (NPV) can be derived by dividing the number of patients without disease and a negative test result by the number of all patients with a negative test result. Testing will yield a maximum amount of information in patients with maximum uncertainty on the presence of the target condition (i.e., in patients with a pretest probability of having this target condition between 30% and 70%). If the physician estimates the pretest probability of disease to be very high (e.g., 90%), testing is not likely to change this probability significantly. The same applies to conditions when the pretest probability is estimated to be very low.

It is important to realize in which setting the diagnostic test is used. As noticed before, the sensitivity and specificity may depend on the spectrum of disease in the population tested. In addition, the PPV and NPV are dependent on the prevalence of disease. This is illustrated in Tables 5-2 and 5-3. Assuming that the sensitivity and specificity are constant in the populations represented in both tables, it is clear that the PPV

TABLE 5-1. A 2 × 2 Contingency Table and Test Characteristics That Can Be Calculated From This Table

	Disease +	Disease –	Total
Test +	A	B	A+B
Test –	C	D	C+D
Total	A+C	B+D	A+B+C+D

Sensitivity = A/(A+C); *specificity* = D/(B+D); *positive predictive value* = A/(A+B); *negative predictive value* = D/(C+D); *accuracy* = (A+D)/(A+B+C+D); *prevalence* = (A+C) / (A+B+C+D).
Likelihood ratio of a positive test = (A/(A+C)) / (B/(B+D)) = sensitivity / (1 − specificity)
Likelihood ratio of a negative test = (C/(A+C)) / (D/(B+D)) = (1 − sensitivity) / specificity
Kappa = (observed agreement − expected agreement) / (1 − expected agreement), where observed agreement = (A + D) / (A + B + C + D) and expected agreement = (A+B) × (A+C)/(A+B+C+D) + (C+D)*(B+D)/(A+B+C+D).
Pre-test odds = (A+C) / (1 − (A+C)) = pre test probability / (1− pre test probability)
Post test odds = LR × pre-test odds
Post test probability = post test odds / (post test odds + 1)

TABLE 5-2. Example of Influence of Prevalence of Disease on Positive and Negative Predictive Values

	Disease +	Disease –	Total
Test +	90	10	100
Test –	10	90	100
Total	100	100	200

Sensitivity and specificity 90%, prevalence 100/200 (50%), PPV 90%, NPV 90%.

TABLE 5-3. Example of Influence of Prevalence of Disease on Positive and Negative Predictive Values

	Disease +	Disease −	Total
Test +	90	100	190
Test −	10	900	910
Total	100	1000	1100

Sensitivity and specificity 90%, prevalence 100/1100 (9%), PPV 47%, NPV 99%.

and NPV change with the prevalence of the disease. In the first example, the probability of disease changes from 50% to 90% after a positive test result, whereas in the second example the probability of disease changes to only 47% after positive testing.

A disadvantage of the use of sensitivity and specificity is that it requires dichotomization by choosing a certain cut-off point. This implies a loss of information, which can be reduced by constructing a receiver operating characteristic (ROC) curve. In such a curve the true-positive rate (TPR, or sensitivity) is plotted on the vertical axis and the false-positive rate (FPR, or 1 minus the specificity) on the horizontal axis. By calculating the TPR and FPR for several cut-off points, a ROC curve can be constructed. An example is given in Figure 5-1 that represents a ROC curve of ankle/brachial index

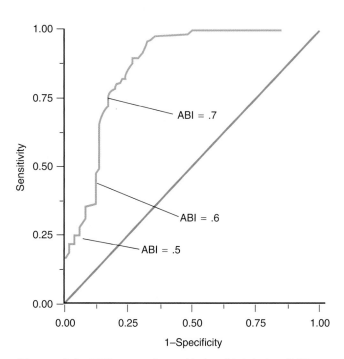

Figure 5-1. *ROC curve for ankle-brachial index (ABI) vs. arteriography for assessment of peripheral arterial occlusive disease.*

(ABI) versus angiography as reference standard for the presence of lower extremity arterial disease. Varying the cut-off point for ABI as presence of arterial disease induces changes in the respective sensitivity and 1 minus the specificity. From the curve it can be seen that there is a trade-off between the TPR and FPR because the increase of one leads to a decrease of the other.

The area under the ROC curve (AUC) can be calculated and is a measure of the discriminatory power of the test. An AUC that equals 0.5, represented by the diagonal line from the lower left-hand to the upper right-hand corner in Figure 5-1, indicates that the test has no discriminatory power at all. In contrast, an AUC that equals 1 signifies perfect discriminatory power. Another possibility of ROC curve analysis is that the AUC can be used to compare the diagnostic performance of different tests.[10]

From the ROC curve, the cut-off point can be chosen that serves the clinical question best. If the test is performed to detect every patient with the disease, because the consequences of a false-negative test are catastrophic, a high sensitivity is needed. A high sensitivity, and as a result a high NPV, is also required if the test is used to rule out disease. When a high PPV is required because the consequences of false-positive testing may be harmful, a high specificity is needed. In practice, the cut-off point that lies closest to the upper left corner of the ROC-curve will be chosen most often.

Likelihood Ratios

As shown in the previous paragraph, the dichotomization of a test leads to a loss of information. Another way to reduce information loss is to calculate likelihood ratios. The likelihood ratio of a positive test (LR +) is the ratio of patients with a true-positive test result to the number of patients with a false-positive test result (see Table 5-1). Similarly, the likelihood ratio of a negative (LR−) test is the ratio of patients with a false-negative test result to the number of patients with a true-negative test result. To decide whether a likelihood ratio is "good" again depends on the conditions in which the test is used. Typically, a LR + greater than 1 indicates that the test has some discriminatory power, which increases with the magnitude of the LR. Similarly, with regard to LR−, values moving toward 0 indicate that the test can accurately identify patients without the target condition.

For dichotomous outcomes, calculation of LRs may not seem particularly helpful to prevent information loss; however, in case of more categories, additional information can be gained. Table 5-4 shows the number of patients with positive, negative, and nondiagnostic test results compared with the reference standard. It turns out that a nondiagnostic test result occurs two times more often in patients with the target condition than in patients without this condition. This information would not have been available if the patients with a nondiagnostic test result had been left out of the analysis, or had been added to one of the other test outcomes.

Another advantage of the use of LRs is that they facilitate the calculation of post-test probabilities by means of Bayes' theorem. This theorem postulates that the post-test probability can be calculated by the following formula:

Post-test odds = LR × pretest odds (see Table 5-1).

From this it follows that:

Post-test probability = post-test odds/(post-test odds + 1).

Although calculating post-test probabilities in this way may not seem easy, it carries the advantage of calculating the probability of disease by simply multiplying the LR of different tests used sequentially. This is true under the condition that all tests are independent of each other. The Evidence-Based Medicine Working Group has developed a nomogram that facilitates calculation of the post-test probability if the pretest probability and LR are known.[11]

Reproducibility

Assessment of reproducibility includes determination of agreement on test results by the same investigator (intraobserver variation) and among other investigators (interobserver variation). It seems natural to start the development and evaluation of a diagnostic test by the determination of its reproducibility. This is, however, the ideal situation, because the introduction of a test in clinical practice often precedes a thorough evaluation of interobserver and intraobserver agreement. Assessment of reproducibility is essential to be able to judge whether the test can be used in different settings. Even more important is that good reproducibility of a test is a prerequisite for good discriminatory power. Although the relationship between reproducibility and diagnostic accuracy can be expressed mathematically,[12] it intuitively is clear that inconsistent classification as diseased or nondiseased by the same or different observers causes imperfect diagnostic accuracy.

Finally, it should be realized that variation might not only depend on observers but can also be caused by equipment-related or environmental factors.

Categorical Data

The intra- and interobserver variation of tests with dichotomous or categorical classifications can be expressed as kappa (κ) values. Kappa is a commonly used measure of agreement beyond chance between two or more observers (for calculation of κ, see Table 5-1). The κ value ranges from 0 to 1 and can be interpreted as poor (κ 0 to 0.2), fair (κ 0.2 to 0.4), moderate (κ 0.4 to 0.6), good (κ 0.6 to 0.8), and perfect agreement (κ 0.8 to 1.0).[13] The κ statistic can also be calculated for more than two categories, assuming that there is a qualitative relationship between each category. In such a case, a weighted κ value is calculated (weighted because full agreement gets full credit and partial agreement only partial).

The significance of the κ statistic is limited in situations with an extreme distribution and an already high agreement beyond chance. In this case the possible agreement beyond chance becomes low with only moderate κ values as a result. This is illustrated in Tables 5-5 and 5-6. Although there is absolute agreement in 20/23 (87%) cases, the κ value indicates good agreement in Table 5-5 and only moderate agreement in Table 5-6. It is not uncommon to express the agreement between two different diagnostic tests as κ values. As explained before, it is more informative to report the sensitivity and specificity of the test or other measures that allow calculation of post-test probabilities.

Continuous Data

The association between continuous data measured by two observers or tests is often presented as their corre-

TABLE 5-4. Example of Likelihood Ratios

	Positive +	Negative –	Nondiagnostic	Total
Disease +	25	5	10	40
Disease –	5	30	5	40

LR+ = (25/40) / (5/40) = 5
LR– = (5/40) / (30/40) = 0.17
LR? = (10/40) / (5/40) = 2

TABLE 5-5. Example of Dependence of Kappa on Distribution

	Test +	Test –	Total
Test +	10	2	12
Test –	1	10	11
Total	11	12	23

κ = 0.74

TABLE 5-6. Example of Dependence of Kappa on Distribution

	Test +	Test –	Total
Test +	18	2	20
Test –	1	2	3
Total	19	4	23

κ = 0.50

lation, or as a linear regression coefficient. Such analyses are less appropriate for diagnostic research because they do not take into account a systematic difference between the observers or different tests. In addition, although the correlation or regression coefficient may be highly significant, it is important to realize that the magnitude of the association (or the explanation of variance of the dependent variable by the independent variable) equals r^2, which in practice is often disappointingly small. For instance, a highly significant correlation coefficient of 0.5 means that only 25% of the variation is explained by the independent variable. Finally, statistical analysis only makes sense when these continuous data follow the normal distribution. In case of a skewed distribution, logarithmic transformation should precede such analyses.

Several better methods are available to express the agreement between observers for continuous data. One is the calculation of the intraclass correlation coefficient (ICC). The ICC expresses the strength of linear correlation between two measurements corrected for systematic bias. The higher the systematic difference, the lower the ICC, which ranges between –1 and 1. One possible reason for the limited use of the ICC may be that it is not automatically calculated by commercially available statistical software.

Because Fleis and Cohen demonstrated that the ICC is mathematically equivalent to the simple and weighted κ statistic,[14] its value can be interpreted likewise. From this follows that the ICC, like κ, is also influenced by extreme distributions. In addition, a study can show high ICCs whereas cross tabs and κ show the opposite, as in a study of interobserver variation in duplex scanning of infrainguinal bypass grafts.[15]

Another method to express the agreement between two observers for continuous data has been developed by Bland and Altman.[16] An example from a study on the reproducibility of various tools for assessment of lower extremity arterial disease is shown in Figure 5-2.[17] On the vertical axis, the difference in measurement performed by two observers is plotted against the mean of the same measurement. In this way it can be observed if the difference in measurement is dependent on the magnitude of the value on the x-axis. In addition, a systematic difference between measurements by both observers can be detected when the regression line differs from the horizontal line through zero.

Methodological Assessment of Diagnostic Research

The methodology of diagnostic research has only recently started to gain attention. Partly because of changing standards over time, the methodologic quality of many studies can be best characterized as mediocre not only in vascular research[18,19] but in general.[20] Some aspects

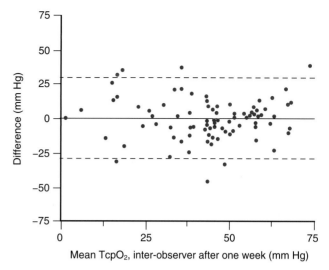

Figure 5-2. *Bland and Altman plot of interobserver assessment of TcPO$_2$ measurements.*

of the validity of studies on diagnostic tests discussed here may help the reader better appreciate the clinical value of diagnostic tests.

Internal Validity

Internal validity relates to design-related systematic errors or bias that may affect study outcomes. Several elements in study design are essential in order to reduce systematic errors or bias. These include a prospective design, an adequate spectrum of disease, a consecutive series of patients, and blinding. Retrospective studies can overestimate the diagnostic accuracy because the reasons for patients to have undergone both the test under study and the reference test are usually unclear. It may be that the reference test was only performed in patients with an equivocal test under study. In addition, selection bias may occur in retrospective studies by a systematic dropout of patients or by certain reasons to include patients. Prospective studies have the advantage of minimizing selection bias by including a consecutive series of patients and by accounting for patients who for some reason could not be included in the study.

Studies can be designed as cohort or case-control studies. In cohort studies, patients with a relevant spectrum of disease are included. In case-control studies, test results are compared in patients who definitely have the disease and in those who definitely have not. Because only the extremes of the disease spectrum are included, the diagnostic accuracy of the test will be overestimated.

Failure to use blinding is also likely to influence the study results. The interpretation of the reference test with knowledge of the results of the test under study may be biased by this knowledge. Vice versa, the interpretation of the test under study may be influenced by knowledge of the reference test result.

Verification bias looms when the decision to perform the reference test is at least partially influenced by the result of the test under study. The sensitivity will be overestimated in studies designed as such. This can be illustrated by the very high sensitivity of duplex scanning in patients referred for percutaneous transluminal angioplasty (PTA) of the superficial femoral artery.[21,22] Patients were probably likely to be referred for angiography and PTA only if duplex scanning identified lesions suitable for PTA. From these studies it remains unclear how many patients had suitable lesions that were not identified by duplex scanning.

In a systematic review of studies on diagnostic tests, Lijmer and colleagues found that the diagnostic performance was overestimated in studies designed as case-control studies when different reference tests were used, when blinding was inadequate, when no cut-off criteria for the test under study were described, and when the study population was not described in sufficient detail.[23]

External Validity

To be able to translate study results to one's own practice it is essential to judge the generalizability or external validity of a study. First, the setting in which the study was performed influences the study results. Vascular patients evaluated in an outpatient setting of a general practitioner compose a different spectrum of disease than patients evaluated in a tertiary center. In addition, a clear description of patient demographics may clarify whether the patients represent those seen in one's own practice. Another important aspect is knowledge on referral patterns before patients entered the study. This is often difficult to judge because from most publications it remains unclear which tests were already performed before patients entered the study protocol. Special attention should be given to studies that include asymptomatic contralateral limbs or arteries in their results. This is commonly encountered in studies evaluating noninvasive modalities for assessment of carotid artery stenosis in symptomatic patients. Studies designed as such will report an artificially high specificity because the majority of normal contralateral carotid arteries will be detected with the modality that is studied.

Finally, adequate description of details on how the diagnostic test was performed (to permit replication), which cut-off values were used, and how nondiagnostic results were dealt with complete the assessment of external validity. A full list of criteria for methodologic assessment of diagnostic research can be found on the Web page of the Cochrane Methods Group of Screening and Diagnostic Tests (www.cochrane.org).

Analysis

Any article on diagnostic tests should at least report the sensitivity and specificity of the test or report its likeli-hood ratios. The calculation of the precision of estimates of diagnostic accuracy has been given little attention so far, but is very important. The 95% confidence interval (CI) around a point estimate for the sensitivity and specificity should be reported as its upper and lower boundary. Rothwell and colleagues have provided an example of the diagnostic accuracy of duplex scanning for detection of a stenosis greater than 70% in the internal carotid artery.[19] They calculated that in a population of 600 patients with a 20% prevalence of 70% to 99% stenosis and a sensitivity of 90%, DS would detect 108 of 120 stenoses. The lower 95% confidence interval limit of the sensitivity in this case, however, is only 75%, which they considered unacceptable. The issue of underpowered studies is not unique for noninvasive carotid artery assessment. In a meta-analysis of studies evaluating MRA for assessment of lower extremity arterial disease, the median sample size was only 25 patients.[24] The diagnostic accuracy in these studies obviously has wide confidence intervals.

Reporting

Ideally, 2 × 2 contingency tables are provided in the original studies to enable the reader to make additional calculations and to be informed on the prevalence of target conditions. Unfortunately, this is not common practice for all medical journals. To improve the standards of design and reporting of diagnostic research, the Standards for Reporting of Diagnostic Accuracy (STARD) steering committee has recently published a guideline (www.consort-statement.org/stardstatement.htm). This includes a 25-item checklist that can be used for methodologic assessment and to appreciate the applicability of the findings for clinical practice.[25]

Systematic Reviews of Diagnostic Research

Analogous to studies evaluating the effectiveness of therapy, meta-analysis is a powerful tool to obtain the best available estimates of the diagnostic accuracy of a test in the absence of large studies. The methodology of systematic reviews and meta-analyses of diagnostic research is still evolving. In short, literature retrieval, methodologic assessment according to the criteria described in the previous sections, data extraction, and data synthesis follow principles similar to the systematic reviews of studies of effectiveness. It is important to determine the presence of heterogeneity among the different studies; this can be caused by differences in study population, design, or technical aspects, or by variation in cut-off points between studies. In case of homogeneity among studies, the diagnostic accuracy can be estimated by calculating a pooled sensitivity and specificity. In case of heterogeneity, summary ROC (SROC) curves can be constructed. These curves differ from the standard ROC curve in that the SROC curve is defined by the data from the original studies and cannot be plotted beyond these limits. A shortcoming of SROC curves is that they cannot be used to determine the optimal cut-off point of a diagnostic test. It is possible, however, to determine differences between the diagnostic performance of several modalities. This is illustrated in the study by de Vries and colleagues, who found a significantly better performance of color duplex scanning compared with conventional duplex scanning for assessment of lower extremity arterial disease.[26] The authors could compare 3D contrast-enhanced (CE) MRA with 2D time-of-flight (TOF) MRA for assessment of the lower extremity arteries (Fig. 5-3).[24]

Guidelines

Current clinical practice is increasingly based on the use of evidence-based guidelines. A guideline can be described as a "systematically developed statement to assist practitioner and patients in decisions about appropriate health care for specific clinical circumstances." The Evidence-Based Medicine working group has suggested a classification for the levels of evidence for the evaluation of diagnostic modalities, together with the strength of recommendation for their use in clinical practice (see suggested readings). This classification is presented in Table 5-7.

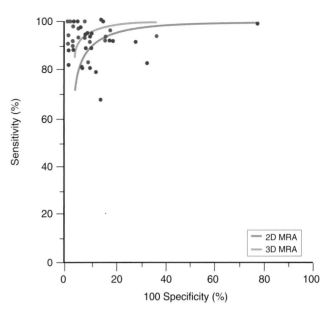

Figure 5-3. Example of Summary ROC curve for 2D TOF MRA and 3D CE MRA compared with arteriography for assessment of lower extremity arterial disease.

Assessing the Clinical Value of Diagnostic Tests

Previous discussions were about evaluating the diagnostic accuracy of a test; however, diagnostic accuracy alone does not tell us about the clinical relevance of the

---

TABLE 5-7. **Grades of Recommendation and Levels of Evidence for Diagnostic Tests**

Grade	Level	Description
A	Level 1a	SR (with homogeneity) of Level 1 diagnostic studies, or a CPG validated on a test set
A	Level 1b	Independent blind comparison of an appropriate spectrum of consecutive patients, all of whom have undergone both the diagnostic test and the reference standard
A	Level 1c	Extremely high sensitivity and specificity
B	Level 2a	SR (with homogeneity) of Level >2 diagnostic studies
B	Level 2b	Any of the following: • Independent blind or objective comparison • Study performed in a set of nonconsecutive patients, or confined to a narrow spectrum of study individuals (or both), all of whom have undergone both the diagnostic test and the reference standard • A diagnostic CPG not validated in a test set
B	Level 3	Independent blind comparison of an appropriate spectrum, but the reference standard was not applied to all study patients
C	Level 4	Reference standard was unobjective, unblended, or not independent
D	Level 5	Expert opinion without explicit critical appraisal, not based on physiology, bench research, or "first principles"

CPG = clinical practice guideline.

test. The patient and physician may be more interested in how a test result and subsequent treatment can improve the patient's health status than in the diagnostic truth. This implies that the clinical value of the test is also dependent on the availability of an effective treatment. In a meta-analysis of MRA, performed predominantly in patients with claudication, the authors found a high diagnostic accuracy for 3D CE MRA, with a statistically significant 4% difference in Q-point (where sensitivity equals specificity in the SROC curve), compared with 2D TOF MRA.[24] The clinical significance of this difference cannot be determined without taking into account possible differences in treatment and patient outcomes depending on a work-up based on either or both MRA modalities.

The lack of clear clinical relevance of diagnostic testing can also be illustrated by follow-up with duplex scanning after carotid endarterectomy for early detection of a restenosis. Although a postoperative duplex scan may be used as self-assessment, there is no evidence that reoperation for an asymptomatic restenosis benefits the patient. In addition, despite an increase in costs, there is no gain in quality of life.[27] Hence, the clinical relevance of follow-up with duplex scanning is debatable. Some methods to analyze the clinical value of diagnostic tests and to compare different test and treatment strategies are mentioned briefly in the following section.

Diagnostic Before-After Study

The before-after study design, introduced by Guyatt and colleagues, can be used to estimate the effect of additional testing.[28] In brief, the physician establishes a diagnosis (e.g., based on ankle/brachial index measurements in diabetic patients suspected of peripheral arterial disease). Then the results of a second diagnostic modality (e.g., toe pressures) are revealed, after which the diagnosis is re-established.[29] Both diagnoses can be filled in the 2×2 contingency table, and the shift in classifications can be seen. In addition, both classifications can be compared to a reference standard (e.g., angiography) and the difference in diagnostic accuracy can be established. In this way information is gained on whether additional diagnostic testing improves the physician's accuracy of assessment and patient management. The advantage of this strategy is that it is easy to perform within a short time. A limitation of this design is that, although it is suited to estimate the effect of additional testing, it cannot compare the outcome of different test and treatment strategies. Observed differences between two strategies may be the result of many confounding factors and need not necessarily be related to differences in test properties.

Decision Analysis

In a decision analysis, data on the prevalence of disease, the performance of diagnostic tests, and the expected benefits and harm of a treatment are combined to compare different test and treatment strategies. Differences between strategies can be expressed as utilities, quality adjusted life years (QALYs), costs, and cost-effectiveness. The study by Visser and colleagues is an example of a cost-effectiveness analysis of patients with intermittent claudication having a work-up and subsequent treatment based on duplex scanning, MRA, or iaDSA.[30] Differences in diagnostic accuracy of all modalities, complications of the tests, consequences of missing some lesions, and consequences of overtreatment were explored in the analysis. Surprisingly, they conclude that the differences in costs and clinical outcome between each diagnosis and treatment strategy are small.

The strength of decision analysis is limited by conflicting or missing data about the accuracy of diagnostic tests or about the benefits and harms of different treatment modalities.

Randomized Trials

Randomization is commonly used to study the effect of different treatment modalities. In contrast, randomized controlled trials to study the effects of different diagnostic test strategies are rare. However, there is a growing interest in the theoretical and practical aspects of such studies. As mentioned previously, diagnostic trials should not only include the diagnostic strategy but should also evaluate a test and treatment strategy in terms of relevant health outcome or clinical endpoints. One example from vascular surgery practice is the uncertainty about the clinical significance of duplex surveillance programs for early detection of asymptomatic stenosis after peripheral bypass surgery. A randomized trial by Lundell and colleagues indicated that surveillance and subsequent intervention in case of a stenosis improved patency rates after 3 years follow-up.[31] However, the study insufficiently focused on clinically relevant end-points (e.g., quality of life or limb salvage rates), which was a reason to embark on a larger randomized trial.[32]

It is beyond the scope of this chapter to further discuss the various designs for randomized diagnostic trials, each of which has its own advantages and limitations. Although the thorough evaluation of a test and treatment strategy is desirable to be able to fully appreciate its additional clinical value, randomized trials may be limited by the rapid developments in imaging technology: By the time a trial is completed, the technology may be outdated. An interesting new flexible study design that offers the possibility to incorporate rapid advances in imaging technology into the study may help to overcome this limitation.[33]

Conclusions

This chapter has provided an overview of the various aspects of diagnostic testing, in particular those available to the vascular patient. For added information on these tests, see the publications listed in Suggested Readings.

REFERENCES

1. McGee SR, Boyko EJ: Physical examination and chronic lower-extremity ischemia. A critical review. Arch Int Med 158:1357–1364, 1998.
2. Lederle F, Simel DL: Does this patient have abdominal aortic aneurysm? JAMA 281:77–82, 1999.
3. Sauve JS, Laupacis A, Ostbye T, et al: Does this patient have a clinically important carotid bruit? JAMA 270:2843–2845, 1993.
4. Sniderman K, Morse SS, Straus EB: Comparison of intra-arterial digital subtraction angiography and conventional filming in peripheral arterial disease. J Can Assoc Radiol 37:76–82, 1986.
5. Baum RA, Rutter CM, Sunshine JH, et al: Multicenter trial to evaluate vascular magnetic resonance angiography of the lower extremity. JAMA 274:875–880, 1995.
6. Kwok Y, Kim C, Grady D, et al: Meta-analysis of exercise testing to detect coronary artery disease in women. Am J Cardiol 83:660–666, 1999.
7. Coffi SB, Ubbink DT, Zwiers I, et al: The value of the peak systolic velocity ratio in the assessment of the haemodynamic significance of subcritical iliac artery stenoses. Eur J Vasc Endovasc Surg 22:424–428, 2001.
8. Aly S, Sommerville K, Adiseshiah M, et al: Comparison of duplex imaging and arteriography in the evaluation of lower limb arteries. Br J Surg 85:1099–1102, 1998.
9. Larch E, Minar E, Ahmadi R, et al: Value of color duplex sonography for evaluation of the tibioperoneal arteries in patients with femoropopliteal obstruction. A prospective comparison with anterograde intra-arterial digital subtraction angiography. J Vasc Surg 25:629–636, 1997.
10. Hanley JA, McNeil BJ: The meaning and use of the area under a receiving operating characteristic (ROC) curve. Radiology 143:29–36, 1982.
11. Guyatt G, Rennie D (eds): User's Guides to the Medical Literature. Chicago: AMA Press, 2002.
12. Quinn MF: Relation of observer agreement to accuracy according to a two-receiver signal detection model of diagnosis. Med Decis Making 39:207–215, 1989.
13. Altman DG: Practical Statistics for Medical Research. London: Chapman and Hall, 1995.
14. Fleis JL, Cohen J: The equivalence of weighted kappa and the intraclass correlation coefficient as measures of reliability. Educ Psychol Meas 33:613–619, 1973.
15. Gomes MER, de Graaff JC, van Gurp JA, et al: Interobserver variation in duplex scanning of infrainguinal arterial bypass grafts. Eur J Vasc Endovasc Surg 25:224–228, 2003.
16. Bland JM, Altman DG: Statistical methods for assessing agreement between two methods of clinical measurement. Lancet i:307–310, 1986.
17. De Graaff JC, Ubbink DTh, Legemate DA, et al: Interobserver and intraobserver reproducibility of peripheral blood and oxygen pressure measurements in the assessment of lower extremity arterial disease. J Vasc Surg 33:1033–1040, 2001.
18. Sostman HD, Beam CA: Evaluation of the quality of clinical research studies of magnetic resonance angiography: 1991–1994. J Magn Reson Imaging 6:33–38, 1996.
19. Rothwell PM, Pendlbury ST, Wardlaw J, et al: Critical appraisal of the design and reporting of studies of imaging and measurement of carotid stenosis. Stroke 31:1444–1450, 2000.
20. Reid MC, Lachs MS, Feinstein AR: Use of methodological standards in diagnostic test research: Getting better but still not good. JAMA 274:645–651, 1995.
21. Whyman MR, Gillespie I, Ruckley CV, et al: Screening patients with claudication from femoropopliteal disease before angioplasty using Doppler colour flow imaging. Br J Surg 79:907–909, 1992.
22. Davies AH, Magee TR, Parry R, et al: Duplex ultrasonography and pulse-generated run-off in selecting claudicants for femoropoliteal angioplasty. Br J Surg 79:894–896, 1992.
23. Lijmer JG, Mol BW, Heisterkamp S, et al: Empirical evidence of design-related bias in studies of diagnostic tests. JAMA 282:1061–1066, 1999.
24. Koelemay MJW, Lijmer JG, Stoker J, et al: Magnetic resonance angiography for evaluation of lower extremity arterial disease: A meta-analysis. JAMA 285:1338–1345, 2001.
25. Bossuyt PM, Reitsma JB, Bruns DE, et al: Towards complete and accurate reporting of studies of diagnostic accuracy: The STARD initiative. BMJ 326:41–44, 2003.
26. de Vries SO, Hunink MGM, Polak JF: Use of summary ROC curves as a technique for meta-analysis of the diagnostic performance of duplex ultrasonography in peripheral arterial disease. Acad Radiol 3:361–369, 1996.
27. Post PN, Kievit J, van Baalen JM, et al: Routine duplex surveillance does not improve the outcome after carotid endarterectomy: A decision and cost utility analysis. Stroke 33:749–755, 2002.
28. Guyatt GH, Tugwell PX, Feeney DH, et al: The role of before-after studies in the evaluation of therapeutic impact of diagnostic technology. J Chronic Dis 39:295–304, 1986.
29. Ubbink DT, Tulevski II, den Hartog D, et al: The value of noninvasive techniques for the assessment of critical limb ischaemia. Eur J Vasc Endovasc Surg 13:296–300, 1997.
30. Visser K, Kuntz KM, Donaldson MC, et al: Pretreatment imaging work-up for patients with intermittent claudication: A cost-effectiveness analysis. J Vasc Interv Radiol 14:53–62, 2003.
31. Lundell A, Lindblad B, Bergqvist D, et al: Femoropopliteal-crural graft patency is improved by an intensive surveillance program: A prospective randomized study. J Vasc Surg 21:26–34, 1995.
32. Kirby PL, Brady AR, Thompson SG, et al: The Vein Graft Surveillance Trial: Rationale, design and methods. VGST participants. Eur J Vasc Endovasc Surg 18:469–474, 1999.
33. Hunink MGM, Krestin GP: Study design for concurrent development, assessment, and implementation of new diagnostic technology. Radiology 222:604–614, 2002.

SUGGESTED READINGS

Sackett DL, Haynes RB, Guyatt GH, et al: Clinical Epidemiology. A Basic Science for Clinical Medicine. Boston: Little, Brown & Co., 1991.
Knottnerus A (ed): The Evidence Base of Clinical Diagnosis. London: BMJ books, 2002.
Guyatt G, Rennie D (eds): User's Guides to the Medical Literature. Chicago: AMA Press, 2002.

Chapter 6

Principles of Ultrasound Physics and Instrumentation: An Overview

KIRK W. BEACH

Ultrasound physics have not changed since the beginning of time. Our understanding of ultrasound physics has evolved, however, and there is some disagreement. Ultrasound instrumentation has not changed much since the beginning of medical ultrasound, about half a century ago, at least not in concept. The introduction of transistors and solid state circuits, and of digital circuits and software, have simplified the tasks conceived in the early days of diagnostic medical ultrasound development. Advances in technology have allowed the progression from one-dimensional imaging to two-dimensional imaging to three-dimensional imaging. Advances in technology have also simplified and speeded the process of "demodulating" ultrasound echoes to create B-mode and color Doppler displays. By constantly sharing observations and insights, and by discussing the subject, a deeper understanding of the diagnostic process evolves. Formal math can sometimes offer insight. The mathematical concepts in this chapter use methods taught in high school, so it seems that they should be understandable with a single reading. However, like poetry, each time the equations are read, new meanings appear.

There is still a great deal left to comprehend about ultrasound physics, the physics of bloodflow, and the biology of vascular diseases. As these topics are better understood, the still-unresolved issues of ultrasound safety and of proper diagnostic criteria can be approached. The evolution of thought is a partnership between examiners, who have the opportunity to observe the processes firsthand; and the developers, who try to convert the wisdom of the examiners into better instruments. Medical ultrasound diagnostic methods are expected to change as much in the next 50 years as they have in the last 50 years.

Introduction

Pulse-echo ultrasound imaging is based on radar principles. The analogies between current two-dimensional color Doppler imaging and modern television weather reporting are striking. Like the Doppler, weather radar shows where the moving reflectors of rain are located, measuring the lateral speed, which is caused by the wind. Diagnostic medical Doppler systems are used to measure the speed of bloodflow.

The term *imaging* will be used here to refer to all methods of interrogating the body with active ultrasound and providing an output, whether that output is a picture, sound, feeling, taste, smell, direct connection to the nervous system of the examiner, or for the automatic control of some therapy device.

Ultrasound Propagation Through Tissue

Ultrasound is a mechanical wave. Ultrasound passes through tissue like light passes through foggy air. Tissue is like foggy air because the cells in tissue scatter ultrasound just as the water droplets in fog scatter light. For ultrasound imaging, the ultrasound beam is collimated like a laser beam that shines as a thin line through tissue. At least that is what we think; the ultrasound beam is more like a flashlight beam, with a brighter central region, pretty well directed, but with some ultrasound heading off to the sides in "sidelobes." In the central region, some zones are brighter and some zones are dimmer. We believe that the ultrasound beam passes along one line into tissue and that the reflections pass back along the same path; however, the ultrasound beam is bent by refraction and reflection, like the flashlight. The beam also has a focus, like a flashlight beam.

Think of the ultrasound beam as light coming from the bulb in a flashlight by way of a focusing device. In the flashlight, the focus is provided by the reflector; in ultrasound, the focus is provided by a rubber or plastic lens or by an electronic beam former acting on a segmented transducer array. Continuing the flashlight analogy, the ultrasound echo is similar to light that is reflected by an object and returns through the focus system and back to the source. In the flashlight, the majority of the light that returns to the lightbulb has been directed there by the reflector. Of course, if the lightbulb is on and emitting light when the reflected light (echo) returns, the bulb can't detect the reflection. So for the "flashlight" system to work, the flashlight is turned on for a brief period, then it is turned off, allowing the bulb to become a detector of light so that the echoes can be received. This would be a "radar" operated with light rather than with radio waves. The same job can be done with ultrasound.

Although the "light radar" would work, it is hard to operate because light travels so fast (300,000,000 meters/second compared to the ultrasound speed of 1500 meters/second). Radio waves travel the same speed as light, so radar waves travel 200,000 times as fast as ultrasound. Ultrasound will travel through the liver and back 150 millimeters each way in 200 microseconds; radar (radio) waves would return from a reflector 30 kilometers away in the same time. If you replace the ultrasound transducer on your scanner with a radar antenna, you can look through walls at the buildings around you. At 5 MHz, the wavelength of RADAR waves is 60 meters (λ = C/F, 60 meters/cy = (300,000,000 meters/s)/ (5,000,000 cy/s)). Because buildings are spaced at intervals between 20 meters (house) and 100 meters (commercial), spanning the wavelength of 5 MHz radar, individual houses may not be resolved, but city blocks would be.*

Because the wavelength of 5-MHz ultrasound is 0.3 mm (300 μm), and the size of a cell is about 10 μm, individual cells cannot be resolved with ultrasound; however, blood vessels can be. Even though it appears that blood cells can be seen in blood vessels, each disk-shaped erythrocyte is about 8 μm in diameter and 2 μm thick, and the spacing is about 5 μm, so individual erythrocytes cannot be resolved with ultrasound frequencies below 300 MHz, having a wavelength of 5 μm ([1500 μm/μs] / [300 cycles/μs], λ = C/F). Even rouleaux (stacks of erythrocytes) are only 20 μm long and cannot be resolved.

The speed of ultrasound propagation through tissue can be derived from simple equations of mechanics such as force = mass × acceleration (F = m × a). To develop

---

*A "light radar" system has been used to see the ossicles in the middle ear behind the eardrum. With continuous wave light (like a normal lightbulb), the reflection from the eardrum is so bright that reflections of light from the ossicles cannot be seen. By flashing the light for 10 picoseconds (0.01 nanoseconds = 0.000 01 microseconds), and waiting for 200 picoseconds until the reflections from the eardrum have passed from a depth of 30 mm before looking at the reflected light, the light coming from the ossicles can be seen. Of course, pulsed lasers and electronic shutters are needed to operate in these very short times.

the math, the tissue is treated like a stack of blocks. Each block is much smaller than the wavelength of sound, so each theoretical block is about the dimension of the smallest cell, about 1 micron (μm = micrometer). The mass "m" is the volume multiplied by the density of the tissue "ρ." As an ultrasound wave passes through tissue, the tissue shakes like an earthquake is passing. Each block of tissue moves back and forth along the direction of wave propagation. This is called a longitudinal wave. The shaking velocity of each block will be called "v," the molecular velocity. The distance that the block moves from the resting location will be called "δ," the molecular displacement. The wave is moving along the direction "x" in time "t." The tissue strain in calculus terms is $s = d\delta/dx$. In calculus terms, the molecular velocity is $v = d\delta/dt$ and $a = dv/dt = d^2\delta/dt^2$.

The force "F" on the block comes from a pressure gradient in tissue (Fig. 6-1), a change in pressure with distance along the direction of wave propagation. Pressure changes above and below atmospheric pressure are caused by changes in tissue strain, $p = K \times s$ where K is the stiffness of the tissue and s is the strain. The pressure gradient, in calculus terms is $d(p)/dx = K \times ds/dx = K \times d^2\delta/dx^2$.

Setting the acceleration force equal to the pressure gradient force yields the following:

$$K \times d^2\delta/dx^2 = \rho \times d^2\delta/dt^2$$

where the properties of the tissue are as follows:

- $d^2\delta/dx^2$ is tissue distortion as the ultrasound wave passes through the tissue.
- $d^2\delta/dt^2$ is tissue acceleration as the ultrasound wave passes through tissue.
- K is the stiffness or spring constant of the tissue.
- δ is the displacement of molecules and cells of the tissue as the wave passes.

- x is the distance along the ultrasound beam path.
- t is the time after the wave begins the journey through tissue.
- ρ is the density of the tissue, the mass per volume.

The density determines whether the tissue will float. Fat floats, muscle sinks, but both fat and muscle densities are near the density of water. Fat has a density lower than water, muscle has a density higher than water.

Using differential calculus, if we make "δ" a function of the variable (x-Ct), then using the chain rule from calculus, the equation can be simplified with the substitutions:

$$d^2\delta/dx^2 = \delta$$
$$d^2s\delta/dt^2 = C^2 \times \delta$$

Using calculus notation, the equation becomes as follows:

$$K \times \delta = \rho \times C^2 \times \delta$$

which solves to

$$K = \rho \times C^2$$

C has units of cm/sec, like velocity. To understand C, think of a wave traveling on the ocean. The shape stays the same, over time, but the position changes. C makes the connection between position and time: C is the velocity of the wave. If a log is floating in the water, the wave passes by without moving the log. The log moves with the water molecules. The velocity of the log is like molecular velocity, "v."

The speed of ultrasound in tissue is dependent on the properties of tissue (density and stiffness) and is *not* dependent on the properties of the ultrasound, at least at low ultrasound intensities where these equations apply.

$$C = SQRT(K/\rho)$$

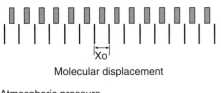

Molecular displacement

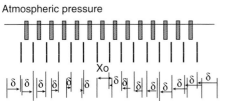

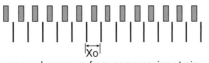

Increased pressure from compression strain

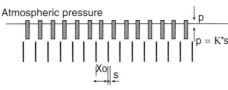

Compression strain gradient causes pressure gradient

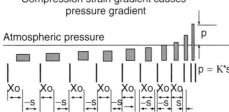

Figure 6-1. Tissue strain and forces.

C is the speed of ultrasound in tissue that you find stated, but not explained, in ultrasound physics books. The speed of ultrasound in tissue is a property of the stiffness and the density of the tissue. In stiffer tissue like bone, ultrasound speed is higher. In denser tissue, the ultrasound speed is lower. The reason that the speed is low in fat (low density) is that fat is not stiff.

From the definition of stiffness, tissue pressure $P = Po + p = Po + K \times d\delta/dx$, where "p" is the tissue pressure fluctuation above or below atmospheric pressure. As the ultrasound wave passes through tissue, the tissue molecules vibrate back and forth. Because "δ" is the normal position of the tissue molecules, $d\delta/dt$ is the molecular velocity which is called "v."

Equation 1 can be integrated with calculus as follows:

$$K \times d\delta/dx = (\rho/C) \times d\delta/dt$$

Substituting values into the equation yields the following:

$$p = (\rho \times C) \times v$$

So, as an ultrasonic wave passes, the tissue pressure fluctuation is *always* proportional the instantaneous oscillatory velocity of the molecules. The ratio between the pressure fluctuation and the velocity fluctuation is a constant. That constant is called "impedance" and its symbol is "Z."

$$Z = p/v = (\rho \times C) = SQRT(K \times \rho)$$

Like ultrasound velocity, impedance is a property of stiffness and density: Impedance increases when either stiffness or density increases. So, if density is constant, then ultrasound impedance "Z" is proportional to ultrasound velocity "C."

Acoustic impedance in tissue is dependent on the properties of tissue and is *not* dependent on the properties of the ultrasound (at least at low ultrasound intensities).

If the density of tissue is higher, but the stiffness is the same, the acoustic impedance is higher but the speed of ultrasound is lower. If the stiffness of the tissue is higher but the density is the same, then both the speed of ultrasound and the impedance of the tissue are higher.

The fascinating result is that the shape of the disturbance (i.e., the shape of the ultrasound wave, the frequency, the amplitude) is not part of the solution to the equation. Any wave shape will propagate the speed "C" through tissue and the ratio of p/v (Z) will be determined by the tissue.

The Role of Impedance

The speed of ultrasound in tissue is used to determine the depth of the reflector causing an ultrasound echo, so that an image of that reflector can be placed in the correct location on the ultrasound image. An ultrasound echo occurs when the ultrasound burst encounters a location where the acoustic impedance changes.

The acoustic impedance is the ratio of the molecular pressure fluctuation to the molecular velocity fluctuation. When the ultrasound wave encounters an impedance change, as the wave passes from one tissue into another, the ratio of the molecular pressure fluctuation "p" to the molecular velocity fluctuation "v" must be different in the second tissue than it was in the first tissue (that is what impedance means). However, the product of the two is the ultrasound intensity, which must be conserved. Suppose that the impedance is 2% higher in the second material than in the first material: then the pressure fluctuation could go up by 1% and the velocity fluctuation could go down by 1%, making the ratio 2% higher and the product (intensity) unchanged. That seems OK.

But there is one other requirement: The pressure fluctuation in the second material must equal the pressure fluctuation in the first material at the boundary, and the velocity fluctuation in the second material must equal the velocity fluctuation in the first material. If this were not true, then the tissue would tear at the boundary. This is called a "boundary condition."

This problem can be resolved by fabricating a new wave that adds pressure and velocity to the molecules. The only wave that will make the boundary conditions work is a reflected wave. The incoming wave is described by "p1" and "v1," the transmitted wave is described by "p2" and "v2," and the reflected wave is described by "pr" and "vr."

If the wave passes from material 1 to material 2, and the reflected wave travels "back" in material 1, then all of the following equations must be true.

For impedance relations:

$$p1/v1 = Z1$$
$$p2/v2 = Z2$$
$$pr/vr = Z1$$

For boundary conditions:

$$p1 + pr = p2$$
$$v1 - vr = v2$$

The sign change ($+pr$, $-vr$) is because the reflected wave is traveling backwards. The result is that the amplitude of the new reflected wave is:

$$pr/p1 = (Z2 - Z1)/(Z2 + Z1)$$

And the ratio of the intensities is:

$$Ir/I1 = (Z2 - Z1)^2/(Z2 + Z1)^2$$

Every time that an ultrasound wave encounters a change in acoustic impedance, there is a reflection. The remaining transmitted wave, if the ultrasound speeds are different, bends according to Snell's law. In addition, some of the longitudinal wave motion is converted into shear wave motion, which is rapidly converted to heat.

Impedance has units of pressure divided by velocity:

$$(dynes/cm^2)/(cm/sec) = (dyne \times sec) / (cm^3)$$

Because $Z = \rho C$, the units are $(gm/cm^3) \times (cm/sec) = gm / (cm^2 \times sec)$

From $F = m \times a$ the conversion $1 = (dyne \times sec^2)/(gm \times cm)$ can be used to show that $(dyne \times sec) / (cm^3) = gm / (cm^2 \times sec)$.

The accepted units of measure for impedance are called Rayls after Lord Rayleigh (1842–1919) (Table 6-1). The unit is defined in the MKS metric system as follows:

$$Rayl = Kilogram/(meter^2 \times second) = (N \times s)/ (M^3)$$

Computing Ultrasound Intensity

Ultrasound intensity has units of Watts/cm^2. The instantaneous intensity is the molecular pressure multiplied by the molecular velocity. The units work out as follows:

Energy (joules) = force (newton) × distance (meter)
Power (watt) = energy/time (watt/second) = force (newton) × distance/time (meter/second)
Power (watt) = force (newton) × velocity (meter/second)
Intensity (Watt/cm^2) = power/area (watt/cm^2) = force/area (newton/cm^2) × velocity (meter/second)
Intensity (watt/cm^2) = molecular pressure (newton/cm^2) × molecular velocity (meter/second)

The most common ultrasound waveshape for the molecular pressure and velocity fluctuations is the sine wave. A sine wave is usually expressed in the trigonometric form:

$$p = pmax \times \sin(2\pi Ft)$$

or

$$v = vmax \times \sin(2\pi Ft)$$

where F is the ultrasound frequency (Hz or cycles/second), which is multiplied by 2π to convert it to radians per second.

For a sine wave, the averaged intensity of ultrasound is I = (1/2) × pmax × vmax. Using the possible substitution of Z for either pmax or vmax:

$$I = (1/2) pmax^2 / Z = (1/2) \times vmax^2 \times Z$$

Intensity is proportional to amplitude squared.

The ultrasound intensities used in medical diagnostic ultrasound are *not* "low intensities," and therefore ultrasound does not follow these equations.

So why do we learn the equations if medical ultrasound does not behave this way? Because we can learn from the equations, and understanding these equations is a starting point for learning about nonlinear propagation.

The ultrasound impedance of tissue is near 1.5×10^5 (d s)/(cm^3) = 1.5×10^5 gm/(cm^2 s).

When pmax is equal to atmospheric pressure (10^6 dyne/cm^2), the pressure in tissue doubles during the compression phase of the ultrasound wave and drops to 0 during the decompression half cycle of the wave. The intensity when pmax = 1 atm is Isptp = 0.333 Watts/cm^2. Isptp meant spatial peak temporal peak intensity. Let's explore the methods of computing intensity (Table 6-2).

The spatial average temporal average is the value that has been traditionally quoted. The value of 100 mW/cm^2 SATA was in common use as the maximum intensity for diagnostic ultrasound in 1976 when the Medical Devices Act gave the Food and Drug Administration authority to regulate medical devices. According to the act, any intensity value used in diagnostic medical ultrasound equipment before 1976 is considered safe unless there is evidence of harm. New diagnostic ultrasound instruments with intensities under that level can be brought to market by filing a 510K application stating that the new ultrasound instrument is equivalent to a "pre-enactment" system. Ophthalmic ultrasound instruments used intensities below 17 mW/cm^2 before 1976, so ophthalmic examinations are limited to that level until a manufacturer files a new device applica-

TABLE 6-1. **Ultrasound Impedance of Tissues**

Tissue	Impedance	Impedance	Impedance
Fat	1.38 MegaRayls	1.38×10^6 N s / M^3	1.38×10^5 gm/(cm^2 s)
Muscle	1.65 MegaRayls	1.65×10^6 N s / M^3	1.65×10^5 gm/(cm^2 s)
Blood	1.62 MegaRayls	1.62×10^6 N s / M^3	1.62×10^5 gm/(cm^2 s)
Bone	7 MegaRayls	7×10^6 N s / M^3	7×10^5 gm/(cm^2 s)
Water	1.48 MegaRayls	1.48×10^6 N s / M^3	1.49×10^5 gm/(cm^2 s)

TABLE 6-2. Intensity Measures

Label	Abbreviation	Meaning	Typical Value
Spatial peak temporal peak	Isptp or SPTP	Cavitation	30W/cm²
Spatial average temporal peak	Isatp or SATP		10W/cm²
Spatial peak temporal average	Ispta or SPTA		300 mW/cm²
Spatial average temporal average	Isata or SATA	Heating	100 mW/cm²
Thermal index	TI	Heating	1
Mechanical index	MI	Cavitation	1

tion (NDA) for ophthalmic ultrasound showing that higher levels are safe in the eye. Only the heating of tissue is considered a safety issue in the paragraph above.

However, during an ultrasound examination, the ultrasound is only transmitted for 1 microsecond every 100 microseconds or so. Therefore, even if the temporal average intensity is below 100 mW/cm², the peak intensities can be 100 times that high because it is on for such a short time. Recently there has been concern that the high peak intensities might be hazardous because of cavitation. This will be discussed later in the chapter.

We've computed the tissue pressure fluctuation at an Isptp (intensity) of 0.333 Watts/cm² when the tissue pressure fluctuation is 1 atmosphere. It is also instructive to compute the tissue velocity fluctuation at that intensity. One atmosphere of pressure is 10^6 d/cm². Using the definition of impedance ($Z = pmax/vmax$) and $pmax = 1$ atm $= 10^6$ d/cm², the maximum tissue molecular velocity $vmax = 6$ cm/s. At a frequency of 5 MHz, the maximum acceleration is 2 megameters/s² maximum tissue molecular acceleration, and 2 nanometers maximum molecular displacement. The maximum displacement is on the order of molecular size, but the maximum acceleration is 200,000 times the acceleration of gravity. That seems large, but it only lasts for 0.1 microsecond.

If you are wondering what this means, nobody knows. If you want to think that ultrasound is safe, remember that the cells jiggle only 2 nanometers. If you want to think that ultrasound is dangerous, then remember that tissues accelerate at 200,000 times the acceleration of gravity. But ultrasound machines transmit 100 mW/cm² SPTA; during the ultrasound burst, the SPTP is 10,000 mW/cm², so the accelerations are 10 times as large as we just calculated. (If pmax is 10 times higher, then $pmax^2$ is 100 times higher. Remember $I = [1/2] pmax^2 / Z$). Although 2 million times the acceleration of gravity sounds scary, nobody knows how to interpret this number.

Harmonic Waves

The discussion of ultrasound waves in tissue is all nice theory, but a complete understanding of ultrasound during imaging isn't so easy. If the ultrasound intensity is greater than 333 mW/cm², the tissue molecular pressure drops to *below 0*, an impossible situation. Of course the Ispta (temporal average) in medical diagnostic instruments is held below 0.100 Watts/cm² to avoid excess heating of the tissues. But the Isptp (temporal peak) value is 100 times as large because the ultrasound is only on for 1% of the time (duty factor = 0.01). So, during the transmission of a short ultrasound burst, the instantaneous intensity Isptp = 10 Watts/cm², and the peak pressure pmax = 5.5 atmospheres. The peak positive pressure is 6.5 atmospheres and the peak negative pressure is −4.5 atmospheres. Because this is impossible, the linear equations of wave propagation above don't work and nonlinear equations must be used. Of course, we will use the linear equations improperly later to compute the mechanical index as if the equations apply to this case. We will do this because the nonlinear equations are too difficult.

The spring expressions, $K \times d^2s/dx^2$ and $P = Po + p = Po + K \times ds/dx$ are not valid for these high intensities used in diagnostic ultrasound (i.e., greater than 300 mW/cm² Isptp). When the tissue is stretched so far, K is not a constant any longer. There are lots of everyday examples of the stiffness (also called the spring constant) failing. Stretch a rubber band between your hands. If you pull a little harder, the rubber band will lengthen. If you reduce the pull, the rubber band will shorten. However, if you reduce the pull to 0 so that the rubber band shortens to its flaccid length, you cannot reduce the force further, so the spring constant K no longer works. If you pull the rubber band to the maximum length, pulling harder does not lengthen the rubber band, but might break it. This is the other limit to K. So, for a rubber band, if $X = Xo + x$ is the length of the rubber band and Xo is the flaccid length of the rubber band, then the force on the rubber band, $f = K \times x$, and is valid from $x = 0$ to $x$max. If you try to stretch the rubber band beyond $x$max, you can apply a large f, with no increase in length, and then the rubber band breaks. Blood vessel walls follow the same rules. The circumference of an empty vein might be 3 cm, so the venous pressure stays near 0 as the vein fills until the cross section changes from flat to a circle 1 cm in diameter. If it fills further, the pressure increases rapidly.

Some people explain what happens with Isptp intensities above 300 mW/cm^2 by saying that the ultrasound speed increases in compression and decreases in decompression. Whatever happens, the result is that the tissue takes some energy out of the original frequency and converts it into double the ultrasound frequency or triple the ultrasound frequency. The result is harmonic waves, the addition of double and triple frequencies to the ultrasound. These higher harmonic frequencies help decrease the negative pressure. The high-pressure portion of the wave becomes sharper and steeper, whereas the low pressure portions of the wave flatten out. This is similar to the ocean wave that crests and breaks as it approaches the shoreline. The presence of harmonics is a way to explain the change in shape. An FFT frequency spectrum of the sharpened wave contains harmonic frequencies. In addition to flattening the negative pressure regions, the harmonics also increase attenuation of the wave because attenuation is proportional to frequency. This lowers the intensity of the ultrasound by converting the energy into heat. Of course, the harmonic frequencies are also scattered by the tissue, so they can be received by the transducer if the transducer is sensitive to them. This is the basis of harmonic imaging.

Because harmonics form best where the intensities of the fundamental frequency are highest, the harmonics are most likely to be scattered from the center of the ultrasound beam pattern. Harmonic waves can be used for imaging and for Doppler.

Harmonic waves form because the ultrasound intensities used in diagnostic ultrasound are so high that ultrasound propagation is nonlinear. Nonlinear means that the waves don't follow the linear (simple) equations above.

However, harmonic imaging requires a trick. Ultrasound transducers are not sensitive at twice the natural ultrasound frequency of the transducer ($2 \times$ Fo). By using a broadband transducer and lowering the transmit frequency to 0.7, the natural frequency ($0.7 \times$ Fo), then the strongest harmonic generated by tissue, is double that or $1.4 \times$ Fo, still below the frequency $2 \times$ Fo at which the transducer is not sensitive. Unfortunately, the third harmonic ($3 \times [0.7 \times$ Fo]) is close to the $2 \times$ Fo at which the transducer is not sensitive ($3 \times 0.7 = 2.1 \sim 2.0$).

Ultrasound Attenuation

As an ultrasound burst passes through tissue, a fraction of the energy in the burst is converted to heat and a fraction is converted to reflected or scattered ultrasound. The original burst, traveling in the original direction, becomes progressively weaker. The easiest way to think about attenuation is that you can find a slab of tissue that will attenuate the energy of the burst to half of the original energy. For the same tissue, a thicker slab will attenuate the ultrasound more, leaving the burst with lower energy. If a slab of muscle 1 cm thick attenuates the energy of a 3-MHz ultrasound burst by 50% to 50%, then a slab of muscle 2 cm thick will attenuate the ultrasound energy by 75% to 25% and a slab of muscle 3 cm thick slab will attenuate the ultrasound by 87.5% to 12.5%. The remaining ultrasound burst energy, after attenuation, has an exponential relationship to depth. Attenuation can be computed in: (1) deciBels (dB), based on factors of 10 in energy; (2) Nepers, based on factors of "e" in amplitude; (3) half amplitude; or (4) half energy levels.

The rate of attenuation is proportional to ultrasound frequency. In the example above, doubling the ultrasound frequency from 3 MHz to 6 MHz results in doubling of the ultrasound attenuate rate. So for 6-MHz ultrasound, a 1 cm thick slab of muscle will attenuate the ultrasound burst energy to 25% and 2 cm of muscle will attenuate the ultrasound burst energy to 6.25%.

The easiest way to compute attenuation is to remember that in average soft tissue, half of the ultrasound power will have been scattered or converted to heat after 20 wavelengths of tissue penetration. The attenuation is lower in fat (34 wavelengths to half power) and higher across muscle fibers (6 wavelengths to half power). With older ultrasound systems, we can get echoes back from a "perfect" reflector at a depth of 200 wavelengths average tissue; the best ultrasound systems of the future will never be able to get echoes back from a perfect reflector that is 400 wavelengths deep. That limit is because of the intrinsic ultrasound noise emitted by tissue. At 5-MHz ultrasound, with a wavelength of 0.3 mm, 200 wavelengths is 6 cm. For Doppler measurements, the echogenicity of blood is poor, only about 1/1,000,000 of the 5-MHz echo power reflects from blood. So, at 5-MHz, Doppler studies are limited to about 2 cm with older systems. Newer systems with better electronics may get 5-MHz Doppler signals from 4 cm deep or more.

Lower ultrasound frequencies are able to get signals from deeper in tissue because the lower attenuation at those frequencies means that echoes returned from those depths are likely to be stronger. One factor working against this is that reflectors smaller than the ultrasound wavelength (like blood cells) are not good reflectors. According to the Rayleigh theory of wave scattering* from small reflectors, the scattered intensity increases with the forth power of the ratio of scatterer size to wavelength. So for higher ultrasound frequencies with shorter wavelengths, the scattering from red blood cells increases. If a 6-MHz Doppler replaces a 3-MHz Doppler, except for the attenuations problem, the 6-MHz Doppler will receive echoes from blood that are 16 times greater than echoes using a 3-MHz Doppler. However, the addition of attenuation, which is twice as great for 6-MHz ultrasound as for 3-MHz ultrasound, does diminish the benefit of using a higher ultrasound frequency to take advantage of Rayleigh scattering. Taking the two factors together, 5-MHz ultrasound gives the strongest Doppler signal from carotid arteries 2 cm deep under fat and muscle (carotid arteries); 2-MHz ultrasound gives the strongest echo from renal arteries 10 cm deep under muscle and fat (renal arteries).

---

*The third Lord Rayleigh, whose name was John William Strutt, became Lord Rayleigh when he inherited the title from his father. Both the impedance unit Rayl and Rayleigh scattering of ultrasound from blood cells are credited to him.

Ultrasound Burst

Although it is possible to listen for ultrasound naturally produced in the body (the emission intensity is about 0.01 picoWatts/cm^2), in this discussion, all ultrasound imaging begins by sending a burst of sound into the body and listening for the echoes returning from tissues. The transmitted ultrasound is called a burst, rather than a pulse, because the burst may contain few or many cycles of ultrasound (Fig. 6-2). For good depth resolution in B-mode imaging, the burst is short (0.5 microseconds); for Doppler, the burst is long (1 to 10 microseconds); in the extreme of continuous-wave Doppler, ultrasound is transmitted continuously.

Ultrasound Propagation in Tissue

The ultrasound passes into the body traveling at a speed of about 1.5 millimeter per microsecond (1.5 mm/µs, Table 6-3). At that speed, the ultrasound can travel the 150 mm across your head in 100 µs. An echo from the far skull takes another 100 µs to return to the trans-

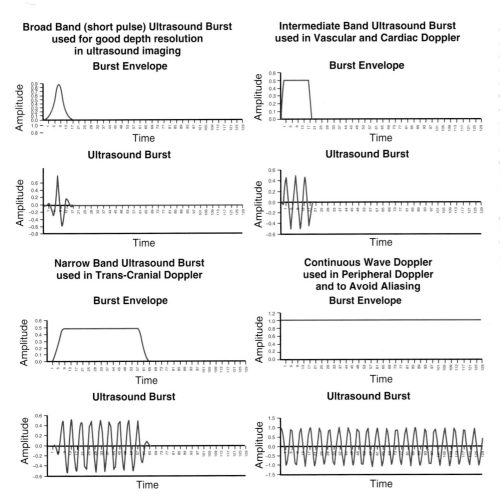

Figure 6-2. Ultrasound transmit bursts. Longer transmit bursts are called narrow band because the frequency of the long burst can be measured accurately with low variance. Shorter transmit bursts allow improved depth resolution, but the frequency cannot be accurately defined. These bursts are called broadband. Longer transmit bursts allow higher transmit energy in the burst when mechanical index or temporal peak power is limited. Upper graph is the "envelope" of each burst; the lower graph is the radio frequency (RF) ultrasound burst sent to the transducer.

TABLE 6-3. Speed and Impedance of Ultrasound in Tissues

Tissue	Speed (mm/μs)	Impedance (KiloRayls)
Air	0.33	0.0004
Fat	1.45	1.38
Water (25 °C)	1.48	1.48
Liver	1.54	1.65
Blood	1.57	1.62
Muscle	1.58	1.65
Cartilage	1.65	
Bone	4	7

mitting transducer for a total round trip time of 200 μs. Any echo that returns after a 200 μs trip comes from a reflector at a one-way distance of 150 mm (Table 6-4). We expect that the trip is straight, along a selected ultrasound line, so information from that echo is displayed as if it came from a known direction and depth. All of the caution in these statements is because we know that ultrasound propagation in tissue is more complicated: the ultrasound path is bent by refraction and reflection, and those complications result in image distortions called artifacts.

Of course, in tissues where the speed is not 1.5 mm/μs (see Table 6-3), the depth display (see Table 6-4) is distorted by the percent error in speed. The depth errors occur in both depth distance between the ultrasound transducer and the reflector, and in the depth distance between two reflectors in tissue. For example, when measuring the thickness of the temporal bone during transtemporal ultrasound brain imaging, a bone layer of 4 mm thickness will appear to be 1.5 mm thick on the ultrasound image. Ultrasound can do a 4-mm each way round trip in bone in 2 microseconds, and ultrasound can do a 1.5-mm each way round trip in soft tissue in

TABLE 6-4. Reflector Depth vs. Echo Time, Maximum Pulse Repetition Frequency, and Doppler Aliasing Frequency

Depth	Time	PRF	Aliasing
0.75 mm	1 μs	1 MHz	500 KHz
3 mm	4 μs	250 KHz	125 KHz
30 mm	40 μs	25 KHz	12.5 KHz
60 mm	80 μs	12.5 KHz	6.25 KHz
150 mm	200 μs	5 KHz	2.5 KHz

2 microseconds. The two round trips look the same to the ultrasound scanner because both last 2 microseconds. Such effects may be important in ultrasound-guided biopsy in fatty breast, where a tumor that is 58 mm deep appears to be 60 mm deep on the image because the engineers designing the ultrasound system do not provide a control to adjust the image scale for different ultrasound speeds.

With this information, in about 1950, medical diagnostic ultrasound imaging began.

B-Mode Ultrasound Imaging

By transmitting a short burst of ultrasound into tissue along a line and measuring the time for an echo to return, the depth of the reflector causing that echo can be determined (Fig. 6-3). There are two features of the echo which are important: (1) the strength of the echo; and (2) the phase of the echo. Phase is used for Doppler velocity detection and will be discussed later. The strength (amplitude) of the echo is used for B-mode (brightness mode) imaging. The echo strength is determined by acoustic impedance changes in tissue and by attenuation of the ultrasound as it passes through tissue. To infer the tissue type represented at specific locations in the image, it is common to display the echo strength after adjusting for attenuation.

Ultrasound attenuation occurs because some of the energy of the ultrasound burst is scattered in all directions and because other energy is converted to heat in each part of the tissue. The strength (amplitude) of the burst decreases with time (depth) in the tissue, and echoes from deeper depths are weaker than echoes from shallow tissues. If the amount of attenuation in the tissue is known, then the ultrasound instrument can adjust the strength of those echoes from deeper tissue by amplifying them more than the echoes from shallow tissue. This adjustment of the echo strength is called compensation for attenuation. The amount of amplification is called gain. Because the depth of the reflector is proportional to the time that it takes for the echo to return, the amplification is called time gain compensation (TGC) or depth gain compensation (DGC) or time gain control or depth gain control. This control is adjusted by the examiner to make the image look right. Of course, it is possible for the examiner to "paint" features into the image by adjusting the TGC control.

Doppler Ultrasound Imaging

Doppler methods are designed to identify the speed of moving tissue rather than the tissue type. Doppler methods are similar to M-mode (see Figure 6-3, Panel

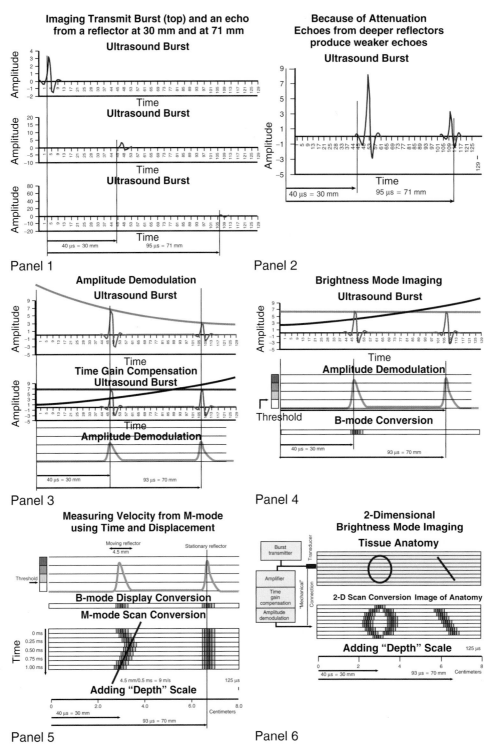

Figure 6-3. *Ultrasound echo strength imaging modes:* **Panel 1,** *A broadband ultrasound transmit burst (upper row) is followed in 40 μs by an echo from a reflector at 30 mm deep and another echo at 95 μs from a reflector at 71 mm deep. Using the given value for the speed of ultrasound in tissue and accounting for the round trip, the instrument displays the 40 μs echo at a depth of 30 mm and the 95 μs echo at a depth of 71 mm.* **Panel 2,** *Both echoes enter the ultrasound system via a single signal path. The 71-mm echo has a smaller amplitude than does the 30-mm echo. Although the smaller amplitude could be caused by reflection from a smaller impedance difference at 71 mm deep, the examiner assumes that the difference is caused by attenuation.* **Panel 3,** *The examiner adjusts the TGC control (violet line) to make the two echo amplitudes appear equal, and the signal is routed to the demodulator where the echo amplitude is measured (green line).* **Panel 4,** *The echo amplitude can be divided into sections representing echo strength. Four divisions are shown here representing four gray levels. Modern ultrasound instruments divide the echo strength into 256 gray levels even though the examiner can only differentiate about 16. These gray level values, as a function of depth, are stored in the scan converter computer memory.* **Panel 5,** *If the ultrasound transducer beam pattern is held stationary, and the process is repeated over moving tissue like the heart, and the results are displayed along adjacent lines, each below the last, an M-mode (motion mode) display is generated. The speed of the moving structure can be measured. It is the slope of the line, the change in depth with change in time.* **Panel 6,** *If the tissue is stationary, and the process is repeated while the ultrasound beam pattern is moved from location to location in the tissue, and the resultant echo patterns are shown along corresponding lines on the image, a two-dimensional B-mode image display is generated.*

5). As in M-mode, to measure the speed of moving blood or other tissue, a series of ultrasound pulse-echo cycles are directed along a stationary ultrasound beam pattern. In contrast to M-mode, when measuring the speed of bloodflow, there is no large reflector that can be seen after amplitude demodulation. So the motion detection must occur using the undemodulated radio frequency (RF) signal (Fig. 6-4).*

Radio station WWV in Fort Collins, Colorado, operated by the National Institute of Standards and Technologies broadcasts radio signals on 2.5-MHz, 5-MHz, 10-MHz, 15-MHz, and 20-MHz bands providing time signals, weather and geophysical alerts, and global positioning system status reports. If you try to use a conventional ultrasound instrument in Fort Collins at one of these frequencies, it is possible that the WWV transmitter will cause interference in your image. Ultrasound instrument manufacturers shield the case and cables of the ultrasound instrument to avoid this interference. Damage to the cables (e.g., like that caused by rolling a wheel over the scanhead cable) will defeat the shielding and allow interference.

Although amplitude demodulated ultrasound echo signals can resolve motions of a fraction of a millimeter (mm), measurement of changes in phase of the RF echo can resolve motions of a fraction of a micron (micrometer, μm), 1000 times better than with the amplitude demodulated echo used in M-mode.

Although time domain methods (see Figure 6-4, Panels 6, 7, and 8) are advocated as being resistant to aliasing, in practice, the echoes are so complicated that the correct echo match cannot usually be found, so the methods work about as well as Doppler, but they take more computing power. Therefore, few ultrasound instruments have used time domain methods.

Each new echo from a pulse-echo cycle (PEC) taken along a single beam pattern gives new information about tissue motion. A pair of echoes can identify which voxels contain moving tissue. Echoes from a third PEC are required to separate strong echoes bouncing off blood vessel walls from the weak echoes representing moving blood. The vessel wall echoes are called "clutter" by the engineers. Because each echo contains noise, more pulse-echo cycles (longer ensembles) are needed to separate the noise from the bloodflow and the wall motion. Most two-dimensional color Doppler systems use 8 pulse-echo cycles (PECs) per ensemble. At a pulse repetition frequency (PRF) of 10 KHz suitable for examinations up to 75 mm deep (see Table 6-4), an ensemble of 8 PECs requires 0.8 milliseconds to acquire.

Color-flow systems represent the velocity in each voxel as a single value represented by a color selected from a color scale (red to blue). If the velocity has some fluctuation, then the variance may be added by adding green to the color.

If the sample volume contains turbulent bloodflow, many velocities should be measured in a voxel. The number of measurements that can be made is equal to the ensemble length. For each spectrum in a spectral waveform, an ensemble of 128 PECs is usually used, allowing a new spectrum of 128 frequency tests to be displayed representing data gathered over 12.8 milliseconds. Some 78 spectra, each representing 12.8 milliseconds, are displayed each second to form a spectral waveform (Fig. 6-5).

Because so much data are displayed about a single sample volume in the spectral waveform, data are not displayed about other sample volumes. The alternative is to display velocity data for many sample volumes, showing a single velocity for each sample volume as color (Fig. 6-6).

Both color Doppler and spectral Doppler are subject to aliasing. A pulsed Doppler cannot differentiate between different possible velocities separated by twice the velocity corresponding to the Nyquist frequency.* In Figure 6-7, Panel 1, pairs of possible Doppler frequency waveforms, separated by twice the Nyquist frequency, are displayed.

By knowing from hemodynamics that the frequencies should be connected to form a smooth waveform, a proper-appearing waveform can be selected (see Fig. 6-7, Panel 2).

Aliasing Computation

If a Doppler signal is aliased, the correct velocity can be computed. Remember that as the wave leaves one edge of the spectral waveform, it enters the other edge, so both edges represent the same frequency and velocity (Fig. 6-8).

Doppler Equation

If the blood is flowing parallel to the axis of the visualized vessel, then the Doppler frequency scale, which is measured, can be converted into a velocity scale by using the Doppler equation (Fig. 6-9).

---

*The echo is called a radio frequency signal because it is radio frequency. If the ultrasound transducer plug were connected to an antenna wire strung out the window rather than to an ultrasound transducer in contact with a patient, then the antenna would send a radio signal at a frequency above the AM broadcast band (0.55 MHz to 1.6 MHz) but below the FM broadcast band (88 to 108 MHz).

---

*Harry Nyquist was a physicist at Bell Laboratories around 1920. He figured out the rules for sampling and aliasing while developing methods of sampling telephone conversations to combine 20 conversations on a single trans-Atlantic telephone cable circuit.

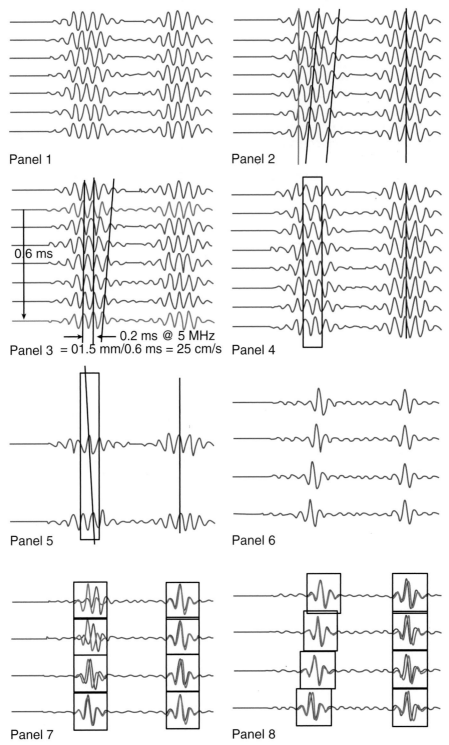

Panel 1

Panel 2

0.6 ms

0.2 ms @ 5 MHz

Panel 3   = 01.5 mm/0.6 ms = 25 cm/s   Panel 4

Panel 5

Panel 6

Panel 7

Panel 8

Figure 6-4. *Doppler velocity measurement. To perform Doppler measurements, usually between 8 and 120 pulse-echo cycles are used and analyzed as a group. In this figure, 8 pulse-echo cycles are used. This group is called an ensemble. The ensemble length is 8.* **Panel 1**, *A shallow echo representing a moving structure and a deep echo representing a stationary echo are shown. The envelopes of the echoes of both echoes appear stationary.* **Panel 2**, *By tracking the RF peaks from echo to echo, the phase change can be measured.* **Panel 3**, *With a pulse repetition frequency (PRF) of 10 KHz, seven successive echoes span 0.6 milliseconds. A tissue motion of 0.15 mm toward the ultrasound transducer means a tissue velocity of 25 cm/s.* **Panel 4**, *Modern digital ultrasound instruments divide the depth into segments called voxels and look at the echoes from one voxel to see if the phase is stationary or moving.* **Panel 5**, *If the time interval between two pulse-echo cycles is too long for the velocity in the tissue under study, the displacement of the tissue represented in the sample volume may be greater than 0.125 wavelengths of ultrasound in tissue. If so, the phase will move too far between observations to be properly tracked. In that case, when the analysis system selects the lowest possible phase shift, the measurement is low and often in the opposite direction. This is called aliasing.* **Panel 6**, *The time domain method is an alternate ultrasonic velocity measurement system that is resistant to aliasing. It differs from Doppler by using a short broadband transmit burst resulting in shorter echoes.* **Panel 7**, *By comparing the echoes in a voxel that come back at different times, voxels containing stationary reflectors can be differentiated from those containing moving reflectors.* **Panel 8**, *When a voxel containing moving reflectors is detected, then a model of the echo is moved in depth until a match is found and the velocity computed from the time delay detected.*

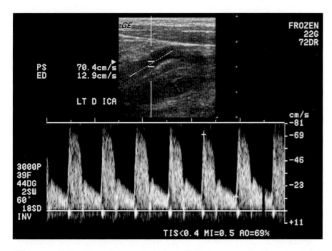

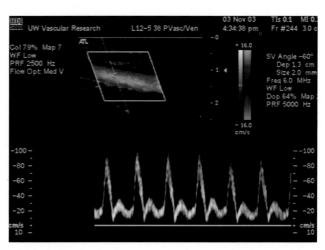

Figure 6-5. *Two-dimensional brightness-mode image with Doppler spectral waveform. The Doppler is operating at a PRF of 3 KHz, allowing the sample gate to be located at any depth shallower than 250 mm. The 3-KHz PRF allows frequencies between +1.5 KHz and −1.5 KHz to be displayed. The texture of the spectral broadening in the spectral waveform is formed by the results of about 50 spectra per second, each displaying the intensity of each of 60 Doppler frequencies (50 × 60 = 3000).*

Figure 6-6. *Color-Flow Image. The spectral waveform at the bottom displays all of the velocities in the sample volume over a period of 4 seconds, showing velocities in both systole and diastole. The color-flow image shows the velocities at about 40 locations on each of 20 color Doppler ultrasound beam pattern lines, 800 locations in all. The color bar shows a velocity range from −16 cm/s to +16 cm/s, a 32 cm/sec range that is different from the −10 cm/s to +100 cm/s on the spectral waveform (a 110 cm/sec range). After removing the adjustment for the Doppler examination angle (60 degrees, cos[60°] = 0.5), the spectral waveform velocity range is −5 cm/s to +50 cm/s. The PRF for the spectral Doppler is higher than for the color Doppler, and the color Doppler velocity is not adjusted for Doppler angle. A baseline shift has been applied to the spectral waveform display by the examiner to show high aliased velocities continuous with the low unaliased velocities. The color-flow image is aliased in the center of the vessel. Notice the color change from red to orange to cyan, going off one end of the color scale and onto the other. If this had been reverse flow, the color sequence in the image would have been red to black to blue to cyan.*

Unfortunately, in nearly all arteries, the normal blood velocities are not parallel to the axis of the artery. Instead the flow is helical, like the flow down the drain of a washbasin (Fig. 6-10). Thus, the measured Doppler velocity can only be used for the empirical classification of arteries and veins into disease categories based on experience.

In cardiology, where Doppler signals are always acquired using a Doppler angle of 0 degrees, the measured

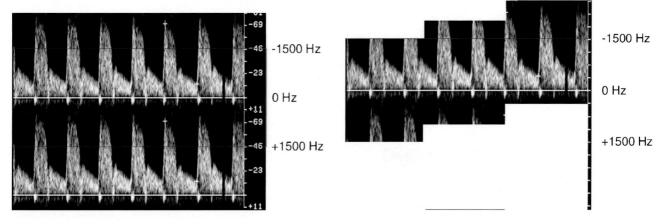

Figure 6-7. *Doppler aliasing, redisplayed with baseline shift. Because a Doppler system can't really tell if the echo phase has shifted by 360 degrees plus the measured shift, or 360 degrees minus the measured shift, the possible spectral waveforms could be stacked as one manufacturer did (left). A simple Doppler display (right) shows the Doppler frequency values displayed between the upper and lower Nyquist lmit frequency values at + and −1.5 KHz. The Nyquist limit is half the PRF. In this case, the PRF is 3 KHz. The frequencies representing high velocities away from the transducer appear on the lower part of the display where flow toward the transducer should appear. The examiner recognizes that this display is aliased and moves the aliased portion of the display to a corresponding region representing flow away from the transducer. This control is usually called baseline shift.*

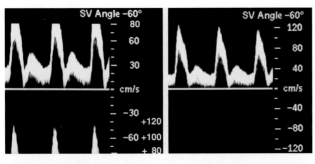

Figure 6-8. *Aliasing computation. Notice the addition of velocity labels at the edge of the velocity scale. Both the higher PRF waveform at the right and the scale adjusted waveform at the left demonstrate peak systolic angle adjusted velocities of 118 cm/s.*

blood velocity is commonly used for the computation of both cardiac output and for the computation of Bernoulli pressure drop across a stenotic valve. Both measurements have been validated by gold standard cardiac catheterization methods. However, in vascular studies where Doppler data can be acquired only at Doppler examination angles between 40 degrees and 70 degrees, attempts at computing validated arterial and venous flow rates and pressure drops have failed. Even a simple test of taking velocity data at an angle of 40 degrees and at 60 degrees from the same location usually leads to an angle adjusted velocity value taken at 60 degrees, about 40% higher than the value taken at 40 degrees. This "error" in the Doppler equation is not caused by faulty math but by the incorrect assumption that blood flows parallel to the vessel axis.

The systematic increase of angle adjusted blood velocity measurements as the Doppler examination increases is a source of variability in facilities that do not use a constant Doppler examination angle in peripheral arteries. The question of which angle is most accurate appears regularly on the e-mail discussion service, UVM Flownet < UVMFLOWNET@LIST.UVM.EDU > .

Evidence of helical flow is easy to demonstrate with color-flow imaging (Fig. 6-11). By placing the view to the artery in cross section, the helical flow can be demonstrated.

Ultrasound Instrumentation

The evolution of diagnostic ultrasound pulse-echo ultrasound instruments since 1950 has been based on the adoption of advances in electronics rather than advances in concepts. Vacuum tubes were in common use in 1950. The invention of the transistor by John Bardeen and Walter Brattain in 1947 led to commercial pocket-sized transistor radios by 1960 and pocket-sized transistorized continuous-wave (CW) Doppler ultrasound systems before 1970. The availability of inexpensive digital memory for computer systems around 1975 started the development of the modern computerized two-dimensional ultrasound imaging system.

The "all analog systems" constructed before 1975 changed in performance as analog components dried out, corroded, became fouled with dust, and otherwise deteriorated. This deterioration caused continuous shifts in instrument performance such as the display of time seen as distance on the viewing screen. Because of this, the use of alignment targets and phantoms was constantly required to readjust the instrument to compensate for drifting analog electronic components. The introduction of digital circuits, and later programmed microprocessors and computers, eliminated the instabilities of analog systems. It also eliminated the need for alignment targets and phantoms, although these are still discussed because of tradition and because these devices are useful teaching tools. It is important to understand the difference between analog and digital processing.

In ambulation, compare a ramp to a staircase. The ramp is like an analog circuit, the staircase is like a digital

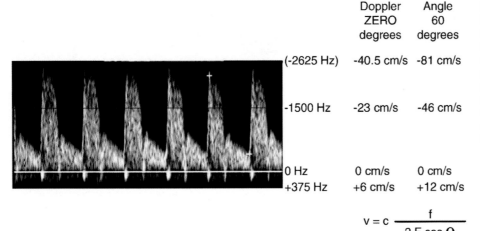

	Doppler ZERO degrees	Angle 60 degrees
(-2625 Hz)	-40.5 cm/s	-81 cm/s
-1500 Hz	-23 cm/s	-46 cm/s
0 Hz	0 cm/s	0 cm/s
+375 Hz	+6 cm/s	+12 cm/s

Figure 6-9. *Doppler equation. If the examiner aligns the Doppler cursor parallel to the axis of the vessel during the examination, the Doppler equation is applied automatically by modern duplex Doppler instruments, converting the measured frequency scale into velocity and shrinking that scale according to the inverse cosine of the Doppler examination angle.*

$$v = c \; \frac{f}{2 \, F \cos \Theta}$$

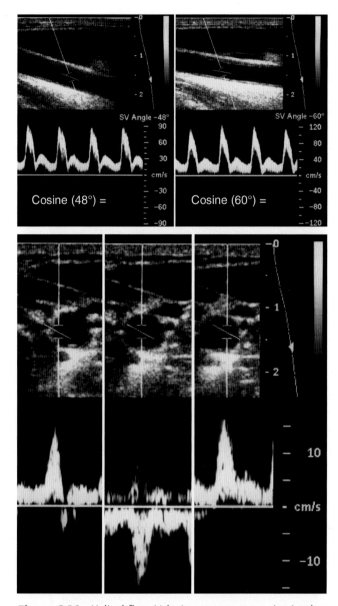

Figure 6-10. *Helical flow. Velocity measurements* (top) *taken from the middle right common carotid artery at two angles have the same Doppler frequencies, resulting in differing angle adjusted velocities. Velocity waveforms* (bottom) *taken from a perpendicular cross section at the same mCCA location show the dual helical velocities of 13 cm/s, which may be the cause of the failure of the two angle adjusted Doppler measurements to agree.*

circuit. You can number the stairs on the staircase and define exactly your elevation by the stair number. You can place a ruler on the ramp, but you cannot exactly define all possible locations on a ramp. If something is on a particular stair of the staircase, you know exactly the elevation. Even if an earthquake shakes the object around a little (system noise), it is still on the stair and still at a known elevation. If the object were on a ramp, a little shaking would change the elevation. However,

if there are 20 stairs, only 20 elevations are possible, so a very small elevation change is not possible. On the ramp, there is no elevation change too small to be allowed. So, analog has the advantage that very small differences can be differentiated. Digital has the advantage that each step is defined and resistant to noise.

Analog processing of ultrasound echoes in early ultrasound instruments allowed subtle differences in gray scale to be displayed. When digital scan converter memories were introduced in 1977, the digital memory could only store and display 16 shades of gray, about the same as the eye can detect. Although that should be OK, often the examiner viewing an image will want to adjust the display after storing in the memory. For example, the brightness of two tissues might be 4.1 and 4.4 on a scale of 16. If there are 64 brightness levels stored instead of 16, then the two tissues could be resolved. On a 16 level scale the 4.1 tissue would be at 4/16 and the 4.4 tissue would be at 4/16, the same. On a 64 level scale, the 4.1 tissue would be at 16/64 and the 4.4 tissue would be at 18/64. By converting the display for viewing by eye (which only sees 16 gray levels), you can choose to show stored levels 1/64 through 12/64 as 1/16 and 20/64 through 64/64 as 16/16. Then you can spread the stored level range 13/64 to 19/64 over the display levels 2/16 to 15/16. If you do, then the 4.1 is greater than 16/64 is greater than 8/16 and the 4.4 is greater than 18/64 is greater than 12/61, so it would be easy for the eye to differentiate them. This process is called post processing; it provides flexibility for improving the display of the image.

As digital systems have improved, digital processing has taken over more components of ultrasound imaging systems. The major improvement of digital processing is to increase the number of values that are allowed. In early image memories, only 4 bits (binary digits) were available to record the brightness of each pixel (spot on the image screen corresponding to a memory location in the scan converter). These 4 bits could store 16 levels of gray. Some systems call 0 = white and 15 = black, others use the inverse (Table 6-5).

The improvement to 6 bit memories allowed 64 levels of gray. Increasing to 8 bits allowed 256 levels of gray. Now, 16 bit memories are common. That allows 65,000 levels of gray. Of course, only 256 levels of gray are used. The rest of the values are for color in the image.

The components of an ultrasound system, whether analog, digital, or software, are similar. Figure 6-12 shows the components of a basic system to display an ultrasound image. The transducer is not coupled to the patient, so the burst energy is trapped in the transducer, causing only a rapidly decaying oscillation in the transducer and no echo from the patient.

The echoes returned from the patient's anatomy can be demodulated to display echo strength and then scan converted to form an image (Figs. 6-13 through 6-18).

Real-Time Imaging

Generating an ultrasound image takes time. Although different parts of the image are gathered at different times, generally the image acquisition proceeds from left to right. The effect of this orderly progression can introduce effects in the image that could be mistaken for physiology or anatomy. Figure 6-19 shows a series of two-dimensional color Doppler images gathered from a single cardiac cycle. By displaying the ECG, the relationship between the spectral waveform and the time of image acquisition can be seen.

Note that in Frame 2 the highest "color velocities" (aliased) are on the right, taken later in the image nearer to peak systole. Note that in Frame 3 the highest "color velocities" (aliased) are on the left, taken earlier in the image near to peak systole. Although the horizontal dimension in a two-dimensional ultrasound image is supposed to be lateral dimension, the lateral dimension also contains time (Fig. 6-20).

Text continued on page 68

TABLE 6-5. **Binary Numbers**

4-Bit Binary Number	Hexidecimal Number	Decimal Number
0000	0	0
0001	1	1
0010	2	2
0011	3	3
0100	4	4
0101	5	5
0110	6	6
0111	7	7
1000	8	8
1001	9	9
1010	a	10
1011	b	11
1100	c	12
1101	d	13
1110	e	14
1111	f	15

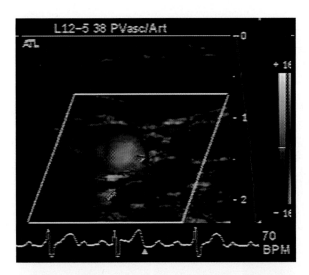

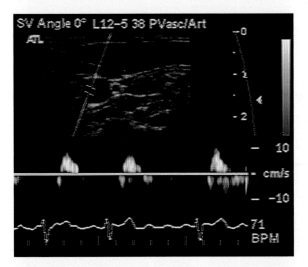

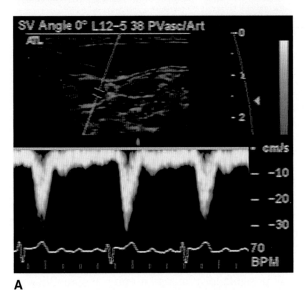

A

Figure 6-11. **A**, *Color Doppler demonstration of helical velocities in the common carotid artery. Notice that the systolic peak of velocity waveform on the left occurs after the ECG T-wave, but the systolic peak of velocity waveform on the right occurs before the ECG T-wave.*

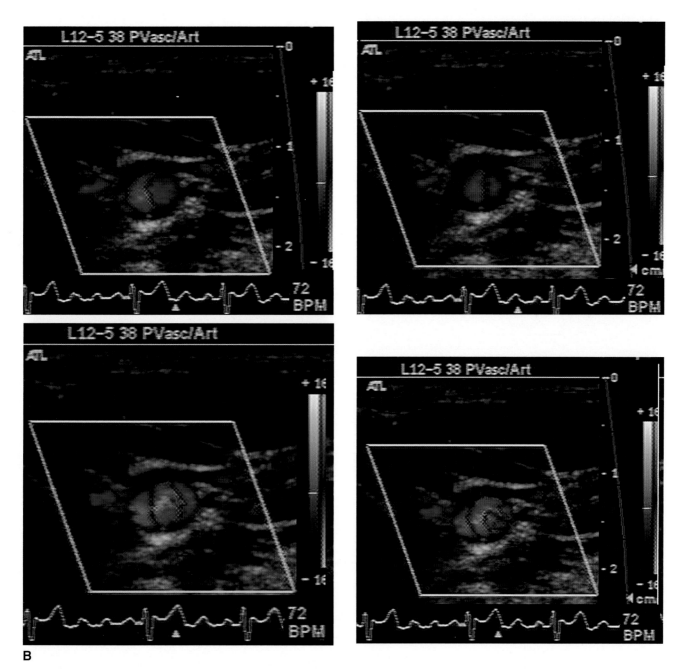

B

Figure 6–11. **B**, *The helical shape of the waveform changes with angle of view and time in the cardiac cycle. Notice that the scan plane is perpendicular to the common carotid artery axis, as verified by the intima-media thickness image on the deep side of the artery.*

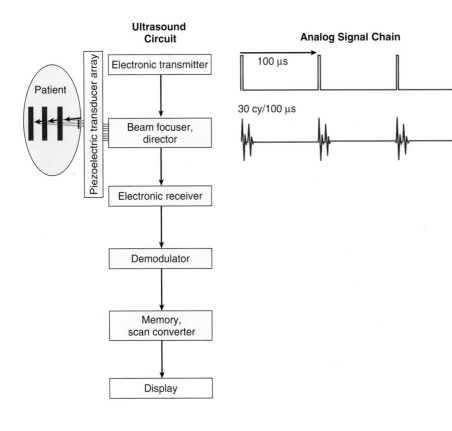

Figure 6-12. *Ultrasound system not coupled to a patient. The transmit impulse causes an oscillation in the transducer, seen as an oscillating voltage. The frequency of oscillation is higher if a thinner transducer is used. Because the energy loss from the transducer into the patient is not present, the transducer oscillates, producing bright echoes at the superficial edge of the image.*

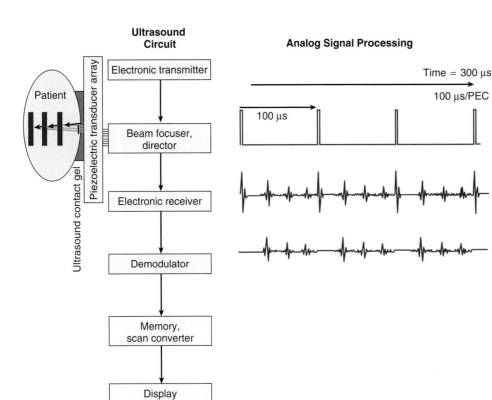

Figure 6-13. *Ultrasound system showing RF echoes from three reflectors, each at a different depth in the patient. Transducer oscillation stops more quickly (transducer is damped) because most of the ultrasound burst energy is going into the patient. The echoes are at the same frequency as the natural oscillation of the transducer based on its thickness. In the patient, there are three reflectors. Echoes from each of the three reflectors are seen after each transmit burst. The receiver has removed the transmit bursts from the signal.*

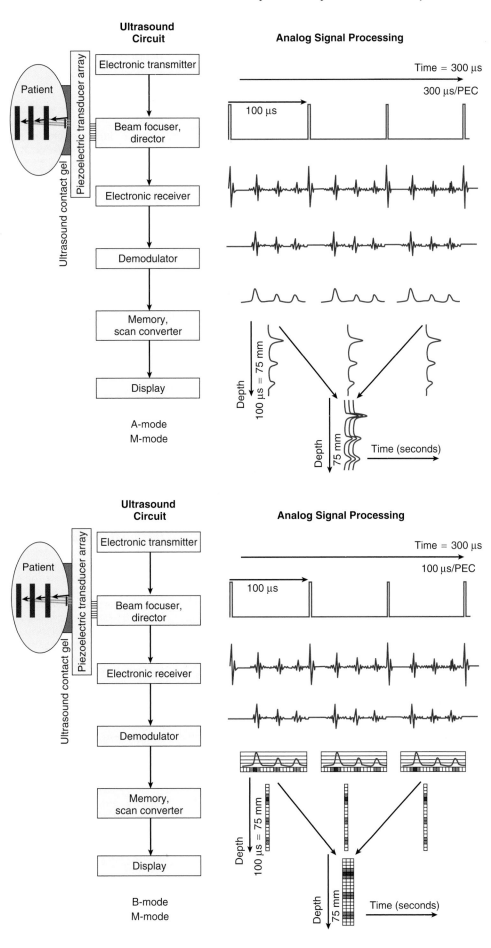

Figure 6-14. *Ultrasound M-mode (motion mode) display showing the amplitude as A-mode (amplitude mode). The receiver has removed the high voltage transmit burst from the signal. Amplitude demodulation preserves the echogenicity of the three tissue structures in the patient. Motion would appear as an upward or downward drift of the peaks on the lower display.*

Figure 6-15. *Ultrasound M-mode (motion mode) display showing the amplitude as B-mode (brightness mode). Motion would appear as an upward or downward drift of the reflectors on the lower display*

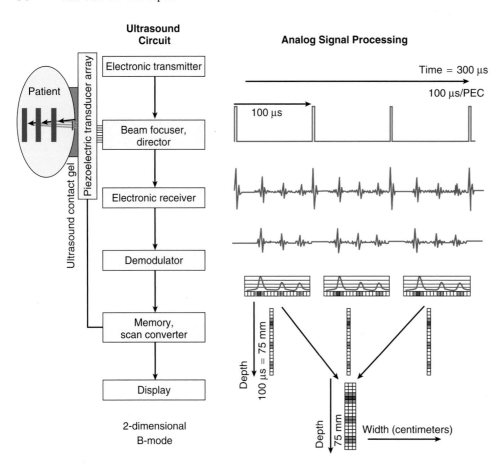

Figure 6-16. *Two-dimensional ultrasound B-mode display. Notice that the only difference between an M-mode system and a two-dimensional system is the signal path from the beam former to the memory/scan converter to deliver the position information to the memory, which will deliver it to the display.*

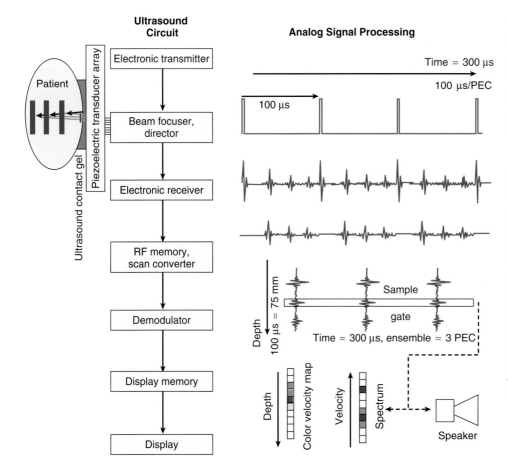

Figure 6-17. *Pulsed Doppler ultrasound system. The spectral waveform and the sound from the speaker represents the blood velocity at the selected sample depth. The three pulse-echo cycles represent an ensemble. A spectral waveform usually uses an ensemble of 128 pulse-echo cycles to display 128 frequencies (velocities) on a spectrum. The spectral waveform and audio output displays the Doppler signal from a single depth and single lateral location, called a voxel or Doppler sample volume. The lateral dimension on the spectral waveform is time (seconds). A color Doppler image usually uses an ensemble of eight pulse-echo cycles to display a color representing a single velocity. A different velocity is computed for each depth. Adjacent lines can represent either time (color M-mode) or lateral dimension (2-D color display).*

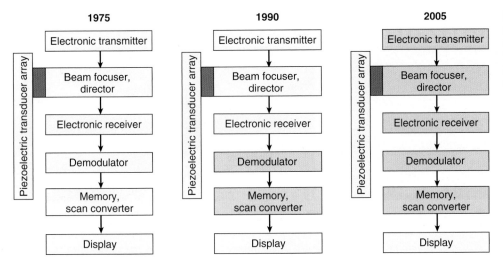

Figure 6-18. History of introduction of digital devices in ultrasound systems. Shaded devices are digital. Now the entire ultrasound system is a computer with software.

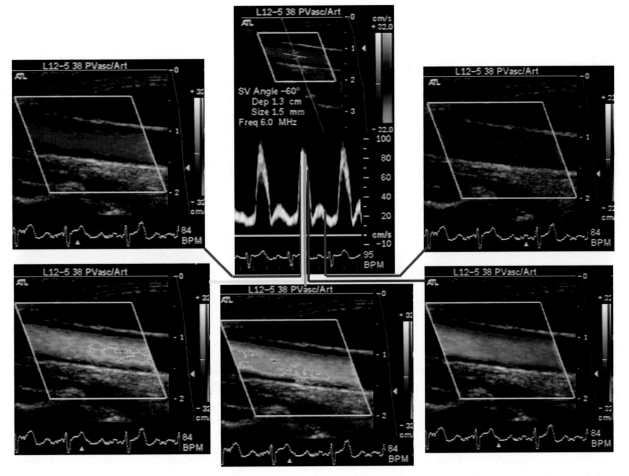

Figure 6-19. A sequence of color Doppler images. Each image takes about 40 milliseconds to acquire. **Frame 1** (upper left), systolic velocity upslope. **Frame 2** (lower left), presystolic velocity peak. **Frame 3** (lower center), postsystolic peak. **Frame 4** (lower right), systolic downslope. **Frame 5** (upper right), mid-diastole.

2 Methods of Flow Visualization

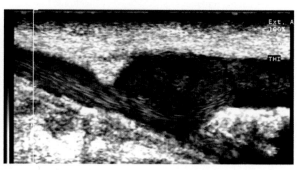

Scan Line Speed = 100 cm/s ---->

Blood Velocity = 100 cm/s ------------->

Figure 6-20. Flow tracing in the proximal anastomosis of a vein graft. These images are formed by the ultrasound scan lines proceeding from left to right. Although the color Doppler image is beautiful, the B-mode image is remarkable. In the B-mode image at the right, the scan lines move across the 30-mm wide linear array scanhead in 30 milliseconds, proceeding at 1 mm/ms = 1 m/s = 100 cm/s, which is equal to the blood velocity. The streaks are formed by groups of erythrocytes arranged by chance such that they produce a strong echo. These are not formed structures in blood. The effect is achieved by using a long complex transmit burst matched to a demodulation filter to emphasize speckle. This is similar to what is called B-flow. The effect is only seen when the blood velocity matches the ultrasound scan velocity. Reversing the scanhead eliminates the streaks.

Text continued from page 62

Ultrasound Beam Former

The ultrasound scanhead has two tasks: (1) to direct the ultrasound beam pattern into the tissue to be imaged; and (2) to focus the ultrasound beam at a depth of interest. In early systems, the focusing was performed by using a transducer that is concave or has a lens attached. The directing was done by pointing the transducer by hand or by using an electric motor. These two processes were called mechanical focusing and mechanical directing of the ultrasound beam. Poor focusing leads to loss of lateral resolution in the ultrasound image.

Around 1975, many ultrasound transducers were directed by hand. One group of instruments was called "static B-scanners." The sonographer developed the art of making good ultrasound images by "painting" the image into memory. Echoes obtained with the ultrasound beam pattern perpendicular to surfaces were bright and gave a pleasing image. Static Doppler scanners were also popular between 1975 and 1980. These instruments tracked the position of the ultrasound transducer and marked the image at the corresponding location when an arterial Doppler signal was detected. Friends became competitors making the Arteriograph, DopScan, and EchoFlow.

Beginning in 1970, ultrasound transducers were mounted on motorized wheels or oscillators. These systems flourished until about 1995, when most were replaced by segmented array transducers. Some scanheads used a combination of electronic beam forming and mechanical directing of the beam pattern. The most

popular is the annular array that uses concentric ring transducer elements arranged like a Bull's-eye target to allow electronic focusing of the transducer combined with mechanical directing of the beam pattern. This was called an annular array. The other popular combined system, recently released, is a three-dimensional B-mode imaging system that uses an electronic array to direct the ultrasound beam pattern in one direction and a mechanical actuator to direct the ultrasound beam in the other direction.

Between 1975 and 2003, transducer arrays evolved to direct and focus the ultrasound beam pattern. Early linear array transducer scanheads used a row of single independent transducers to form an image. Each ultrasound line was formed by a different ultrasound transducer. This is called a low-density array. Each element is focused separately.

The focus of an ultrasound beam can be controlled to the end of the near field (also called the Fresnel zone). The depth of the near field (L) is:

$$L = D^2 / (4X \lambda)$$
$$L = R^2 / (\lambda)$$

where D is the diameter or width of the transducer (R is the radius of the transducer). For a carotid ultrasound examination to a depth of 20 mm using an ultrasound wavelength of 0.3 mm (5 MHz), the width of the transducer must be at least 6 mm.

The width of the transducers in a low-density array must be 6 mm for a 5-MHz carotid scanhead to a depth of 2 cm; and a width of 20 mm for a 3-MHz abdominal scanhead to a depth of 10 cm. The ultrasound line spacing can be no closer than the transducer width, so a low-density array has limited lateral resolution. By 1980, linear transducer arrays were constructed that had closely spaced transducer elements that could work together to make an aperture spanning a group of transducer elements. The ultrasound beam pattern could be directed along many lines within one plane. Now transducers arrays are segmented in two directions so that ultrasound beams can be directed along lines in three-dimensional space.

In order to use the elements of an array to direct an ultrasound beam, the time of transmission from each transducer element must be controlled within a few nanoseconds. By introducing a 6-nanosecond delay between two transducers spaced at 0.5 mm, an ultrasound beam can be tilted about 1 degree. Controlling the time in nanoseconds is not easy.

Linear array transducers move the ultrasound beam pattern to parallel locations by using a new transmit/receive aperture for each selected beam pattern. Phased array transducers tilt the ultrasound beam pattern to new angular locations by adjusting the relative time of transmission for each transducer element and inserting an equivalent delay to the echoes received by each transducer, before the echo signals are combined. Sounds originating from locations other than the selected beam pattern are suppressed by destructive interference. To tilt an ultrasound beam by 45 degrees using a transducer 14 mm wide requires a progressive time delay between the transducers amounting to a total delay of 6 microseconds from one edge of the aperture to the other.

Ultrasound Scanning Considerations

Modern ultrasound scanners automate most of the examiner controls so that the examiner can direct attention to the important issues of the patient and the pathology. In older systems, the examiner can turn down the receiver gain, dimming the B-mode image, and turn up the transmit power to make it bright. This reduces the noise in the image but exposes the patient to more ultrasound intensity. Because the instruments are designed not to exceed safe limits, this is not an issue.

In Figures 6-10 and 6-11, the importance of using a consistent Doppler examination angle was illustrated. There is also an angle issue with B-mode imaging of blood vessels. The resolution of ultrasound images is about equal to the wavelength of ultrasound in the depth direction but is much greater (poorer) in the lateral direction, where electronic focusing is possible; and greater (poorer) still in the thickness direction, where the focus is fixed by the plastic lens on the scanhead face. This unequal resolution in three-dimensions is called anisotropic resolution. The most obvious effect on vascular ultrasound scanning is the measurement of the intima-media thickness (IMT) (Fig. 6-21).

To visualize the IMT, the scan lines must be perpendicular to the vessel wall. The line appears brighter if the curvature of the ultrasound wavefronts matches the curvature of the wall. The wavefront curvature can be changed by changing the focus of the transducer.

Effect of Imaging Angle on B-mode

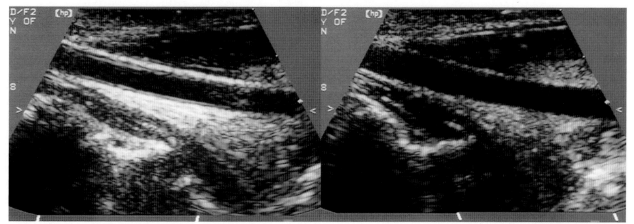

Jean Primozich

Figure 6-21. *Anisotropic resolution and the intima-media thickness. With the ultrasound scan lines tilted to the left (**left panel**), perpendicular to the artery wall, the double line of Pignoli representing the intima-media thickness (IMT) can be easily appreciated. With the ultrasound scan lines tilted to the right (**right panel**), not perpendicular to the artery wall, the double line of Pignoli (DLP) representing the IMT cannot be seen.*

Although common carotid IMT measurement is a popular surrogate for coronary artery atherosclerosis, agreement on IMT evaluation is not as easy as agreement on Doppler criteria. In a blinded study of reader variability of IMT presence and thickness between Gene Strandness, Jean Primozich, and the author, there was no agreement on which images demonstrated a DLP, so agreement on where to measure and what to measure was hopeless. The project was abandoned.

Ultrasound Safety Considerations

Both the American Institute of Ultrasound in Medicine (AIUM) and the United States Food and Drug (and devices) Administration (FDA) agree that ultrasound is safe. Or, at least, that diagnostic ultrasound is safe. Or, at least, safe or at least not very dangerous if you use it with caution and set the output power to as low as reasonably allowable (ALARA).

It is true that you can cauterize tissue with ultrasound. Surgical ultrasound systems have been under development since 1950; now several companies are attempting to promote the ablation of tumors, or at least entire prostates, with high intensity–focused ultrasound (HIFU). HIFU may be used for the ablation of breast tumors and uterine fibroids, and for the sealing of arterial leaks after arterial catheter procedures. HIFU intensities exceed 1000 Watts/cm^2. These intensities can raise tissue temperature 25 °C per second, boiling a region of tissue the size of a grain of rice in 2.5 seconds. Cautery can be done to depths of several centimeters noninvasively without damaging the intervening tissues.

Diagnostic ultrasound examinations can raise tissue temperature. Temperature elevations less than 1 °C are thought to be safe. In Figure 6-5, the TIS is less than 0.4. The TIS is the thermal index and predicts that if the examination is performed, the temperature of the examined tissue will rise no more than the thermal index in °C. In this case, the expected temperature rise is computed to be less than 0.4 °C. Similar temperature rises are found during noninvasive MRI examinations. The volume of tissue heated during an MR examination is much larger than the volume of tissue heated during an ultrasound examination. The ultrasound thermal index is computed from the spatial peak temporal average intensity. It includes the effect of the blood perfusion carrying heat away. If the patient does not have a fever, and if the temperature rise caused by the ultrasound examination is not expected to increase the temperature of local tissue up to a "fever" temperature, the examination is considered to have no thermal hazard.

It is true that if, during a fetal ultrasound examination, ultrasound is directed at the ear, the fetus will move "out of the way." Fetuses may be able to hear high audible frequencies of 20 KHz, but they cannot hear ultrasound

frequencies of 3 MHz. However, during an ultrasound B-mode examination, the pulse repetition frequency (PRF) along each line is about 30 Hz. And if the color Doppler is used, ensembles of 50-KHz PRF are added to the mix. Ultrasound can push tissue. This is called radiation pressure. Diagnostic ultrasound pulses probably push tissue a couple of microns with each ultrasound burst. Therefore, a color Doppler ultrasound system may be vibrating the oval window of the ear with an amplitude of a few microns and a frequency of 5 KHz (PRF), which would be easily heard by the fetus.

Sometimes transcranial ultrasound examinations include an examination of the ophthalmic artery through the eye. Transcranial Doppler instruments, in order to penetrate the skull, often operate at higher output levels than regular Dopplers. As the eye causes little attenuation, the ultrasound intensities at the retina may be higher than the legally allowable 17 mW/cm^2 for ophthalmic ultrasound.

Diagnostic ultrasound examinations can cause cavitation, or little "explosions" in tissue. The most likely time for this to happen is if air or a gas is present. One example is the use of ultrasound contrast agents. Ultrasound contrast agents consist of tiny bubbles (4 μm in diameter) containing a fluorocarbon (safe) housed in a surfactant of unknown composition (unknown safety). Contrast bubbles can also be made from agitated saline. These bubbles are 20 microns in diameter and will not pass through the capillaries of the lung, so they are useful for detecting cardiac shunts when the agitated saline is injected intravenously. When ultrasound is applied to these bubbles, enhanced echoes are generated at the fundamental frequency and harmonic echoes are generated. If the spatial peak temporal peak intensity is high, the bubbles cavitate, break, and damage capillaries. As the bubbles break, they enhance contrast on color-flow images but show diminished contrast on two-dimensional real-time B-mode ultrasound. So, for B-mode contrast imaging, the examiner must set the MI to the lowest possible value. The mechanical index (MI; in Figure 6-5 the MI is 0.5) indicate a moderate chance of bubble breaking during the examination.

The MI is considered to be an indicator of whether cavitation will occur. MI is the peak negative pressure of the ultrasound wave computed from the spatial peak temporal peak intensity divided by the square root of the ultrasound frequency. During ultrasound examinations with contrast agents, the contrast agents seem to vanish. If the imaging is done at low MI, the agents don't vanish, but at high MI they do vanish. During the 1 millisecond required to acquire a color Doppler ensemble, the contrast bubbles may vanish. It usually takes about 0.5 milliseconds for them to disappear. The color Doppler processor will see this change and report it as bloodflow. Color Doppler at high MI is used to detect contrast agent when it is otherwise difficult to see. By extinguishing the contrast agent with high MI and then imaging the influx of new contrast agent with low MI, perfusion measurements can be done. Cardiac gated interrupted imaging is used to visualize contrast agents because new contrast bubbles can enter the image plane during the time between images and capillary refilling can be measured.

It is possible to perform a diagnostic ultrasound examination that causes verifiable harm to a patient because of cavitation. *Do not do this examination.* There is evidence that capillary damage can occur at high MI in the presence of contrast agent. High MI occurs at low frequency and high intensity. Transcranial Doppler uses relatively high intensity to penetrate the skull and uses low frequency, so the MI should be high. Use an ultrasound contrast agent during the examination. Examine the ophthalmic artery through the eye, with the transcranial Doppler and with the power on high. Remember that the acceptable intensity for eye examinations is 17 mW/cm^2, 1/6 the intensity allowed for other tissues. If the cavitating contrast agent does damage small blood vessels, it is possible that a bleed into the vitreous humor of the eye will occur, causing the patient to see a red cloud immediately. Of course, the small bubbles of the commercial contrast agents might not cause overt bleeds into the vitreous. However, if you use agitated saline as the contrast agent, and the patient has a right-to-left cardiac shunt, these large bubbles will be in the arterial circulation. It is common to look for them through the temporal bone with a transcranial Doppler. If you look for them in the ophthalmic artery, approaching through the eye, the low attenuation of the lens and the vitreous will provide high MI in the vessels of the retina, and these larger bubbles may be stuck in the retinal arterioles. *Do not do this examination* on humans, but this might be an opportunity to show a critical hazard associated with diagnostic ultrasound.

Diagnostic levels of ultrasound have been shown to increase the permeability of membranes including the blood-brain barrier and the skin. Inventors have suggested the use of ultrasound to allow the delivery of insulin through the skin, to allow the easy entry of antibiotics and antipsychotic medications through the blood-brain barrier, and to ease the entry of genetic material into target cells during gene therapy. This raises the possibility that ultrasound may enhance the transport of pathogens across secure membrane barriers. The effect may be increased if contrast agents are present. Ultrasound may allow pathogens to cross the placenta or the blood-brain barrier in patients with acute or chronic viral diseases. This possibility has not been investigated.

Although ultrasound, without doubt, is safe, it is important to continue discussions about potential hazards to ensure that any hazards are identified and explored at the earliest possible opportunity.

SUGGESTED READINGS

Health Protection Branch, Minister of National Health and Welfare: Safety Code 23, Guidelines for the Safe Use of Ultrasound, Part I: Medical and Paramedical Applications. Environmental Health Directorate: Ottawa, Canada K1A OK9, 80-EHD-59.

Stewart HF, Stratmeyer M: An Overview of Ultrasound, Theory, Measurement, Medical Applications, and Biological Effects. Bureau of Radiological Health, U.S. Department of Health and Human Services, Public Health Service, Food and Drug Administration, Rockville, MD, July 1982.

The Heart and Electrical Hazards in Directions in Cardiovascular Medicine (vol III). Hoechst Pharmaceuticals, Inc. 1973.

Evans DH, McDicken WN: Doppler Ultrasound: Physics, Instrumentation, and Clinical Applications, 2nd ed. Chichester: John Wiley, 1989.

Fish P: Physics and Instrumentation of Diagnostic Medical Ultrasound. Chichester, NY: John Wiley & Sons, 1990.

Hedrick WR, David L, Hykes D, et al: Ultrasound Physics and Instrumentation, 3rd ed. St. Louis: Mosby, 1995.

Hedrick WR, David L, Hykes D, et al: Ultrasound Physics and Instrumentation, Practice Examinations. St. Louis: Mosby, 1995.

Kremkau FW: Diagnostic Ultrasound: Principles and Instruments, 6th ed. Philadelphia: WB Saunders, 2002.

McDicken WN: Diagnostic Ultrasonics: Principles and Use of Instruments, 2nd ed. New York: John Wiley, 1981.

Powis RL, Powis WJ: Thinkers Guide to Ultrasonic Imaging. Baltimore: Lippincott Williams & Wilkins, 1982.

Powis RL, Schwartz RA: Practical Doppler Ultrasound for the Clinician. Baltimore: Williams & Wilkins, 1991.

Wells PNT: Advances in Ultrasound Techniques and Instrumentation. New York: Churchill Livingstone, 1993.

Zagzebski JA: Essentials of Ultrasound Physics. St. Louis: Elsevier 1996.

American Institute of Ultrasound in Medicine, www.aium.org/

American Registry of Diagnostic Medical Sonographers, www.ardms.org/

American Society of Echocardiography, www.asecho.org

Australasian Society for Ultrasound in Medicine, www.asum.com.au/

The British Medical Ultrasound Society, www.bmus.org/

Cardiovascular Credentialing International, www.cci-online.org/

Society for Vascular Ultrasound, www.svunet.org/

World Federation for Ultrasound in Medicine and Biology, www.wfumb.org/

Chapter 7

B-Flow and Power Doppler in Vascular Imaging

PHILLIP J. BENDICK

Introduction

B-mode imaging was combined with pulsed Doppler frequency analysis in the mid-1970s to provide anatomic feedback on the actual site of flow measurement without regard for the actual visualization of the flow itself. Throughout the 1980s, flow was "visualized" by discrete sampling of specific sites by placing the pulsed Doppler sample volume at regions of interest. When color Doppler imaging was introduced in the late 1980s, this allowed for the first time the qualitative analysis of bloodflow characteristics over a larger region of interest. Throughout the 1990s, technology continually improved the quality of color Doppler displays such that it has become as widely used as gray scale imaging for the evaluation of patients with vascular disease. Despite this widespread use, however, color Doppler imaging does have its disadvantages and limitations. Color Doppler displays use an overlay technique that results in a significant loss of spatial resolution in the image and that often obscures anatomic features of interest by overwriting the gray scale information. Signal processing for color Doppler imaging is necessarily more complex than that for gray scale and results in loss of frame rate and an inability to view rapidly changing flow phenomena in real time. At the other extreme, very low pulse repetition frequencies are needed to detect slow flows, causing further decreases in the image frame rate. And, as the name implies, it is still a Doppler technique and subject to all the same limitations as any other pulsed Doppler system (e.g., significant aliasing and loss of flow information at Doppler angles near 90 degrees because of too small a Doppler frequency shift). To overcome these limitations, power Doppler imaging and, more recently, the direct B-mode imaging of bloodflow have been developed to provide more sensitive direct imaging of bloodflow hemodynamics.

Power Doppler Imaging

Power Doppler imaging, although still a Doppler-dependent technique, displays ultrasound signal amplitude or intensity rather than the Doppler frequency shift information.[1-3] Similar to color Doppler imaging, each scan line in the defined region of interest is divided into small pixels. When a series of ultrasound echoes for a single scan line return to the probe and ultrasound machine, they are compared to a reference signal to detect the presence or absence of any Doppler frequency shift for each pixel. If a frequency shift is detected for a pixel, rather than create a display based on the magnitude of the frequency shift (as color Doppler imaging does), the total amplitude or intensity of the returned signal within that pixel is calculated and displayed using a color map, typically with bright yellow as high intensity and darkening toward purplish-brown or black for low amplitude/intensity signals. The resulting image displayed is relatively independent of flow velocities. By repetitive sampling of multiple transmissions along a single scan line, power Doppler imaging is particularly sensitive to slow flows such as are seen in the venous system, in vessels of small lumen caliber, near the vessel walls, or in vessels downstream from near total occlusions (Fig. 7-1). For high-speed flows, because signal amplitude/intensity is displayed and not the frequency shift, there is no aliasing associated with power Doppler images. Flow with Doppler angles near 90 degrees can also be displayed more reliably with power Doppler imaging so long as a small Doppler shift can be detected (Fig. 7-2). Pixel size for power Doppler images tend to be smaller than that for color Doppler imaging as well; this allows a better definition of vessel continuity and of the vessel lumen-wall interface.

As with all things related to Doppler and ultrasound, however, there are disadvantages associated with power Doppler imaging that must be considered. It is still a Doppler technique, so a frequency shift must be detected to produce a display; at 90 degrees, when no Doppler

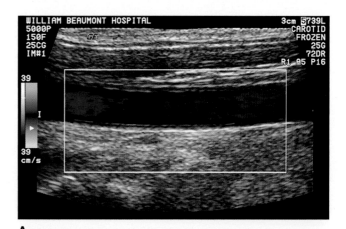

A

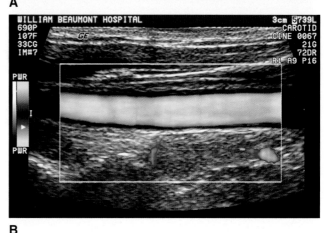

B

Figure 7-2. **A**, *Color Doppler image of a normal common carotid artery with the flow direction very nearly at 90 degrees to the direction of the Doppler ultrasound beam, resulting in a very poor display of flow information.* **B**, *Power Doppler image of the same vessel at the same Doppler angle showing the ability of power Doppler to provide flow information even under these extreme conditions.*

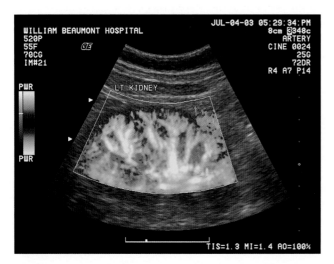

Figure 7-1. *Power Doppler image of a kidney showing flow in the major segmental arteries as well as distally out through the arcuate arteries and into the interlobular arteries to the edges of the cortex indicative of normal perfusion.*

frequency shift is present, there will be no power Doppler display, though this is less sensitive to this limitation than is color Doppler imaging. Because of the need for multiple pulse transmissions along a single scan line, the frame rate for power Doppler imaging is also very slow, especially when the system is optimized for detecting slow flows. Improved sensitivity to low speed motion can be a disadvantage if there is significant tissue motion as well as bloodflow in the region of interest; these cause severe imaging artifacts. Flow direction is not displayed in a power Doppler image, but this is rarely a significant drawback and, in fact, helps improve the display of vessel continuity in tortuous vessels.

B-Mode Imaging of Bloodflow

More recently, by adapting technology developed for radar systems, it has become possible to use B-mode gray scale to directly image bloodflow (e.g., B-flow, GE Ultrasound, Milwaukee, WI). The ability to image bloodflow simultaneously with tissue using B-mode ultrasound relies heavily on technology only recently available in duplex ultrasound instruments: Very high frequency digital signal processing, wide bandwidth, and high dynamic range combine to provide the necessary spatial, temporal, and contrast resolution. In addition to these features, the two adaptations from radar technology that have been applied to the signal processing of the ultrasound system are pulse compression, using coded excitation, and signal equalization filtering.[4-6]

Pulse compression allows the use of a short duration (wideband) transmit pulse to maintain high spatial resolution. This single transmit pulse is coded into a longer sequence of pulses to put more energy into the transmitted ultrasound signal. By using digital electronics this code can be made completely random, pseudorandom, or repetitive in nature; of most importance, the coding can be optimized in terms of length and pulse sequences for the particular application and tissue depth. The same code used for transmission is then applied in the receiver, or "decoder," to correlate with the return echoes and provide pulse compression once again into a single pulse. The effects of pulse compression are to restore the original spatial resolution of the single wideband transmit pulse while keeping as much of the transmitted energy as possible in the received signal so that the very weak echoes from the blood can be processed along with stronger tissue-based echoes.

The equalization filter is then used to extract the very much weaker echoes from the blood along with the relatively strong tissue-based echoes. For repetitive coded transmit sequences, the stream of acoustic backscatter data from each sequence is decoded with pulse compression and fed into a memory buffer. For each pair of sequences the filter subtracts a fraction of the second signal from the first. If, for example, a fraction of 1.0 is used, all of the stationary echoes in the first signal would be subtracted entirely, eliminating from that signal the information corresponding to large but stationary tissue-based echoes. Because the blood was flowing, the parts of the two signals corresponding to blood would be slightly different (i.e., slightly decorrelated) and not subtract completely, leaving a signal related to bloodflow at the filter output, which is then sent on for conventional B-mode processing and display with the original B-mode frame rates and spatial resolution. In practice, some fraction less than 1.0 would be used in the equalization filter so that B-mode tissue-based echoes are displayed simultaneously and with approximately the same intensity as the echoes related to the bloodflow (Fig. 7-3A). This allows the display of tissue characteristics essentially in real time, at frame rates of 30 to 40 per second, which are comparable to conventional B-mode imaging. Neither axial resolution nor temporal resolution are sacrificed as they are with color or power

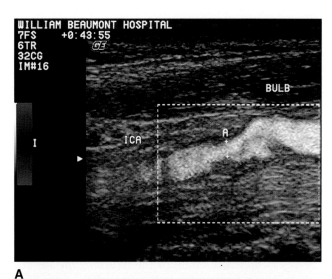

A

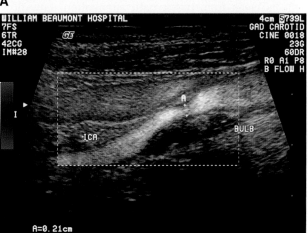

B

Figure 7-3. **A**, *B-flow image of the carotid bifurcation and proximal ICA showing qualitative bloodflow characteristics independent of bloodflow angle to the ultrasound beam, as well as providing a clear image of the surrounding tissue and the blood–vessel wall interface, including a plaque ulceration. Measured minimum vessel lumen diameter (A) was 2.5 mm.* **B**, *B-flow image of a mildly stenotic lesion at the origin of the ICA with the hypoechoic gray scale plaque characteristics preserved and evidence of the point of maximum flow velocity seen as a brightening of the B-flow image just past the point of maximum narrowing (A).*

Doppler imaging, which use multiple, longer duration (narrowband), transmitted pulses. These high frame rates with virtually real-time imaging of the flow stream potentially provide a more reliable map of the true direction of the flow throughout the cardiac cycle, which is not possible with slower frame rate flow imaging techniques. B-mode imaging of bloodflow offers the additional advantage that it is not Doppler dependent in any fashion, with no significant loss of signal intensity for flows at 90 degrees to the ultrasound beam (see Fig. 7-3A). B-flow image brightness does vary slightly with flow speed relative to the ultrasound probe (which is somewhat angle dependent) because successively transmitted signals decorrelate more rapidly at higher flow speeds. This feature translates into the maximum velocity flow jet appearing brighter in the gray scale image than the surrounding flows, allowing direct visualization in real time of the site of peak flow velocity (Fig. 7-3B).

Clinical Applications of Flow Imaging: Power Doppler

Power Doppler imaging has proved most useful clinically in those situations where flow speeds are very low, the vessel lumen is small, or the returning ultrasound echo is weak from tissue path attenuation. Low flow speeds such as those seen in the venous system or in small peripheral vessels are readily displayed by power Doppler imaging (see Figure 7-1), providing a qualitative image of overall perfusion.[7] In larger vessels, power Doppler imaging has proved helpful in situations of low flow such as that seen in Figure 7-4, which shows a proximal internal carotid artery dissection ending in a complete vessel occlusion approximately 2 cm past the vessel origin. Transcranial duplex ultrasound has also benefited from power Doppler imaging because the echoes returning through the acoustic windows of the skull are very weak and often of insufficient strength for color Doppler image processing. Because a Doppler shift can be detected in these signals, power Doppler imaging has proved to be much more reliable in displaying the intracranial vessels of the circle of Willis and allowing placement of the spectral Doppler sample volume.[8-10] Power Doppler imaging has also been used to evaluate the cerebral sinuses and the internal cerebral veins.[11]

Because of its improved ability to image the lumen–vessel wall interface, power Doppler has also been utilized for three-dimensional (3-D) vascular ultrasound.[12-16] For adequate reconstruction of ultrasound data into a 3-D image, good edge and border detection are necessary to discriminate the patent lumen of the vessel from surrounding tissue. (Fig. 7-5). Studies have shown that qualitative features of organ perfusion and vascular obstructive disease can be readily identified from such 3-D images (Fig. 7-6A). Artifacts commonly encountered in angiography (e.g., vessel overlap) are easily eliminated with 3-D vascular ultrasound because the resulting images can be manipulated to view the vessels from virtually any angle. It has also been possible to accurately measure anatomic data (e.g., the length and severity of stenoses) from the 3-D images of the carotid artery bifurcation; atherosclerotic plaque features such as surface ulceration are more easily identified from a 3-D image than from its 2-D counterparts[17] (Fig. 7-6B).

Clinical Applications of Flow Imaging: B-Flow

The direct B-mode imaging of flow is a new technology and has not been evaluated as extensively in clinical situations as have color Doppler and power Doppler imaging. It has been evaluated at both ends of the velocity spectrum, however, with useful applications in clinical situations of low flow (e.g., in the portal vein or in cases of venous insufficiency) and in high flow (e.g., in the evaluation of arterial stenoses).[18-21] Because gray scale information is preserved along with visualization of the flow stream, the venous valve leaflets of patients with venous insufficiency can be observed in real time to

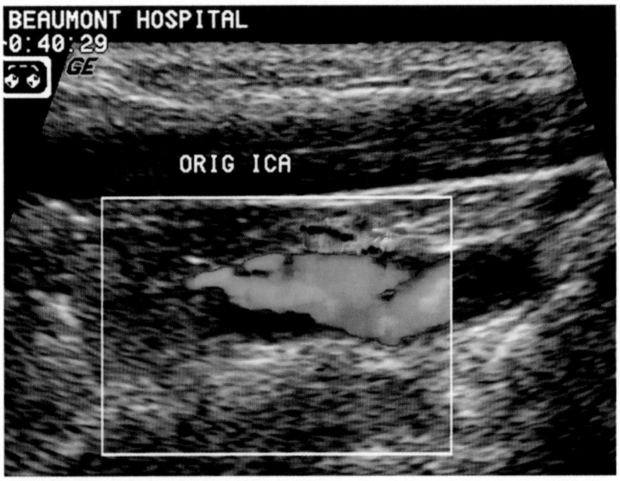

Figure 7-4. *Power Doppler image of the proximal internal carotid artery showing the long gradual taper of the lumen to a complete occlusion approximately 2 cm beyond the origin, characteristic of a dissection.*

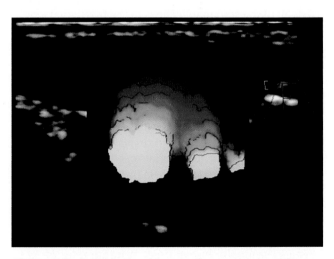

Figure 7-5. *3-Dimensional image of a normal carotid artery bifurcation region using power Doppler imaging to show the patent lumen. Even the superior thyroid branch off the proximal ECA can be seen.*

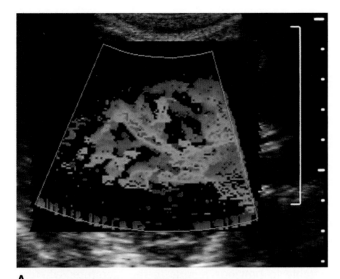

A

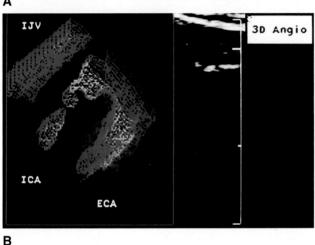

B

Figure 7-6. **A**, *3-Dimensional image of the upper pole of a normal kidney using power Doppler imaging, taking advantage of its ability to detect slow flows in small vessels so that renal perfusion out to the interlobular arteries can be seen.* **B**, *3-Dimensional image of an ulcerated plaque at the origin of the ICA. Spatial resolution and low flow sensitivity of power Doppler imaging make it possible to clearly see the ulceration just past the origin of the ICA.*

evaluate their behavior during periods of reflux flow. In patients with chronic venous disease secondary to previous deep vein thrombosis, B-flow offers a better means to image chronic thrombus, with simultaneous imaging of the degree of recanalization (antegrade flows) and post-thrombotic insufficiency (reflux flows).

A number of applications have been evaluated in the diagnosis of carotid artery atherosclerotic disease. Appropriate indications for carotid endarterectomy have been clarified since publication of the results of randomized trials such as the North American Symptomatic Carotid Endarterectomy Trial (NASCET) and the Asymptomatic Carotid Atherosclerosis Study (ACAS).[22–24] These and similar studies also confirmed the morbidity of diagnostic

carotid artery angiography, with stroke rates as high as 1.2% attributable just to the angiographic procedure. This has led to an increased reliance on preoperative duplex ultrasound as the sole determinant of the degree of stenosis of atherosclerotic lesions. The author and colleagues have evaluated the preoperative duplex ultrasound capabilities of B-flow in assisting in two areas: (1) placement of the Doppler sample volume more precisely within the maximum flow jet and (2) angle correction parallel to the actual bloodflow. The goal was to determine whether these modifications in technique provide a more accurate categorization of stenosis[25] (Fig. 7-7). Spectral Doppler velocity measurements were taken with angle correction made parallel to the vessel walls and using either conventional gray scale imaging or color Doppler imaging to place the Doppler sample volume at the site of the suspected maximum flow jet near the point of minimal lumen diameter. An additional spectral Doppler velocity measurement was obtained using B-flow to position the Doppler sample volume within the maximum flow jet and to correct the Doppler angle parallel to the imaged bloodflow rather than parallel to the vessel walls.

No significant differences were seen in the Doppler angle between the two techniques. The mean difference in angle was 0.4 ± 3.0 degrees (p > 0.20). Eighteen of the 20 vessels evaluated had a Doppler angle very near 60 degrees for both techniques (within ± 3 degrees). One vessel had both measurements taken at a Doppler angle of 51 degrees. One vessel had conventional Doppler done at an angle of 49 degrees, with a B-flow-assisted Doppler angle of 60 degrees. For this last vessel, conventionally measured velocities were PSV = 131 cm/sec and EDV = 44 cm/sec versus B-flow-assisted

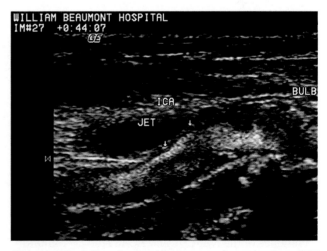

Figure 7-7. *B-flow image of a severe (greater than 80% diameter) stenosis at the origin of the ICA clearly showing the flow jet adjacent to and parallel to the upper wall of the vessel. A short segment of increased brightness highlights the point of maximum flow velocity, aiding accurate placement of the spectral Doppler sample volume.*

velocities of PSV = 167 cm/sec and EDV = 59 cm/sec. Both of these sets of velocity measurements place the degree of narrowing between 30% and 50% diameter reduction. These data showed that the great majority of vessels (90%) could be evaluated at very nearly 60 degrees with no significant effect of correcting along the direction of flow as seen in the B-flow image. "Parallel to the vessel walls" appears to be a reliable, and certainly reproducible, technique for Doppler angle correction.

Significant differences were seen in measured velocities, both for peak systole and end diastole. The relative change in peak systolic velocities (ratio of B-flow-assisted velocity to conventionally measured velocity) was 1.23 +/- 0.21 (p < 0.005) and in end-diastolic velocities was 1.29 +/- 0.18 (p < 0.005). In 19 of 20 vessels, B-flow-assisted velocities were higher than the conventionally measured velocities, with a mean increase in absolute velocities of 40 +/- 36 cm/sec for peak systole and 13 +/- 11 cm/sec for end-diastole. In eight vessels the higher B-flow-assisted velocities increased the category of stenosis. In four vessels the category merely increased from <30% to 30% to 50% diameter narrowing. In three vessels the category increased from 30% to 50% to 50% to 70%, and in one vessel the category increased from 50% to 70% to greater than 70% diameter stenosis. No changes in category of stenosis were seen in the other 12 vessels despite higher B-flow-assisted measured velocities in 11 of these.

An additional area of investigation has been an attempt to improve on the overall accuracy of preoperative duplex ultrasound by making direct measurements of minimum residual lumen diameter, using the B-flow image to determine the site of maximum stenosis. Previous efforts to do so from B-mode images of atherosclerotic lesions have largely been unsuccessful because of the effects of the complex heterogenicity of the lesions on the image and the small residual lumens to be measured, which for a >60% diameter stenosis are characteristically less than 2 to 2.5 mm. Garra and colleagues compared the results of duplex ultrasound–derived percent stenosis using anatomic measurements of the minimum lumen diameter from B-flow images (using the ACAS/NASCET method of comparing the lumen to the normal distal ICA diameter) to angiography. They found agreement of percent stenosis within +/- 10% in 40 of 40 vessels; agreement within +/- 5% was seen in 18 of 40 vessels.

In the author's own laboratory, validated spectral Doppler velocity criteria were used to grade stenoses as greater or lesser than 60% diameter reduction using the techniques of the NASCET and ACAS study.[26] Minimum residual lumen diameter measurements were made at the point of maximal narrowing using the B-mode image, a color Doppler image, a power Doppler image, and the B-flow display to guide placement of the measurement cursors. To calculate percent diameter reduction a final measurement was made of the distal ICA lumen diameter. Twenty-seven patients had preoperative duplex ultrasound spectral Doppler velocity findings indicative of greater than 60% diameter stenosis, and visual inspection of the operative specimen confirmed the presence of a significant atherosclerotic lesion. In 25 cases (93% sensitivity), direct measurements from the B-flow image correlated with these findings in predicting a greater than 60% diameter stenosis. In the remaining two cases the measurements from the B-flow image indicated minimum residual lumen diameters of 2.5 and 2.7 mm, which corresponded to 50% to 60% diameter reductions. (In six patients in whom preoperative angiography was done, the B-flow data correlated in all cases.) The sensitivity of B-mode imaging alone to greater than 60% diameter stenosis in this patient group was 53%, comparable to previous reports in the literature; whereas the sensitivity of color Doppler imaging was only 44%, and that of power Doppler imaging was 55%.

A second area of investigation has been in lower extremity arterial examinations for vein graft surveillance. B-flow has proved helpful in identifying segments of graft stenosis. Segments of increased flow velocity and flow jets are readily identified using B-flow. With the simultaneous high-resolution imaging of the surrounding tissue, the cause for the narrowing is typically also identified at the same time, whether it is intimal hyperplasia, a fibrotic retained valve, or recurrent atherosclerotic disease (Fig. 7-8). Preliminary results on a small number of patients have thus far shown promise for B-flow as a rapid means of evaluating bypass graft hemodynamics qualitatively throughout the entire course of the graft and of reliably identifying segments needing more quantitative (i.e., spectral Doppler velocity measurements) examination.

Conclusions

Power Doppler imaging and the direct B-mode imaging of bloodflow are proving to be clinically valuable adjuncts to the standard duplex ultrasound examination for vascular disease. They provide a sensitive means of directly imaging the flow field in a variety of settings, from very slow flows in the venous system to high velocity jets in arterial stenotic disease. Qualitative hemodynamics can be readily assessed from these images, leading to more accurate quantification of any flow disturbances present. Power Doppler imaging and B-flow will not replace the quantitative spectral Doppler velocity measurements for severity of stenoses, but they do provide additional information reinforcing the velocity findings and give an improved anatomic view of the characteristics of the lesion involved, further diminishing any reliance on more invasive testing such as angiography.

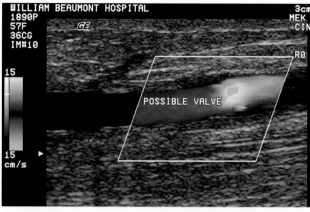

A

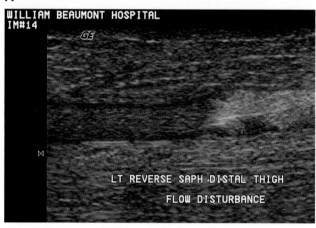

B

Figure 7-8. **A,** *Conventional color Doppler image of a lower extremity in situ vein bypass graft at a site of flow disturbances. Color Doppler overlay prevents any imaging of the possible anatomic cause of the flow disturbances.* **B,** *B-flow image of the same site of the in situ vein graft taking advantage of the preservation of gray scale spatial and contrast resolution to clearly show the echogenic fibrotic retained valve and the resulting flow disturbances.*

REFERENCES

1. Bude RO, Rubin JM: Power Doppler sonography. Radiology 200:21–23, 1996.
2. Rubin JM, Bude RO, Carson PL, et al: Power Doppler US: A potentially useful alternative to mean frequency-based color Doppler US. Radiology 190:853–856, 1994.
3. Chen JF, Fowlkes JB, Carson PL, et al: Autocorrelation of integrated power Doppler signals and its application. Ultrasound Med Biol 22:1053–1057, 1996.
4. O'Donnell M: Coded excitation systems for improving the penetration of real-time phased array imaging systems. IEEE Trans UFFC 39:341–351, 1992.
5. Welch LR, Fox MD: Practical spread spectrum pulse compression for ultrasonic tissue imaging. IEEE Trans UFFC 45:349–355, 1998.
6. Bendick PJ, Newhouse VL: An ultrasonic random signal flow measurement system. J Acoust Soc Am 56:860–865, 1974.
7. Bude RO, Rubin JM, Adler RS: Power versus conventional color Doppler sonography: Comparison in the depiction of normal intrarenal vasculature. Radiology 192:777–780, 1994.
8. Kenton AR, Martin PJ, Evans DH: Power Doppler: An advance over colour Doppler for transcranial imaging? Ultrasound Med Biol 22:313–317, 1996.
9. Baumgartner RW, Schmid C, Baumgartner I: Comparative study of power-based versus mean frequency-based transcranial color-coded duplex sonography in normal adults. Stroke 27:101–104, 1996.
10. Postert T, Meves S, Bornke C, et al: Power Doppler compared to color-coded duplex sonography in assessment of the basal cerebral circulation. J Neuroimaging 7:221–226, 1997.
11. Baumgartner RW, Nirkko AC, Muri RM, et al: Transoccipital power-based color-coded duplex sonography of cerebral sinuses and veins. Stroke 28:1319–1323, 1997.
12. Lyden PD, Nelson TR: Visualization of the cerebral circulation using 3-dimensional transcranial power Doppler ultrasound imaging. J Neuroimaging 7:35–39, 1997.
13. Bendick PJ, Brown OW, Hernandez D, et al: Three-dimensional vascular imaging using Doppler ultrasound. Am J Surg 176:183–187, 1998.
14. Bendick PJ, Glover JL: Three-Dimensional Vascular Imaging Using Doppler Ultrasound. In Yao JST, Pearce WH (eds): Modern Vascular Surgery. New York: McGraw-Hill, 2000.
15. Bendick PJ: Three-Dimensional Vascular Imaging and Three-Dimensional Color Power Angiography Imaging. In AbuRahma AF, Bergan JJ (eds): Noninvasive Vascular Diagnosis. London: Springer-Verlag, 2000.
16. Carson PL, Moskalik AP, Govil A, et al: The 3D and 2D color flow display of breast masses. Ultrasound Med Biol 23:837–849, 1997.
17. Eliasziw M, Streifler JY, Fox AJ, et al: Significance of plaque ulceration in symptomatic patients with high-grade carotid stenosis. North American Symptomatic Carotid Endarterectomy Trial. Stroke 25:304–308, 1994.
18. Weskott HP: B-flow—A new method for detecting blood flow. Ultraschall Med 21:59–65, 2000.
19. Furuse J, Maru Y, Mera K, et al: Visualization of blood flow in hepatic vessels and hepatocellular carcinoma using B-flow sonography. J Clin Ultrasound 29:1–6, 2001.
20. Pellerito JS: Current approach to peripheral arterial sonography. Radiol Clin North Am 39:553–567, 2001.
21. Umemura A, Yamada K: B-mode flow imaging of the carotid artery. Stroke 32:2055–2057, 2001.
22. North American Symptomatic Carotid Endarterectomy Trial Collaborators: Beneficial effect of carotid endarterectomy in symptomatic patients with high-grade carotid stenosis. N Engl J Med 325:445–453, 1991.
23. Executive Committee for the Asymptomatic Carotid Atherosclerotic Study: Endarterectomy for asymptomatic carotid artery stenosis. JAMA 273:1421–1428, 1995.
24. North American Symptomatic Carotid Endarterectomy Trial Collaborators: Benefit of carotid endarterectomy in patients with symptomatic moderate or severe stenosis. N Engl J Med 339:1415–1425, 1998.
25. Doverspike GA, Bechtel G, Burr M, et al: Accuracy of Doppler sample volume placement and angle correction for stenotic lesions of the carotid artery. Proceedings of the 24th Annual Conference, Society of Vascular Technology, Pittsburgh, PA, 2001.
26. Doverspike GA, Bendick PJ: Direct B-mode imaging of blood flow to complement spectral Doppler velocities for the evaluation of carotid atherosclerotic disease. Proceedings of the 23rd Annual Conference, Society of Vascular Technology, Orlando, FL, 2000.

Part Two

Imaging the Body

CEREBROVASCULAR DISEASE

Chapter 8

Vascular Diagnosis in Carotid Disease

JULIE ANN FREISCHLAG • JENNIFER HELLER

- Angiography
- Duplex Sonography
- Transcranial Doppler (TCD)
- Computed Tomographic Angiography (CTA)
- Magnetic Resonance Angiography (MRA)
- Conclusions

As technology advances, physicians have witnessed a meteoric influx of innovative methods to diagnose both normal and abnormal processes. The choice for the best study is dependent on many factors including cost, patient risk, accuracy, reproducibility, and accessibility. This chapter reviews the evolution of diagnostic imaging modalities for the extracranial circulation and outlines an algorithm to assist in formulating a treatment plan.

Angiography

Since the advent of the first carotid angiogram in 1927 by Moniz, the angiogram has been considered the "gold standard" study for the diagnosis for carotid disease. Indeed, investigators in the North American Symp-tomatic Carotid Endarterectomy Trial (NASCET), the Asymptomatic Carotid Atherosclerotic Study (ACAS), and the European Carotid Surgery Trial (ECST) all utilized the angiogram to determine diagnostic criteria to establish standard of care.[1-3]

The angiogram provides extensive information about the circulation from the aortic arch through the intracranial circulation. Concomitant pathologic processes such as tandem lesions, siphon stenoses, intracranial masses, and arteriovenous malformations are easily delineated. In addition, anatomic information such as the level of the carotid bifurcation, carotid kinks, and carotid coils can be obtained and may influence the preoperative and intraoperative management (Fig. 8-1).

The angiogram is an invasive procedure, however, and as such it carries with it a myriad of complications. Allergic reactions from the contrast media range from a minor response to an anaphylactic and possibly fatal event. Arterial injuries include hematoma, embolization, thrombosis, dissection, and rupture. Contrast nephropathy, both reversible and permanent requiring dialysis, has been documented. The most dreaded complication of the procedure is the stroke risk.

The ACAS reported a 1.2% stroke rate.[2] Even higher iatrogenic embolic stroke rates have been observed in patients with bilateral, high-grade, internal carotid artery stenoses; and in those patients with symptomatic carotid disease (i.e., patients with crescendo transient ischemic attacks [TIAs] or stroke-in-evolution).[4,5]

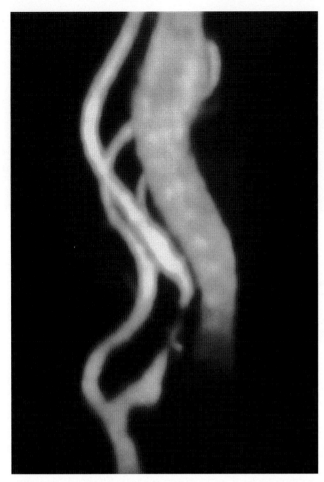

Figure 8-1. CT Angiogram of the carotid bifurcation revealing a severe ICA stenosis.

Based on the advantages and limitations of this procedure, it is prudent to construct a diagnostic plan or a set of patient criteria based on a risk benefit analysis of the angiogram. In order to devise such a plan, another study must be deemed as accurate as the angiogram, or certainly be associated with less risk. These criteria best fit the duplex ultrasound.

Duplex Sonography

Noninvasive imaging became available in the 1960s with the inception of the device by Miyazaki and Kato, who were the first to describe the use of Doppler equipment for extracranial cerebrovascular disease. However, it took decades to produce a streamlined and perfected noninvasive imaging technique: duplex sonography. Duplex ultrasound is actually composed of two sets of functions: B-mode imaging and Doppler gray scale. Color duplex is the most recent addition to the sonographic armamentarium. Color duplex sonography improves visualization of the flow divider at the carotid bifurca-

tion. It also aids in visualization of reversal of vertebral flow and internal carotid artery occlusion[6] (Fig. 8-2).

The duplex ultrasound has significant advantages. The examination is extremely cost effective; the machine is easily accessible. Although operator dependent, there are accreditation courses available to both credential and recertify registered vascular technicians and their laboratories. Because duplex sonography is noninvasive, there are none of the risks associated with the angiogram.

When compared with angiography for internal carotid artery stenoses greater than 70%, duplex ultrasonography has been estimated to have sensitivities ranging from 80% to 100% and specificities of 68% to 99%.[7-14] Limitations of the duplex are related to operator technique. Underestimation of disease can be seen in the presence of tortuous arteries and in large plaques where angle determination can be difficult. In the presence of contralateral occlusion, stenosis can be overestimated.

Although certain investigators have suggested that such complex anatomic abnormalities cannot be adequately visualized with the duplex, experienced registered vascular technicians may provide information otherwise unattainable.

Certain characteristics that may be difficult to assess by duplex include a long internal carotid artery plaque, a small internal carotid artery diameter, redundancy of the internal carotid artery, kinks, coils, or a high carotid bifurcation. Wain and colleagues prospectively examined patients to evaluate such difficult carotid anatomic characteristics.[15] They obtained excellent sensitivity rates between 80% to 100%, and specificities ranged from 56% to 100%.

However, these rates are clearly influenced by the quality of the vascular laboratory. Intersocietal Commission for the Accreditation of Vascular Laboratories (ICAVL) accreditation is the first important step. More-

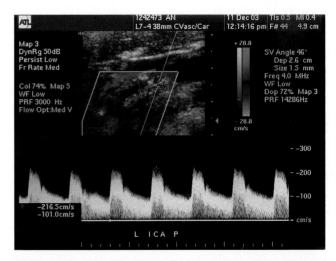

Figure 8-2. Color duplex of the internal carotid artery and carotid bifurcation with velocities consistent with high-grade stenosis.

over, it is imperative that the laboratory be adequately supervised with regular quality control and with continuing medical education for the registered vascular technicians. It is essential to maintain high standards and to ensure that objective criteria exist with which to base a management plan. It is only in this setting that the duplex ultrasound may be used with impunity. It is also only in this setting that the carotid duplex may be utilized as the sole imaging study with which to base medical or surgical management.

Transcranial Doppler (TCD)

In 1982, the first clinical report on the transcranial Doppler was published by Aaslid, Markwalder, and Nornes.[16] The TCD is a noninvasive imaging technique that permits visualization of the intracranial circulation through pulsed wave insonation of bone windows: the transtemporal, the transorbital, and the suboccipital. The TCD delineates a myriad of intracranial pathology such as intracranial mass lesions and arteriovenous malformations. In addition, the TCD can measure intracranial collateral pathways of the intracranial circulation. This information may be helpful not only to document collateral flow but also to measure stenosis of the extracranial carotid artery. Some centers utilize the TCD as an intraoperative monitor during carotid endarterectomy using it to detect a shunt requirement and to detect embolic phenomenon.[17]

However, the TCD has some limitations. Insonation of the middle cerebral artery is inadequate or even impossible in some patients because of insufficient ultrasound transmission through the skull. Furthermore, the accuracy and reliability of TCD have been questioned, with error introduced both by operator technique as well as by measurement errors caused by the dynamic flow changes in these insonated vessels. The TCD is used as an adjunctive diagnostic modality; however, its utility as a dominant tool to measure carotid disease has yet to be established.

Computed Tomographic Angiography (CTA)

Conventional tomographic angiography was developed by Kalendar in 1989 as a new modality with which to visualize the arterial anatomy. Spiral CT power cables were replaced with sliprings, which allowed the x-ray tube to be rotated continuously. The rapid and continuous rotation of the scanner enabled a patient to be advanced through the machine without stopping, significantly decreasing the examination time. To obtain arterial images, a single bolus of contrast is injected intra-venously. This is followed by a precisely timed image display and computer-assisted generation of postprocessing arterial images. The technical advantages provided by spiral technology have significantly improved the ability of CT to image the vascular system. The technique is noninvasive, and therefore there is no risk of arterial or neurologic complications associated with its use.[18] Sensitivities of CTA in evaluation of internal carotid artery stenoses of 70% or greater range from 67% to 100%. Specificities in the same category of stenosis range from 84% to 100%.[19-23]

Although CTA does provide good results in parts of the arterial circulation, there remain significant drawbacks to its use in the diagnosis of carotid disease. CTA has been used less commonly for evaluating carotid artery stenosis. Although CTA can evaluate the carotid artery wall and characterize the morphology of the carotid plaque, calcification remains a problem. Unfortunately, calcification of the carotid artery bifurcation is common, and mural calcification often completely obscures the arterial lumen. Furthermore, although CTA is a noninvasive technique, the examination still requires a large amount of contrast, and in some cases, even more than conventional angiography.[24]

At this time there are no sufficient data with large numbers to advocate this study; therefore CTA is neither recommended as the single imaging modality nor as a confirmatory study to diagnose extracranial carotid disease.

Magnetic Resonance Angiography (MRA)

Magnetic resonance imaging uses the energy of an electromagnetic field to create different atomic signals in soft tissues. Two techniques are utilized to image the arterial system: (1) time of flight (TOF); and (2) phase contrast pulse sequences. Although TOF images may be generated in either two or three dimensions, three-dimensional TOF images are preferred in the intracranial circulation because this technique is less sensitive to artifacts caused by turbulent flow (Fig. 8-3).

Gadolinium, the MRA contrast agent of choice, enhances arterial imaging because of the increased contrast between blood and the surrounding soft tissues.

Gadolinium is not nephrotoxic and is administered as a single intravenous bolus injection. A new advancement in MRA technology is contrast enhanced magnetic resonance imaging (CEMRA), which has resulted in a significant reduction of flow void artifacts, elimination of inplane flow defects, and improved spatial resolution.[25] Borisch and colleagues utilized the CEMRA and reported a sensitivity of 95% and a specificity of 79% for evaluation of carotid stenoses of 70% or greater.[26]

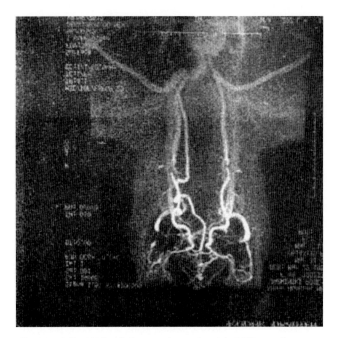

Figure 8-3. MRA of the aortic arch with RICA moderate to severe stenosis.

In 2000, Back and colleagues[27] prospectively determined that the MRA is an acceptable substitute for the conventional angiogram. The investigators utilized the MRA as a modality with which to supplement inconclusive duplex sonograms. They reported a sensitivity rate of 100% and a specificity of 77% for carotid stenoses 75% or greater. Similar sensitivities in the range of 92% to 100% and specificities in the range of 75% to 100% for internal carotid artery stenoses of greater than 70% have been reported.[28-32]

There are many advantages to the MRA. The MRA provides images of both the brain parenchyma as well as the intra- and extracranial circulation. The examination is noninvasive and does not require ionizing radiation. As previously described, sensitivities and specificities in many studies demonstrate the MRA to be an excellent noninvasive alternative to the conventional angiogram.

The MRA is, however, very sensitive to motion, and severe image degradation occurs with even slight movement. In addition, patients with pacemakers, metallic clips, or orthopedic devices should not be studied with this modality. Small numbers of patients may be unable to proceed with this study because of severe claustrophobia. Anatomic limitations of the study are mainly caused by overestimation of stenoses as a result of hemodynamic turbulance and the current limitations of MRA technology. It is expected that as the technique continues to evolve, this drawback may be resolved. Despite its limitations, MRA is an excellent noninvasive modality that may be used as an adjunct to the duplex as a confirmatory or supplementary imaging study.

Conclusions

The advancement of technology brings not only the refinement of older methods but also the introduction of new modalities. This precept holds true for the evolution of imaging the carotid circulation. Vascular surgeons now have a wide armamentarium of studies from which to choose. However, it is essential to tailor imaging studies to meet the needs of the patient while appreciating the particular strengths and weaknesses of local hospital resources.

The advantages of each of these imaging studies may vary from one institution to another. Duplex sonography, without ICAVL accreditation and quality assurance, cannot be considered a sole imaging study for carotid disease. Similarly, a lack of radiologic resources may retard technologic growth, thereby preventing state-of-the-art imaging and interpretation. One cannot blindly utilize an MRA as a confirmatory study in this setting. Therefore, to construct a diagnostic algorithm, it is prudent to review the individual risk factors of the patient, as well as to understand the strengths and limitations of the facility and the quality of the imaging products.

The risk-to-benefit ratio of a procedure is crucial for maintaining safe outcomes in the vascular surgical population. Market-driven forces and rising health care costs all contribute to the need for cost containment. The Internet age has brought knowledge to every computer screen, enabling patients to become enamored with new technology that may not be suitable for their disease.

The following is a list of factors that would describe the ideal imaging study to diagnose carotid disease: low cost, low patient risk, high accuracy, highly reproducible, and easily accessible. Obviously, based on the authors' review, there is no device that can provide all of these characteristics.

Therefore, the risks and benefits associated with each procedure must be evaluated and applied to a diagnostic approach that will afford the patient and the physician with a reliable plan.

In an ICAVL-accredited laboratory that practices regular quality control, the duplex sonogram should be utilized as the primary imaging modality for screening, diagnosis, and postoperative surveillance. Indeed, once accuracy and quality assurance have been documented, the duplex should be the sole imaging study before endarterectomy. If MRA technology is available, this noninvasive study is ideal as a confirmatory noninvasive examination.

Certainly, the MRA may over-read a lesion, or in circumstances in which the diagnosis remains inconclusive, the angiogram may be required as a third examination. If MRA technology is not available, the angiogram may be required as a second stage of diagnostic imaging. In these cases, it would be ideal to aggressively pursue methods to make the vascular laboratory a more powerful resource, thereby decreasing use of the invasive angiogram. Although the CTA may continue to evolve, current data do not support its use as a superior method to the MRA.

The establishment of a gold standard is difficult to achieve because expertise and resources vary between centers. It is therefore the responsibility of the practitioner to evaluate the outcomes of resources available and to delineate a plan that will meet the standards of any diagnostic test (i.e., low risk, high accuracy, reproducible results, and optimal patient care).

REFERENCES

1. North American Symptomatic Carotid Endarterectomy Trial Collaborators: Beneficial effect of carotid endarterectomy in symptomatic patients with high grade stenosis. New Engl J Med 325:445–453, 1991.
2. Endarterectomy for asymptomatic carotid artery stenosis: Executive Committee for the Asymptomatic Carotid Atherosclerosis Study. JAMA 273:1421–1428, 1995.
3. European Carotid Surgery Trialists' Collaborative Group: MRC European Carotid Surgery Trial: Interim results for symptomatic patients with severe (70–99%) or with mild (0–29%) carotid stenosis. Lancet 337:1235–1243, 1991.
4. Dion JE, Gates DC, Fox AJ, et al: Clinical events following neuroangiography: A prospective study. Stroke 18(6):997–1004, 1987.
5. Theodotu BC, Whaley R, Mahaley MS: Complications following transfemoral cerebral angiography for cerebral ischemia: Report of 159 angiograms and correlation with surgical risk. Surg Neurol 28(2):90–92, 1987.
6. Sumner DS: Use of color-flow imaging technique in carotid artery disease. Surgical Clinics of North America 70(1):201–211, 1990.
7. Mittl RL, Broderick M, Carpenter JP, et al: Blind-reader comparison of magnetic resonance angiography and duplex ultrasonography for carotid artery bifurcation stenosis. Stroke 25:4–10, 1994.
8. Anderson CM, Saloner D, Lee RE, et al: Assessment of carotid artery stenosis by MR angiography: comparison with xray angiography and color-coded Doppler ultrasound. Am J Neuroradiol 13:989–1003, 1992.
9. Riles TS, Eidelman EM, Litt AW, et al: Comparison of magnetic resonance angiography, conventional angiography, and duplex scanning. Stroke 23:341–346, 1992.
10. Turnipseed WD, Kennell TW, Turski PA, et al: Magnetic resonance angiography and duplex imaging: Noninvasive tests for selecting symptomatic carotid endarterectomy candidates. Surgery 114:643–648, 1993.
11. Turnipseed WD, Kennell TW, Turski PA, et al: Combined use of duplex imaging and magnetic resonance angiography for evaluation of patients with symptomatic ipsilateral high-grade carotid stenosis. J Vasc Surg 17:832–839, 1993.
12. Young GR, Humphrey PR, Shaw MD, et al: Comparison of magnetic resonance angiography, duplex ultrasound and digital subtraction angiography in the assessment of extracranial internal carotid artery stenosis. J Neurol Neurosurg 57:1466–1478, 1994.
13. White JE, Russell WL, Greer MS, Whittle MT: Efficacy of screening MR angiography and doppler ultrasonography in the evaluation of carotid artery stenosis. Am Surg 60:340–348, 1994.
14. Spartera C, Morettini G, Marino G, et al: Detection of internal carotid artery stenosis. Comparison of 2D-MR angiography, duplex scanning, and arteriography. J Cardiovasc Surg 34:209–13, 1993.
15. Wain RA, Lyon RT, Veith FJ, et al: Accuracy of duplex ultrasound in evaluating carotid artery anatomy before endarterectomy. J Vasc Surg 27:235–244, 1998.
16. Aaslid R, Markwalder TM, Nornes H: Noninvasive Doppler ultrasound recording of flow velocity in the basal cerebral arteries. J Neurosurg 57:769, 1982.
17. Visser GH, Wieneke GH, van Huffen, et al: The use of preoperative transcranial Doppler variables to predict which patients do not need a shunt during carotid endarterectomy. Eur J Vasc Endovasc Surg 19:226–232, 2000.
18. Heller JA, Kent KC: Sequential Helical Computed CTA. In Cameron JL (ed): Current Surgical Therapy, 7th ed. Philadelphia: Mosby, 2001, pp 790–795.
19. Magarelli N, Scarabino T, Simeone AL, et al: Carotid stenosis: A comparison between MR and spiral CT angiography. Neuroradiology 40:367–373, 1998.
20. Verhoek G, Costello P, Ee Wk, et al: Carotid bifurcation CT angiography: Assessment of interactive volume rendering. J Comput Assisted Tomogr 23:590–596, 1999.
21. Marcus CD, Ladam-Marcus VJ, Bigot JL, et al: Carotid arterial stenosis: Evaluation at CT angiography with the volume-rendering technique. Radiology 211:775–780, 1999.
22. Leclerc X, Godefroy O, Lucas C, et al: Internal carotid arterial stenosis: CT angiography with volume rendering. Radiology 210:673–682, 1999.
23. Anderson GB, Ashforth R, Steinke DE, et al: CT angiography for the detection and characterization of carotid artery bifurcation disease. Stroke 31:2168–2174, 2000.
24. Heller JA, Kent KC: Sequential helical computed CTA. In Cameron JL (ed): Current Surgical Therapy, 7th ed. Philadelphia: Mosby, 790–795, 2001.
25. Cosottini M, Pingitore A, Puglioli M, et al: Contrast-enhanced three-dimensional magnetic resonance angiography of atherosclerotic internal carotid artery stenosis as the noninvasive imaging modality in revascularization decision making. Stroke 34(3):660–668, 2003.
26. Borisch I, Horn M, Butz B, et al: Preoperative Evaluation of Carotid Artery Stenosis: Comparison of contrast-enhanced MR angiography and duplex sonography with digital subtraction angiography. Am J Neuroradiol 24:1117–1122, 2003.
27. Back MR, Wilson JS, Rushing G, et al. Magnetic resonance angiography is an accurate imaging adjunct to duplex ultrasound scan in patient selection for carotid endarterectomy. J Vasc Surg 32:429–440, 2000.
28. Serfaty JM, Chirossel P, Chevallier JM, et al: Accuracy of three-dimensional gadolinium-enhanced MR angiography in the assessment of extracranial carotid artery disease. Am J Roentgenol 175:455–463, 2000.
29. Johnson MB, Wilkinson ID, Wattam J, et al: Comparison of Doppler ultrasound magnetic resonance angiographic techniques and catheter angiography in evaluation of carotid stenosis. Clin Radiol 55:912–920, 2000.
30. Scarabino T, Carriero A, Giannatemp GM, et al: Contrast-enhanced MR angiography (CE MRA) in the study of the carotid stenosis: Comparison with digital subtraction angiography (DSA). Neuroradiol 26:87–91, 1999.
31. Leclerc X, Martinat P, Godefroy O, et al: Contrast-enhanced three-dimensional fast imaging with steady-state prescession (FISP) MR angiography of supraaortic vessels; preliminary results. Am J Neuroradiol 19:1405–1413, 1998.
32. Sardanelli F, Zandrino F, Parodi RC, et al: MR angiography of internal carotid arteries: Breath-hold Gd-enhanced 3D fast imaging with steady-state precession versus unenhanced 2D and 3D time-of-flight techniques. J Comput Assisted Tomogr 23:208–215, 1999.

Chapter 9

Cerebral Vascular Color-Flow Scanning Technique and Applications

NICOS LABROPOULOS • VICTOR ERZURUM
• MAUREEN K. SHEEHAN • WILLIAM H. BAKER

Diagnostic duplex ultrasonography (DUS) of the cerebral vasculature has evolved significantly over the past decade. The noninvasive nature of DUS makes this testing modality more attractive than the "gold standard" of angiography. If the diagnosis of significant carotid stenosis can be accurately made with DUS, the risk of stroke inherent in carotid angiography (1.2% in the Asymptomatic Carotid Atherosclerosis Study[1]) could be avoided. Currently, many patients (90% at the authors' institution) undergo carotid endarterectomy based solely on a duplex

examination. Whichever method is used to diagnose carotid stenosis, the clinician must remember that the test results determine the patient's need for carotid endarterectomy. In this chapter, carotid endarterectomy is used exclusively as the therapy for cervical carotid stenosis. Carotid angioplasty and stenting (CAS) is currently being evaluated as an equivalent therapy. When (or if) CAS is proven to have equipoise, the clinician should include both therapies in the therapeutic algorithm.

Indications for Testing

Symptomatic Patients

Randomized, multicenter, prospective trials have documented the efficacy of carotid endarterectomy (CE) in reducing stroke in symptomatic carotid stenosis. The North American Symptomatic Carotid Endarterectomy Trial (NASCET) showed a clear benefit of CE for patients with 70% to 99% carotid stenosis who present with transient ischemic attack (TIA) and/or nondisabling stroke.[2] Carotid atherosclerosis may either reduce flow by obstructing the lumen of the internal carotid artery

(ICA) or by embolizing to the intracranial arteries. The carotid arteries lead to the anterior cerebral, middle cerebral, and ophthalmic arteries. Thus, the patient will present with contralateral monoparesis (arm or leg), hemiparesis (arm and leg), aphasia (dominant hemisphere), or ipsilateral transient monocular blindness (amaurosis fugax). In this group there was a 65% relative risk reduction in ipsilateral stroke at 2 years. Similarly, those symptomatic patients in NASCET with a 50% to 69% carotid stenosis showed a 29% relative risk reduction in ipsilateral stroke at 5 years.[3] Based on these results, CE is indicated for patients with symptomatic 70% to 99% carotid stenosis and in selected symptomatic patients with 50% to 69% carotid stenosis at centers with low morbidity associated with CE. For this reason, all patients with carotid or hemispheric TIA or nondisabling stroke who potentially may benefit from carotid endarterectomy should undergo carotid imaging. This test should be performed even in the absence of carotid bruit because analysis of NASCET data revealed over one third of patients with high-grade carotid stenosis lacked a carotid bruit.[4]

Patients may also present with symptoms such as dizziness or light-headedness, but these symptoms are nonspecific and, in the absence of other evidence, cannot be assumed to be caused by carotid stenosis. Other symptoms such as cranial nerve dysfunction (e.g., dysphasia, double vision, or blurred vision) and drop attacks are more likely to be vertebral basilar in location. However, testing in these patients, as well as in asymptomatic patients with computed tomographic (CT) or magnetic resonance (MR) infarcts, is indicated to rule out cervical cerebral vascular disease.

Asymptomatic Patients

The Asymptomatic Carotid Atherosclerosis Study (ACAS) documented a 53% relative risk reduction in any ipsilateral stroke and any perioperative stroke/death at 5 years when comparing CE with medical management for asymptomatic carotid stenosis greater than 60%.[1] The absolute risk reduction was from 11% to 5%. This has led to increased performance of CE in patients with asymptomatic carotid stenosis; however, controversy continues regarding who best to screen for asymptomatic carotid stenosis. Routine screening of all patients is unlikely to be cost-effective, and most physicians have adopted a selective approach. The most commonly used selection criteria will be reviewed.

Carotid bruit can be expected in up to 8.2% of patients over 75 years of age.[5] These bruits have been associated with up to a three-times increased risk of stroke in a population-based prospective cohort study.[6] In a prospective natural history study of duplex scanning for asymptomatic carotid bruit, Roederer and colleagues from the University of Washington showed 36% of imaged carotids had a greater than 50% stenosis.[7] Importantly, in a follow-up report, this group reported on progression of disease in patients initially diagnosed with carotid stenosis by screening for carotid bruit.[8] Some 21% of patients with greater than 50% stenosis progressed to 50% to 79% stenosis, and 27% of patients with 50% to 79% stenosis progressed to greater than 80% stenosis at 7 years. These data support the concept of carotid duplex screening for carotid bruit, and regular follow-up of those patients with carotid disease not severe enough to warrant surgery. The measurement of percent stenosis using imaging alone is fraught with hazard. Image angle, vessel tortuoisity, differing flow velocities, and patterns of flow all contribute to this inaccuracy. The Stanford laboratory requires at least a 50% stenosis by image to establish a diagnosis but relies on flow velocities to categorize the narrowing.[9] Others have reasonable accuracies using the image alone, but at this time flow measurements, not image alone, should be used as the definitive diagnostic criteria.

Patients harboring a near-total occlusion will have a reduced flow (i.e., the peak systolic velocity [PSV] may be reduced rather than elevated). The distal ICA may be diminutive (string sign) with likewise reduced flow. Total occlusion obviously has no flow at or past the point of occlusion, with the exception of very few reported cases that had ICA branches. In the past, arteriography was recommended for an ultrasound diagnosis of total occlusion because of inaccuracies of black and white imaging. With the advent of color-flow imaging, the accuracy of a total occlusion diagnosis is excellent. Mansour and colleagues from Southern Illinois University (SIU) confirmed 64 of 65 ultrasound-diagnosed occlusions by angiography.[10] Twenty-six of thirty string signs were correctly diagnosed. Moneta and colleagues reported no false-positive or false-negative duplex examinations for ICA occlusions.[11] Thus, the diagnosis of total occlusion using color-flow duplex is now accurate. Confirmatory angiography is rarely required.

Patients with severe congestive heart failure who have reduced cardiac indices will have reduced PSV in their carotid arteries.[12] This reduced flow may mask a significant stenosis. If imaging identifies a severe stenosis, but flow criteria do not cross the diagnostic threshold, angiography may be required. Patients with a contralateral occlusion may have increased flows in their remaining patent ICA. Intuitively, if a flow to the brain is to be maintained and flow is zero in one carotid artery, flow in the opposite carotid artery must be increased. A multi-institutional study in 1988 identified a 45% stenosis using a PSF of 5500 Hz with an overall accuracy of 92.2%.[13] If the patient had a contralateral ICA occlusion, a threshold of 8500 Hz was required to achieve this same accuracy. Whereas others suggest a contralateral severe stenosis leads to diagnostic inaccuracy, Hayes and colleagues could verify this only in patients with a contralateral occlusion.[13] Recent studies have shown that contralateral stenosis affects the diagnostic accuracy. This was evident in patients with bilateral carotid stenosis that underwent CE in one side and were retested by DUS. It was shown that the velocities in the unoperated side were usually decreased after CE.[14,15]

Significant carotid stenosis can exist in the absence of cervical bruit. For this reason, recommendations for carotid duplex scanning have been made based on specific risk factors such as age, hypertension, smoking, coronary artery disease (CAD), and peripheral vascular disease (PVD).[16] In one study conducted in a veteran population aged more than 50 years,[17] significant carotid stenosis was present in 17.5% of patients with CAD, tobacco abuse, and PVD and 0% of patients with none of these risk factors. The authors suggested aggressive surveillance in patients with multiple risk factors. Claudication and decreased ankle-brachial index have both been found to be predictive of carotid artery disease.[18] In particular, in patients without a cervical bruit, the presence of age greater than 68 years, hypertension, PVD, and prior cardiac surgery have been correlated with an incidence of significant carotid stenosis as high as 45%.[19] By focusing carotid duplex screening for asymptomatic carotid stenosis on patients with cervical bruits or multiple risk factors, screening protocols, which are most cost-effective, can be established for the early identification of high-risk lesions and prevention of stroke.

Carotid duplex scanning has also been recommended as a screening tool for patients undergoing noncarotid surgery and for patients at risk for atherosclerosis. Patients with asymptomatic carotid stenosis undergoing coronary artery bypass graft (CABG) have been shown to have an increased risk of perioperative stroke.[20,21] In a prospective evaluation of 1087 patients undergoing CABG at Washington University Medical Center, 17% of patients had carotid lesions greater than 50% and 5% had lesions greater than 80. Some 83% of patients had minimal or no stenosis. Major predictors of a greater than 50% stenosis were PVD, female sex, previous TIA or stroke, hypertension, and left main coronary disease. Patients with none of these major predictors would be expected to have a 5% chance of a 50% carotid stenosis. In a similar study, Ascher and colleagues[22] examined the results of carotid duplex scanning in 3708 patients who underwent cardiovascular surgery. They found age greater than 60 years to be a major predictor of concomitant significant carotid disease. Patients younger than 60 years had a 1% chance of significant carotid disease, whereas patients older than 60 years had a 6.7% chance. The presence of the risk factors of hypertension, diabetes mellitus, and smoking increased the risk of significant stenosis to 3% for patients younger than 60 years and 14.4% for patients older than 60 years. Based on this data, duplex scanning pre-CABG can be recommended, either selectively based on risk factors or routinely in all elderly patients.

Finally, carotid duplex scanning has been used as a surveillance tool for carotid restenosis. Widely varying protocols exist for the follow-up of patients after CE. Routine duplex surveillance has been criticized as unnecessary and expensive.[23,24] Conclusive data about the benefit (or lack thereof) of carotid surveillance post-CE is absent. It is likely carotid duplex scanning for surveillance post-CE will continue to be a common indication until more definitive data are available, given the quoted restenosis rates (which can be as high as 19.7%).[24] In contrast, there are data to support carotid duplex surveillance of the contralateral carotid artery after ipsilateral CE because progression of the disease requiring surgery has been noted in substantial numbers.[25,26] Ricotta and colleagues reported progression from less than 50% stenosis to greater than 50% stenosis in 10.1% of patients followed.[25] The optimal frequency of this surveillance is open to speculation, but biennial examinations have been suggested.[26]

Methodology (Testing Procedure)

After a short history to record relevant symptoms and risk factors, the examination starts by measuring blood pressure in both arms. A blood pressure differential of 20 mmHg or more is considered abnormal and indicates a brachiocephalic or a subclavian/axillary artery stenosis. Blood pressure variability is common in nervous, tense patients, and any blood pressure differential should be verified by a repeat examination at the end of the testing procedure.

The patient is made comfortable in the supine position. The head is turned away from the examiner but not to an extreme degree. Coupling gel is applied liberally over the course of the carotid artery, which in general parallels the easily seen anterior border of the sternocleidomastoid artery.

The thyroid gland and internal jugular vein are seen, and the common carotid artery is identified. Varying the depth, focus, and gain settings maximizes the image. The common carotid artery is visualized just above the clavicle and followed to the carotid bifurcation. The widened carotid bulb indicates the origin of the ICA. Both the internal and external carotid arteries should be identified. Usually the carotid bifurcation is located comfortably below the mandible. Abnormal anatomic variation of this bifurcation should be noted. This is especially important if the carotid duplex examination is the sole diagnostic test before proceeding with surgical endarterectomy.

A sagital scan is also obtained. Again, the examination is begun low in the neck and continued up to the angle of the mandible. The scan head may be placed anterior, medial, or posterior to the sternocleidomastoid muscle to maximize the image and flow tracings. There should be wall-to-wall color flow. Any luminal or wall abnormalities are noted. Velocity measurements are taken with an angle of insonation of 60 degrees. Usually these are taken in the proximal and distal common carotid artery (CCA), one in the external carotid artery (ECA); two or three in the ICA (i.e., proximal, middle, and distal); and one in the vertebral. The ICA is followed as far cephalad as possible. In patients with a significant carotid plaque, the distal extent of the plaque should be noted. For example, if the plaque ends at the distal bulb, and a centimeter or so of normal ICA can be identified, this should be noted. If the carotid plaque continues posteriorly cephalad into the ICA, this likewise should be noted. These two different variations in pathology are extremely important to the operating surgeon.

The vertebral arteries will be noted posterior to the common carotid artery between the vertebral bodies. In some laboratories an effort will be made to identify the vertebral arteries low in the neck as they arise from the subclavian artery. The tortuous course of these arteries makes diagnosis of a stenosis quite difficult. Regardless, flows should be noted to be antegrade (the same direction as normal carotid flow) or retrograde. Absent flow indicates an occluded artery.

Diagnostic Criteria

The normal common carotid artery has flow characteristics of both the internal and external carotid arteries (Fig. 9-1). The PSV in both the left and right common carotid arteries should be equal. An increased PSV indicates a stenosis; a decreased PSV indicates a proximal severe stenosis. The precise numeric criteria of a diagnosis of proximal cervical carotid disease have not

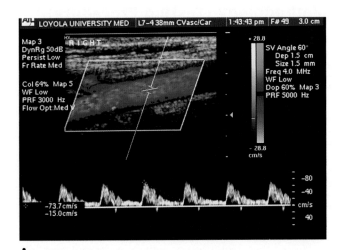

A

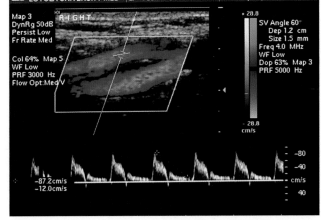

B

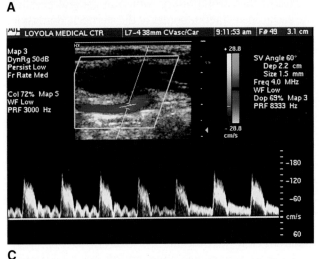

C

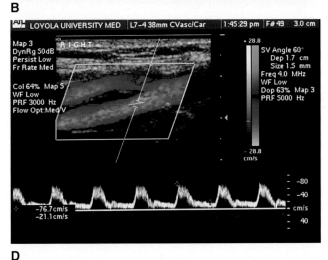

D

Figure 9-1. *Normal waveforms from the carotid arteries.* **A,** *The CCA has a waveform that represents a high (ECA) and a low (ICA) resistance arterial tree.* **B,** *The ECA has a high resistance as shown by the reverse flow component and the low end-diastolic velocity. It is smaller than the ICA and it has branches. Identification of the branches is the best way to separate the two arteries.* **C,** *Temporal tapping should be used as an adjunct to this method or when unable to identify the branches coming off the ECA. This is particularly useful in cases like this one, where the ECA is internalized because of ICA occlusion.* **D,** *The ICA has a low-resistance flow pattern as seen by the absence of the reversed flow and the high end-diastolic velocity. Unlike the ECA it has no branches in the cervical region, with the exception of very few case reports.*

been established. There should be an absence of disturbed flow as indicated by a clear window under the systolic peak. The ICA should have a similar flow pattern with forward flow seen in both systole and diastole (see Fig. 9-1). The external carotid artery in general has a slightly increased peak systolic velocity (see Fig. 9-1). Forward flow is not seen in diastole because the external carotid artery supplies a relatively high resistant vascular bed, much like any artery supplying muscle.

The presence or absence of atherosclerosis within the carotid system should be noted. The measurement of intimal medial thickness is covered elsewhere and will not be reviewed here (see Chapter 14). However, not only the presence or absence of plaque should be evaluated, but also its morphologic characteristics such as irregularity, echogenicity, and calcification (Fig. 9-2).

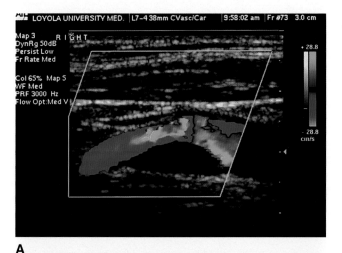

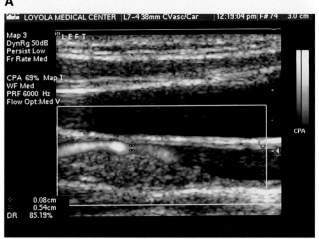

*Figure 9-2. Examples of an echolucent and an echogenic plaque. **A**, This is an echolucent plaque in the ICA from a patient who presented with ipsilateral amaurosis fugax. **B**, Echogenic plaque in the ICA of an asymptomatic patient with ipsilateral neck bruit. For more information on the plaque morphology, see Chapter 12.*

Different laboratories will either record the entire examination on tape or produce hard copy for review. Both are satisfactory and should allow the interpreting physician ample material to make a proper diagnosis. In the authors' laboratory, it is established that a peak systolic velocity of greater than 250 cm/sec is indicative of a greater than 60% diameter stenosis (Fig. 9-3). These statistics were established by comparing duplex ultrasonography to angiography as qualification for the ACAS. Other criteria follow.

Other Interpretations and Quality Assurance

To ensure that patients who may benefit from operation are accurately differentiated from those who may not, the accuracy of DUS in diagnosing significant carotid stenosis must first be determined. Most diagnostic laboratories simply use the well-established criteria of others to diagnose severe carotid stenosis. Roederer and colleagues from the University of Washington established diagnostic criteria based on a comparison of arteriograms and ultrasound studies.[27,28] Criteria were established to categorize the carotid lesion as less than 50%, 50% to 79%, and 80% to 99% stenotic. The amount of residual lumen was compared to the wall of the carotid bulb as seen on ultrasound. After the original publication of NASCET,[2] which emphasized the importance of a greater than 70% diameter stenosis compared to a 50% to 69% stenosis, the original Strandness criteria were modified to identify patients at greatest risk of future stroke. In addition, ACAS identified asymptomatic patients with a greater than 60% stenosis to be at risk.[1] Furthermore, both ACAS and NASCET compared the residual lumen to the narrower distal ICA rather than the wider carotid bulb used by the University of Washington group. Clearly, new guidelines were in order.

DUS is operator- and machine-dependent. Laboratories acknowledge to be excellent have, after similar ultrasound and angiographic comparisons, established a variety of differing criteria. To diagnose a greater than 70% stenosis, most laboratories use the PSV; however, the threshold velocity varies from 210 to 340 cm/sec. The University of Oregon found that in ICA PSV/CCA PSV greater than 4.0 was more accurate than a PSV of 325 cm/sec.[29] Southern Illinois University (SIU) found that a combination of PSV of 130 cm/sec and end-diastolic velocity (EDV) of 100 cm/sec was better than either PSV (210 cm/sec) or EDV (100 cm/sec) alone.[30,31] Stanford combined PSV, EDV, PSVICA/CCA, and the image to establish their diagnostic scheme.[9] Criteria to diagnose a greater than 50% and greater than 60% stenosis are likewise varied.[32,33] The results are more accurate when a single cutoff point for stenosis is used, or when a broad category is used rather than a small range of stenosis (e.g., 60% to 69%).[33] At Loyola, during the authors' entrance into ACAS, it was established that a PSV of greater than 250 cm/sec was the best threshold to diagnose a greater than 60% diameter stenosis. Because of a paucity of arteriograms, the authors' accuracy statistics have not been updated since the early 1990s. Recently, two review papers analyzed the diagnostic accuracy of DUS in detecting ICA stenosis when compared with angiography.[34,35] The first study showed that 18/22 papers who matched their criteria had a sensitivity ranging from 80% to 100%, and 20/22 had a specificity of the same range.[34] The second study compared 70% to 99% stenosis to greater than 70%, and occlusion to patent ICA.[35] The pool-weighted sensitivity and 95% CI were 86% (84% to –89%) and 96% (94% to –98%). The pool-weighted specificity and 95% CI were 87% (84% to –90%) and 100% (99% to –100%).

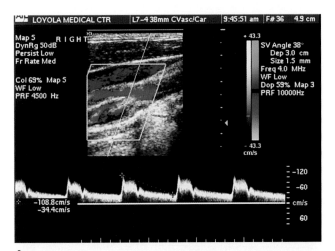

A

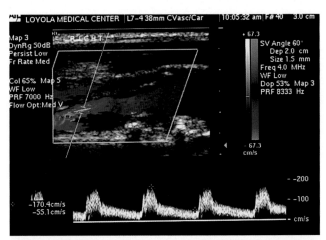

B

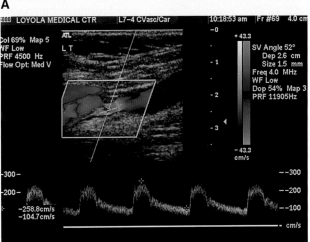

C

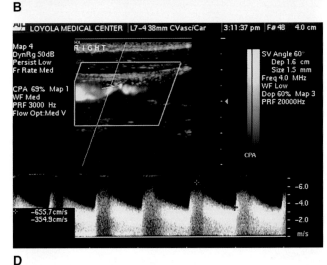

D

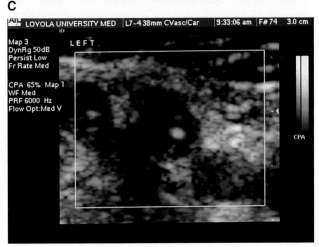

E

Figure 9-3. *Various degrees of stenosis in the ICA.* **A,** *Echogenic plaque in the proximal ICA producing greater than 50% stenosis.* **B,** *ICA producing 50% to 79% stenosis. The ICA/CCA PSV was 2.3, indicating a stenosis at the lower end of this range.* **C,** *Significant stenosis at the origin of the ICA. Both the PSV and EDV are elevated, indicating a greater than 60% stenosis according to the authors' criteria because the PSV is greater than 250 cm/sec.* **D,** *Tight stenosis in the ICA in an asymptomatic patient with ipsilateral neck bruit. This is greater than 80% stenosis because the EDV is greater than 130 cm/sec.* **E,** *Subtotal occlusion of the ICA with a string sign and very low flow velocities in a patient with recent ipsilateral TIAs.*

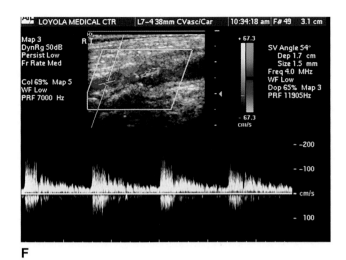

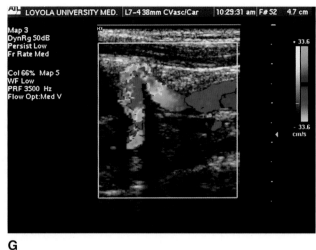

F

G

Figure 9-3, cont'd. **F,** *Poststenotic turbulence, which is seen after significant stenosis.* **G,** *Stenosis may occur in the absence of a plaque from a kink. The aliasing indicates the significant stenosis at the site of the kink. The PSV was 230 cm/sec and the EDV was 60 cm/sec at an angle of insonation at 0 degrees.*

Planimetric Evaluation

Measuring diameter and percent area stenosis has advantages over velocity measurements. Different velocity criteria have been utilized to determine the degree of carotid stenosis. In a recent study it was shown that velocity criteria were not equivalent in different centers.[36] In addition, area and diameter, in contrast to velocity measurements, are not sensitive to contralateral stenosis or occlusion, ipsilateral proximal or distal stenosis or occlusion, or cardiac output or cardiac arrhythmia. Recent studies have tested the accuracy and practicality of area and diameter measurements with promising results (Fig. 9-4).[37-41] Tri-axial and area measurements are hindered when heavy calcification or significant tortuosity cause inadequate imaging of the affective stenosis. Previous studies have reported poor imaging caused by heavy calcification in as much as 10% of carotids.[37,42] This is not a problem for the velocity measurements because the highest velocities are seen at the exit of the stenosis. These methods complete each other and should be used together.

Other Vessels and Special Cases

There has not been much work done in validating detection of stenosis or occlusion by DUS in ECA and CCA. Both these arteries are graded as normal, less than 50%, greater than 50% diameter stenosis, and occlusion. Regarding the ECA there is one study with magnetic resonance angiography comparison in 60 carotid bifurcations; it shows that a PSV greater than 250 cm/sec was the best cut-off for determining greater than 60%

stenosis (Fig. 9-5). A PSV less than 150 cm/sec was associated with less than 50% stenosis.[43] Another study on 707 normal and stenotic ECAs showed that a PSV ratio of ECA to ICA greater than 2.0 indicates a greater than 50% stenosis.[44] It was also shown that ipsilateral ICA stenosis greatly affects the ECA velocities. Increased velocities and internalization of the ECA may be seen in carotid body tumors; in paragangliomas and other masses fed by the ECA; in local inflammation (e.g., thyroid and parotid glands); and when the ICA has a tight stenosis or occlusion.

CCA occlusion has been demonstrated by ultrasound in several reports, particularly when the ICA is open through retrograde flow in ECA (Fig. 9-6).[45] Evaluation of CCA stenosis is limited. In the authors' institution the best cutoff value is a poststenotic to prestenotic PSV ratio of greater than 2.0 (unpublished data). Asymmetrical velocities in the CCA indicate proximal stenosis (CCA or brachiocephalic artery) or ICA stenosis or occlusion. Usually the EDV is less than 12 cm/sec and there is an EDV difference of greater than 10 cm/sec compared with the normal side.[46] Low velocities in both the CCA and ICA may be seen after recanalization of previously occluded ICA (Fig. 9-7).[47,48] Occasionally, when there is internalization of the ECA, this may not be true. In general, low EDV indicates a high resistance distal to the measurement and a significant stenosis or occlusion can be suspected. In cases of trauma or in patients that have no atherosclerotic disease but low EDV[46,49] that is asymmetrical to the other side, dissection or thrombosis of the distal ICA should be ruled out. In the absence of trauma, dissection in the CCA is an extension of the aortic dissection. Such dissection may involve the ICA. There are two lumens, a real and a false one, with opposite flow direction (Fig. 9-8). The false lumen sometimes is thrombosed.

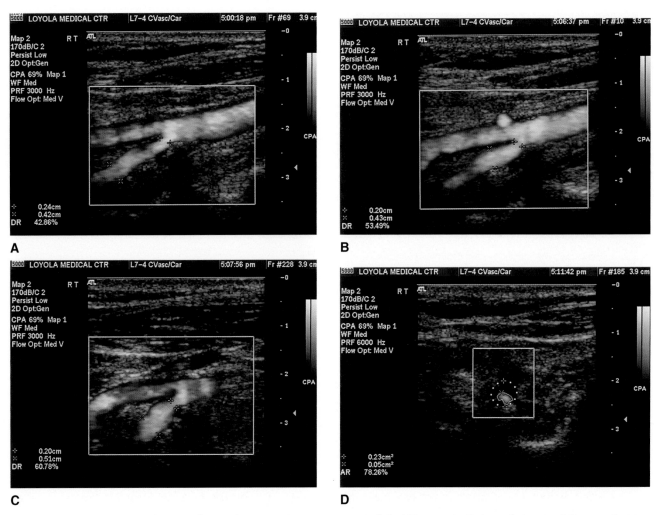

Figure 9-4. *Planimetric evaluation of carotid stenosis. **A**, Anterior view of the ICA stenosis; **B**, lateral view; and **C**, posterior view of the same lesion. The stenosis was measured by the NASCET method, and the average of the three views was calculated (43 + 53 + 61 = 52%). The velocities in this patient corresponded with the planimetric measurements (PSV = 170 cm/sec and EDV = 53 cm/sec). **D**, The area stenosis of the same lesion was evaluated as well.*

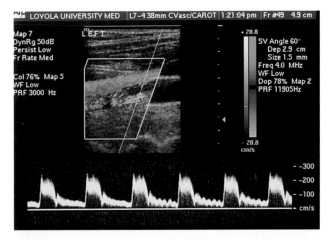

Figure 9-5. *Significant ECA stenosis in a symptomatic patient from the contralateral side. Both the PSV and EDV are elevated, indicating a greater than 50% stenosis. The exact grade cannot be calculated because there is no validation for the different degrees of stenosis.*

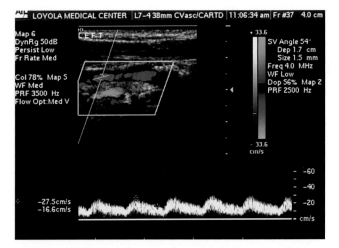

Figure 9-6. *CCA occlusion with the ICA being filled through the ECA. The ECA has reversed flow. Note the opposite colors between the ECA (blue) and the ICA (red).*

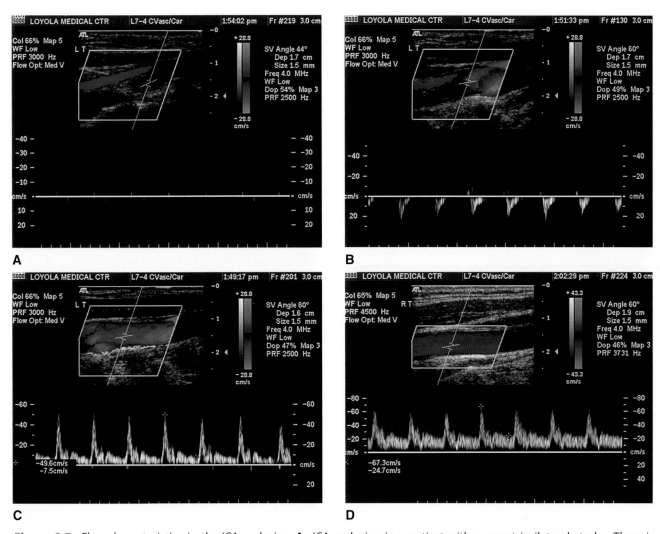

Figure 9-7. *Flow characteristics in the ICA occlusion.* **A,** *ICA occlusion in a patient with a recent ipsilateral stroke. There is absence of flow in the ICA and there is flow reversal as seen by the blue color at the beginning of the occlusion.* **B,** *Low velocities in the CCA with an EDV of less than 12 cm/sec.* **C,** *The velocities in the ECA are unaffected in this case. In some patients the ECA is internalized.* **D,** *The contralateral CCA has normal velocities. The EDV difference between the two sides is greater than 10 cm/sec.*

Carotid aneurysms are rare and are found in the common, external, and internal carotid. The most common location is the carotid bifurcation; this is followed by the ICA and ECA.[50] There is strong association with atherosclerosis, which is present in up to 70% of the cases.[51] There are no strict criteria for the definition of a carotid aneurysm, but the doubling of the diameter is used for its diagnosis. Most of the detected aneurysms are much larger than this cutoff. Pseudoaneurysms are the result of penetrating trauma and occasionally may be seen at an anastomosis or after endarterectomy with a patch. The ultrasound features of large symptomatic human immunodeficiency virus (HIV) related carotid aneurysms are false aneurysms with a wall defect or "blow-out," and to-and-fro pulsatile flow.[52] There is marked wall thickening adjacent to the aneurysm with a hyperechoic "spotting."

Takayasu's arteritis is most often present at the origin and the proximal part of the CCA.[53] It is not associated with atherosclerosis and the patients are usually asymptomatic. When seen by ultrasound is characterized by concentric wall thickening (Fig. 9-9). The velocities are increased, but because of the concentric nature of the lesion there is minimal or no spectral broadening.

Carotid body tumors are slow-growing tumors with unpredictable malignant potential. They are unilateral in 95% of the reported cases. They are fed by the ECA and have very rich vascularization (Fig. 9-10).[54] They most often occur in the fifth decade of life and have been associated with a high altitude.[54] There are three types: type I has minimal attachment to the vessels and has small size; type II it is bit larger and partially encircles the vessels; type III is the largest in size and incorporates both arteries and the vagus nerve.

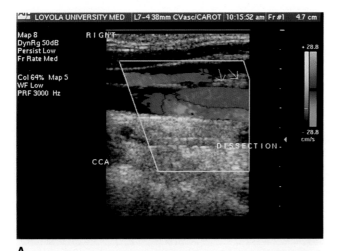

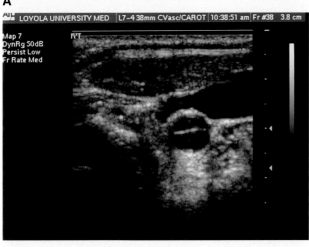

Figure 9-8. **A**, *CCA dissection in a patient with a known aortic dissection. There are two lumens. The false one has a retrograde flow* (blue). **B**, *Cross-sectional view of the CCA showing the two lumens in a patient with dissection.*

Fibromuscular dysplasia is a degenerative primary disease and has no association with atherosclerosis. It is found in many arteries in the body, but its prevalence in consecutive carotid angiograms is around 0.5%.[55] In the carotid arteries it is most often found in the ICA. When it occurs in the proximal ICA it can be diagnosed by ultrasound (Fig. 9-11). It is characterized by a series of stenoses and dilatations with moderate to significant increase in the velocity.

Validation

The ACAS evaluated the performance of 63 devices before the initiation of the study.[36] Only 37 devices were used to enter patients. The majority of devices not used were rejected because their performance was unacceptable. Thirteen of the 63 devices had an excel-

lent sensitivity (80%+) and a PPV of 90%; 32 had a marginal sensitivity (50% to 80%); 9 had poor sensitivity (0% to 50%); and in 9, no threshold could be established. The threshold PSV varied from 150 to 450 cm/sec. If there is this much variation between devices from institutions voluntarily applying to enter a National Institutes of Health (NIH) sponsored study, the variation and inaccuracy of community hospital devices may be even greater. The ACAS was initiated in the late 1980s. Hopefully, 15 years later, our accuracy is somewhat better. Regardless, the need to validate each diagnostic laboratory is obvious.

The standard technique of validating DUS is through comparison to angiography. Each patient must undergo both testing modalities and comparisons made. The DUS criteria routinely examined include PSV, ICA/CCA velocity ratios, and end-diastolic velocities (EDV). The goal for a definitive examination would be a high positive predictive value (PPV) to minimize the number of patients who would undergo an unnecessary operation. In general, a PPV is achieved by missing the diagnosis in some patients with a stenosis (decreased sensitivity). That is, certain patients do not meet the strict criteria required to achieve a high PPV despite the presence of an angiographic stenosis. The laboratory at the authors' institution has a high PPV, and thus diagnostic angiography may be avoided before recommending endarterectomy. In elderly, asymptomatic patients, the few patients underdiagnosed should be at a low risk for stroke.[56] A younger, otherwise healthy patient with a carotid bruit, multiple TIAs, and an atherosclerotic carotid artery on scan, who does not meet the flow criteria of a significant stenosis, should have additional diagnostic studies (e.g., contrast angiography, magnetic resonance angiography, or CT angiography). The patient's physician needs to ensure that a potential stroke-prone lesion is not left untreated.

Other diagnostic laboratories may use DUS as a screening test only. That is, these labs wish to have a high negative predictive value (NPV) so that few patients with a stenosis are underdiagnosed. It is obvious that a high NPV is achieved by decreasing the specificity. Many patients will be overdiagnosed so that few are missed. Thus all patients in this setting will need an additional study before proceeding along the therapeutic algorithm toward endarterectomy.

Ideally, validation of a vascular lab could be performed without subjecting all patients to the inherent risks of angiography. Eckstein and colleagues validated DUS not only with angiography but also using endarterectomy specimens.[57] Some 68 eversion endarterectomy specimens were embedded in a prosthesis, followed by a fixation, and then sectioned. Their combined Doppler standard criteria predicted 70% to 99% ICA stenosis with a sensitivity of 95% and a PPV of 96%; they concluded that 90% of all angiograms were unnecessary. Using tissue specimens as the gold standard has some practical limi-

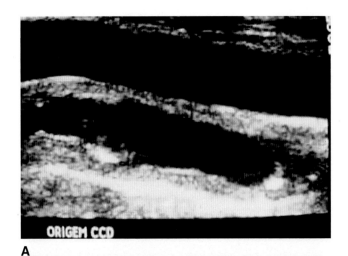

A

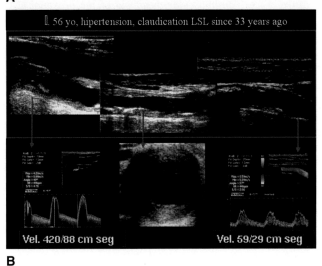

B

Figure 9-9. Common carotid artery stenosis in a 56-year-old female with Takayasu's arteritis **(A)**. The CCA has a significant amount of circumferential plaque **(B)**. The PSV was 420 cm/sec and the PSV ratio across the stenosis was 7.1. (Courtesy of Dr. Carmen Porto, HUPE-UERJ, Rio de Janeiro, Brazil.)

tations because pathology technicians require an intact, noncrushed sample of carotid bifurcation plaque. Specimens obtained by the standard technique are usually unsatisfactory. Specimens obtained by the eversion endarterectomy technique lend themselves to such a study. Ideally, the lumen should be pressurized at the patient's mean blood pressure at the time of fixation. The percent stenosis determined by pathology usually compares the residual lumen to the "normal" lumen at the site of the stenosis, whereas both NASCET and ACAS compare the angiographic residual lumen to the more distal, smaller ICA. A comparison using the specimen will establish a PPV but not a NPV (patients with minimal stenoses do not get operations). At Loyola the authors relied on the surgeon's "eyeball" estimation, which is obviously poorly controlled. The surgeon can clearly differentiate a severe from a not severe stenosis, but assigning percentages is patently inaccurate. Regardless, in the absence of angiography (gold standard), specimen estimation is the best available correlation for accuracy statistics. In fact, at Loyola the few errors discovered have led to minor modifications of technique and interpretation.

An alternative quality control plan would be to have patients tested at two different laboratories, one previously validated and one undergoing validation. Patients with matching diagnostic criteria would be assumed to have the correct diagnosis. Patients with differing stenoses in different laboratories or devices would need an angiogram to arbiter the dispute. This quality control measure would need to be financed by the laboratories (hospitals) because third-party carriers are unlikely to support dual payment of laboratory testing.

A group of experts from different medical specialties met in October 2002 to arrive at a consensus document with regard to the use of DUS in the diagnosis of ICA.[58] Table 9-1 illustrates their recommendations when using

TABLE 9-1. **Current Recommendations for Gray Scale and Doppler Ultrasound for Diagnosis of ICA Stenosis**

	Primary Parameters		Additional Parameters	
Degree of Stenosis	ICA PSV(cm/sec)	Plaque estimate (%)*	ICA/CCA PSV ratio	ICA EDV (cm/sec)
Normal	<125	None	<2.0	<40
<50	<125	<50	<2.0	<40
50-69	125–230	50	2.0–4.0	40–100
70 but less than near occlusion	>230	50	>4.0	>100
Near occlusion	High, low, or undetectable	Visible	Variable	Variable
Total occlusion	Undetectable	Visible, no detectable lumen	Not applicable	Not applicable

* Plaque estimate (diameter reduction) with gray scale and color Doppler ultrasound.
From Grant EG, Benson CB, Moneta GL, et al: Carotid artery stenosis: Gray-scale and Doppler US diagnosis. Society of Radiologists in Ultrasound Consensus Conference. Radiology 229:340–346, 2003.

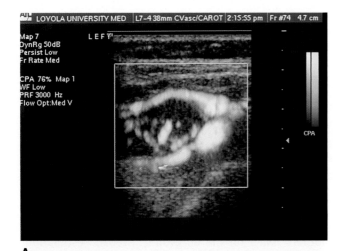

A

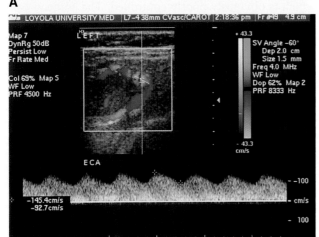

B

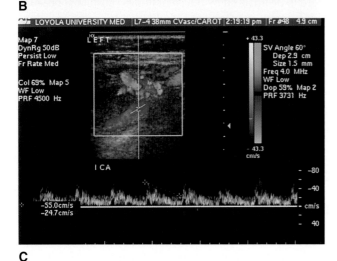

C

*Figure 9-10. Carotid body tumor. **A**, The tumor is located in the bifurcation and is well vascularized. **B**, The ECA very high EDV because it feeds the tumor. **C**, The ICA has normal flow.*

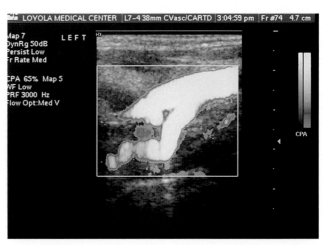

Figure 9-11. Fibromuscular dysplasia of the proximal ICA. This is from a 47-year-old female who had vague cerebrovascular events twice. The proximal ICA has a series of stenoses and dilatations, which is typical for fibromuscular dysplasia. She had mild hypertension controlled with one medication, but her renal arteries were normal.

ment issues were all discussed and suggestions were made. Recommendations were also made for follow-up of patients at high risk or with asymptomatic carotid stenosis (depending on the severity of the stenosis), and research topics were suggested for the future.[58]

Ideally, each center should perform its own validation; however, most centers do not perform internal validation and therefore it was recommended by this panel of experts to use the criteria suggested in Table 9-1.

Conclusions

Carotid duplex ultrasonography is the established method for diagnosing a cervical carotid artery stenosis. In medical centers with a laboratory that has established an excellent positive predictive value, angiography may be avoided before embarking on carotid endarterectomy. These laboratories per force will underdiagnose certain patients with a carotid stenosis. Other laboratories will emphasize the screening aspect of their testing: They will have a less envious positive predictive value. Patients diagnosed by these laboratories will need a confirmatory study to establish that their patients do indeed have a carotid stenosis. The criteria used for diagnosis are variable between laboratories, and each laboratory needs to establish its own criteria. All laboratories, even those with established criteria, need to embark on a continuous quality assurance program.

gray scale imaging and Doppler ultrasound. Technical considerations, diagnostic stratification, imaging and Doppler parameters, Doppler diagnostic thresholds, structure and content of the final report, and quality assess-

REFERENCES

1. Executive Committee for the Asymptomatic Carotid Atherosclerosis Study: Endarterectomy for asymptomatic carotid artery stenosis. JAMA 273:1421–1428, 1995.

2. North American Symptomatic Carotid Endarterectomy Trial Collaborators: Beneficial effect of carotid endarterectomy in symptomatic patients with high-grade stenosis. N Engl J Med 325:445–453, 1991.

3. North American Symptomatic Carotid Endarterectomy Trial Collaborators: Benefit of carotid endarterectomy in patients with symptomatic moderate or severe stenosis. N Engl J Med 339:1415–1425, 1998.

4. Sauve JS, Loaupacis A, Ostbye T, et al: Does this patient have a clinically important carotid bruit? JAMA 270:2843–2845, 1993.

5. Heyman A, Wilkinson WE, Heydan S, et al: Risk of stroke in asymptomatic persons with cervical arterial bruits: A population study in Evans County, Ga. N Engl J Med 302:838–841, 1980.

6. Wiebers DO, Whisnant JP, Sandok BA, et al: Prospective comparison of a cohort with asymptomatic carotid bruit and a population-based cohort without carotid bruit. Stroke 21:984–988, 1990.

7. Roederer GO, Langlois YE, Jager KA, et al: The natural history of carotid arterial disease in asymptomatic patients with cervical bruits. Stroke 15:605–613, 1984.

8. Johnston BF, Verlato F, Bergelin RO, et al: Clinical outcome in patients with mild and moderate carotid stenosis. J Vasc Surg 21:120–126, 1995.

9. Filis KA, Arko FR, Johnson BL, et al: Duplex ultrasound criteria for defining the severity of carotid stenosis. Ann Vasc Surg 16:413–424, 2002.

10. Mansour MA, Mattos MA, Hood DB, et al: Detection of total occlusion, string sign, and preocclusive stenosis of the internal carotid artery by color-flow duplex scanning. Am J Surg 170(2):154–158, 1995.

11. Moneta GL, Edwards JM, Papnicolaou G, et al: Screening for asymptomatic internal carotid artery stenosis: Duplex criteria for discriminating 60% to 99% stenosis. J Vasc Surg 21:989–994, 1995.

12. Hayes AC, O'Connell JB, Baker WH: Cardiac dysfunction and carotid Doppler spectral analysis. J Vasc Tech 11:74–78, 1987.

13. Hayes AC, Johnston KW, Baker WH: The effect of contralateral disease on carotid Doppler frequency. Surgery 103:19–23, 1988.

14. Ray SA, Lockhart SJ, Dourado R, et al: Effect of contralateral disease on duplex measurements of internal carotid artery stenosis. Br J Surg 87(8):1057–1062, 2000.

15. Abou-Zamzam AM Jr, Moneta GL, Edwards JM, et al: Is a single preoperative duplex scan sufficient for planning bilateral carotid endarterectomy? J Vasc Surg 31:282–288, 2000.

16. Clase CM, Cina CS: Medical management versus investigate and operate strategy in asymptomatic carotid stenosis: A decision analysis. J Vasc Surg 36:541–546, 2002.

17. Fowl RJ, Marsch JG, Love M, et al: Prevalence of hemodynamically significant stenosis of the carotid artery in an asymptomatic veteran population. Surg Obst Gyn 172:13–16, 1991.

18. Marek J, Mills JL, Harvich J, et al: Utility of routine carotid duplex screening in patients who have claudication. J Vasc Surg 24:572–579, 1996.

19. Ahn SS, Baker DB, Walden K, et al: Which asymptomatic patients should undergo routine screening carotid duplex scan? Am J Surg 162:180–184, 1991.

20. Berens ES, Kouchoukos NT, Murphy SF, et al: Preoperative carotid artery screening in elderly patients undergoing cardiac surgery. J Vasc Surg 15:313–323, 1992.

21. Faggiola GL, Curl GR, Ricotta JJ: The role of carotid screening before coronary artery bypass. J Vasc Surg 12:724–731, 1990.

22. Ascher E, Hingorani A, Yorkovich W, et al: Routine preoperative carotid duplex scanning in patients undergoing open-heart surgery: Is it worthwhile? Ann Vasc Surg 15:669–678, 2001.

23. Post PN, Kievit J, Baalen JM, et al: Routine duplex surveillance does not improve the outcome after carotid endarterectomy. Stroke 33:749–755, 2002.

24. Strandness DE: Screening for carotid disease and surveillance for carotid restenosis. Sem Vasc Surg 14:200–205, 2001.

25. Ricotta JJ, DeWeese JA: Is routine carotid ultrasound surveillance after carotid endarterectomy worthwhile? Am J Surg 172:140–143, 1996.

26. Iafrati MD, Salamipour H, Young C, et al: Who needs surveillance of the contralateral carotid artery? Am J Surg 172:136–139, 1996.

27. Roederer GO, Langlois YE, Chan ATW, et al: Ultrasonic duplex scanning of the extra cranial carotid arteries: Improved accuracy using new features from the common carotid artery. J Cardiovasc Ultrasonography 1:373–380, 1982.

28. Roederer GO, Langlois YE, Jager GA, et al: A simple spectral parameter for accurate classification of severe carotid artery disease. Bruit 8:174–178, 1984.

29. Moneta GL, Edwards JM, Chitwood RW, et al: Correlation of North American Symptomatic Carotid Endarterectomy Trial (NASCET) angiographic definition of 70% to 90% internal carotid stenosis with duplex scanning. J Vasc Surg 17:152–159, 1993.

30. Hood DB, Mattos MA, Mansour MA, et al: Prospective evaluation of new duplex criteria to identify 70% internal carotid artery stenosis. J Vasc Surg 23:254–262, 1996.

31. Faught WE, Mattos MA, van Bemmelen PS, et al: Color-flow duplex scanning of carotid arteries: New velocity criteria based on receiver operator characteristic analysis for threshold stenoses used in the symptomatic and asymptomatic carotid trials. J Vasc Surg 19:818–828, 1994.

32. Kuntz KM, Polak JF, Whittemore AD, et al: Duplex ultrasound criteria for the identification of carotid stenosis should be laboratory specific. Stroke 28:597–602, 1997.

33. Grant EG, Duerinckx AJ, El Saden SM, et al: Ability to use duplex ultrasound to quantify internal carotid artery stenoses: Fact or fiction? Radiology 214:247–252, 2000.

34. Long A, Lepoutre A, Corbillon E, et al: Critical review of non- or minimally invasive methods (duplex ultrasonography, MR- and CT-angiography) for evaluating stenosis of the proximal internal carotid artery. Eur J Vasc Endovasc Surg 24:43–52, 2002.

35. Nederkoorn PJ, van der Graaf Y, Hunink MG: Duplex ultrasound and magnetic resonance angiography compared with digital subtraction angiography in carotid artery stenosis: A systematic review. Stroke 34:1324–1332, 2003.

36. Schwartz SW, Chambless LE, Baker WH, et al: Consistency of Doppler parameters in predicting arteriographically confirmed carotid stenosis. Asymptomatic Carotid Atherosclerosis Study Investigators. Stroke 28:343–347, 1997.

37. Jmor S, El-Atozy T, Griffin M, et al: Grading internal carotid artery stenosis using B-mode ultrasound (in vivo study). Eur J Vasc Endovasc Surg 18:315–322, 1999.

38. Pan XM, Saloner D, Reilly LM, et al: Assessment of carotid artery stenosis by ultrasonography, conventional angiography, and magnetic resonance angiography: Correlation with ex vivo measurement of plaque stenosis. J Vasc Surg 21:82–89, 1995.

39. Beebe HG, Salles-Cunha SX, Scissons RP, et al: Carotid arterial ultrasound scan imaging: A direct approach to stenosis measurement. J Vasc Surg 29:838–844, 1999.

40. Bendick PJ, Brown OW, Hernandez D, et al: Three-dimensional vascular imaging using Doppler ultrasound. Am J Surg 176:183–187, 1998.

41. Guo Z, Fenster A: Three-dimensional power Doppler imaging: A phantom study to quantify vessel stenosis. Ultrasound Med Biol 22:1059–1069, 1996.

42. Arbeille P, Desombre C, Aesh B, et al: Quantification and assessment of carotid artery lesions, degree of stenosis, and plaque volume. J Clin Ultrasound 23:113–124, 1995.

43. Ascer E, Gennaro M, Pollina RM, et al: The natural history of the external carotid artery after carotid endarterectomy: Implications for management. J Vasc Surg 23:582–585, 1996.

44. Paivansalo MJ, Siniluoto TM, Tikkakoski TA, et al: Duplex US of the external carotid artery. Acta Radiol 37:41–45, 1996.

45. Belkin M, Mackey WC, Pessin MS, et al: Common carotid artery occlusion with patent internal and external carotid arteries: Diagnosis and surgical management. J Vasc Surg 17:1019–1027, 1993.

46. Androulakis AE, Labropoulos N, Allan R, et al: The role of common carotid artery end-diastolic velocity in near total or total internal carotid artery occlusion. Eur J Vasc Endovasc Surg 11:140–147, 1996.

47. Camporese G, Verlato F, Salmistraro G, et al: Spontaneous recanalization of internal carotid artery occlusion evaluated with color-flow imaging and contrast arteriography. Int Angiol 22:64–71, 2003.

48. Meves SH, Muhs A, Federlein J, et al: Recanalization of acute symptomatic occlusions of the internal carotid artery. J Neurol 249:188–192, 2002.

49. Kremer C, Mosso M, Georgiadis D, et al: Carotid dissection with permanent and transient occlusion or severe stenosis: Long-term outcome. Neurology 60:271–275, 2003.

50. Jerry Goldstone: Aneurysms of the Extracranial Carotid Artery. In Rutherfod R (ed): Vascular Surgery, 5th ed. Philadelphia: WB Saunders, 2000.

51. Zwolak RM, Whitehouse WM Jr, Knake JE, et al: Atherosclerotic extracranial carotid artery aneurysms. J Vasc Surg 1:415–422, 1984.

52. Woolgar JD, Ray R, Maharaj K, et al: Colour Doppler and grey scale ultrasound features of HIV-related vascular aneurysms. Br J Radiol 75:884–888, 2002.

53. Johnston SL, Lock RJ, Gompels MM: Takayasu arteritis: A review. J Clin Pathol 55:481–486, 2002.

54. Westerband A, Hunter GC, Cintora I, et al: Current trends in the detection and management of carotid body tumors. J Vasc Surg 28:84–92, 1998.

55. Schneider PA, Rutherfod R: Extracranial fibromuscular arterial dysplasia. In Rutherfod R (ed): Vascular Surgery, 5th ed. Philadelphia: WB Saunders, 2000.

56. Howard G, Baker WH, Chambless LE, et al: An approach for the use of Doppler ultrasound as a screening tool for hemodynamically significant stenosis (despite heterogeneity of Doppler performance). A multicenter experience. Stroke 27:1951–1957, 1996.

57. Eckstein HH, Winter R, Eichbaum M: Grading of internal carotid stenosis: Validation of Doppler/duplex ultrasound criteria and angiography against endarterectomy specimen. Eur J Vasc Endovasc Surg 21:301–310, 2001.

58. Grant EG, Benson CB, Moneta GL, et al: Carotid artery stenosis: Gray-scale and Doppler US diagnosis. Society of Radiologists in Ultrasound Consensus Conference. Radiology 229:340–346, 2003.

Chapter 10

Alternative Imaging Techniques for Extracranial Carotid Occlusive Disease

GRETCHEN SCHWARZE • JENNIFER K. GROGAN • HISHAM BASSIOUNY

Introduction

In the majority of cases, patient selection for carotid endarterectomy or stent angioplasty of the carotid bifurcation is considered when clinically significant extracranial internal carotid artery (ICA) stenoses are detected by color duplex ultrasound (CDU). A priori, an accredited vascular lab with the necessary quality control measures is essential for the accurate determination of the degree and nature of the ICA stenosis. However, several clinical scenarios exist in which alternate imaging techniques are needed to provide greater anatomic detail and resolution of the extra- and intracranial vasculature to determine whether intervention is indeed indicated for the ICA stenosis in question. In this chapter the indications and the added value of alternate imaging modalities in the management of carotid bifurcation disease are discussed.

Indications for Alternate Imaging

Internal Carotid Pseudo-occlusion

A staccato Doppler flow signal with a minimal or an absent diastolic flow component by CDU evaluation is highly suggestive of near or total occlusion of the extracranial ICA or of severe distal ICA siphon disease. Differential diagnosis when staccato signal is found on CDU includes ruptured unstable carotid plaque, hypertensive dissection, and fibromuscular dysplasia. Further investigation of such CDU findings with digital subtraction or magnetic resonance arteriography is advised to diagnose and treat the underlying condition. In patients presenting with a recent transient ischemic attack or nondisabling stroke who are being considered for revascularization, additional imaging is necessary to further determine patency of distal ICA beyond CDU suspicion of a cervical string sign. Establishing a disease-free distal ICA is essential for a satisfactory hemodynamic outcome and long-term patency following revascularization. Figure 10-1 demonstrates the velocity profiles of a patient with a cervical string sign by CDU; and the subsequent angiogram, which showed an ICA dissection.

Carotid Plaque Disruption

Although velocity criteria for high-grade stenosis form a reliable basis for investigation and possible intervention, the role of plaque structural morphology has lagged behind as an important biologic variable when treating patients with significant carotid disease. Studies of carotid endarterectomy specimens have indicated that plaque ulceration and even proximity of plaque necrotic core to the lumen are associated with clinical ischemic events.[1,2] The presence and degree of plaque echoluceny as determined by duplex ultrasound appears to correlate with structural features that connote plaque instability and predisposition to ischemic events.[3,4] Hence, a moderate nonstenotic yet highly echolucent internal carotid plaque should be considered as the culprit lesion in the absence of other sources of thromboembolism (e.g., cardiac, arch, or intracranial disease). Unfortunately, duplex ultrasound is not reliable for detection of plaque ulceration.[5,6] Multiplanar digital subtraction

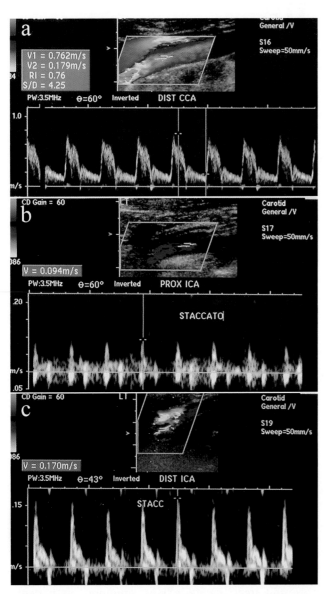
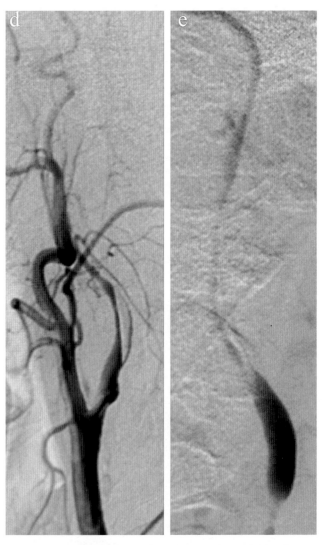

Figure 10-1. *CDU findings in ICA pseudo-occlusion. There is significant decrease in peak systolic velocity with marked reduction of diastolic flow (staccato flow signal) in the proximal ICA (PSV = 0.1 m/sec) (**B**) and distal ICA (PSV = 0.2 m/sec) (**C**) compared with CCA (PSV = 0.8 m/sec) (**A**). Corresponding selective left ICA arteriogram demonstrating a string sign in the mid ICA with delayed clearance of the contrast column (**D** and **E**).*

arteriography is potentially helpful to uncover subtle plaque surface irregularity or ulceration, and it also helps in selecting patients for further intervention. Other imaging techniques continue to evolve for the assessment of plaque structural components that underlie plaque instability. These include spiral computed tomography (CT) and magnetic resonance imaging (MRI) for the delineation of such features as calcification, necrosis, intraplaque hemorrhage, and fibrous cap integrity; however, these have yet to be investigated in prospective natural history trials.

Carotid Bifurcation Thrombus

Freely floating thrombus involving the carotid bifurcation, visualized by CDU in a patient presenting with a TIA, stroke in evolution, or fixed stroke, is an alarming finding. Characteristically, this unusual event is encountered in relatively younger individuals with minimal if any atherosclerotic plaque formation at the carotid bifurcation. Along with a thorough evaluation for the source of the embolic material, the persistence of thrombus should be confirmed before intervention by serial CDU evaluation or arteriography because some thrombi will lyse with systemic anticoagulation.

Fibromuscular Dysplasia and Arteridities

Atypical diffuse or tandem stenoses involving the common and internal carotid arteries may represent nonatherosclerotic occlusive disease. Because of the skip nature of the disease, conventional CDU velocity criteria for atherosclerotic ICA stenosis do not apply for this type of pathology. Such conditions typically involve longer segments of the carotid and other arterial segments such as the renal arteries and aortic arch branches. Precise delineation of the disease extent by alternate imaging is essential if intervention is contemplated.

Carotid Body Tumors

CDU is unique in identifying carotid body tumors. A carotid body tumor is easily recognized by the presence of a speckled color filling of a vascular mass splaying the carotid bifurcation (Fig. 10-2). Contrast-enhanced spiral CT helps delineate the extent of the tumor and the degree of carotid arterial encasement as defined in the Shamblin classification.[7] MRI may have more specific signal characteristics and better delineation of neurovascular structures than CT.[8] To date, MRI has not been shown to be adequately sensitive for detecting tumor feeder arteries.[9] Arteriographic study of the carotid body tumor vascularity provides additional information regarding the vascular supply of the tumor and the level of the carotid bifurcation if preoperative coil embolization is contemplated before resection. Such anatomic detail is helpful in surgical planning (e.g., for resection with or without carotid bifurcation reconstruction).

Vertebrobasilar Insufficiency

Patients with symptomatic posterior fossa ischemia who have either demonstrable vertebral artery flow reversal or evidence of vertebral stenosis and occlusion by duplex must undergo further detailed assessment of the vertebrobasilar anatomy and the integrity of the circle of Willis, preferably with digital subtraction arteriography as a first choice or with MRI/A.

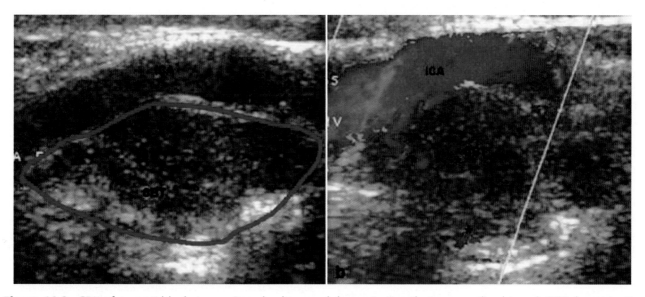

Figure 10-2. CDU of a carotid body tumor. B-mode ultrasound demonstrating the tumor outlined in red. CDU demonstrating color speckling, indicated by the asterisks.

Recurrent Carotid Stenosis

In most instances, early recurrent carotid stenosis is asymptomatic by virtue of the benign natural history of the underlying intimal hyperplastic response.[10] Recurrent stenosis discovered after many years of carotid intervention is most commonly attributed to de novo atherogenesis. With the advent of stent/angioplasty as a novel treatment of ICA stenoses, increased rigidity and reduced vessel compliance results in relative increases in peak systolic flow velocity measurements.[11,12] New criteria are being reported for what constitutes a hemodynamically significant in-stent restenosis.[13] Thus far, accurate classification of the degree of in-stent restenosis by CDU has not been established. When clinically indicated (e.g., with symptomatic or contralateral occlusion), the suspect lesion should be further evaluated with arteriography to determine the precise degree of stenosis and the feasibility of an endovascular approach.

Intracranial Pathology

Patients with history or symptoms suggestive of intracranial cerebral pathology (e.g., aneurysms and arteriovenous malformations) are best investigated with CT, MR, or arteriography; or with a combination of these as determined by the pathologic entity in question.

The above clinical scenarios highlight the significant value of alternate imaging in further refining our diagnostic skills and for assigning patients to medical therapy or intervention. However, carotid and vertebral CDU, when performed and interpreted in a skilled accredited vascular laboratory, remains the primary screening method for patients with possible carotid bifurcation disease.

Alternate Imaging Modalities

Computed Tomography Angiography

Computed tomography angiography (CTA) has only recently been regarded as a valuable test for carotid artery stenosis. Although use of CTA for carotid disease is not widespread, CTA is a powerful tool with potential broad applications. CTA is usually performed using a timing bolus technique. This requires intravenous injection of approximately 120 mL of iodinated contrast. Motion or interference artifact from dental amalgam may limit full visualization of the carotid lesion in question. Patient positioning with elevation of the jaw, a shoulder harness, and instructions to avoid swallowing help limit these technical difficulties.

The study of carotid stenosis with CTA imaging has been slow to gain acceptance because of the paucity of data validating accuracy and because of the limited knowledge regarding the attributes of this modality for providing information regarding the severity of luminal reduction. CTA analysis of ICA stenosis is generally expressed as lumenal area reduction at the location of maximum ICA plaque burden. This is in distinction from digital subtraction angiographic (DSA) estimates of ICA stenosis, in which maximum lumenal reduction is calculated by diameter measurements at the stenosis relative to the diameter of a normal segment of the distal ICA (as reported in the North American Symptomatic Carotid Endarterectomy Trial [NASCET] and Asymptomatic Carotid Atherosclerosis Study [ACAS] studies).[14] Some authors who recommend CTA have advocated the use of back-calculating diameter reduction from the luminal area reduction, which is the parameter that is typically expressed. Cinat and colleagues demonstrated a curvilinear relationship between area stenosis by CTA and diameter reduction by DSA. They showed that an area reduction of 80% by CTA corresponded to a DSA stenosis of greater than 60%, which is significant by NASCET criteria (Fig. 10-3).[15] An added value for CTA is the feasibility of three-dimensional (3-D) image reconstruction with commercially available software and the current generation of CT scanners (Fig. 10-4). Three-dimensional reconstruction is advantageous in providing more reliable information regarding plaque geometric configuration and structure, and luminal dimensions.

Limitations of CTA include a lack of widespread familiarity with image processing techniques and a difficulty in assessing timing and direction of intracranial collateral filling in the presence of occlusive disease.

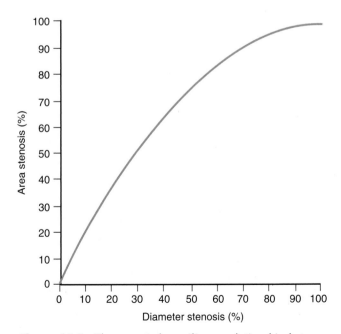

Figure 10-3. The expected curvilinear relationship between diameter reduction (as measured by arteriography) and area reduction (as measured by CTA). (From Journ Vasc Surg)

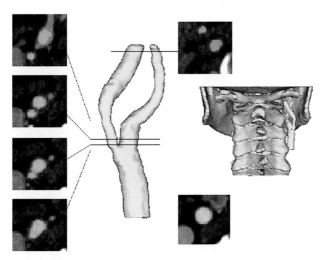

Figure 10-4. Three-dimensional reconstruction of SCT images of the carotid bifurcation in a patient with a 60% to 70% symptomatic right ICA stenosis.

However, CTA is easy to perform and is associated with few risks. Unlike DSA, arterial access is not required, and there is no associated risk of a cerebral vascular accident. Image quality rivals that of DSA when the examination is performed with a high-speed helical scanner programmed to generate thin (1.25-mm interval) slices for 3-D reconstruction.

More importantly, CTA can provide additional information about conformation and composition of carotid plaque, which may help differentiate stable and unstable plaques. Certainly, CTA can easily distinguish calcified plaque from soft or lipid-laden plaque. Figure 10-5 shows spiral CT cross-section images of plaques with variable degrees of calcification, as measured by computer-assisted morphometry with color density scale analysis. These plaque structural features may prove helpful in predicting possible plaque rupture and in stratifying patients at increased risk for stroke and in need of intervention.

Magnetic Resonance Angiography

Magnetic resonance angiography is a more widely used alternative imaging technique; it is more commonly used for evaluation of carotid disease than is CTA. Two techniques are used; time-of-flight imaging (TOF), which is a flow-dependent technique; and contrast-enhanced MRA (CE-MRA), which is a filling-dependent technique comparable to the technique of CTA.

TOF is a technique widely used to establish the diagnosis of carotid stenosis. This technique is optimized to minimize the signal from stationary tissue, thereby

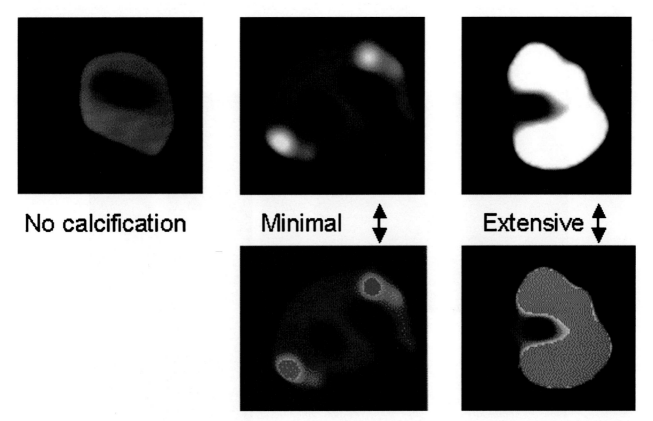

Figure 10-5. Ex vivo SCT cross-section images of plaques with variable degrees of calcification. Calcification area was measured using computer-assisted morphometry with color density scale analysis (calcified regions in the 0 to 100 range vs. noncalcified regions in the 100 to 250 range).

increasing relative signal from the fresh spins delivered to the volume by bloodflow from outside the imaging volume.[16] There are two modes of TOF, 2-D and 3-D. The 2-D time of flight is more sensitive to slower flow, whereas 3-D TOF depicts a wide range of flow velocities, and as such has greater accuracy than 2-D in defining internal and external carotid artery morphology.[16] Because this imaging is flow dependent, there is some distortion of the carotid anatomy with high-grade lesions or in lesions with turbulent flow. TOF spins may remain in imaging volume long enough to see numerous pulses and become saturated, thereby causing loss of signal within vessel lumen and an inability to depict the vessel contiguous with the lesion.[16] This can lead to overestimation of the degree of stenosis. Thus an MRA that demonstrates no evidence of disease at the carotid bifurcation is quite accurate. A normal MRA is highly specific for the absence of carotid atherosclerotic disease.

CE-MRA utilizes flow-independent anatomic information. This technique provides a more accurate assessment of stenosis and visualization of ulcerated plaques. There may be some technical difficulty in capturing the timing bolus, but a variety of approaches have been developed to overcome this. The use of a test bolus and automatic detection by the scanner to detect the arrival of the contrast material greatly assists in optimizing timing for contrast enhancement.[17,18] A principal advantage of CE-MRA is that the shorter imaging time (less than 25 seconds) increases accuracy secondary to a decreased risk of motion artifact. Figure 10-6 shows the excellent resolution and 3-D geometry that is possible with CE-MRA.

The ability to use MRA as a diagnostic tool for carotid stenosis has unfortunately been limited by lack of expertise and lack of familiarity with the test. In centers where the test is widely used, it can provide valuable additional data to the CDU findings. Furthermore, MRA is not associated with ionizing radiation or ionic contrast, and as such is quite safe for most patients. Additionally, information about the cerebral circulation, including patency of the carotid siphon and MCA, can be obtained simultaneously.

There are several limitations to MRI. Some patients are unable to tolerate the lengthy procedure because of claustrophobia or health problems. This can sometimes be overcome with coaching and sedation. Patient motion and surgical clips can cause artifacts, making results difficult to interpret. Additionally, small carotid lumens and tortuous vessels can be interpreted as occlusion or severe stenosis. Finally, the test is expensive, which limits its utilization as a screening method.

More advanced techniques are now being evaluated for visualization of atherosclerotic plaque and vessel wall. These methods include standard CE-MRA and TOF obtained with specialized surface carotid coils to increase the signal-to-noise ratio (Fig. 10-7). Additional techniques include 3-D bright blood MRA and 2-D spin echo and fast-spin echo methods. Important developments are also being made in the postprocessing of MRI. Algorithms have been developed that allow calcu-

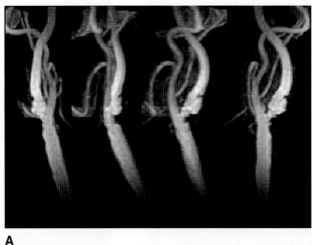

A

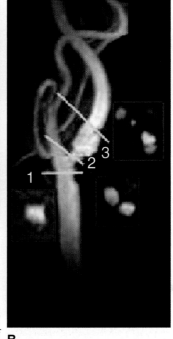

B

Figure 10-6. Contrast-enhanced MRA study of a patient with moderate disease at the origin of the internal carotid artery. **A,** The anatomy of the bifurcation is well displayed in maximum intensity projection (MIP) images (four different projection angles were selected for display here). **B,** Multi-planar reformats show the complexity of the shape of the residual lumen: level 1, the distal CCA with small invaginations; level 2, the level of the maximum stenosis showing ICA and ECA; and level 3 in the mid ICA, which has the shape of a figure 8.

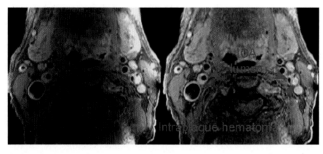

Figure 10-7. Cross-sectional slice of the proximal ICA using high-sensitivity surface coil MRI. The residual lumen is black with enhancement of an intraplaque hematoma underlying an intact fibrous cap.

lation of vessel lumen dimensions, wall thickness, and even composition and distribution of tissue components.[19,20,21] Data obtained from these techniques demonstrate good correlation with ex vivo plaque morphology (Fig. 10-8).

Digital Subtraction Angiography

Although digital subtraction angiography (DSA) is considered the "gold standard" for cerebrovascular imaging, it may be soon supplanted by less invasive imaging modalities such as CTA and MRI. In a single examination, DSA provides a complete evaluation of the aortic arch and the extracranial and intracranial cerebrovascular systems. Additionally, DSA is advantageous in defining the timing and direction of filling between the left and right hemisphere and between the anterior and posterior circulation. This is helpful in diagnosing anterior or posterior circulation watershed ischemia related to occlusive disease involving the aortic arch and its branches.

Guidelines for operative intervention from both NASCET and ACAS are based on luminal diameter reduction as diagnosed by DSA. Before the NASCET study, diameter reduction criteria were often based on a theoretical estimate of the size of the nondiseased lumen. Given the inherent inaccuracy and tendency to overestimate the degree of stenosis using such estimates, NASCET defined the degree of carotid stenosis in relation to the actual measurement of the lumen of the normal ICA distal to the carotid stenosis. This method is widely accepted as standard in North America, and as such is the basis for operative intervention in both asymptomatic and symptomatic patients with carotid disease.[22,23]

Although the risk of cerebral arteriography is relatively low, it is significantly greater than with CTA and MRA. Although the stroke risk has been quoted as high as 1% in the NASCET trial, in practice the CVA/TIA risk from carotid angiography is closer to 0.5%.[24] Additionally, the risk of femoral sheath hematoma, while low with the 5 French sheath required for angiography,

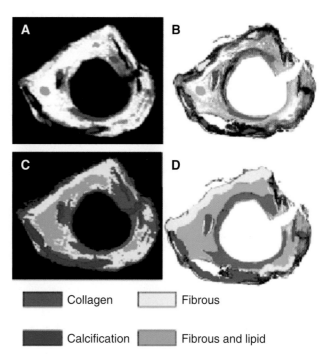

Collagen   Fibrous

Calcification   Fibrous and lipid

*Figure 10-8. MR images are acquired (**A**) and the corresponding histological section is digitized (**B**), and registered with the MR image. Based on histology, a representative region for each plaque component is selected. Training regions for collagen (red), fibrous plaque (yellow), calcification (blue), and fibrous plaque mixed with lipid (green) are shown in **A** and **B**. Based on MR properties of these training regions, each pixel in the MR image is classified. Classification results are shown in **C**. Manual segmentation of the histology image by a pathologist is shown in **D**, and this segmentation can then be compared with classification algorithm results **C** on a pixel-by-pixel basis. (From Demarco JK, Rutt BK, Clarke SE: Carotid plaque characterization by magnetic resonance imaging: Review of literature. Top Magn Reson Imaging 12(3)205–217, 2001.)*

is still 0.1% to 0.5%.[25] Additionally, in comparison to MRA in which there is no ionic contrast or ionizing radiation, DSA puts the patient at some risk for renal insufficiency and radiation hazards.

Finally, DSA provides accurate information regarding the lumen of the carotid artery but fails to provide any information about plaque composition, the vessel wall, or surrounding cervical structures.

Research/Future Directions

The future holds great promise for both CTA and MRI/A, as it does for continued positive evolution in both software and hardware technology. The ability to perform a single study that would accurately assess the cerebral vascular anatomy, the brain parenchyma, and the degree of plaque stability is soon forthcoming. Findings from these imaging modalities will further refine our judgment in treating patients with carotid bifurcation atherosclerosis.

REFERENCES

1. Zukowski AJ: The correlation between carotid plaque ulceration and cerebral infarction seen on CT scan. J Vasc Surg 1(6):782–786, 1984.
2. Bassiouny HS, Sakaguchi Y, Mikucki SA, et al: Juxtalumenal location of plaque necrosis and neoformation in symptomatic carotid stenosis. J Vasc Surg 26(4):585–594, 1997.
3. Sabeti M, Tegos T, Nicolaides A, et al: Hemispheric symptoms and carotid plaque echomorphology. J Vasc Surg 31:39–49, 2000.
4. Langsfeld M, Gray-Weale AC, Lusby RJ: The role of plaque morphology and diameter reduction in the development of new symptoms in asymptomatic carotid arteries. J Vasc Surg 9(4):548–557, 1989.
5. O-Leary DH, Holen J, Ricotta JJ, et al: Carotid bifurcation disease: Prediction of ulceration with B-mode ultrasound. Radiology 162:523–525, 1987.
6. Sitzer M, Wolfram M, Jorg R, et al: Color-flow Doppler-assisted duplex imaging fails to detect ulceration in high-grade internal carotid artery stenosis. J Vasc Surg 24:461–465, 1996.
7. Swartz JD, Korsvik H: High-resolution computed tomography of paragangliomas of the head and neck. J Comp Tomog 8(3):197–202, 1984
8. Win T, Lewin JS: Imaging characteristics of carotid body tumors. Am J Otolaryngol 16(5):325–328, 1995.
9. Van den Berg R, Wasser MN, van Gils AP, et al: Vascularization of head and neck paragangliomas: Comparison of three MR angiographic techniques with digital subtraction angiography. Am J Neuroradiol 21(1):162–170, 2000.
10. Strandness DE Jr: Screening for carotid disease and surveillance′ for carotid restenosis. Semin Vasc Surg 14(3):200–205, 2001.
11. Ringer AJ, German JW, Guterman LR, et al: Follow-up of stented carotid arteries by Doppler ultrasound. Neurosurgery 51:639–643, 2002.
12. Robbin ML, Lockhart ME, Weber TM, et al: Carotid artery stents: Early and intermediate follow-up with Doppler ultrasound. Radiology 205:749–756, 1997.
13. Lal BK, Hobson RW, Goldstein J, et al: Carotid artery stenting: Is there a need to revise ultrasound velocity criteria? J Vasc Surg 39(1):58–66, 2004.
14. Eliasziw M, Smith RF, Singh N, et al: Further comments on the measurement of carotid stenosis from angiograms. North American Symptomatic Carotid Endarterectomy Trial (NASCET) Group. Stroke 25(12):2445–2449, 1994.
15. Cinat M, Lane C, Pham H, et al: Helical CT angiography in the preoperative evaluation of carotid artery stenosis, J Vasc Surg 28:290–300, 1998.
16. Phillips CD, Bubash LA: CT angiography and MR angiography in the evaluation of extracranial carotid vascular disease. Radiol Clin North Am 40:783–798, 2002.
17. Kim JK, Farb RI, Wright GA: Test bolus examination in the carotid artery at dynamic gadolinium enhanced MR angiography. Radiology 206(1):283–289, 1998.
18. Wilman AH, Riederer SJ, Huston J 3rd, et al: Arterial phase carotid and vertebral artery imaging in 3-D contrast-enhanced MR angiography by combining fluoroscopic triggering with an elliptical centric acquisition order. Mag Reson Med 40(1):24–35, 1998.
19. Yuan C, Lin E, Millard J, et al: Closed contour edge detection of blood vessel lumen and outer wall boundaries in black-blood MR images. Mag Reson Imag 17:257–266, 1999.
20. Kerwin WS, et al: A quantitative vascular analysis system for evaluation of atherosclerotic lesions by MRI. In MICCAI 4th International Conference 2001. Utrecht, Netherlands.
21. Demarco JK, Rutt BK, Clarke SE: Carotid plaque characterization by magnetic resonance imaging: Review of literature. Top Magn Reson Imaging 12(3):205–217, 2001.
22. Executive Committee for the Asymptomatic Carotid Atherosclerosis Study: Endarterectomy for asymptomatic carotid stenosis. JAMA 273:1421–1428, 1995.
23. North American Symptomatic Carotid Endarterectomy Trial Collaborators: Beneficial effect of carotid endarterectomy in symptomatic patients with high-grade carotid stenosis, N Engl J Med 325:445–453, 1991.
24. Johnston DC, Chapman KM, Goldstein LB: Low rate of complications of cerebral angiography in routine clinical practice. Neurology 57(11):2012–2014, 2001.
25. Lilly MP, Reichman W, Sarazen AA, et al: Anatomic and clinical factors associated with complications of transfemoral arteriography. Ann Vasc Surg 4:264–269, 1990.

Chapter 11

Transcranial Doppler: Technique and Applications

STEPHEN C. NICHOLLS

Introduction

Although transcranial Doppler (TCD) was introduced in 1982 to measure bloodflow velocity in the circle of Willis,[1] its first clinical application was in the detection of cerebral vasospasm following aneurysm rupture.[2] It was not, however, until it became routinely employed to evaluate middle cerebral artery flow velocity in patients undergoing carotid endarterectomy (CEA) that its full potential as a diagnostic and therapeutic tool was established.[3] Initially, the technique was used to evaluate adequacy of middle cerebral artery flow ipsilateral to the clamped internal carotid artery. Later it was used in evaluating postoperative hyperemia, and this included monitoring the effects of pharmacologic interventions aimed at controlling reperfusion injury. Expansion into embolism detection, both in the operating room and in the recovery room, has now enabled clinicians to detect this phenomenon early, institute therapeutic measures, and evaluate the efficacy of such interventions.

The technique may also be used to evaluate vasomotor reserve (VMR) using the CO_2 challenge test; this has expanded its role to the evaluation of cerebrovascular hypoperfusion, enabling assessment of stroke risk and evaluation of the effects of surgical revascularization.

The noninvasive nature of the technique, its ability to supply continuous information in real time, and its ability to make quantifiable physiologic measurements has expanded its utility into areas as diverse as coronary artery bypass, subclavian steal, treatment of arteriovenous malformations, cerebrovascular vasospasm, the evaluation of intracranial pressure by examination of the TCD waveform profile, diagnosis of patent foramen ovale, and evaluation of the efficacy of antiplatelet therapy. This chapter focuses on those areas of particular interest to the vascular surgeon and vascular interventionalist.

Background

The most important factor influencing susceptibility of the brain to ischemia is its severity and duration. Normal cerebral bloodflow is approximately 50 mL/100 g/min, and a critical level appears to exist at 20 mL/100 g/min. Below this level, metabolism begins to decline. If the ischemia is short-lived, or the demand is reduced (e.g., in hypothermia or barbiturate intoxication), lower flow values may be tolerated without sustaining deficit. The ischemic tolerance of neural tissue varies. In regions of marginal perfusion, bloodflow is not homogeneous, and areas of local ischemia may be adjacent to areas of normal perfusion. Furthermore, an embolus or thrombosis that would normally cause no deficit or a temporary deficit may result in permanent deficit if the perfusion pressure is severely reduced.

The aim of intraoperative monitoring is to reduce the incidence of neurologic deficits by identifying ischemia and implementing measures to alleviate it while the situation is still reversible. Hypoperfusion during occlusion may be identified and prevented by insertion of a temporary shunt. Embolic events and postoperative thrombosis cannot be prevented by monitoring, but they may be recognized and treated early. Hyperperfusion, manifested by sustained reactive hyperemia following clamp release, may be identified early and therapeutic measures instituted.

Many techniques have been proposed to determine the adequacy of cerebral perfusion during carotid occlusion.

Monitoring Methods

1. Direct observation. Neurologic assessment during anesthesia provides a sensitive and accurate method. Surgeons utilizing selective shunting and regional anesthesia generally use them in approximately 5% of cases, indicating that the fraction of patients who require shunts is about 10%. Patient and surgeon discomfort, as well that of the anesthesiologist, has limited acceptance of this technique. There occasionally may also be a prolonged delay between clamping and onset of neurologic deficit.

2. Stump pressure. This method has been advocated for years as a reliable and simple measurement of collateral adequacy, and thus indirectly of cerebral bloodflow. The critical level is normally stated to be approximately 50 mmHg at normocapnea, or somewhat lower during hypocapnea or if vasodilating agents such as halothane are used. Stump pressure measurements reflect pressure at a single point in time immediately after clamping. Not surprisingly, other methods including cerebral bloodflow, electroencephalography (EEG), and clinical outcome have shown discrepancies with this method. Stump pressure therefore may be considered a crude method of assessment only.

3. Electroencephalography. Although close correlation between cerebral bloodflow and EEG has been demonstrated, with significant slowing of frequency occurring when cerebral bloodflow is of the order of 16 mL/100 g/min, reports of its reliability have varied, and clamp-related EEG changes occur in approximately 10% to 30% of cases. This oversensitivity, together with a demand for an experienced technician, are considered serious drawbacks, although interpretation is now facilitated by the use of compressed spectral array analysis. Somatosensory-evoked potentials can also be used as an index of cerebral perfusion. The applicability and advantages and disadvantages are similar to those of EEG.

4. Cerebral bloodflow (CBF). CBF may be measured using the xenon 133 clearance technique. Correlation between CBF and EEG has been shown in several studies. Below 10 mL/100 g/min, virtually all patients develop EEG changes. These numbers are in agreement with the threshold for brain infarction suggested by experimental observation and substantiated by endarterectomy series performed without the use of a shunt. CBF measurement provides only an instantaneous measure of perfusion. It is also cumbersome and requires the use of radioisotopes. It is, however, a useful reference against which other modalities may be measured.

5. Cerebral oximetry. This is a noninvasive method for continuous monitoring of intracerebral oxygen saturation. Significant linear correlation is found between oxygen saturation and TCD velocities on cross clamping. The preliminary data are promising but as yet are insufficient to assess the role of cerebral oximetry as a monitoring tool during CEA.

6. Transcranial Doppler. Changes in flow velocity measured in the middle cerebral artery parallel changes in cerebral bloodflow, provided that the vessel diameter, flow profile, and the angle between the ultrasound beam and the vessel remain constant. Although there is significant scatter amongst patients, the continuous and noninvasive monitoring ability of TCD provide real-time information on changes in flow velocity. Recent experience indicates that the ratio of clamp to preclamp flow velocity in the MCA is a reliable indicator of cerebral ischemia during temporary carotid clamping. TCD also monitors shunt patency. TCD appears to represent the most promising intraoperative monitoring technique currently available to determine the need for a shunt. The only large randomized study to look at carotid shunting does not clarify this issue.[4] It included 503 patients, and the morbidity was 4% among the shunted as

well as unshunted patients. However, a small group of 10 patients in the nonshunt group who developed severe EEG changes during clamping were shunted. A more recent study collected data from 1495 procedures in 11 centers that used intraoperative TCD.[5] The incidence of intraoperative stroke was assessed depending on degree of cerebral ischemia during clamping: severe, 0% to 15% of the preclamp velocity in the middle cerebral artery; mild, 16% to 40%; none, greater than 40%. The data showed that unnecessary shunting increased the perioperative risk of stroke 1% vs. 4% (p < 0.001). Furthermore, it indicated that shunting of patients who develop severe ischemia during clamping (as assessed by TCD) lowered the risk of stroke, 19% vs. 0% (p < 0.01). These data suggest that selective shunting is indicated and that selection be based on MCA velocity data acquired during intraoperative TCD monitoring.

Physiology of TCD Monitoring

This is based on several assumptions:

1. The diameter of the insonated cerebral arteries is constant. TCD monitoring may be used to insonate all the major cerebral arteries in a noninvasive and continuous fashion, although velocity in the middle cerebral artery (VMCA) is most commonly measured.[1] Flow velocity is proportional to CBF only when the diameter of the insonated vessel and the angle of insonation remain constant. There is considerable evidence to suggest that major cerebral arteries do not dilate or constrict as vascular resistance changes. A number of validation studies have confirmed the reliability of TCD as an index of CBF[6,7] (Fig. 11-1). Angiographic and CO_2 reactivity studies confirm that changes in CO_2 tension and blood pressure have negligible influence on the diameter of the proximal basal arteries.[8,9] The exception is nitroglycerine, which may cause vasodilatation when administered to healthy volunteers.[10] Intravenous anesthetic agents do not vasodilate or vasoconstrict the basal cerebral arteries.[11] Similarly, commonly used inhalational anesthetics do not dilate the MCA appreciably,[12] although this remains controversial.[13] During steady state anesthetic conditions, changes in the VMCA can be interpreted to mean corresponding changes in cortical CBF.[14,15] The only clinically important situation in which basal cerebral arteries do change diameter is when vasospasm occurs as a complication of subarachnoid hemorrhage. Vasospasm renders the relationship between CBF velocity and CBF volume invalid. As the vessel constricts the bloodflow, the flow velocity increases but CBF

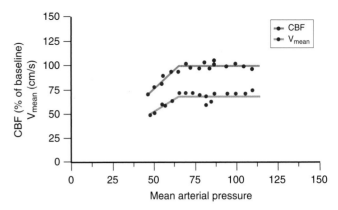

Figure 11-1. Mean middle cerebral artery velocities are a reliable index of cerebral bloodflow over a wide range of mean arterial pressures.

decreases. This increase in flow velocity with constriction of the basal cerebral artery represents one of the most important and established uses of TCD.[16] If a diagnosis of vasospasm is confirmed by angiography, TCD can be used to track patient response to therapy and time course of resolution.

2. Changes in MCA velocity reflect relative changes in CBF. TCD can only give relative indices of CBF. Because vessel diameter varies with individuals, the normal VMCA range is from 35 to 90 cm/sec. Thus, although correlation between absolute flow velocity and CBF in any given population is poor, good correlation has been demonstrated between relative changes in flow velocity and CBF.[6,17] Furthermore, validity of TCD for determination of the lower limit of CBF autoregulation has been established.[18]

3. Pulsatility of flow velocity reflects cerebral vascular resistance. In the absence of stenosis or vasospasm, pulsatility of the flow velocity profile reflects the distal cerebrovascular resistance. Two derived indices have been used to quantify the resistance:

Pulsatility index (PI or Gosling index)
= (Vsys - Vdias)/mean VMCA
Resistance index (RI or Pourcelot index)
= (Vsys - Vdias)/Vsys

TCD in Carotid Endarterectomy

The benefit of prophylactic CEA has been demonstrated in both symptomatic and asymptomatic patients by the NASCET,[19] European,[20] and ACAS[21] trials, but this benefit is contingent on low perioperative neurologic complication rates for the procedure. The combined morbidity/mortality should be below 2% to 4%, as was achieved in the randomized multicenter studies.

There are four mechanisms for neurologic complications resulting from carotid endarterectomy: (1) hypoperfusion with clamping; (2) embolization; (3) perioperative thrombosis; and (4) hyperperfusion syndrome. Hypoperfusion during carotid clamping occurs in a minority of complications, but it is the complication most commonly discussed in the literature because it may be prevented with a temporary indwelling shunt to ensure ipsilateral hemispheric perfusion. Current data suggest that detachment of embolic material from the carotid bifurcation during dissection, during shunt insertion, or upon reopening the endarterectomized vessel may be an important pathogenic factor in perioperative stroke. Postoperative thrombosis at the endarterectomy site is often associated with technical error, and should be minimized with meticulous surgery and judicious use of antiplatelet agents. Sustained reactive hyperemia leading to hyperperfusion and intracerebral hemorrhage (ICH) is thought to account for approximately 10% to 15% of all intraoperative strokes. It is the most difficult of all perioperative complications to prevent. Recent evidence suggests that the relative incidence of ICH is increasing.[22]

The generation of continuous real-time information regarding hemispheric bloodflow by monitoring VMCA makes TCD monitoring well suited to address hypoperfusion, perioperative thromboembolism, perioperative thrombosis, and hyperperfusion syndrome, as well as sustained postoperative intra-arterial embolism.[3]

Prevention of Hypoperfusion During Carotid Clamping

Mean MCA velocities can be used to detect hypoperfusion during cross clamping of the internal carotid artery, and therefore can help determine the need for an indwelling shunt (Fig. 11-2). The validity of selective shunting (as validated by Halsey) has been previously discussed.[5] Correlation between flow velocity changes and electroencephalographic changes appears to be good in several studies.[23,24] The correlation with stump pressure is less consistent, but low stump pressures are generally associated with low flow velocity during cross clamping.[25,26] Perfusion is defined as adequate if the VMCA does not fall below 40% of the preclamp value (i.e., no greater than a 60% drop).[25] TCD can be used as a continuous monitor of shunt function, detecting inadequate perfusion that may be caused by kinking or by thrombosis in the shunt.

Detection of Microembolism

Both air and particulate emboli may be detected by TCD.[3] Validation studies using both in vitro and in vivo models

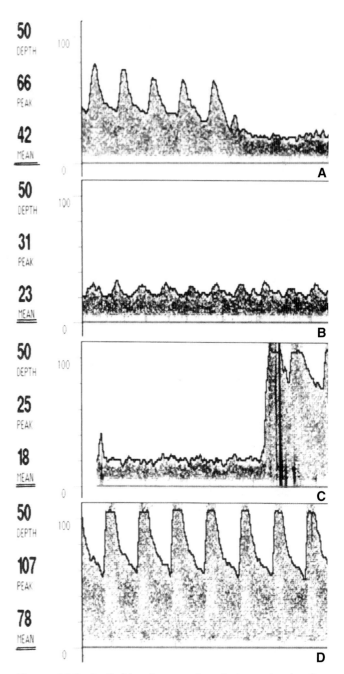

Figure 11-2. **A,** *Sudden decrease in velocity and pulsatility occurs with carotid artery cross clamping. In this case, mean velocity middle cerebral artery is maintained above 40% of preclamp values. Concomitant stump pressure was 55 mmHg. This patient does not require a shunt.* **B,** *A slight increase in flow and pulsatility is noted during cross clamping; this is caused by the recruitment of collaterals.* **C,** *Hyperemic response following release of carotid cross clamp. The high-intensity vertical lines immediately after clamp release are air emboli.* **D,** *Sustained hyperemic response. If this lasts more than 3 to 5 minutes, and is an increase of 100% to 120% over baseline, it is defined as hyperperfusion and should be treated. The response to pharmacologic intervention may then be monitored until normal perfusion has been restored.*

have confirmed that the embolic "signatures" consist of high intensity backscatter energy; these are caused by reflected ultrasound from the emboli, which are of higher density than the surrounding flowing blood. The number of embolic signals found during dissection has been correlated with the occurrence of intraoperative infarcts.[27] Furthermore, the data suggest that embolus counts occurring at a rate of more than 10 per hour in the postoperative period are associated with a significant increased risk of perioperative stroke.[28] Embolism detection represents the most rapidly expanding use of TCD and will be considered in detail in a separate section.

Diagnosis and Treatment of Postoperative Hyperperfusion Syndrome

Following TEA, approximately 1% of patients develop hyperperfusion syndrome that results in cerebral hemorrhage.[29] Studies have demonstrated that hyperemia occurs in patients with high grade stenosis, low stump pressure values, and low flow velocity during cross clamping.[30] Patients who develop hyperperfusion syndrome show sustained elevation of flow velocities after clamp release. The incidence of hyperemia as identified by TCD ranges from 10% to 20%, and the increase in flow velocity can range from 30% to 230%.[31] The findings suggest that there is defective autoregulation in the ipsilateral hemisphere after TEA, because reduction of blood pressure is effective in normalizing the ipsilateral flow velocity and in alleviating the symptoms.

Although hyperperfusion after release of the carotid artery crossclamp is rare, it is a potentially devastating complication.[22,30] In normal patients, ipsilateral flow velocity is transiently elevated following crossclamp release, resulting in a short-lived hyperemic response. In patients with chronic hypoperfusion there is a loss of normal autoregulation with a low vascular impedance distal to the stenosis. These patients may exhibit sustained hyperemia.

If hyperemia persists, symptoms ranging from mild headache to intracranial hemorrhage may develop. Hyperperfusion occurs when there is an increase in velocity of 120% or greater (based on TCD velocity measurements in the ipsilateral MCA) lasting more than 3 to 5 minutes.

Hyperperfusion has been documented as lasting for as little as 3 hours to as long as 12 days. Because, in these situations, bloodflow is completely pressure dependent, it is imperative that systemic arterial bloodflow pressure is strictly controlled postoperatively in these patients (Fig. 11-3). Propofol is a useful agent. Once the patient has been extubated, esmolol may be used.

Diagnosis and Treatment of Perioperative Intimal Flap or Thrombosis

Occlusion of the carotid artery may occur postoperatively because of thrombus formation or as the result of a residual intimal flap. Severely stenotic flaps may be associated with a failure of restoration of normal VMCA. Intraoperative and recovery room monitoring for both microemboli and for normal flow velocities may identify technical problems requiring either administration of antiplatelet agents and/or emergent reoperation.

Use of TCD in Cerebrovascular Revascularization

TCD monitoring is also useful in cerebrovascular surgery other than CEA.[32] It has been used as follows:

1. To assess ipsilateral hemispheric perfusion when the common carotid artery is clamped for carotid subclavian bypass or in vertebral reimplantation. In cases of fetal circulation anatomy, posterior cerebral artery monitoring may also be indicated.

2. For basilar artery monitoring to assess basilar flow when vertebral artery clamped, in the presence of poor or absent posterior communicating arteries, or with stenosis of occlusion of the contralateral vertebral artery.

3. To assess the ipsilateral hemispheric perfusion when there is change in mean arterial pressure (MAP) in patients whose VMR is severely impaired or absent. This is particularly useful in cardiopulmonary bypass when flow is pressure-dependent.

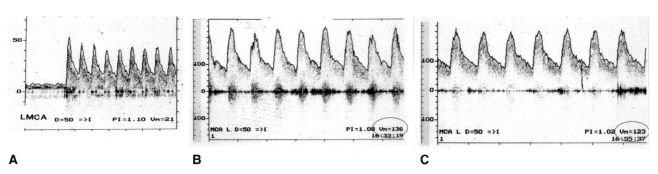

A   **B**   **C**

Figure 11-3. Postoperative reactive hyperemia. **A**, *Normal hyperemic response at clamp release (note mean middle cerebral artery velocity).* **B**, *Sustained hyperemia in the recovery room more than half an hour after clamp release (note mean middle cerebral artery velocity).* **C**, *Hyperemic response controlled with propofol (note mean middle cerebral artery velocity).*

Technical Problems of TCD Monitoring

Incorrect Vessel Identification. This should be a rare occurrence with experienced technologists. An increase in flow velocity after cross clamping would suggest that the posterior cerebral artery (PCA) is being monitored. If the signal disappears completely after cross clamping, but there is backflow from the internal carotid artery, the insonated vessel is most likely the siphon.

Hyperostosis of the Temporal Bone. This may result in an inability to isonate the middle cerebral arteries. Inadequate temporal windows may be encountered in approximately 10% to 15% of patients in an older population.

Vasomotor Reactivity Evaluation of the Cerebral Circulation Using TCD CO_2 Challenge

Patients with cerebral vascular occlusive disease may experience insufficiency because of inadequate CBF. In these patients the compensatory mechanism of the collateral circulation and autoregulation is inadequate to maintain distal perfusion.

The main collateral supply to the cerebral hemispheres is through the anterior and posterior communicating arteries, the circle of Willis; and through the external carotid to internal carotid anastomoses around the eye. Anomalies of the circle of Willis are common, and it is estimated that a symmetrical configuration without hypoplastic or atretic segments is present in only about 50% of the population.[33] Major variants include a fetal (or simian) origin of the posterior cerebral arteries from the internal carotid. In some patients there are anomalies of both the anterior and posterior circulation, with a resultant "isolated" hemisphere that is reliant on the ipsilateral ICA and only small ophthalmic and distant leptomeningeal vessels for collateral flow.

Cerebral autoregulation, first described by Lassen in 1959,[34] enables cerebral bloodflow to be maintained over a wide range of MAP between 50 and 150 mmHg. This is accomplished through vasoconstriction and vasodilatation of the microcirculation. Once the microcirculation is maximally dilated, VMR becomes exhausted and a fall in systemic pressure results in compromised flow. Because vasoconstriction and vasodilatation of the microcirculation can be achieved using varying levels of carbon dioxide (CO_2), the response of the cerebral circulation to hypercapnea and hypocapnea enables estimation of the VMR (Fig. 11-4). In 1966 Bloor and colleagues [35] proposed using the CO_2 challenge test to define hemodynamically significant ICA stenoses and occlusions (Fig. 11-5).

Under conditions of standard TCD monitoring, the patient breathes a gas containing 6% CO_2, 40% oxygen,

and a balance of nitrogen through a mouthpiece attached to a one-way valve. The patient is asked to breathe normally, to hyperventilate, and to hypoventilate, enabling conditions of normal capnea, hypercapnea, and hypocapnea to be assessed while middle cerebral artery velocities are recorded.

Normal values for VM reactivity using the TCD CO_2 challenge were established by Ringlestein and colleagues in 1988[36] (Fig. 11-6). Vasomotor reactivity is expressed as the percent change in MCA velocity from baseline between hypercapnea and hypocapnea. The vasomotor

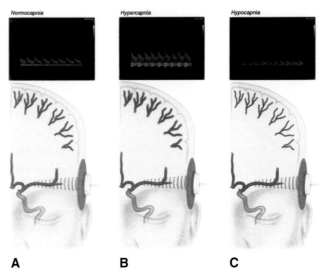

A   **B**   **C**

Figure 11-4. **A,** *Normal vasomotor tone seen in arterioles with normal middle cerebral artery velocities during normocapnia.* **B,** *With inhalation of CO_2 vasodilatation occurs, resistance to flow is lowered and middle cerebral artery velocities increase.* **C,** *During hyperventilation, arterioles vasoconstrict resistance to flow increases and middle cerebral artery velocities decrease.*

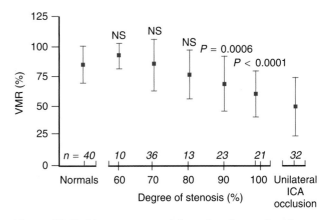

Figure 11-5. *Vasomotor reactivity values in varying degrees of ICA stenosis and occlusion. Where the degree of stenosis reaches 80%, vasomotor reactivity is significantly different from normal (p = 0.053). Even in ICA occlusion, vasomotor reactivity may be normal in individual cases. This is a function of the status of the circle of Willis.*

reactivity may then be divided by the absolute change in end tidal, that is, expired carbon dioxide (ET CO_2). The absolute change in ET CO_2 is the highest CO_2 value during hypercapnea minus the lowest CO_2 value during hypocapnea. This may be then expressed as the percentage change in MCA velocities per mmHg of CO_2. A normal value for total vasomotor reactivity is 86% ± 16%.

Kleiser and Widder, in an analysis of 293 patients with unilateral occlusion of the ICA, found a significant correlation between very low or exhausted CO_2 reactivity and a recent history of ischemic attacks or stroke.[37] In 75 patients they also found a close correlation between hemodynamically caused infarcts demonstrated by cranial CT and an exhausted CO_2 reactivity.

The TCD CO_2 challenge test is therefore a noninvasive, reliable, quantifiable, cost-effective tool that enables identification of patients with abnormal vasomotor reactivity, a known correlate of hypoperfusion-induced stroke. The test also identifies those patients undergoing cerebrovascular revascularization who are at increased risk of reperfusion injury including intracerebral hemorrhage. It constitutes a useful screening test in asymptomatic patients with noncerebral vascular disease who are required to undergo general anesthesia and who may be at risk for cerebral ischemia during systemic hypotension (Fig. 11-7). This is particularly true for patients undergoing coronary artery bypass who are subject to nonpulsatile low pressure flow on bypass. It also enables patients to be assessed postoperatively for the efficacy of a range of cerebral revascularization procedures including not only carotid endarterectomy but also EC/IC bypass and other extracranial cerebrovascular revascularizations (Fig. 11-8).

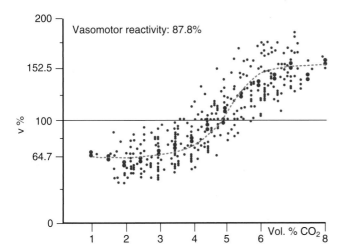

Figure 11-6. Vasomotor reactivity values from 40 individuals. Middle cerebral artery velocities increase with CO_2 inhalation (52%) (upper curve) and decrease with hyperventilation (35%) *(lower curve). The average total change is 87.8%.*

Embolism Monitoring

Background

The ability of Doppler ultrasound to detect gas emboli in flowing blood was first reported in 1968. High-intensity transient signals in the Doppler ultrasound spectrum were presumed to represent air bubbles, the effect being created by their much higher reflectivity compared with the background flowing blood. The phenomenon was described as a practical early warning system in the study of decompression sickness.[38] This led in 1969 to the ultrasonic detection of arterial air embolism during open heart surgery.[39] In 1986, a series of 19 patients monitored with transcranial Doppler ultrasound during CEA was reported.[40] In 17 of the 19 patients, high-amplitude signals were noted to occur when a shunt was inserted. The authors ascribed these high-amplitude signals to turbulent bloodflow or to microscopic air bubbles. It was noted that the signals had no correlation with adverse clinical outcome.

The first report describing Doppler ultrasound signals thought to represent formed element emboli and their correlation with neurologic deficits postoperatively appeared in 1990.[31] This report also defined and differentiated those high intensity transient signals thought to represent solid emboli from those of air bubbles. Microembolic signals (MES) were defined as: (1) transient (i.e., lasting 0.01 to 0.1 second); (2) occurring randomly; and (3) having amplitudes of 10 decibels (dB) or greater than the background Doppler signal. To the ear, signals defined as indicating emboli were harmonic in tone with a chirping or whistling quality, and distinctly different from those indicating probe motion artifacts. Probe motion artifacts did not have a harmonic quality; were coincident with the motion of the probe or electronic switching; and had a noisy "banging" quality with a broad frequency spectrum, the highest energies of which extended to the lowest frequency ranges. Artifacts were invariably bidirectional. In this study, distinction was made between MES thought to represent air emboli (i.e., very high amplitudes up to 60 dB more than the background Doppler signal) and those of particulate or formed element emboli. Of the 91 patients, 35 (38%) demonstrated what were thought to represent air emboli, and these were related to release of cross clamps following arteriotomy closure. MES with similarity to, but with smaller dynamic range than those associated with air bubble emboli (40 dB or less above the background Doppler signal) were noted in 24 patients (26%). They were noted to occur both spontaneously and upon common artery compression, and also during and after surgical dissection in the intact arterial system. These presumed formed element MES were also noted to occur postoperatively. They did not usually cause postoperative symptoms; however, when they persisted for hours they were associated with strokes and cerebral infarction. This study

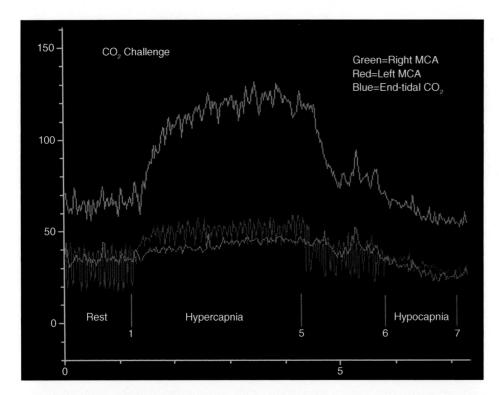

Figure 11-7. Middle cerebral artery (MCA) velocities during a CO_2 challenge test. The time tracing is compressed to show the response throughout normocapnea, hypercapnia, and hypocapnia. The right MCA velocity increases in response to CO_2, whereas the left MCA response is negligible. The left hemisphere is at increased risk of reperfusion injury.

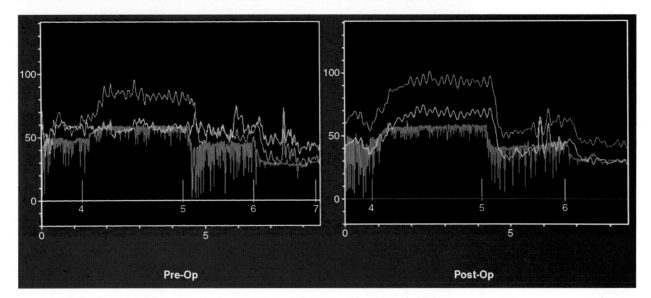

Figure 11-8. The CO_2 challenge test may be used to evaluate VMR and hence hemispheric perfusion in response to cerebral revascularization.

also reported that when MES occurred before surgery, an ulcerated plaque was usually present (Fig. 11-9). These data suggested the ability to detect clinically silent and symptomatic emboli and to demonstrate a mechanism for silent cerebral infarction. The publication of this report suggested intra-arterial embolism could be observed directly by noninvasive means and stimulated much interest in the technique.

One year later, in 1991, the first in vivo experiment was reported.[41] Emboli introduced into a rabbit aorta

(including particulates of clotted whole blood, platelets, atheromatous material, fat, and air) were examined by ultrasound. Over 125 emboli introduced were clearly detected, and it was noted that they caused a Doppler signal of at least 15 dB greater than that of the surrounding blood. Further validation of correlation between MES and air and particulate emboli was reported in another in vivo model (swine) in 1992.[42]

Also in 1992, MES were reported in a series of three patients with recurrently symptomatic extracranial internal

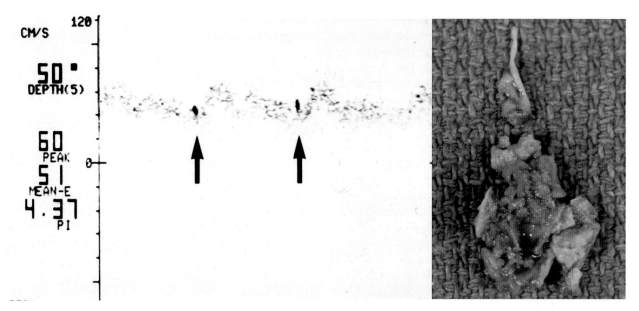

Figure 11-9. *Embolic signals are seen in the MCA waveform of a patient presenting with TIA before carotid endarterectomy. Embolic signals were absent on post-CEA monitoring. Plaque specimen is shown on right.*

carotid artery stenosis or occlusion.[43] Recordings were performed for several hours. Signals were noted only in the territory of the symptomatic internal carotid artery. No emboli were recorded in the internal carotid artery contralateral to the stenosis or the occlusion. MES occurred at a rate of 4.1 per hour. A control group of 10 patients was also monitored. No emboli were found in these subjects. Further correlation between MES and solid emboli (including platelet rich aggregates) was reported using an in vitro model in 1993.[44]

In 1994, TCD embolism monitoring was described as being used in determining both the timing and type of anticoagulation in a series of three patients, two of whom were surgical.[45] The authors concluded that TCD monitoring was able to detect the response of embolism to anticoagulant therapy, and that it was useful in determining the relative efficacy of different regimens, enabling titration of therapy based on embolus counts, and had the potential to eliminate "blind" administration of anticoagulant agents.

In a case report published the same year, heparin was shown to be effective in suppressing MES in a patient presenting with a cerebral infarct.[46]

MES have now been reported in a variety of patient groups with potential embolic sources including carotid stenosis,[47] prosthetic heart valves,[48] myocardial infarction,[49] atrial fibrillation,[50] deep venous thrombosis,[51,52] fat embolism syndrome,[53] cardiopulmonary bypass,[54] carotid angioplasty,[55] and peripheral angioplasty.[56] Most recently there has been direct clinicopathological correlation of MES in the peripheral arterial circulation, where they have been demonstrated to be caused by platelet aggregates.[57]

For the vascular surgeon, particular interest is now focused on postoperative monitoring in carotid endarterectomy, where ongoing embolism has been demonstrated to correlate with neurologic deficits. Correlation of reduction or elimination of such embolization has been demonstrated to confer clinical benefit, and the effects of pharmacologic intervention can be monitored in real time.[58]

Modifications to the basic identification criteria of MES were made in 1995,[59] and a more comprehensive description was published in 1998.[60]

Microembolism Detection in Carotid Endarterectomy

Since the initial report of the detection of emboli in the middle cerebral artery during and in the early postoperative period after CEA,[3] an attempt has been made to correlate the number of microemboli detected in a given period (a rate of microembolism) with postoperative neurologic deficits and silent infarction as demonstrated on brain imaging. Although air embolism is noted to occur commonly during CEA (specifically, when pressure measuring devices are introduced into the internal carotid artery to assess stump pressure and also following release of the clamps after arteriotomy closure), these are now thought to have minimal pathologic consequences. The ability to distinguish between air and particulate emboli has caused some confusion; however, the feature of air emboli that makes them grossly distinguishable from particulates is their large dynamic range (of the order of 60 dB), compared with that of particulates (of the order of 10 dB to 15 dB). Most commercially available machines have been overloaded by signals of such hemodynamic range, and hence air emboli have usually resulted in signals that extend outside the normal velocity waveform of the ultrasound spectrum. Experimental work in animals suggests that this applies to bubbles down to approximately 30 microns in size (i.e., 0.1 microliters or less).[61] Below this size, it is currently impossible to distinguish between large solid emboli and small air emboli.

The first attempt to quantify the number of solid microemboli occurring during CEA that have clinical significance was made in 1995.[62] In patients in whom greater than 10 microemboli were recorded during the procedure, there was a statistically significant relationship with perioperative cerebral complications and with new ischemic lesions on magnetic resonance images of the brain. There was an increased incidence of both intraoperative (p < 0.002) and postoperative (p < 0.02) cerebral complications. Microemboli that occurred during shunting also were also related to intraoperative complications (p < 0.007). It was noted that microembolism did not result in new morphologic changes in postoperative CT scans, although there was a correlation between more than 10 microemboli during dissection and new lesions on postoperative T2-weighted MRI scans (p < 0.005). The authors concluded that surgeons could be guided in the documentation of embolic signals by changing their operative technique with the expectation that a decrease in the incidence of microembolism would result in a decline in the intraoperative stroke rate.

Although the ability to alter operative technique is limited, interest has continued to be focused on postoperative monitoring in the recovery room, a time when most perioperative neurologic events are either noted immediately or observed to evolve. Continuing to monitor in the recovery room has revealed interesting data regarding the occurrence of perioperative events. In a prospective series of 100 patients who underwent endarterectomy with 6-hour postoperative monitoring, dextran 40 infusion was commenced if 25 or more emboli were detected in any 10-minute period.[58] It was noted that 48% of the patients had one or more emboli detected in the postoperative period, the majority of these occurring in the first 2 hours. Only five patients developed sustained embolization requiring administration of dextran. In each of these cases, the embolization was abolished by dextran administration, and during the period of this protocol they recorded a 0% perioperative morbidity and mortality. This compared favorably with their previous postoperative carotid thromboembolic stroke rate, which was 3%. The authors concluded that postoperative embolism monitoring and intervention with dextran in patients who demonstrated sustained high rates of embolization would contribute markedly to an improved perioperative stroke rate.

A lower rate of postoperative microembolism was significant in a report of 65 patients undergoing carotid endarterectomy who were studied at intervals up to 24 hours postoperatively.[63] The study design was open and prospective, with blinded offline analysis of microembolism counts. MES were detected in 69% of the cases during the first hour postoperatively, with counts ranging from 0 to 212 per hour. In seven cases (10.8%), counts were greater than 50 per hour. Five of these seven cases developed ischemic neurologic deficits in the territory of the insonated MCA. It was concluded that frequent signals (greater than 50 MES per hour) occurred in about 10% of cases in the early postoperative phase of endarterectomy, and that they were predictive of the development of ipsilateral focal cerebral ischemia.

The microembolism rate (emboli/hour) that is predictive of ipsilateral cerebral ischemia and that should be used as the threshold for intervention (either pharmacologic or surgical) remains to be elucidated, but it appears even lower rates of embolism are deleterious. In a study analyzing 76 carotid endarterectomy patients retrospectively,[28] only one clinical stroke (1.3%) was noted; however, ipsilateral small areas of silent ischemic change on seven postoperative MRI studies (9%) were noted. Microembolization rates that occurred at a rate of greater than 20 per hour were associated with MRI changes (p < 0.0001). It was concluded that ischemic changes on MRI after endarterectomy are related to postoperative microembolization.

The question remains of what is the best pharmacologic intervention to employ. Although some experience reports complete abolition of embolism with dextran, others have found it to be useful but not completely effective in all cases. In a prospective randomized series of 148 carotid endarterectomy patients utilizing either dextran or placebo,[64] it was noted that in the first postoperative hour there were 118 patients with less than 10 MES per 30 minute recording. Of these, only 3 had ipsilateral TIA, stroke, or stroke-related death, whereas 8 of 22 with greater than 10 MES per 30-minute period had primary events (p < 0.0001). Fifty-eight percent of the patients in the dextran group had no MES, compared with 43% in the placebo group. This difference was statistically significant (p = 0.043). Trends in favor of using dextran during hours 2 to 3, hours 4 to 6, and hours 24 to 36 in the postoperative period were not statistically significant. This study demonstrated that dextran 40 is very effective in reducing the microembolism rate, but it is not successful in all patients. Similar experience has been reported in a series of 79 TCD-monitored carotid endarterectomies in which dextran was also used[65] (Figs. 11-10 and 11-11). Perioperative stroke occurred in two patients in whom dextran only was utilized. These patients had high rates of embolization (greater than 150 emboli per hour). In six other patients who had dextran failure, a IIB-IIIA receptor antagonist (abciximab) was given. In these six patients, abciximab was administered when a persistent rate of greater than 10 emboli

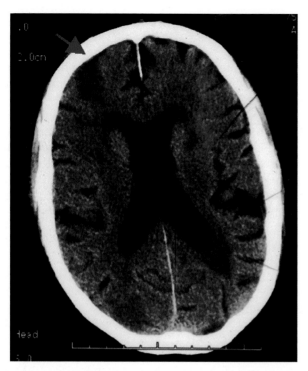

Figure 11-10. Persistent embolic signals in the middle cerebral artery ipsilateral to CEA recorded postoperatively in the recovery room were associated with ipsilateral hemispheric neurologic deficit (upper extremity weakness). At reoperation, embolic signals ceased when the common carotid was reclamped and platelet thrombus was found at the endarterectomy site. Postoperatively on CT a watershed infarct was found in the ipsilateral MCA/ACA territory. The case demonstrated postoperative neurologic deficit caused by platelet embolism from the endarterectomy site.

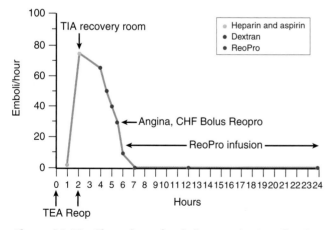

Figure 11-11. Chronology of embolism monitoring of patient in Figure 11-10. High rates of embolism were partially suppressed with dextran; however, the patient developed angina and cognitive heart failure. Complete suppression was achieved with administration of a glycoprotein II_B III_A inhibitor. The patient was on aspirin and the heparin had not been reversed. Some describe this phenomenon as "sticky platelet syndrome."

per hour was recorded while on dextran. No patient in whom embolization was abolished (either by dextran or abciximab) suffered a perioperative stroke.

Transcranial Doppler monitoring has also been used to evaluate S-nitrosoglutathione (NSGO) as adjunctive perioperative antiplatelet therapy.[66] In 12 control patients and 12 experimental patients NSGO was administered from the induction of anesthesia until 2 hours after skin closure. Both groups received standard aspirin and heparin therapy. Dextran was not utilized. The median range of MES detected during the initial 3-hour postoperative recording was markedly reduced in the NSGO group compared with the control group (7.5 vs. 38.5; p = 0.018). This difference persisted until 6 hours after surgery. There were three perioperative events in the control group and none in the NSGO group.

These studies demonstrate that abolition of microembolization following carotid endarterectomy reduces the incidence of both clinical and silent cerebral ischemia. The method demonstrates a quantifiable technique for assessing the efficacy of different anticoagulation regimens in postoperative patients. In the future it can also be expected to provide guidance in determining dosage.

Although the use of balloon angioplasty in the treatment of carotid stenosis is still under evaluation, it is likely to gain increasing acceptance if cerebral embolization can be successfully managed. Cerebral embolization is a major drawback to this technique.[19] It may occur as a result of initial wire and catheter placement, causing dislodgment of atheromatous material during balloon dilatation; or as a result of thrombus formation on the stent. Documenting this problem and the assessment of methods used to control it, whether pharmacologic or mechanical, are best evaluated by TCD monitoring.[67] The role of TCD in carotid stenting is discussed in detail in a separate section.

Embolism Monitoring in the Posterior Cerebral Circulation

Although 25% of brain infarcts involve the vertebrobasilar territory, diagnosis of the etiology of vertebrobasilar insufficiency (VBI) remains imprecise. The location and anatomy of the vertebral arteries and the ill-defined symptom complex of VBI have contributed to the mechanism of cerebral ischemia in vertebrobasilar insufficiency being poorly defined until recently. Current data suggest that embolism is more common than previously suspected.[68]

A recent study evaluated 52 patients presenting with acute or recent vertebrobasilar insufficiency.[69] MES were documented in 10 patients (19.2%) when TCD monitoring of the posterior cerebral artery was performed for a 20-minute period.

The clinical usefulness of embolism monitoring in VBI was demonstrated in a report of four patients in whom embolism monitoring by TCD enabled precise diagnosis of embolism and helped in localization of the embolic source. When these were amenable to surgical management, selection for surgery and decision making for type of surgery were aided. When medical management was selected, the efficacy of the antiplatelet and anticoagulation regimen was able to be assessed. The data suggested a role for embolism monitoring of the vertebrobasilar system by TCD in all patients presenting with vertebrobasilar insufficiency.[70]

Cardiac Surgery

A major concern associated with use of open-heart bypass has been the documentation of a relatively high incidence of both clinical and silent brain infarction and protracted impairment on postoperative psychometric testing.[71] Both phenomena are associated with cerebral embolism. Based on autopsy study, it is estimated that up to 15 million emboli measuring 15 to 70 microns are trapped in cerebral arterioles during the procedure.[72]

Doppler ultrasound has now been used to correlate the rate of microembolization and postoperative cognitive function. In a report of 127 patients, high rates of microembolism (greater than 60 MES) were associated with a higher incidence of central nervous system symptoms including stroke.[73] Cardiac and pulmonary complications and mortality were also higher in the greater than 60 MES group. The authors concluded that intraoperative TCD was useful in assessing operative strategy, the quality of perfusion, and had potential as an indicator for pharmacologic therapy in the operating room. Using a different technique, others have found greater than 100 MES were associated with neurobehavioral deficits.[74]

Microembolism monitoring has also been used to improve the technique of arch cannulation,[75] to introduce neuroprotective agents,[76] and to modify pump components (e.g., filters and tubing). It has also been shown to have predictive value for cerebral ischemia during use of a left ventricular assist device.[77]

Initial concern over the extremely large number of MES seen in the middle cerebral arteries of patients with prosthetic heart valves has now abated. These appear to be caused by cavitation bubbles because they are affected by the oxygen partial pressure.[78,79] This also explains why some investigators have had difficulty documenting reductions in emboli counts with anticoagulation.[80]

Transcranial Doppler monitoring may also be used as a highly sensitive and specific method in the diagnosis of right-to-left shunts. The air microbubbles in an injection of agitated saline administered via an antecubital vein normally do not pass the pulmonary capillaries. In the presence of a right-to-left shunt (e.g., a patent foramen ovale), air MES are detected intracranially several seconds after injection (Fig. 11-12). The technique may be used to assess shunt volume.[81] The method is highly sensitive and specific when compared with transesophageal echocardiography.[82]

Other Uses of TCD

Microembolism monitoring appears to have value in the management of cerebral aneurysms. In a study of 100 patients treated with coil embolization for this condition, microemboli were detected significantly more often in patients who suffered from cerebral ischemia after the procedure.[83] The observation appeared to support the definition of a high-risk group of patients with incomplete embolization or a larger-diameter, broad neck aneurysm. The authors felt that early detection of microemboli after treatment might be an indicator of excessive intraneurysmal thrombus formation and could influence

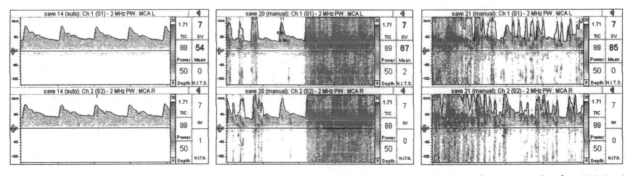

Figure 11-12. *Microembolic signals (air) in the middle cerebral artery of a patient with patent foramen ovale after IV injection of agitated saline.*

the decision for prophylactic treatment with heparin or aspirin.

Fat embolism syndrome is associated with hemorrhagic cerebral infarcts secondary to small vessel occlusion from fat emboli. This occurs spontaneously in the presence of traumatic fractures but is known to be exacerbated by orthopedic procedures.[84] Intramedullary nailing appears to be associated with particularly large numbers of fat globules. In the presence of a patent foramen ovale (PFO), cerebral sequelae may be particularly severe.[85] Embolism monitoring in these patients may be used to guide modification of surgical procedures (as in carotid endarterectomy and coronary bypass) and, by identifying patients with PFO, identify those at particular risk.

In traumatic carotid and vertebral artery injury, MCA monitoring may be used to determine both the hemodynamic effect and embolic potential of these lesions. Their response to antithrombotic and antiplatelet therapy may help to select those patients who require either endovascular or open intervention (Fig. 11-13).

Future Directions

It is apparent that quantification of embolism (i.e., an estimation of "embolus load" or "volume") would be useful to correlate embolic events with potential clinical effects. This requires knowing embolus size as well as frequency. Although embolus detection is sensitive, sizing of emboli remains problematic. Measurements of the embolus-to-blood ratio (EBR) of back-scattered acoustic power, using two different insonation frequencies simultaneously, appears to offer a solution to problems of ultrasound beam refraction artifact and to allow gross discrimination of embolus size; however, application in the clinical setting has yet to be achieved.[86]

Although a consensus regarding what constitutes a true embolic signal is forming, on-line automatic embolus detection will be required in the future. Various efforts have been made in this direction, including neural networks[87] and the use of dual frequency and various signal transformations.[88,89] To date, however, none has been perfected. A Holter system of embolus monitoring in the

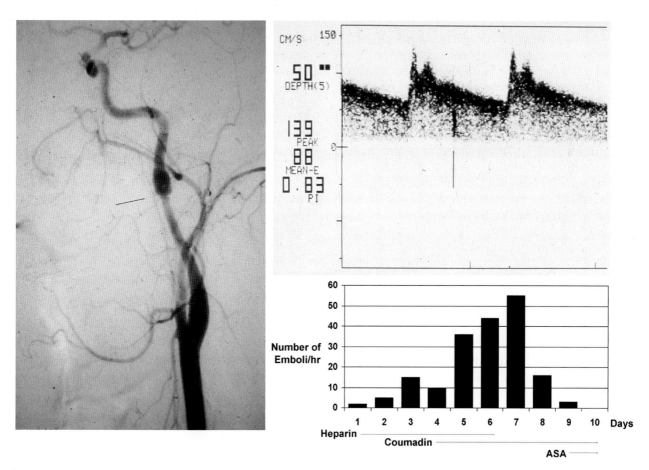

Figure 11-13. Patient was a 26-year-old who sustained carotid injury from a ski pole. Ipsilateral middle cerebral artery embolism was detected and treated with heparin. When persistent embolization was recorded, coumadin was added. Follow-up monitoring recorded persistent embolization that was suppressed with a single dose of aspirin.

absence of an observer will be necessary for the period required to reduce sampling error.

Although in many cases there is a clear-cut relationship between clinical symptomatology and observed embolization, it is clear that silent embolization may occur in many patients with no apparent untoward effects. Presumably this is because of ongoing disaggregation of platelets/fibrinolysis in the presence of an adequate collateral circulation. The status of the collateral circulation is clearly a major determinant of clinical outcome of embolization observed, and greater emphasis on consideration of available collaterals will be fundamental to more clearly defining the clinical significance of ongoing embolization.

Although much observed embolism appears to be "silent," there are two respects in which reconsideration of this apparent "silent" embolization may be interpreted: (1) the observed embolization may indicate a procoagulant or incipient state of more clinically significant embolization; and (2) subclinical embolization may be considered with more concern in the future as imaging techniques are improved. Increasing use of MRI scanning, including diffusion instead of CT scans in acute brain imaging, demonstrates this.

Recent evidence suggests that much observed microembolism consists of platelet aggregates.[57,65,90] Back-scatter characteristics of platelet material can be tested experimentally. If the assumption is made that increased back-scatter energy of a given embolus corresponds to an increase in size, a nomogram of embolus back-scatter energy versus size for platelet emboli should be able to be constructed. This would enable rough estimates of embolus volume delivered to target tissues.

Standardization of equipment and machine settings remains unresolved in current embolus detection. For example, the back-scatter energy of a MES relative to the background flowing blood (embolus-to-blood ratio, or EBR) is related to both instrument gain and sample volume size.[91] Also, some MES may be missed if the time window overlap is insufficient.[92] Both instrument design and data acquisition will need to be standardized to improve the currently large interobserver error.[93] Adoption of the Frankfurt criteria[24] by those reporting embolism and instrument manufacturers can be expected to improve agreement and reproducibility in the future.[94]

Transcranial Doppler in Carotid Artery Stenting (CAS)

As would be expected, the uses of TCD developed for CEA have direct application to CAS. A significant accumulation of TCD monitoring experience with CAS has now been reported.

The Carotid and Vertebral Artery Transluminal Angioplasty Study (CAVATAS) was a randomized prospective trial comparing the safety and efficacy of CEA with carotid PTA with and without stenting. The preliminary report of this trial focused on the transcranial Doppler results.[95] Of 28 patients undergoing either carotid PTA (n = 14) or CEA with shunt (n = 40), CEA was noted to have significantly longer occlusion time (CEA 337 ± 70; PTA 27 ± 10) (p < 0.001); however, there were significantly more embolic signals during PTA; (202 ± 119) than during CEA (52 ± 64) (p = 0.0001). Thus, there was approximately four times the number of microemboli during angioplasty compared with CEA. This difference, however, did not translate into an overall difference in stroke or death rates between the two groups.

In the Leicester trial,[96] a prospective randomized study also confirmed that carotid artery stenting (CAS) generates significantly more embolic particles than does CEA. Although the trial was stopped early, 17 patients were randomized before suspension. There were 10 CEA procedures without complication, but 5 of 7 undergoing CAS had stroke (p = 0.03). The median number of microembolic signals during CEA was 12 (range, 0 to 26), whereas the median number during CAS was 284 (range, 151 to 379) (p = 0.015).

Jordan and colleagues[97] reported 105 patients undergoing 112 procedures (CAS, n = 40; CEA, n = 75), all of whom had TCD monitoring. The CAS procedures had a mean of 74 microembolic signals per stenosis (range, 0 to 398), whereas CEA had a mean of 8.8 microembolic signals per stenosis (range, 0 to 102) (p = 0.0001). Although there were four neurologic events in the CAS group and one neurologic event in the CEA group, this was not significant (p = 0.08). This study therefore demonstrated that CAS was associated with eight times the rate of microemboli compared with CEA.

The introduction of cerebral protection devices during CAS results in a reduction of the number emboli, particularly of the larger sizes, which are more clinically significant. However, these devices do not eliminate all embolization with the device deployed. Embolization also occurs during predilatation of the lesion. TCD monitoring may also be used to observe embolization after the procedure and, as in CEA, to guide the use of antiplatelet agents.

TCD monitoring appears to serve the same function in CAS as in CEA with respect to cerebral reperfusion. Meyers and colleagues[98] reported on 140 patients undergoing CAS; of these, 7 (5%) developed clinical or radiologic manifestations of cerebral hyperperfusion. Six of these patients demonstrated ipsilateral hemispherical edema, and two of these developed ICH. These data would suggest the role of TCD in managing postprocedural cerebral hyperperfusion may be even greater in CAS than in CEA.

In summary, TCD monitoring serves the same function in CAS as in CEA and has now characterized both differences and similarities between the two techniques.

It is able to assess hemispheric perfusion during balloon occlusion, to monitor for microembolization during manipulation, and to diagnose and guide the treatment of reperfusion. It also has the ability to compare the efficacy of the various protection devices.

REFERENCES

1. Aaslid R, Markwalder TM, Nornes H: Noninvasive transcranial Doppler ultrasound recording of flow velocity in basal cerebral arteries. J Neurosurg 58:769–774, 1982.
2. Aaslid R, Huber P, Nornes H: A transcranial Doppler method in the evaluation of cerebrovascular spasm. Neuroradiology 28:11–16, 1986.
3. Spencer MP, Thomas GI, Sauvage LR, et al: Detection of middle cerebral artery emboli during carotid endarterectomy using transcranial doppler. Stroke 21:415–423, 1990.
4. Sandmann W, Willeke F, Kolvenbach R: Shunting and Neuromonitoring: A Prospective Randomized Study. In Greenhalgh RM, Hollier LH (eds): Surgery For Stroke. London: WB Saunders, 1993.
5. Halsey JH Jr: Risks and benefits of shunting in carotid endarterectomy. The International Transcranial Doppler Collaborators. Stroke 23:1583–1587, 1992.
6. Bishop C, Powell S, Rutt D, et al: Transcranial Doppler measurement of middle cerebral artery bloodflow velocity: A validation study. Stroke 17:913–915, 1986.
7. Lindegaard K, Lundar T, Froysaker T, et al: Variations in middle cerebral artery bloodflow investigated with noninvasive transcranial blood velocity measurements. Stroke 18:1025–1030, 1987.
8. Huber P, Handa J: Effect of contrast material, hypercapnia, hyperventilation, hypertonic glucose, and papaverine on the diameter of the cerebral arteries: Angiographic determination in man. Investigational Radiology 2:17–32, 1967.
9. Giller CA, Bowman G, Dyer H, et al: Cerebral arterial diameters during changes in blood pressure and carbon dioxide during craniotomy. Neurosurgery 32:737–741, 1993.
10. Dahl A, Russell D, Nyberg-Hansen R, et al: Effect of nitroglycerin on cerebral circulation measured by transcranial Doppler and SPECT. Stroke 20:1733–1736, 1989.
11. Schregel W, Schafermeyer H, Muller C, et al: The effect of halothane, altentanil, and propofol on bloodflow velocity, blood vessel cross section, and blood volume flow in the middle cerebral artery. Anaesthetist 41:21–26, 1992.
12. Lam AM, Matta BF: Isoflurane does not dilate the middle cerebral artery appreciably. Anesthesia and Analgesia 80:S262, 1995.
13. Schregel W, Schaefermeyer H, Sihle WM, et al: Transcranial Doppler sonography during isoflurane/N20 anaesthesia and surgery: Flow velocity, "vessel area," and "volume flow." Can J Anaesth 41:607–612, 1994.
14. Bissonette B, Leon J: Cerebrovascular stability during isoflurane anaesthesia in children. Can J Anaesth 39:128–134, 1992.
15. Lam AM, Mayberg TS, Eng CC, et al: Nitrous oxide-isoflurane anesthesia causes more cerebral vasodilation than an equipotent dose of isoflurane in humans. Anesth Analg 78:462–468, 1994.
16. Aaslid R, Huber P, Nornes H: Evaluation of cerebrovascular spasm with transcranial Doppler ultrasound. J Neurosurg 60:37–42, 1984.
17. Dahl A, Russell D, Nyberg-Hansen R, et al: A comparison of regional cerebral bloodflow and middle cerebral artery bloodflow velocities: Simultaneous measurements in healthy subjects. J Cereb Bloodflow Metab 12:1049–1054, 1992.
18. Larsen FS, Olsen KS, Hansen BA, et al: Transcranial Doppler is valid for determination of the lower limit of cerebral bloodflow autoregulation. Stroke 25:1985–1988, 1994.
19. North American Symptomatic Carotid Endarterectomy Trial Collaborators. Beneficial effect of carotid endarterectomy in symptomatic patients with high-grade carotid stenosis. N Engl J Med 325:445–453, 1991.
20. European Carotid Surgery Trialists' Group, MRC European Carotid Surgery Trial: Interim results for symptomatic patients with cerebral carotid stenosis and with mild carotid stenosis. Lancet 1:1235–1243, 1991.
21. Executive Committee for the Asymptomatic Carotid Atherosclerosis Study. JAMA 273:1421–1428, 1995.
22. Ouriel K, Shortell CK, Illig KA, et al: Intracerebral hemorrhage after carotid endarterectomy: Incidence, contribution to neurologic morbidity, and predictive factors. J Vasc Surg 1:82–87; discussion 87–89, 1999.
23. Jansen C, Briens EM, Eikelboom BC, et al: Carotid endarterectomy with transcranial Doppler and electroencephalographic monitoring. A prospective study in 130 operations. Stroke 24:665–669, 1993.
24. Steiger HJ, Schaffler L, Liechti S, et al: Results in microsurgical carotid artery endarterectomy. Schweiz Med Wochenschr 119:555–560, 1989.
25. Spencer MP, Thomas GI, Moehring MA: Relation between middle cerebral artery bloodflow velocity and stump pressure during carotid endarterectomy. Stroke 23:1439–1445, 1992.
26. Kalra M, al Khaffaf H, Farrell A, et al: Comparison of measurement of stump pressure and transcranial measurement of flow velocity in the middle cerebral artery in carotid surgery. Ann Vasc Surg 8:225–231, 1994.
27. Jansen C, Ramos LM, van-Heesewijk JP, et al: Impact of microembolism and hemodynamic changes in the brain during carotid endarterectomy. Stroke 25:992, 1994.
28. Cantelmo NL, Babikian VL, Samaraweera RN, et al: Cerebral microembolism and ischemic changes associated with carotid endarterectomy. J Vasc Surg 27:1024–1031, 1998.
29. Piepgras DG, Morgan MK, Sundt TM, et al: Intracerebral hemorrhage after carotid endarterectomy. J Neurosurg 68:532–536, 1988.
30. Jansen C, Sprengers AM, Moll FL, et al: Prediction of intracerebral hemorrhage after carotid endarterectomy by clinical criteria and intraoperative transcranial Doppler monitoring. Eur J Vasc Surg 8:303–308, 1994.
31. Jorgensen LG, Schroeder TV: Defective cerebrovascular autoregulation after carotid endarterectomy. Eur J Vasc Surg 7:370–379, 1993.
32. Nicholls SC, Newell DW: Use of TCD monitoring in revascularization of the vertebral artery. 10th International Symposium on Cerebral Hemodynamics, Munich, Germany, August 1996. Cerebrovascular Diseases 6(Suppl 3):18, 1996.
33. Toole JF: Applied Anatomy and Rmbroyology of the Brain Arteries. In Toole JF (ed): Cerebrovascular Disorders. New York: Raven Press, 1990.
34. Lassen NA: Cerebral bloodflow and oxygen consumption in man. Physiol Rev 39:183–238, 1959.
35. Bloor BM, Asli RP, Nugent GR, Majzoub HS: Relationship of cerebrovascular reactivity to degree of exracranial vascular occlusion. Circulation 28(Suppl II):33–34, 1966.
36. Ringelstein EB, Sievers C, Ecker S, et al: Noninvasive assessment of CO_2-induced cerebral vasomotor response in normal individuals and patients with internal carotid artery occlusions. Stroke 19:963–969, 1988.
37. Kleiser B, Widder B: Doppler CO_2 Test in Carotid Artery Occlusions: Prospective and Retrospective Results. In Schmiedek P, Einhaupl KM, Kirsch H (eds): Stimulated Cerebral Flow. Berlin: Springer, 1992.
38. Spencer MP, Campbell SD, Sealey JL, et al: Experiments on decompression bubbles in the circulation using ultrasonic and electromagnetic flowmeters. J Occup Med 11:238–244, 1969.
39. Spencer MP, Lawrence GH, Thomas GI, et al: The use of ultrasonics in the determination of arterial aeroembolism during open heart surgery. Ann Thorac Surg 8:489–497, 1969.

40. Padayachee TS, Gosling RG, Bishop CC, et al: Monitoring MCA blood velocity during carotid endarterectomy. Br J Surg 73:78–100, 1986.

41. Russell D, Madden KP, Clark WM, et al: Detection of arterial emboli using Doppler ultrasound in rabbits. Stroke 22:253–258, 1991.

42. Nicholls SC, Glickerman DJ, Lam AM: Cerebral embolism transcranial Doppler monitoring in the swine model (abstract). Stroke 23:473, 1992.

43. Siebler M, Sitzer M, Steinmetz H: Detection of intracranial emboli in patients with symptomatic extracranial carotid artery disease. Stroke 23:1652–1654, 1992.

44. Markus H, Brown MM: Differentiating between different pathological cerebral embolic materials using transcranial Doppler in an in vitro model. Stroke 24:1–5, 1993.

45. Nicholls SC, Newell D: Use of transcranial Doppler embolism monitoring in determination of anticoagulation regimens (abstract). Cerebrovascular Diseases 4:21, 1994.

46. Siebler M, Nachtman A, Siebler M: Anticoagulation monitoring and cerebral microemboli (letter). Lancet 344:555, 1994.

47. Siebler M, Nachtman A, Sitzer M, et al: Cerebral microembolism and the risk of ischemia in asymptomatic high grade internal carotid artery stenosis. Stroke 26:2184–2186, 1995.

48. Sliwka U, Georgiadis D: Clinical correlations of Doppler microembolic signals in patients with prosthetic cardiac valves. Stroke 28:1203–1207, 1997.

49. Kitzman DW, Tegeler C, Barber CC, et al: Detection of carotid microemboli following acute myocardial infarction (abstract). Circulation 88:I-223, 1993.

50. Georgiadis D, Lindner A, Manz M, et al: Intracranial microembolic signals in 500 patients with potential cardiac or carotid embolic source and in normal controls. Stroke 28:1203–1207, 1997.

51. Nicholls SC, O'Brien JK, Sutton MG: Venous thromboembolism: Detection by duplex scanning. J Vasc Surg 511–516, 1996.

52. Valdueza JM, Harms L, Doepp F, et al: Venous microembolic signals detected in patients with cerebral sinus thrombosis. Stroke 28(8):1607–1609, 1997.

53. Forteza AM, Koch S, Romano JG, et al: Transcranial Doppler detection of fat emboli. Stroke 30:2687–2691, 1999.

54. Clark RE, Brillman J, Davis DA, et al: Microemboli during coronary artery bypass grafting: Genesis and effect on outcome. J Thorac Cardiovasc Surg 109:249–257, 1995.

55. Markus HS, Clifton A, Buckenham T, et al: Carotid angioplasty: Detection of embolic signals during and after the procedure. Stroke 25:2403–2406, 1994.

56. Al-Hamali S, Baskerville P, Fraser S, et al: Detection of distal emboli in patients with peripheral arterial stenosis before and after iliac angioplasty: A prospective study. J Vasc Surg 29:345–351, 1999.

57. Nicholls SC, Smith W: Peripheral arterial embolization: Doppler ultrasound diagnosis. J Vasc Surg 31:811–814, 2000.

58. Lennard N, Smith JL, Dumville J, et al: Prevention of postoperative thrombotic stroke after carotid endarterectomy: The role of transcranial Doppler ultrasound. J Vasc Surg 26:579–584, 1997.

59. Consensus Committee of the Ninth Cerebral Hemodynamic Symposium: Basic identification criteria of Doppler microembolic signals. Stroke 26:1123, 1995.

60. Ringelstein EB, Droste DW, Babikian VL, et al (International Consensus Group on Microembolic Detection): Consensus statement on microembolic detection by transcranial Doppler ultrasound. Stroke 29:725–729, 1998.

61. Nicholls SC, Glickerman D, Lam A, et al: Cerebral air embolus detection by transcranial Doppler monitoring (abstract). Stroke 24:510, 1993.

62. Ackerstaff RGA, Jansen C, Moll FL, et al: The significance of microemboli detection by means of transcranial Doppler ultrasonography monitoring in carotid endarterectomy. J Vasc Surg 21:936–939, 1995.

63. Levi CR, O'Malley HM, Fell G, et al: Transcranial Doppler detected cerebral microembolism following carotid endarterectomy: High microembolic signal loads predict postoperative cerebral ischaemia. Brain 120(Pt 4):621–629, 1997.

64. Levi CR, Chambers BR, Bladin CF, et al: 10% Dextran 40 reduces microembolic signals after carotid endarterectomy (abstract). Stroke 31:322, 2000.

65. Nicholls SC, Olson A, Moore A, et al: TCD evaluation of antiplatelet therapy for postoperative thromboembolism in carotid endarterectomy (abstract). Stroke 31(1):323, 2000.

66. Molloy J, Martin JF, Baskerville PA, et al: S-Nitrosoglutathione reduces the rate of embolization in humans. Circulation 98:1372–1375, 1998.

67. Crawley F, Stygall J, Lunn S, et al: Comparison of microembolism detected by transcranial Doppler and neuropsychological sequelae of carotid surgery and percutaneous transluminal angioplasty. Stroke 31:1329–1334, 2000.

68. Caplan LR, Tettenborn B: Embolism in the Posterior Circulation. In Bergner R, Caplan LR (eds): Vertebrobasilar Arterial Disease. St. Louis: Quality Medical Publishing, 1992.

69. Koennecke HC, Mast H, Trocio SS, et al: Microemboli in patients with vertebrobasilar ischemia. Stroke 28:593–596, 1997.

70. Nicholls SC, Newell D, Byrd S, et al: Embolization in the Posterior Circulation: TCD Diagnosis. In Klingelhofer J, Bartels E, Ringelstein E (eds): New Trends in Cerebral Hemodynamics and Neurosonology. Amsterdam: Elsevier, 1997.

71. Taylor KM: Brain damage during cardiopulmonary bypass. Ann Thorac Surg 65(4 Suppl):S20–S26; discussion S27–S28, 1998.

72. Moody DM, Bell MA, Challa VR, et al: Brain microemboli during cardiac surgery or aortography. Ann Neurol 59:1304–1307, 1990.

73. Clark RE, Brillman J, Davis DA, et al: Microemboli during coronary artery bypass grafting: Genesis and effect on outcome. J Thorac Cardiovasc Surg 109:249–257, 1995.

74. Hammon J, Stump DA, Kon ND, et al: Risk factors and solutions for the development of neurobehavioral changes after coronary artery bypass grafting. Ann Thorac 63:1613–1618, 1997.

75. Borger MA, Taylor RL, Weisel RD, et al: Decreased cerebral emboli during distal aortic arch cannulation: A randomized clinical trial. J Thorac Cardiovasc Surg 118:740–745, 1999.

76. Arrowsmith JE, Harrison M, Newman SP, et al: Neuroprotection of the brain during cardiopulmonary bypass. Stroke 29:2357–2362, 1998.

77. Nabavi DG, Georgiadis D, Mumme T, et al: Clinical relevance of intracranial microembolic signals in patients with left ventricular assist devices. Stroke 27:891–896, 1996.

78. Kaps M, Hansen J, Weiher M, et al: Clinically silent microemboli in patients with prosthetic heart valves are predominantly gaseous and not solid. Stroke 28:322–325, 1997.

79. Georgiadis D, Wenzel A, Lehman D, et al: Influence of oxygen ventilation on Doppler microemboli signals in patients with artificial heart valves. Stroke 28:2189–2194, 1997.

80. Sturzenegger M, Beer JH, Rihs F, et al: Monitoring combined antithrombotic treatments in patients with prosthetic heart valves using transcranial doppler and coagulation markers. Stroke 26:63–69, 1995.

81. Schwarze JJ, Sander D, Kukla C, et al: Methodological parameters influence the detection of right to left shunts by contrast transcranial Doppler ultrasonography. Stroke 30:1234–1239, 1999.

82. Klotzch C, Janssen G, Berlit P: Transesophageal echocardiography and contrast TCD in the detection of patent foramen ovale: Experiences with 111 patients. Neurology 44:1603–1606, 1994.

83. Klotzch C, Nasher HC, Henkes H, et al: Detection of microemboli distal to cerebral aneurysms before and after therapeutic embolization. Am J Neuroradiol 19:1315–1318, 1998.

84. Herndon JH, Bechtol CO, Crickenberger DP: Use of ultrasound to detect fat emboli during total hip replacement. Acta Orthop Scand 46:108–118, 1975.

85. Edmonds CR, Barbut D, Hager D, et al: Comparison of cerebral embolization during total hip arthroplasty and coronary bypass surgery (abstract). Ann Thorac Surg 64:924, 1997.

86. Moehring MA, Ritcey JA: Sizing emboli in blood using pulsed Doppler ultrasound. IEEE Transactions on Biomedical Engineering 43:572–588, 1996.

87. Kemeny V, Droste DW, Hermes S, et al: Automatic embolus detection by a neural network. Stroke 30:807–810, 1999.

88. Brucker R, Russell D: Improved discrimination of microembolic events by combining dual frequency Doppler with wavelet transformation (abstract). Cerebrovasc Dis 9:37, 1999.

89. Aydin N, Padyachee S, Markus HS: The use of the wavelet transform to describe embolic signals. Ultrasound Med Biol 25:9538, 1999.

90. Goertler M, Baeumer M, Kross R, et al: Rapid decline of cerebral microemboli of arterial origin after intravenous acetylsalicyclic acid. Stroke 30:66–69, 1999.

91. Droset DW, Markus HS, Brown M: The effect of different settings of ultrasound pulse amplitude, gain and sample volume on the appearance of emboli: Studies in a transcranial Doppler model. Cerebrovasc Dis 4:152–156, 1994.

92. Markus H: Importance of time window overlap in the detection and analysis of embolic signals. Stroke 26:2044–2047, 1995.

93. Markus HS, Ackerstaff R, Babikian V, et al: Intercenter agreement in reading Doppler embolic signals: A multicenter international study. Stroke 28:1307–1310, 1997.

94. Evans DH: Cerebral embolism and Doppler ultrasound. Cardiovasc Dis 9:189–191, 1999.

95. Crawley F, Clifton A, Buckenham T, et al: Comparison of hemodynamic cerebral ischemia and microemboic signals detected during CEA and carotid angioplasty. Stroke 28:2460–2464, 1997.

96. Naylor AR, Bolia A, Abbott RJ, et al: Randomized study of carotid angioplasty and stenting vs. CEA: A stopped trial. J Vasc Surg 28:326–334, 1998.

97. Jordan WD, Voellinge DC, Doblar DD, et al: Microemboli detected by TCD monitoring in patients during carotid angioplasty vs. CEA. Cardiovasc Surg 7:33–38, 1999.

98. Meyers PM, Higashida RT, Phatouros CC, et al: Cerebral hyperfusion syndrome after percutaneous transluminal stenting of the craniocervical arteries. Neurosurgery 47:335–343, 2000.

Chapter 12

Evaluation of Carotid Plaque Morphology

ANDREW N. NICOLAIDES • MAURA GRIFFIN • STAVROS K. KAKKOS • GEORGE GEROULAKOS • EFTHYVOULOS KYRIAKOU

Introduction

Carotid bifurcation disease has two main clinical manifestations: (1) asymptomatic bruits; and (2) cerebrovascular syndromes, such as amaurosis fugax, transient ischemic attacks (TIAs), and stroke, which are often the result of plaque erosion or rupture with subsequent thrombosis producing occlusion or embolization.[1,2] Internal carotid artery stenosis, the main consequence of atherosclerotic disease of the carotid bifurcation, remains the single preventable cause of ischemic stroke. Recent studies involving angiography; high-resolution ultrasound; thrombolytic therapy; plaque pathology; coagulation studies; and, more recently, molecular biology, have implicated atherosclerotic plaque rupture as a key mechanism responsible for the development of acute coronary syndromes and cerebrovascular events.[3–5]

Atherosclerotic plaques consist of a lipid-rich core and a fibrous cap that separates the core from the lumen. The lipid-rich core contains T cells and lipid-laden macrophages (foam cells), which are derived from blood monocytes.[3] T cells produce interferon-γ, which suppresses the production of collagen by the smooth muscle cells[4] and stimulates the macrophages to produce metalloproteinases (e.g., stromelysins, gelatinases, and collagenases), which digest existing collagen and other extracellular matrix components. In addition, foam cells produce tissue factor, which stimulates thrombus formation when in contact with blood after plaque rupture.

Rupture-prone plaques tend to have a large lipid core, a thin fibrous cap, few smooth muscle cells, and an abundance of macrophages.[5] Ruptured plaques heal or enlarge by incorporating the thrombus formed on their surface. Some thrombi grow and occlude the lumen or produce emboli. Whether a thrombus will occur or enlarge depends on the local bloodflow and the hypercoagulable state.

Conventional arteriography has been used for several decades to investigate the presence and severity of internal carotid artery stenosis. Because it is invasive and carries a 1.2% risk of stroke, it cannot be repeated frequently. In addition, angiography provides little information on plaque structure. The development and continuing technical improvement of noninvasive, high-resolution vascular ultrasound has enabled us to study the presence; rate of progression (or regression); and, most importantly, the consistency of plaques. A number of ultrasonic characteristics of unstable (vulnerable) plaques have been determined,[6-9] and populations or individuals at increased risk for cardiovascular events can now be identified.[10] In addition, high-resolution ultrasound has enabled us to identify the different ultrasonic characteristics of unstable carotid plaques associated with amaurosis fugax, TIAs, stroke, and different patterns of computed tomography (CT) brain infarction.[6-8] This information has provided new insight into the pathophysiology of the different clinical manifestations of extracranial atherosclerotic cerebrovascular disease by using noninvasive methods.

This chapter highlights the advances of high-resolution ultrasound in carotid plaque characterization and their clinical importance.

The Need for B-Mode Image Normalization: Description of the Method

High-resolution ultrasound provides information not only on the degree of carotid artery stenosis but also on the characteristics of the arterial wall including the size and consistency of the atherosclerotic plaque. Different classifications according to plaque consistency have been proposed in the literature, resulting in considerable confusion. For example, plaques containing medium or high-level uniform echoes were classified as homogenous by Reilly[11]; these correspond closely to Johnson's dense and calcified plaques,[12] to Gray-Weale's type 3 and 4,[13] and to Widder's type I and II plaques[14] (i.e., echogenic or hyperechoic).

The most popular and most commonly used ultrasonic plaque classification is based on the Gray-Weale classification as modified by Geroulakos[15] in 1993. It is defined below with examples shown in Figures 12-1 through 12-5.

- Type 1: Uniformly echolucent plaques with or without a thin fibrous cap (see Fig. 12-1)
- Type 2: Predominantly echolucent plaques with less than 50% echogenic areas (see Fig. 12-2)
- Type 3: Predominantly echogenic plaques with less than 50% echolucent areas (see Fig. 12-3)

- Type 4: Uniformly echogenic plaques (see Fig. 12-4)
- Type 5: Heavily calcified plaques that cannot be classified accurately because of acoustic shadow (see Fig. 12-5)

A recent consensus on carotid plaque characterization suggested that echodensity should reflect the overall

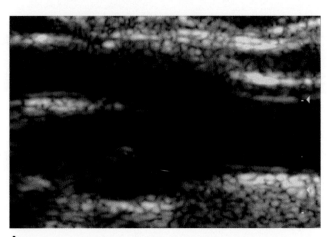

A

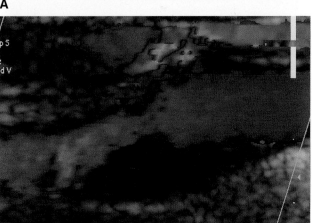

B

*Figure 12-1. Uniformly echolucent plaque, without (**A**) and with (**B**) the color Doppler.*

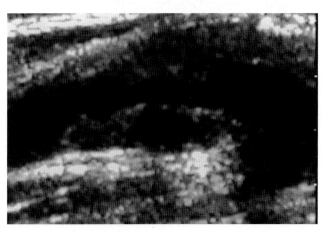

Figure 12-2. Type 2: Predominantly echolucent plaque with less than 50% echogenic areas.

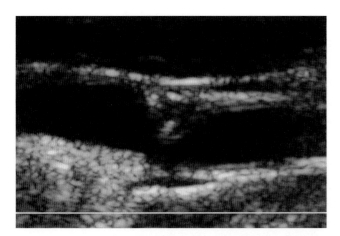

Figure 12-3. Type 3: Predominantly echogenic plaque with less than 50% echolucent areas.

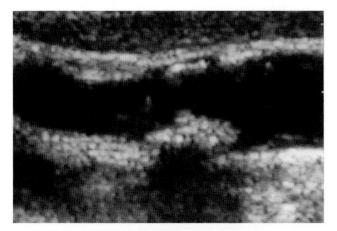

Figure 12-4. Type 4: Uniformly echogenic plaque.

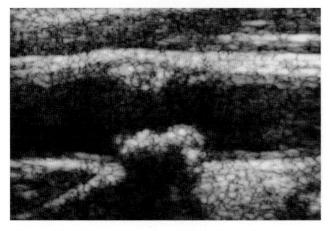

Figure 12-5. Type 5: Heavily calcified plaque that cannot be classified accurately because of acoustic shadow.

brightness of the plaque, with the term hyperechoic referring to echogenic plaques and the term *hypoechoic* referring to echolucent plaques.[16] Plaque echodensity should be compared with reference structures: for hypoechoic plaques, the blood; for isoechoic plaques, the

sternomastoid muscle; and for hyperechoic plaques, the bone of the adjacent cervical vertebra.

There is enough evidence published to support the potential clinical usefulness of ultrasonic plaque characterization. Patients with hypoechoic carotid plaques are at increased risk for stroke. Polak has recently investigated the association between stroke and internal carotid artery plaque echodensity.[17] In his study, plaques were subjectively characterized as hypoechoic, isoechoic, or hyperechoic in relation to the surrounding soft tissues. The stroke rate for hypoechoic plaques was 2.78 times higher than that for isoechoic and hyperechoic plaques. The authors suggested that quantitative methods of grading carotid plaque echomorphology (e.g., computer-assisted plaque characterization, developed by our group) might be more precise in determining the association between hypoechoic (echolucent) plaques and the incidence of stroke.

Computer-assisted plaque characterization involves processing of digitized B-mode images of plaques taken from a duplex scanner with fixed instrument settings including gain and time control. The median of the frequency distribution of gray values of the pixels within the plaque (gray scale median or GSM) is used as the measurement of overall plaque echodensity. In a personal computer (PC), the gray levels of the pixels are usually coded on a scale of 0 to 255 (0 = black, 255 = white) for an 8-bit image (2^8 = 256 shades of gray). Early work by our team has demonstrated that plaques with a GSM of less than 32 (i.e., hypoechoic plaques) are associated with a fivefold increase in the prevalence of silent brain infarcts on CT-brain scans.[18] Similar results were obtained by another team, but the cut-off point for the GSM was 50 instead of 32.[19] Soon it became apparent that ultrasonic image normalization was necessary so that images captured under different instrument settings, from different scanners, by different operators, and through different peripherals (e.g., video or magneto-optical disk) could be made comparable.

As a result, a method has been developed to normalize images by means of digital image processing using blood and adventitia as the two reference points.[20] With the use of commercially available software (e.g., Adobe Photoshop version 3.0 or later) and the histogram facility, the GSM of the two reference points (blood and adventitia) in the original B-mode image is determined. Algebraic (linear) scaling of the image is performed with the curves option of the software so that in the resultant image the GSM of blood equals 0 to 5 and that of the adventitia equals 185 to 195. Thus, brightness of all pixels in the image, including those of the plaque, becomes adjusted according to the two reference points. This results in a significant improvement in the comparability of the ultrasonic tissue characteristics.[21,22] The various steps in image normalization are shown in Figure 12-6. Accurate selection of the appropriate areas of blood and adventitia for image normalization and

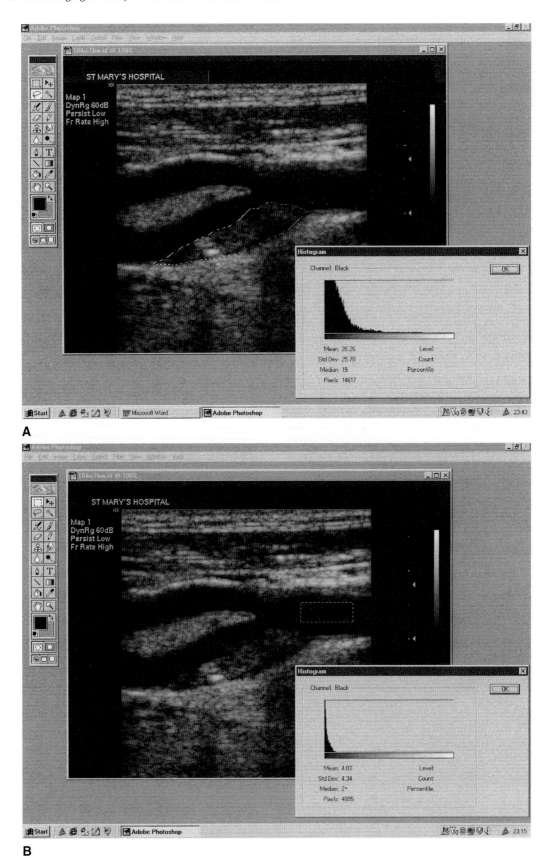

Figure 12-6. **A**, *Before normalization. Histogram of plaque pixels (area of interest) and gray scale median of 19.* **B**, *Histogram and gray scale median 2 of pixels representing blood.*

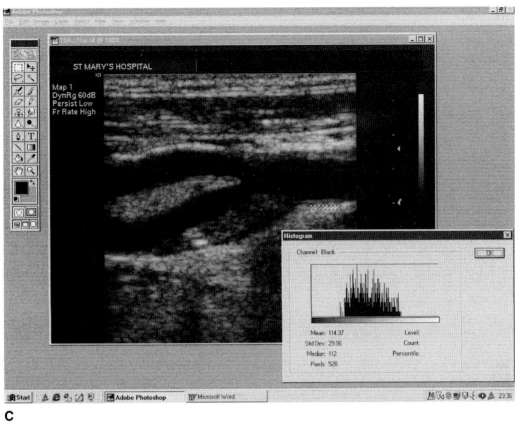

C

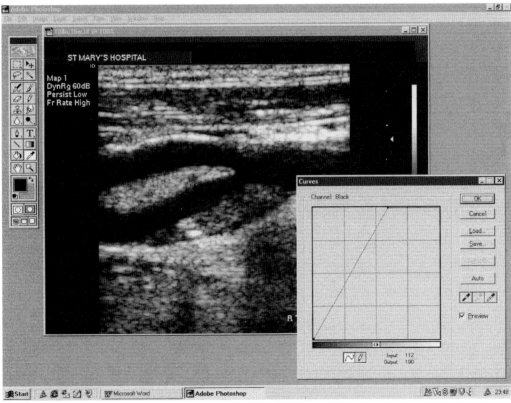

D

Figure 12-6, cont'd. **C**, *Histogram and gray scale median 112 of pixels of adventia. Inset shows sampling of middle two fourths of adventitia after magnification.* **D**, *Linear scaling using the curves facility of Adobe Photoshop. No change has been made in the blood reference point, but gray level of 112 has been changed to 190 (arrow points at horizontal line representing gray level of 190).*

Continued

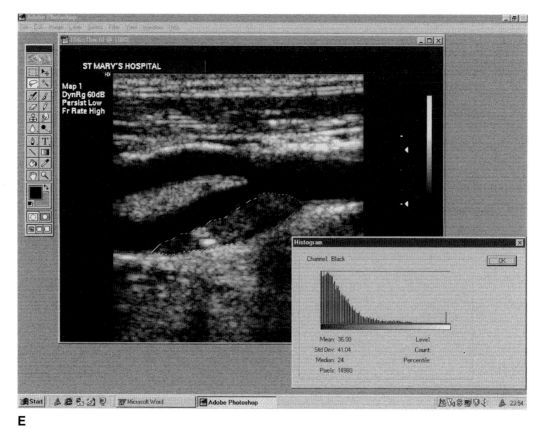

E

Figure 12-6, cont'd. **E,** *After normalization. Histogram of plaque pixels (area of interest) and gray scale median of 24.*

the avoidance of areas of acoustic shadow in the selection of the plaque area are imperative.

Although image normalization can compensate for moderate changes in overall gain or time gain compensation curve (TGC) settings, it cannot do so in extreme situations when practically the whole image, including blood, is white (very high gain); or very dark, when there is lack of information (very low gain). Thus for best results the following duplex settings are recommended: maximum dynamic range, low persistence, and high frame rate. A high-frequency linear array transducer (ideally, 7 to 10 MHz) should be used. A high dynamic range ensures a wide range of gray scale values. High frame rate ensures good temporal resolution. In addition to these presets, the TGC should be positioned vertically through the lumen of the vessel because there is little attenuation of the ultrasound beam as it passes through blood. The overall gain should be adjusted to give optimum image quality (i.e., bright echoes with minimum noise in the blood). It should be increased until there is noise in the blood, and then reduced slowly until there are black areas in the lumen. A linear postprocessing curve should also be used; and finally, where possible, the ultrasound beam should be at 90 degrees to the arterial wall.

The above guidelines should result in the following:

- An area of noiseless blood
- A hyperechoic area of adventitia in the vicinity of the plaque
- Visualization of the extent and borders of the plaque (It is here that color or power Doppler can provide further information about plaque outline.)

Pitfalls of Image Normalization

There are three major causes that would lead to inaccuracy in the normalization process. As already stated, it is imperative that certain prerequisites should be observed in order that the ideal image for this process is captured.

Excess Noise in the Vessel Lumen

Too much noise within the lumen of the vessel does not allow the operator to assess the gray levels of blood. If normalization is attempted it results in an overall darker image. This could result in the loss of information from the plaque itself, especially in the case of a thin fibrous cap.

Plaque or Adventitia Not at 90 Degrees to Ultrasound Beam

When a plaque is not captured at 90 degrees to the ultrasound beam it becomes hard to delineate its borders clearly; therefore, one can easily underestimate its size and components, which in turn, leads to erroneous pixel numbers and GSM values.

Absence of Well-Defined Adventitia on Captured Image

A lack of well-defined adventitia adjacent to the plaque often results in an image that is too bright after normalization. This overcompensation will, in turn, result in falsely high GSM values.

Thus, to summarize, if normalization is to achieve the desired reproducible effect, it is essential to follow these prerequisites:

- One must be able to identify a plaque and its outline clearly

- Provide an image with an area of noiseless blood

- Ensure there is a segment of adventitia adjacent to the plaque that is clearly visible and at right angles to the ultrasound beam

- Use color mapping, especially with very echolucent plaques

Training is both important and necessary. Where possible, the individual performing the scans should be familiar with the normalization technique because understanding the steps involved in this process will result in the acquisition of images that contain all the essential ingredients that will allow normalization with reproducible results.

Reproducibility Studies

Three major reproducibility studies have been performed in order to establish the validity of the method of image normalization and the value of GSM measurements.[20-22] These studies have demonstrated that the GSM of a plaque after image normalization is a highly reproducible measurement that can be used in natural history studies of asymptomatic carotid atherosclerotic disease, aiming to identify patients at higher risk for stroke. The first reproducibility study[20] has shown that image normalization reduces significantly the GSM difference when using different scanners, multifrequency linear array probes, and storage media (e.g., videotape and magneto-optical disk). Interobserver variability in normalizing B-mode images obtained from a single scanner (i.e., HDI 3000, Advanced Technology Laboratories, Bothell, WA) revealed a mean GSM difference of $-1 + 6.3$ (limits of agreement by the Bland and Altman method $+ 2SD = 12.6$). This has enabled us to define the limits of experimental error so that this method can be used

to identify real changes in the echodensity of the atherosclerotic plaques in longitudinal studies using high-resolution ultrasound. The second study[21] assessed the interobserver, interscanner, and the gain variability before and after normalization, in terms of plaque echotexture. The results indicated that normalization reduced the interscanner and gain-level variability, allowing the demonstration of a significantly lower GSM of the symptomatic plaques from the asymptomatic ones. Such a demonstration was not possible before normalization. The third study[22] confirmed the above and demonstrated that the median GSM of plaques associated with ipsilateral nonlacunar silent CT-brain infarction was 14, whereas that of plaques not associated with infarcts was 30 ($p = 0.003$).

It has already been pointed out that training is essential if the level of reproducibility reported above is to be achieved. Training is necessary not only in the use of the software but also in the appropriate scanning technique. For an experienced ultrasonographer, training requires 2 days.

Plaque Texture Features Other Than Overall Echodensity

Plaque Classification

The rationale of plaque classification as described above has been the expectation and hope to determine a relationship between plaque features and symptoms. The problems encountered have been the lack of uniformity in definition, variability in operator experience (especially with gain settings), and the quality of the equipment. It has now become possible to improve the reproducibility of plaque characterization by doing image normalization, plaque gray scale contouring, and using a slightly modified definition of the Geroulakos classification. After image normalization pixels in the range of 0 to 25 are given a pixel gray value of 0, pixels in the range of 26 to 51 are given a value of 26 and so on, so that an image of a contoured plaque is achieved (10 contours in total). A contoured plaque is easier to be classified visually. Figure 12-7 shows the effect of contouring on plaques.

The Geroulakos classification[15] can now be redefined in terms of pixels and gray levels, which makes it amenable to classification by computer.

- Type 1: Hypoechoic plaques in which less than 15% of the pixels have a gray scale greater than 25

- Type 2: Mainly hypoechoic plaques in which 15% to 50% of the pixels have a gray scale greater than 25

- Type 3: Mainly hyperechoic plaques in which 51% to 85% of the pixels have a gray scale greater than

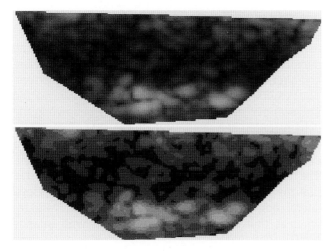

Figure 12-7. Effect of contouring. Digitized plaque before (above) *and after* (below) *contouring.*

25 (or 15% to 50% of the pixels have a gray scale less than 25)

- Type 4: Hyperechoic plaques in which more than 85% of the pixels have a gray scale greater than 25 (or less than 15% of the pixels have a gray scale less than 25)
- Type 5: Plaques with extensive calcification and acoustic shadowing so that it is impossible to visualize or assess the substance of the plaque. In

plaques with small areas of calcification, the area of acoustic shadowing is not included in the area of plaque selected for image analysis.

Table 12-1 shows the classification of 988 carotid plaques of patients in the ACSRS natural history study before image normalization using the original Geroulakos classification; and after image normalization, when the modified Geroulakos classification was used. It can be seen that using the original classification, 120 plaques were type 1; 258 were type 2; 286 were type 3; 155 were type 4 and 169 were type 5. After image normalization and reclassification, there was a marked change. For example, of the 120 plaques originally classified as type 1, only 54 (45%) remained as type 1; 43 (36%) became type 2; 12 (10%) became type 3; 10 (8.3%) became type 4; and 1 (0.8%) became type 5. The changes in classification resulted in a low kappa statistic of 0.215.

The distribution of neurologic events (atrial fibrillation [AF], TIAs, and strokes) that occurred during follow-up in relation to the type of plaque before and after image normalization are shown in Tables 12-2 and 12-3, respectively. Before image normalization, 61 of the 92 events (66%) were associated with plaque types 2 and 3. After image normalization, 83 of the 92 events (90%) were associated with plaque types 2 and 3. These findings emphasize the importance of image normalization and may explain the lack of definitive conclusions from studies performed in the past.

TABLE 12-1. The Distribution of Ipsilateral Plaque Types in 988 Patients Before and After Image Normalization (Kappa 0.215)

Plaque Type After Image Normalization (New Geroulakos Classification)		1	2	3	4	5	Total
Plaque Type Before Image	1	54 (45%)	43 (36%)	12 (10%)	10 (8.3%)	1 (0.8%)	120 (100%)
Normalization (Old	2	33 (13%)	147 (57%)	54 (21%)	20 (7.8%)	4 (1.6%)	258 (100%)
Geroulakos Classification)	3	13 (4.5%)	81 (28%)	114 (40%)	64 (22%)	14 (5%)	286 (100%)
	4	4 (3%)	37 (24%)	41 (26%)	59 (38%)	14 (9%)	155 (100%)
	5	3 (2%)	32 (19%)	72 (43%)	46 (27%)	16 (10%)	169 (100%)
	Total	107 (11%)	340 (34%)	293 (30%)	199 (20%)	49 (5%)	988 (100%)

TABLE 12-2. Distribution of Ipsilateral Neurologic Events That Occurred During Follow-Up, in Relation to Type of Plaques Before Image Normalization

Ipsilateral Neurologic Events		Absent	Present	Total
Ipsilateral Plaque Type	1	114	6 (5%)	120 (100%)
	2	222	36 (14%)	258 (100%)
	3	261	25 (8.7%)	286 (100%)
	4	140	15 (9.7%)	155 (100%)
	5	159	10 (5.9%)	169 (100%)
	Total	805	92 (9.3%)	988 (100%)

TABLE 12-3. **Distribution of Ipsilateral Neurologic Events That Occurred During Follow-Up In Relation to Type of Plaques After Image Normalization**

Ipsilateral Neurologic Events		Absent	Present	Total
Ipsilateral Plaque Type	1	100	7 (6.5%)	107 (100%)
	2	293	47 (13.8%)	340 (100%
	3	257	36 (12.3%)	293 (100%)
	4	198	1 (0.5%)	199 (100%)
	5	48	1 (2.0%)	49 (100%)
	Total	806	92 (9.3%)	988 (100%)

Homogeneity/Heterogeneity

The consensus on carotid plaque characterization has suggested that measurements of texture should not be confused with measurements of echodensity.[16] The term *homogenous* should refer to plaques of uniform consistency, irrespective of whether they are predominantly hypoechoic or hyperechoic (Fig. 12-8). The term *heterogenous* should be used for plaques of nonuniform consistency (i.e., having both hypoechoic and hyperechoic areas; Fig. 12-9). Although O'Donnell in 1985[23] and Aldoori in 1987[24] proposed this otherwise simple classification, there has been a considerable degree of diversity in terminology used by others.

Leahy defined heterogenous plaques as those that contained echolucent areas, and homogenous plaques as those with uniform consistency suggestive of sclerotic plaques.[25] Sterpetti defined heterogenous plaques as those that contained mixed high-, medium-, and low-level echoes; and homogenous plaques as those having uniformly high- or medium-level echoes.[26] Langsfeld defined heterogenous plaques as those that were either predominantly echolucent with a thin "eggshell" cap of echogenicity, or echogenic plaques with substantial areas of echolucency.[27] AbuRahma defined heterogenous plaques as those composed of a mixture of hyperechoic, isoechoic, and hypoechoic areas.[28] The authors who used the above definitions indicated that heterogenous plaques were more commonly symptomatic, or tended to become symptomatic during follow-up more often than did homogenous plaques. In all these studies the uniformly or near-uniformly echolucent plaques that were relatively rarely seen tended to be included within the heterogenous group.

The authors' group has attempted to devise measurements such as heterogeneity index by measuring the GSM difference between the most echogenic and most echolucent plaque areas,[29] or to measure the relative ratio between echogenic and echolucent areas.[20,30] Their studies indicated that symptomatic plaques had large black areas and thus tended to be not only heterogenous but more hypoechoic than asymptomatic plaques. It became obvious that an objective measurement of heterogeneity that could be adopted universally was lacking.

It is now realized that heterogenous plaques are more likely to be associated with symptoms than homogenous (i.e., uniformly echolucent or uniformly echogenic) plaques. However, heterogenous plaques that have large black areas and thus a low GSM are even more likely to give rise to symptoms, especially if the black areas are close to the lumen[8,9] (see the following).

More recently, Pedro and colleagues[8,9] divided plaques subjectively after image normalization according to the ultrasonographic uniformity of plaque echostructure appearance. When it was regular and uniform, the plaque was classified as homogenous; if identification of areas of different echogenicity was possible, the lesion was classified as heterogenous and the presence of hypo- and hyperechogenic areas located in relation to its lumen surface was noted. Symptomatic plaques had a lower GSM and a more common plaque surface disruption than did asymptomatic plaques, irrespective of whether they were homogenous (odds ratio 8.9; 95% CI 2.3 to 32.9) or heterogenous (odds ratio 6.2; 95% CI 2.6 to 14.8). However, a juxtaluminal location of an echolucent region (Fig. 12-9C) was more common in symptomatic heterogenous plaques than in asymptomatic heterogenous plaques (odds ratio 6.8; 95% CI 1.8 to 21.2). On the basis of these findings, plaques could be classified into symptomatic or asymptomatic with an accuracy close to 80%. This is the first time a combination of several ultrasonic features determined after image normalization has been used to assess plaque stability.

Ultrasonic Plaque Ulceration

The association between maroscopic plaque ulceration and the development of embolic symptoms (e.g., AF, TIAs, and stroke) and signs such as silent infarcts on CT brain scans has been described by many authors.[2,31–34] However, the ability to identify plaque ulceration using ultrasound has been questioned. Reports in the literature show that the sensitivity of ultrasound in predicting ulceration ranges from less than 30% to greater than 90%.[11,14,35–41] It is interesting that the sensitivity is high (77%) when the stenosis is less than 50%, and it is low (41%) when the stenosis is greater than 50%. This

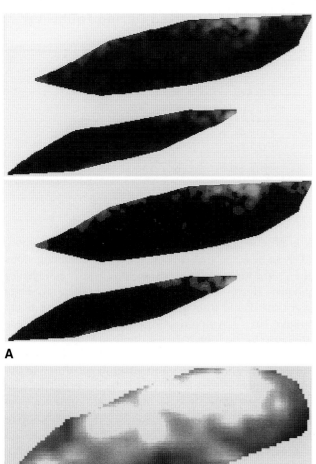

A

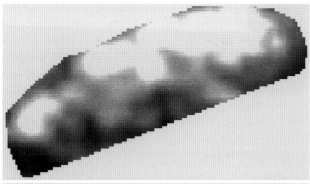

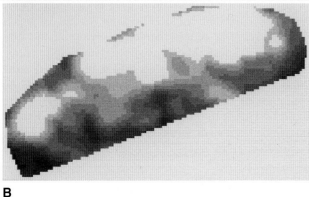

B

Figure 12-8. **A,** *Homogenous plaque uniformly echolucent (hypoechoic) type 1 plaque.* **B,** *Uniformly echogenic (hyperechoic) type 4 plaque.*

indicates that ulceration is much easier to detect in the presence of mild stenosis, when the residual lumen and plaque surface are more easily seen, than with severe stenosis, when the residual lumen and the surface of the plaque are not easily defined because they are not always in the plane of the ultrasound beam. In a series

of 17 carotid plaques, a new promising approach has been to use three-dimensional ultrasound to study plaque surface configuration.[42] The results of large series are awaited.

Two recent studies involving relatively large numbers have investigated plaque surface characteristics and the type of plaque in relation to symptomatology. The first one was a retrospective analysis of 578 symptomatic patients (242 with stroke and 336 with TIAs) recruited for the B-scan Ultrasound Imaging Assessment Program. A matched case-control study design was used to compare brain hemispheres with ischemic lesions to unaffected contralateral hemispheres with regard to the presence and characteristics of carotid artery plaques. Plaques were classified as smooth when the surface had a continuous boundary, irregular when there was an uneven or pitted boundary, and pocketed when there was a crater-like defect with sharp margins. The results demonstrated an odds ratio of 2.1 for the presence of an irregular surface, and of 3.0 for hypoechoic plaques in carotids associated with TIAs and stroke.[43]

The second study included 258 symptomatic and 65 asymptomatic patients. Carotid plaque morphology was classified according to Gray-Weale,[13] and plaque surface features were assessed. The results demonstrated that plaque types 1 and 2 were more common in symptomatic patients; the incidence of ulceration was 23% in the symptomatic group vs. 14% in the asymptomatic group (p = 0.04).[44]

As far as the authors can tell, prospective natural history studies in which high-resolution ultrasound has been used with carefully designed methodology and criteria for identifying plaque ulceration are lacking. Thus, clinical decisions cannot currently be made on the basis of ultrasonic ulceration. However, if the findings of black areas close to the lumen[8,9] can be substantiated by further studies, then this strong indicator of risk may make the presence or absence of true ulceration as defined by ultrasound unnecessary.

Computer Texture Analysis Using the Distribution of Gray Scale Levels of the Image Pixels

Ultrasonic texture characterization using computer algorithms has been successfully applied to liver images.[45,46] A software package has been developed that can be used to analyze ultrasonic images of plaques. This package has four main modules (Fig. 12-10). The first provides a user-friendly way to normalize images (Figure 12-10A). The second provides a means of calibration and of making measurements in millimeters (Figure 12-10B). The third provides the user with a means of selecting the area of interest (plaque) and saving it as a separate file (Figure 12-10C). The fourth (Figure 12-10D) extracts a number of texture features and saves them on a file for subsequent statistical

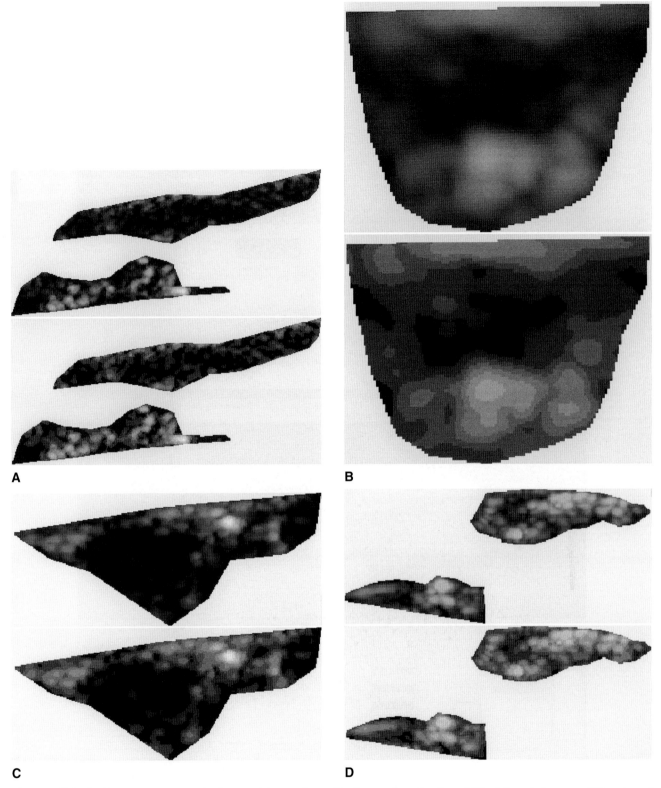

Figure 12-9. **A**, *Heterogenous type 2 plaque without a large black area (greater than 15% of the whole area of the plaque) adjacent to the lumen.* **B**, *Heterogenous type 2 plaque with a black area in the centre of the plaque, not adjacent to the lumen.* **C**, *Heterogenous type 2 plaques with a black area adjacent to the lumen.* **D**, *Homogenous (hyperechoic) type 4 plaque (new Geroulakos classification with a small (less than 15% of total plaque area) close to base of the plaque. Both components of the plaque (anterior and posterior wall) are shown.*

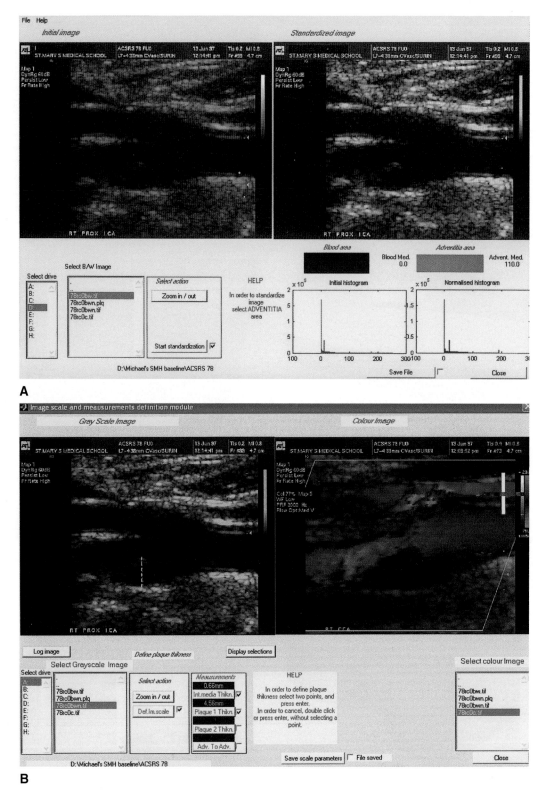

Figure 12-10. **A**, *User-friendly method of image normalization. Original image is on the left. By sampling pixels representing blood and pixels of center of adventitia after magnification, the normalized image is produced on the right. This image can be shared in a database.* **B**, *The measurements module provides a display for both the black and white and the color image. Using the calibration markers, measurements of distance and area can be made in mm and mm².*

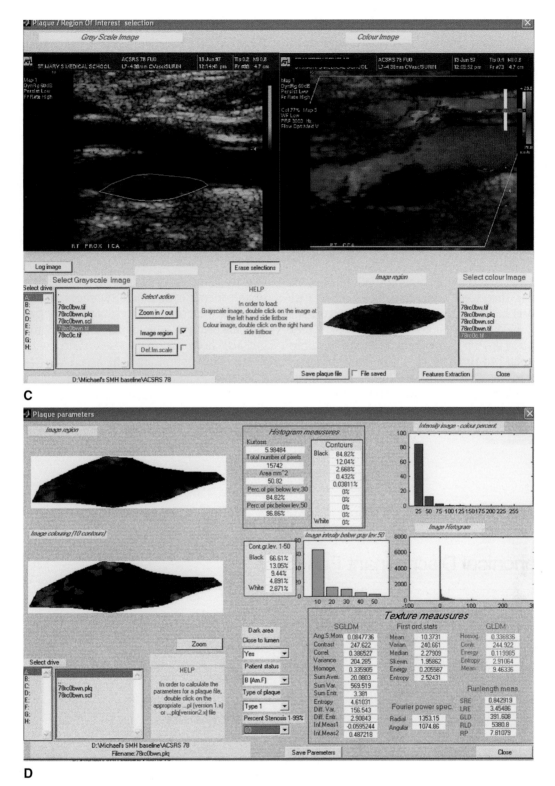

Figure 12-10, cont'd. C, *This module provides the facility for outlining the plaque (area of interest) and saving it in a database as a separate file.* **D**, *This module extracts a large number of well-established standard first-order and second-order statistical features used in image analysis. They can be saved on a database for subsequent analysis. The program allows additional impact on the presence of a dark area adjacent to the lumen, the patient's symptomatology, the type of plaque, and percent carotid stenosis.*

analysis. This package was tested in a cross-sectional study of 409 patients referred to the vascular laboratory for diagnostic duplex scanning. Of these, 242 were asymptomatic, 40 presented with amaurosis fugax, 72 with TIAs, and 55 with stroke. Plaques were classified into three main groups (Fig. 12-11) on the basis of image normalization and six features, three (homogeneity, angular second movement, and correlation) based on the spatial gray level dependence matrix method (SGLDM); plaque type (1–5); GSM; black area close to the lumen (defined as an area with gray scale pixels of less than 25 and greater than 15% of the total plaque area); and using discriminant function analysis. These included a group (left in Fig. 12-11) of asymptomatic plaques, a group (top of Fig. 12-11) of plaques that were asymptomatic or associated with TIAs and stroke, and a group (bottom right of Fig. 12-11) of plaques that were asymptomatic or associated with amaurosis fugax. It can be argued that because all plaques start by being asymptomatic, it is very likely that the group at the top of the figure is that of unstable plaques that tend to produce TIAs and stroke. Similar arguments can be produced for the other groups; however, this methodology and the value of the above six features needs to be tested in prospective natural history studies.

Clinical Significance of Carotid Plaque Echodensity and Structure

The clinical importance of ultrasonic plaque characterization could be focused on two main areas: (1) cross-sectional studies such as the ones described above, aiming to identify the texture features that are associated with stable and unstable plaques and different symptomatology; and (2) prospective natural history studies seeking to identify high- and low-risk groups for ischemic neurologic events.

New Messages From Cross-Sectional Studies

The use of image normalization and analysis has resulted in the identification of differences in carotid plaque structure (in terms of echodensity and degree of stenosis) not only between symptomatic and asymptomatic plaques but also between plaques associated with retinal and hemispheric symptoms.[7] In a series of asymptomatic and symptomatic (i.e., amaurosis fugax, TIAs, and stroke) patients having 50% to 99% stenosis on carotid duplex scan, plaques associated with symptoms were significantly more hypoechoic, with higher degrees of

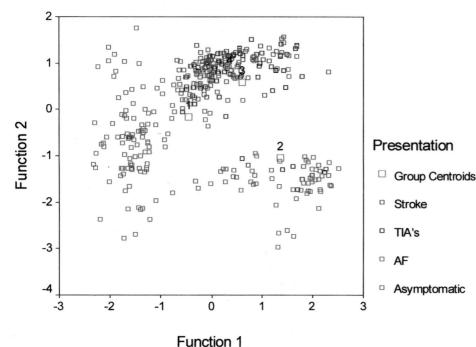

Figure 12-11. Discriminant function analysis of 409 plaques after image normalization (242 asymptomatic, 40 presenting with AF, 72 with TIAs, and 55 with stroke and good recovery). Three main groups of plaques are displayed.

stenosis than those not associated with symptoms (mean GSM = 13.3 vs. 30.5 and mean degree of stenosis = 80.5% vs. 72.2%). Furthermore, plaques associated with amaurosis fugax were hypoechoic (mean GSM = 7.4) and severely stenotic (mean stenosis = 85.6%). Plaques associated with TIAs and stroke had a similar echodensity and a similar degree of stenosis (mean GSM = 14.9 vs. 15.8 and degree of stenosis = 79.3% vs. 78.1%).[6] These findings confirm previous reports, which have shown that hypoechoic plaques are more likely to be associated with symptoms.[15,18-20] In addition, they support the hypothesis that amaurosis fugax has a different pathophysiologic mechanism from that of TIAs and stroke.

Our group has found that GSM separates echomorphologically the carotid plaques associated with silent nonlacunar CT-demonstrated brain infarcts from plaques associated with normal brain scans. The median GSM of plaques associated with ipsilateral nonlacunar silent CT-demonstrated brain infarcts was 14, and that of plaques that were not so associated was 30 (p = 0.003).[22] Additionally, emboli counted on transcranial Doppler (TCD) in the ipsilateral middle cerebral artery were more common in the presence of low-plaque echodensity (low GSM) irrespective of the degree of stenosis. These data support the embolic nature of cerebrovascular symptomatology associated with hypoechoic plaques.[47]

There are several biologic findings explaining the unstable clinical presentation of hypoechoic carotid artery plaques. The authors' group has found an inverse association between carotid plaque GSM and carotid plaque necrotic core volume on histology (r = -35, p = 0.03), which means that plaques with high necrotic core volume have low GSM.[48] In addition, hypoechoic plaques on B-mode imaging have increased macrophage infiltration on histologic examination of the specimen after endarterectomy.[49]

The role of biomechanical forces in the induction of plaque fatigue and rupture has been emphasized.[50-52] In the authors' group of patients, carotid plaques associated with amaurosis fugax were hypoechoic and were associated with very high-grade stenoses. It may well be that the plaques that are hypoechoic and homogenous undergo low internal stresses, and therefore do not rupture but progress to tighter stenosis with poststenotic dilatation, turbulence, and platelet adhesion in the poststenotic area, resulting in the eventual production of showers of small platelet emboli. Such small platelet emboli may be too small to produce hemispheric symptoms but are detected by the retina. In contrast, plaques associated with TIAs and stroke were less hypoechoic and less stenotic than those associated with amaurosis fugax. These plaques are hypoechoic but more heterogenous, undergoing stronger internal stresses. Therefore they may tend to rupture at an earlier stage (i.e., lower degrees of stenosis), producing larger particle debris

(plaque constituents or thrombi) that deprives large areas of the brain of adequate perfusion.

Natural History Studies

The first study to show the value of ultrasonic characterization of carotid bifurcation plaques in asymptomatic patients was done by Johnson in the early 1980s.[12] In that study, hypoechoic carotid plaques, in comparison with the hyperechoic or calcified ones, increased the risk of stroke during a follow-up period of 3 years; this effect was prominent in patients with carotid stenosis more than 75% (estimated by cross-sectional area calculations and spectral analysis) because stroke occurred in 19% of them. None of the patients with calcified plaques developed a stroke.

A second study, performed in the 1980s by Sterpetti,[26] has shown that the severity of stenosis (i.e., lumen diameter reduction greater than 50%, which he defined as hemodynamic) and the presence of a heterogenous plaque were both independent risk factors for the development of new neurologic deficits (TIA and stroke). Some 27% of the patients with heterogenous plaques and hemodynamically significant stenosis developed new symptoms. Unfortunately, that study involved mixed cases because 37% of the patients had a history of previous neurologic symptoms (mainly hemispheric ones). History of these neurologic symptoms was a risk factor for the development of new neurologic symptoms during the follow-up period, although this was found only in the univariate analysis. Because no subgroup analysis was performed, no conclusion can be drawn regarding stroke in asymptomatic or symptomatic patients.

A third study, published in the 1980s by Langsfeld, confirmed that patients with hypoechoic plaques (type 1, predominantly echolucent raised lesion, with thin "eggshell" cap of echogenicity; and type 2, echogenic lesions with substantial areas of echolucency) had a twofold risk of stroke. Their 15% risk was compared with the 7% risk of those having hyperechoic plaques (type 3, predominately echogenic with small area of echolucency deeply localized and occupying less than a quarter of the plaque; and type 4, uniformly dense echogenic lesions).[27] Patients with greater than 75% stenosis were also at increased risk; however, the overall incidence of new symptoms was low, in contrast with the previous studies, perhaps because only asymptomatic patients were included in that study. Based on their results, the authors proposed an aggressive approach in those patients with greater than 75% stenosis and heterogenous plaques. There is some confusion regarding the interchangeable use of the terms *heterogenous* and *hypoechoic* in their article. Additionally, the authors raised the point that it is important for each laboratory to verify its ability to classify plaque types. The same group in another study published 4 years later reported a 5.7% annual vessel event rate (TIA and stroke) for echolucent carotid plaques vs. 2.4% for the echogenic ones (p = 0.03).[53] Again, because the numbers were relatively small, TIAs and strokes were grouped together; a clear message about the occurrence of stroke in the absence of warning symptoms was lacking.

Given the fair interobserver reproducibility for type 1 plaques, the use of reference points was proposed: anechogenicity to be standardized against circulating blood, isoechogenicity against sternomastoid muscle, and hyperechogenicity against bone (cervical vertebrae). A similar method was used in the late 1990s by Polak,[17] who investigated the association between stroke and internal carotid artery plaque echodensity in 4886 asymptomatic individuals aged 65 years or older, who were followed-up prospectively for 48 months. Some 68% of those had carotid artery stenosis, which exceeded 50% in 270 patients. In this study, plaques were subjectively characterized as hypoechoic, isoechoic, or hyperechoic in relation to the surrounding soft tissues. Hypoechoic plaques causing stenoses 50% to 100% were associated with a significantly higher incidence of ipsilateral, non-fatal stroke than were iso- or hyperechoic plaques of the same degree of stenosis (relative risk, 3.08). The authors of this study suggested that quantitative methods of grading carotid plaque echomorphology (e.g., computer-assisted plaque characterization) might be more precise in determining the association between hypoechoic (echolucent) plaques and the incidence of stroke.

The Tromsø study, conducted in Norway in 223 subjects with carotid stenosis greater than 35%, also found that subjects with echolucent atherosclerotic plaques have increased risk of ischemic cerebrovascular events independent of degree of stenosis.[54] The authors give no details on their patients' neurologic histories. The adjusted relative risk for all cerebrovascular events in subjects with echolucent plaques was 4.6 (95% CI 1.1 to 18.9), and there was a significant linear trend (p = 0.015) for higher risk with increasing plaque echolucency. Ipsilateral neurologic events were also more common in patients with echolucent or predominantly echolucent plaques (17.4% and 14.7%, respectively). The authors concluded that evaluation of plaque morphology in addition to the grade of stenosis might improve clinical decision making and differentiate treatment for individual patients, and that computer-quantified plaque morphology assessment, being a more objective method of ultrasonic plaque characterization, may further improve this.

This method was recently used by Grønholdt,[55] who found that echolucent plaques causing a greater than 50% diameter stenosis were associated with an increased risk for future stroke in symptomatic (n = 135) but not asymptomatic (n = 111) individuals. Echogenicity of carotid plaques was evaluated with high-resolution B-mode ultrasound and computer-assisted image processing. The mean of the standardized median gray scale values of the plaque was used to divide plaques into echolu-

cent and echorich. Relative to symptomatic patients with echorich 50% to 79% stenotic plaques, those with echorich 80% to 99% stenotic plaques, echolucent 50% to 79% stenotic plaques, and echolucent 80% to 99% stenotic plaques had relative risks of ipsilateral ischemic stroke of 3.1 (95% CI 0.7 to 14), 4.2 (95% CI 1.2 to 15), and 7.9 (95% CI 2.1 to 30), equivalent to absolute risk increase of 11%, 18%, and 28%, respectively. The authors suggested that measurement of echolucency, together with degree of stenosis, might improve selection of patients for carotid endarterectomy. The relatively small number of asymptomatic individuals was probably the reason why plaque characterization was not helpful in predicting risk in the asymptomatic group.

Future Perspectives: The ACSRS Study

The methodology of computer-assisted carotid plaque characterization with B-mode image normalization is now being applied in a prospective multicenter international natural history study of asymptomatic carotid stenosis with stroke as the primary end-point. The aim of the Asymptomatic Carotid Stenosis and Risk of Stroke (ACSRS) Study[56] is to identify a high-risk subgroup that has an ipsilateral stroke rate greater than 4% (ideally, greater than 7%) based on clinical risk factors and the findings of the noninvasive investigations, mainly ultrasonic carotid plaque characterization (echodensity and texture) in addition to degree of stenosis. In addition, a low-risk subgroup with an ipsilateral stroke rate of less than 1% should be identified. This study will provide evidence about the importance of ultrasonic carotid plaque characterization in the prediction of cerebrovascular events (i.e., stroke, TIAs, and amaurosis fugax). The identification of the high- and low-risk groups may eventually provide better indications on selection of patients, not only for carotid endarterectomy but also for carotid artery stenting.

Data of computerized texture analysis of plaques in the ACSRS study are not yet available; however, some preliminary results based on image normalization, subsequent plaque classification using the redefined Geroulakos classification, and the presence of a black area close to the lumen in relation to all ipsilateral hemispheric events that have occurred during follow-up (6 to 72 months) are available (Table 12-4).

Table 12-4 shows that the presence of a black area adjacent to the lumen of the vessel identifies a group of 533 plaques that became associated with 85 (92%) of the 92 neurologic events that occurred during follow-up (event rate of 16%). Only 7 events occurred in the group of 455 plaques that did not have any black areas adjacent to the lumen (event rate of 1.5%) (odds ratio 9.6; 95% CI 4.4 to 21.1).

TABLE 12-4. **The Distribution of Neurologic Events in Relation to Plaque Types and the Presence of Black Area Adjacent to the Lumen (After Image Normalization)**[*]

Black Area Adjacent to Lumen		Absent	Present	Total
Plaque Type	1	_____	7/107 (6.5%)	7/107 (6.5%)
	2	0/29 (0%)	47/311 (15%)	47/340 (13.8%)
	3	5/179 (2.8%)	31/114 (27%)	36/293 (12.3%)
	4	1/198 (0.5%)	0/1 (0%)	1/199 (0.5%)
	5	1/49 (2%)	_____	1/49 (2%)
	Total	7/455 (1.5%)	85/533 (16%)	92/988 (9.3%)

*Events are in the numerator; event rates are shown as percentages.

A black area adjacent to the lumen in type 2 and 3 plaques identifies a group of 425 plaques that became associated with 78 (85%) of the 92 neurologic events that occurred during follow-up (event rate of 18.3%). Only 14 events occurred in the group of the remaining 563 plaques (event rate of 2.5%) (odds ratio 13.5; 95% CI 7.6 to 24.3).

Conclusions

Carotid ultrasound, apart from being a valuable diagnostic tool, provides useful information on the natural history of carotid artery atherosclerosis. The high resolution of modern equipment and our ability to normalize images has provided the basis for reproducible plaque characterization features that can identify unstable plaques. The identification of a high-risk group of patients based on ultrasonic features other than stenosis should lead to a better selection of patients for carotid endarterectomy or stenting. Novel applications, like algorithms and software identifying patients at high risk of stroke, are expected to become available on duplex scanners in the near future.

REFERENCES

1. Gutstein DE, Fuster V: Pathophysiology and clinical significance of atherosclerotic plaque rupture. Cardiovasc Res 41:323–333, 1999.
2. Zukowski AJ, Nicolaides AN, Lewis RT, et al: The correlation between carotid plaque ulceration and cerebral infarction seen on CT scan. J Vasc Surg 1:782–786, 1984.
3. Libby P: Molecular basis of acute coronary syndromes. Circulation 91:2844–2850, 1995.
4. Clinton S, Underwood R, Hayes L, et al: Macrophage-colony stimulating factor gene expression in vascular cells and human atherosclerosis. Am J Pathol 140:301–316, 1992.
5. Davies MJ, Richardson PD, Woolf N, et al: Risk of thrombosis in human atherosclerotic plaques: Role of extracellular lipid, macrophage and smooth muscle cell content. Br Heart J 69:377–381, 1993.
6. Sabetai MM, Tegos TJ, Nicolaides AN, et al: Hemispheric symptoms and carotid plaque echomorphology. J Vasc Surg 31:39–49, 2000.

7. Tegos TJ, Sabetai MM, Nicolaides AN, et al: Patterns of brain computed tomography infarction and carotid plaque echogenicity. J Vasc Surg 33:334–339, 2001.
8. Pedro LM, Pedro MM, Goncalves I, et al: Computer-assisted carotid plaque analysis: Characteristics of plaques associated with cerebrovascular symptoms and cerebral infarction. Eur J Vasc Endovasc Surg 19:118–123, 2000.
9. Pedro LM, Fernandes E, Fernandes J, et al: Ultrasonographic risk score of carotid plaques. Eur J Vasc Endovasc Surg 24:492–498, 2002.
10. Belcaro G, Nicolaides AN, Laurora G, et al: Ultrasound morphology classification of the arterial wall and cardiovascular events in a 6-year follow-up study. Arterioscler Thromb Vasc Biol 16:851–856, 1996.
11. Reilly LM, Lusby RJ, Hughes L, et al: Carotid plaque histology using real-time ultrasonography: Clinical and therapeutic implications. Am J Surg 146:188–193, 1983.
12. Johnson JM, Kennelly MM, Decesare D, et al: Natural history of asymptomatic carotid plaque. Arch Surg 120:1010–1012, 1985.
13. Gray-Weale AC, Graham JC, Burnett JR, et al: Carotid artery atheroma: Comparison of preoperative B-mode ultrasound appearance with carotid endarterectomy specimen pathology. J Cardiovasc Surg 29:676–681, 1988.
14. Widder B, Paulat K, Hachspacher J, et al: Morphological characterization of carotid artery stenoses by ultrasound duplex scanning. Ultrasound Med Biol 16:349–354, 1990.
15. Geroulakos G, Ramaswami G, Nicolaides A, et al: Characterization of symptomatic and asymptomatic carotid plaques using high-resolution real-time ultrasonography. Br J Surg 80:1274–1277, 1993.
16. deBray JM, Baud JM, Dauzat M on behalf of the Consensus Conference: Consensus concerning the morphology and the risk of carotid plaques. Cerebrovasc Dis 7:289–296, 1997.
17. Polak JF, Shemanski L, O'Leary DH, et al for the Cardiovascular Health Study: Hypoechoic plaque at US of the carotid artery: An independent risk factor for incident stroke in adults aged 65 years or older. Radiology 208:649–654, 1998.
18. El-Barghouty N, Geroulakos G, Nicolaides AN, et al: Computer assisted carotid plaque characterization. Eur J Vasc Endovasc Surg 9:389–393, 1995.
19. Biasi GM, Mingazzini P, Baronio L, et al: Carotid plaque characterization using digital image processing and its potential in future studies of carotid endarterectomy and angioplasty. J Endovasc Surg 5:240–246, 1998.
20. El-Atrozy T, Nicolaides A, Tegos T, et al: The effect of B-mode image standardization on the echodensity of symptomatic and asymptomatic carotid bifurcation plaques. Int Angiol 17:179–186, 1998.
21. Tegos TJ, Sabetai MM, Nicolaides AN, et al: Comparability of the ultrasonic tissue characteristics of carotid plaques. J Ultrasound Med 14:399–407, 2000.

22. Sabetai MM, Tegos TJ, Nicolaides AN, et al: Reproducibility of computer-quantified carotid plaque echogenicity. Stroke 31:2189–2196, 2000.

23. O'Donnell TF Jr, Erdoes L, Mackey WC, et al: Correlation of B-mode ultrasound imaging and arteriography with pathologic findings at carotid endarterectomy. Arch Surg 120:443–449, 1985.

24. Aldoori MI, Baird RN, Al-Sam SZ, et al: Duplex scanning and plaque histology in cerebral ischaemia. Eur J Vasc Surg 1:159–164, 1987.

25. Leahy AL, McCollum PT, Feeley TM, et al: Duplex ultrasonography and selection of patients for carotid endarterectomy: Plaque morphology or luminal narrowing? J Vasc Surg 8:558–562, 1988.

26. Sterpetti AV, Schultz RD, Feldhaus RJ, et al: Ultrasonographic features of carotid plaque and the risk of subsequent neurologic deficits. Surgery 104:652–660, 1988.

27. Langsfeld M, Gray-Weale AC, Lusby RJ: The role of plaque morphology and diameter reduction in the development of new symptoms in asymptomatic carotid arteries. J Vasc Surg 9:548–557, 1989.

28. AbuRahma AF, Thiele SP, Wulu JT Jr: Prospective controlled study of the natural history of asymptomatic 60% to 69% carotid stenosis according to ultrasonic plaque morphology. J Vasc Surg 36:1–6, 2002.

29. El-Barghouty N, Nicolaides A, Bahal V, et al: The identification of high-risk carotid plaque. Eur J Vasc Surg 11:470–478, 1996.

30. Tegos TJ, Stavropoulos P, Sabetai MM, et al: Determinants of carotid plaque instability: Echoicity vs. heterogeneity. Eur J Vasc Endovasc Surg 22:22–30, 2001.

31. Persson AV, Robichaux WT, Silverman M: The natural history of carotid plaque development. Arch Surg 118:1048–1052, 1983.

32. Seager JM, Klingman N: The relationship between carotid plaque composition and neurological symptoms. J Surg Res 43:78–85, 1987.

33. Sterpetti AV, Hunter WJ, Schulz RD: Importance of ulceration of carotid plaque. J Cardiovasc Surg 32:154–158, 1991.

34. Eliasziw M, Streifler JY, Fox JA: Significance of plaque ulceration in symptomatic patients with high-grade stenosis. Stroke 25:305–308, 1994.

35. Fisher GG, Anderson DC, Farber R, et al: Prediction of carotid disease by ultrasound and digital subtraction angiography. Arch Neurol 42:224–227, 1985.

36. O'Leary DH, Holen J, Ricotta JJ, et al: Carotid bifurcation disease: Prediction of ulceration with B-mode ultrasound. Radiology 162:523–525, 1987.

37. Comerota AJ, Katz ML, White JV, et al: The preoperative diagnosis of the ulcerated carotid atheroma. J Vasc Surg 11:505–510, 1990.

38. Farber R, Bromer M, Anderson D, et al: B-mode real-time ultrasonic carotid imaging: Impact on decision-making and prediction of surgical findings. Neurology 34:541–544, 1984.

39. Ricotta JJ: Plaque characterization by B-mode scan. Surg Clin North Am 70:191–199, 1990.

40. Goodson SF, Flanigan DP, Bishara RA, et al: Can carotid duplex scanning supplant arteriography in patients with focal carotid territory symptoms? J Vasc Surg 5:551–557, 1987.

41. Rubin JR, Bondi JA, Rhodes RS: Duplex scanning vs. conventional arteriography for the evaluation of carotid artery plaque morphology. Surgery 102:749–755, 1987.

42. Schminke U, Motsch L, Hilker L, et al: Three-dimensional ultrasound observation of carotid artery plaque ulceration. Stroke 31:1651–1655, 2000.

43. Iannuzzi A, Wilcosky T, Mercuri M, et al: Ultrasonographic correlates of carotid atherosclerosis in transient ischemic attack and stroke. Stroke 26:614–619, 1995.

44. Golledge J, Cuming R, Ellis M, et al: Carotid plaque characteristics and presenting symptom. Brit J Surg 84:1697–1701, 1997.

45. Wu Q: Automatic Tumor Detection for MRI Liver Images (PhD Thesis). London, England: Imperial College, 1996.

46. Jirák D, Dezortová M, Taimr P, et al: Texture analysis of human liver. J Magn Reson Imaging 15:68–74, 2002.

47. Tegos TJ, Sabetai MM, Nicolaides AN, et al: Correlates of embolic events detected by means of transcranial Doppler in patients with carotid atheroma. J Vasc Surg 33:131–138, 2001.

48. Sabetai MS, Coker J, Sheppard M, et al: The association of carotid plaque necrotic core volume and echogenicity with ipsilateral hemispheric symptoms. Circulation 104(Suppl 2):671(abstract), 2001.

49. Grønholdt M-LM, Nordestgaard BG, Bentzon J, et al: Macrophages are associated with lipid-rich carotid artery plaques, echolucency on B-mode imaging, and elevated plasma lipid levels. J Vasc Surg 35:137–145, 2002.

50. Richardson PD, Davies MJ, Born GVR: Influence of plaque configuration and stress distribution and fissuring of coronary atherosclerotic plaque. Lancet ii:941–944, 1989.

51. Ku DN, McCord BN: Cyclic stress causes rupture of the atherosclerotic plaque cap. Circulation 88(Suppl 1):1362(abstract), 1993.

52. Glagov S, Bassiouny HS, Sakaguchi Y, et al: Mechanical determinants of plaque modeling, remodeling and disruption. Atherosclerosis 131(Suppl):S13–S14, 1997.

53. Bock RW, Gray-Weale AC, Mock PA, et al: The natural history of asymptomatic carotid artery disease. J Vasc Surg 17:160–171, 1993.

54. Mathiesen EB, Bønaa KH, Joakimsen O: Echolucent plaques are associated with high risk of ischemic cerebrovascular events in carotid stenosis. The Tromsø Study. Circulation 103:2171–2175, 2001.

55. Grønholdt M-LM, Nordestgaard BG, Schroeder TV, et al: Ultrasonic echolucent carotid plaques predict future strokes. Circulation 104:68–73, 2001.

56. Nicolaides AN: Asymptomatic carotid stenosis and risk of stroke. Identification of a high-risk group (ACSRS). Int Angiol 14:21–23, 1995.

Chapter 13

Intraoperative Assessment of Carotid Endarterectomy: Technique and Results

M. ASHRAF MANSOUR

- Arteriography
- Angioscopy
- Transcranial Doppler
- Color-Flow Scanning
- Key Points

Carotid endarterectomy is one of the most commonly performed vascular operations in the United States. Several well-designed, randomized, controlled trials have demonstrated that carotid endarterectomy is superior to medical treatment in patients with either symptomatic or asymptomatic carotid stenosis.[1-3] However, the advantage of carotid endarterectomy over medical therapy alone is dependent on excellent surgical outcomes and minimizing the perioperative stroke and death rates.[3] The technical aspects of carotid surgery have been described in many texts.[4] The aim of carotid endarterectomy is to prevent cerebral ischemia from occurring because of a lesion in the carotid bifurcation. From the technical standpoint, the operation is designed to remove the obstructing lesion and to achieve a satisfactory arterial closure. The immediate and long-term goals are stroke preven-

tion and freedom from recurrent stenosis. This chapter describes the various methods of intraaoperative carotid assessment with emphasis on noninvasive techniques.

Arteriography

For many years, intraoperative completion arteriography was the only diagnostic test performed after carotid operations.[5-9] The test is quite simple to perform. After the endarterectomy is completed, the arterial defect is closed and flow re-established. A sterile 20-mL syringe attached to a 19-gauge butterfly needle is used for the angiogram. About 10 to 15 mL of undiluted contrast agent is injected directly into the common carotid artery proximal to the closure, and a plain radiograph is obtained. Inflow occlusion may be used to enhance the quality of the image. The advantages of intraoperative angiography are that it is a simple, readily available modality with a low complication rate. Its disadvantages are that it requires the use of a potentially nephrotoxic contrast agent, exposes the patient and operating room personnel to ionizing radiation, and is technically inadequate in a significant proportion of patients. Up to 10% of images are considered to be of poor quality or provide no useful information. Furthermore, because the radiographs are static and taken in one plane (in contrast with color-flow scans), they provide no hemodynamic information.[5] Finally, image acquisition is dependent on good timing and skillful radiologic technicians.

In 1967, Blaisdell and colleagues were first to point out that up to 25% of intraoperative angiograms after carotid endarterectomy demonstrated technical flaws.[6] Since then, many authors have shown similar results.[7-9] Roon and Hoogerwerf found that the combined stroke and death rate from carotid endarterectomy can be reduced from 4.5% to 1.3% by routinely performing intraoperative completion angiograms. Abnormal angiograms led to reopening 11 of 535 carotids (2.1%).[7] In another study from the University of Arizona, Westerband and colleagues found angiographic abnormalities in 19% of their patients.[8] They reopened all vessels with severe defects and successfully repaired 30 of 32 defects. They reported a 2.6% stroke rate. Pross and colleagues from UCLA predominantly used completion angiograms in 333 vessels, and in 21 vessels both duplex and angiography were performed. In all, their intraoperative revision rate was 6.3%.[9] They found that the incidence of recurrent stenosis after a normal intraoperative study is quite low at 0.5%. These studies show that intraoperative angiography improves the technical results of carotid endarterectomy by reducing the operative stroke rate and the postoperative recurrent stenosis.

Angioscopy

Angioscopy requires special equipment (i.e., the angioscope and a fiberoptic light source). Prior to completing the arteriotomy closure, and with a distal vascular clamp applied, the angioscope is inserted in the vessel. Continuous irrigation with saline is done to distend the artery and simulate flow conditions while the operator is focused on visualizing the endarterectomy end-point. Flaps, residual atheromas, and clots can be detected and immediately corrected.

A few authors have reported their experiences with angioscopy. Branchereau and colleagues had 102 patients who underwent angioscopy and angiography with a 94% agreement between the two tests.[10] Two additional reports describing the use of angioscopy together with transcranial Doppler are reviewed in the following paragraph.[11,12] Mueller and colleagues performed angioscopy alone in 325 carotids and found technical problems in 16 (5%).[13] Operative revision was necessary in 11, whereas 5 were corrected without major revision. In their hands, angioscopy took less than 3 minutes to perform and had no complications. This technique appears to be quite simple to implement providing that an angioscope is available for use. The necessary turnaround time for equipment sterili-

zation may hamper the use of angioscopy on consecutive cases in a busy hospital.

Transcranial Doppler

Transcranial Doppler (TCD) is an rarely used modality and there are only a few reports describing its benefits. A 2-MHz probe is used to insonate the ipsilateral middle cerebral artery during carotid surgery through a transtemporal window. A plastic probe holder with a special headband or modified helmet is necessary to keep the transducer in place. Monitoring of the middle cerebral artery (MCA) is done continuously from the start of anesthesia to 30 minutes after flow restoration or until the patient is awake. The main role for TCD is to help the surgeon in deciding whether or not to shunt.[11,12] A drop in the MCA velocity to less than 30% is an indication to shunt. Secondary benefits of TCD are monitoring the incidence of microembolization during dissection and clamping, verification of shunt function after it is placed, and aiding in the detection and management of cerebral vasospasm.[14]

In 1996, Gaunt and colleagues compared four different modalities used for quality control after carotid endarterectomy: continuous-wave Doppler, B-mode ultrasound, TCD, and angioscopy.[11] These methods were used on 100 patients. The authors found that a combination of angioscopy and TCD was the most helpful in detection of technical errors leading to perioperative morbidity. Lennard and colleagues attempted to use angioscopy and TCD in 252 patients.[12] They were successful in using the TCD 91% of the time and found that employing two modalities for quality control contributed to lowering the intraoperative stroke risk. In a large study of 1058 patients, Ackerstaff and colleagues found four variables associated with perioperative stroke: (1) TCD-detected microemboli during dissection; (2) wound closure; (3) greater than 90% MCA velocity decrease at cross-clamping; and (4) a greater than 100% increase in pulsatility index after release of the cross-clamp.[14]

It is clear from these studies that TCD provides valuable information during carotid surgery. What precludes its widespread use are issues related to cost (e.g., acquisition of the device, technologist training, and reimbursement) and time for set-up. It should also be remembered that in approximately 5% to 10% of patients, it is impossible to image the MCA because of bone density or other technical barriers.

Color-Flow Scanning

Intraoperative color-flow scanning after arterial reconstruction has gained increasing support from many investigators.[15-19] The vascular literature includes numerous reports describing the utility of this modality as a quality control tool after lower extremity vein bypass, visceral arterial reconstruction, and carotid surgery (see Chapters 26 and 34).

Technique of Intraoperative Carotid CFS

After the endarterectomy is completed and the vessel is closed, flow is re-established. The scanner is brought into the operating room and the 10-5–MHz linear array transducer is placed in a sterile plastic transparent sleeve with a copious amount of acoustic gel at the tip. The authors prefer the hockey stick probe, but other scanner heads can be used.[5,18] A rubber band is placed near the head of the transducer to trap the gel near the scanning surface to provide a good coupling. The surgeon then uses the transducer to scan the operated carotid artery. The transducer is placed in the open wound and longitudinal image acquisition starts in B-mode in the proximal common carotid artery. The transducer is gently advanced on the vessel, scanning both the internal and external carotid arteries. It is sometimes necessary to fill the depths of the wound with sterile saline solution to obtain good contact between the scanner head and the artery. Transverse scanning is also performed along the entire vessel. The operator looks for intimal flaps, loose debris, retained atheroma, or fronds. Platelet clumps or thrombi may also be visualized. Attention should be paid particularly to the proximal and distal end-points of the endarterectomy because technical flaws are often present at those two locations. The external carotid artery stump can also harbor a flap or clot that, if allowed to propagate, may lead to occlusion or embolization into the internal carotid. After imaging the vessel in B-mode, the color flow is turned on and bloodflow characteristics are observed. Any turbulence or mosaic flow should lead to velocity or blood-flow measurement. The authors typically sample velocities from all three vessels because this often serves as a baseline for future postoperative carotid scans. Elevated peak systolic velocities (i.e., over 150 cm/sec) should be clearly investigated. Increased velocities usually signal the presence of a hemodynamically significant stenosis; or less commonly, spasm. If spasm is implicated, the velocity should normalize after intra-arterial injection with papaverine and a few minutes have passed. However, the surgeon should not ignore a residual stenosis because it may be a harbinger for recurrent stenosis or occlusion.[15-26]

The purpose of the intraoperative color-flow scan is to detect any major abnormalities that could possibly lead to a stroke or neurologic event, residual stenosis, or, rarely, intraoperative carotid occlusion. These technical errors can be immediately corrected and intraoperative rescanning should be done to confirm satisfactory results (Fig. 13-1). Minor defects can be ignored because many of them resolve without any further action (Fig. 13-2).[18,19,23,27]

The advantages of intraoperative CFS are that it is a simple and readily available test that provides the surgeon with important information about vessel patency and flow dynamics.[22-26] The disadvantages to intraoperative scanning include the fact that it is operator dependent. The authors have taught residents and fellows surgeons the technique, and many of them become facile with it after a handful of cases. Another logistical problem is bringing the scanner to the operating room. In a busy vascular laboratory, this could translate into a valuable 30 minutes of technologist and machine time that often is not reimbursed by insurance carriers. Before the availability of the small foot-print scanner, the authors encountered some difficulty in reaching the distal aspect of the cervical internal carotid artery near the angle of the mandible, particularly in obese patients with short necks.[18] This led to a virtual blind spot in the test where no image

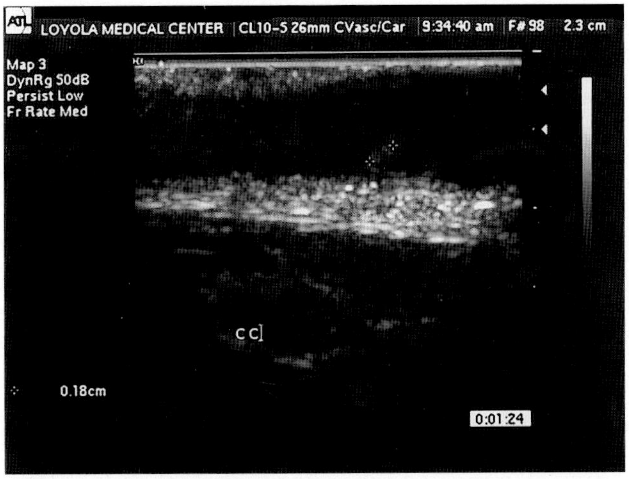

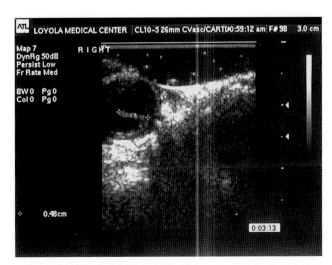

Figure 13-1. *Small 1.8-mm frond in common carotid artery (long view). This small frond was left alone without any adverse sequellae.*

Figure 13-2. *Large frond in common carotid artery (trans view). This large frond was revised and subsequent scan showed it was successfully removed.*

acquisition was possible, and therefore the test was incomplete. Another technical point concerns imaging after sewing the patch. The authors have found that it is quite difficult, if not impossible, to scan through a Dacron or polytetrafluoroethylene (PTFE) patch. To get around this problem, the authors started sewing the patch on the lateral aspect of the vessel, thus freeing up the anterior surface to allow unfettered scanning.

Results of Intraoperative Carotid Color-Flow Scanning

Zierler and colleagues validated the use of pulsed Doppler and real-time spectral analysis as a noninvasive modality to evaluate carotid endarterectomy intraoperatively.[16] Recent reports are summarized in Table 13-1. At Loyola, the authors began performing intraoperative color-flow scans in 1986.[17,18] Over a 12-year period, data was accumulated on 644 carotid endarterectomies performed in 569 patients (Table 13-2). The intraoperative study was completely normal after 466 operations (Table 13-3). Major abnormalities were detected in 20 patients (3.1%), who all underwent immediate revision (Fig. 13-3). Minor abnormalities in 148 vessels (e.g., fronds, proximal

shelf or atheroma, kinks, turbulence, or elevated velocities in the external carotid artery) were not revised (Fig. 13-4). In 10 cases, technical problems led to an unsatisfactory scan. All those cases were in the early learning period. The overall stroke rate was 1.05% in this series. The average follow-up was 34 months. During follow-up, increased velocities, suggesting recurrent stenosis, were noted in eight (5.4%) vessels that had a minor defect intraoperatively. Only one patient needed a reoperation for recurrent stenosis in this latter group (Fig. 13-5). These results are quite similar to those reported by other groups who routinely use intraoperative color-flow scans[16-31] (see Table 13-1). Mays and colleagues found minor abnormalities in 23% of their carotid endarterectomies, and they had an intraoperative revision rate of 10%.[19] Bandyk and colleagues, as well as Sawchuk and colleagues, were able to show that minor defects on intraoperative duplex scan tend to resolve spontaneously with time and lead to no adverse events.[15,23] Most authors agree that a certain amount of clinical judgment is required when performing intraoperative color-flow scans; however, even in experienced hands, there is an intraoperative revision rate of 3% to 10%

TABLE 13-1. Intraoperative Carotid Evaluation: Results of Various Methods

Author, Year	Method	Vessels (n)	Revision rate	Stroke/Death (Percentage)
Bandyk, 1996	CFS	210	5.7%	0
Gaunt, 1996	TCD, angioscopy, CW, B-mode	100	27%	2*
Mueller, 1996	Angioscopy	325	3%	
Papanicolaou, 1996	CFS	86	4.7%	0
Walker, 1996	CFS	50	6%	2
Dykes, 1997	CFS	64	9%	0
Westerband, 1997	Angio	154	21%	2.6
Padayachee, 1998	CFS	106	2.8%	1.9
Seelig, 1999	CFS	102	12.2%	0
Lennard, 1999	TCD, angioscopy	252	5%	
Mansour, 1999	CFS	644	3.1%	1.1
Mays, 2000	CFS	100	10%	1
Panneton, 2001	CFS	155	9%	1.3
Pross, 2001	Angio, CFS	380	6.3%	0.5†
Krug, 2001	CFS & angio	78	3.8%	
Ascher, 2002	CFS, Angio	226	2.7%	0.4

CFS, color-flow scan; TCD, transcanial Doppler; CW, continuous wave.
*2% TIA; †0.5% TIA.

TABLE 13-2. **Patient Characteristics**

	n	Percentage
Carotid endarterectomies	644	100
Right	269	42
Left	333	52
Bilateral	42	6
CEA + CABG	9	1.4
Regional anesthesia	5	0.7
Patients	569	
Men	332	
Women	237	
Age	68 ± 9 years	
Symptomatic	274	43
Asymptomatic	370	57
Preoperative angiogram	202	31

CEA, carotid endarterectomy; CABG, coronary artery bypass graft.

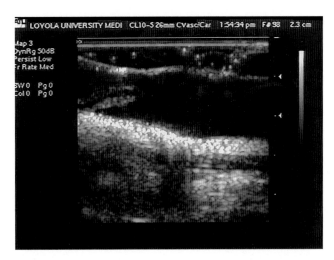

Figure 13-4. *Large flap (long view). This flap requires immediate revision.*

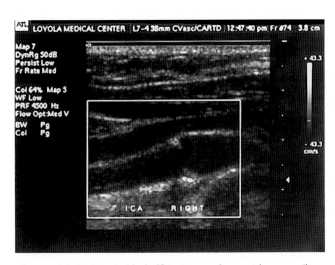

Figure 13-3. *Proximal shelf in internal carotid artery (long view). No revision is required.*

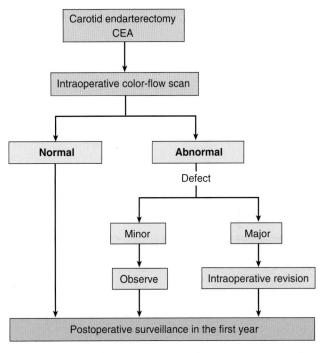

Figure 13-5. *Suggested algorithm for intraoperative color-flow scan during carotid surgery.*

because of major technical flaws at the endarterectomy site (Fig. 13-5).[15,17–19,21–23,25]

Occasionally, cerebral vasospasm will occur immediately after endarterectomy. This can be best demonstrated by TCD, but can also be suspected on intraoperative duplex or angiogram. Ascher and colleagues have used internal carotid artery flow volume measurement in their patients.[32] They observed that a flow volume less than 100 mL/min is abnormal and correlates with postoperative stroke. In these patients, they do not use heparin reversal with protamine and they use Dextran-40 infusion. Others use papaverine or lidocaine to relieve the spasm. The surgeon should make certain that an intracranial internal carotid thrombus is not misdiagnosed as vasospam. In the event of an intracerebral clot, it is still possible to rescue the affected hemisphere with thrombolytics.

Intravascular ultrasound has been very useful in endovascular procedures such as peripheral and coronary angioplasty, as well as endovascular aneurysm repair. Karnik and colleagues used intravascular ultrasound to assess the carotid endarterectomy site in eight patients

TABLE 13-3. Results of Intraoperative Carotid Color-Flow Scanning

Duplex findings	Vessels (n)	Percentage
No abnormality	466	72.5
Minor abnormality (not revised):	148	22.9
Retained atheroma, proximal shelf	56	
Small frond (<3mm)	36	
Kink	7	
Thickened wall	13	
Increased velocity/ turbulence	11	
Other	25	
Major abnormality (revised):	20	3.1
Large frond (>3 mm)	9	
Retained plaque / clot	5	
Distal flap	1	
External carotid flap / turbulence	4	
High frequency	1	
Unsatisfactory study	10	1.5
TOTAL	644	100

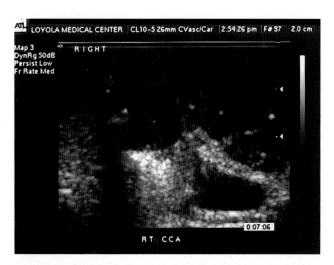

Figure 13-6. *Loose plaque and debris with acoustic shadowing (trans view). This required revision.*

and found it helpful.[33] This modality may play a larger role with carotid angioplasty.

In summary, various methods have been used as quality control tools after carotid surgery. Intraoperative duplex ultrasound provides sensitive and specific real-time images of the operated site and allows the surgeon to correct abnormalities that could lead to adverse neurologic outcomes or recurrent stenosis.

KEY POINTS

- Intraoperative quality control after carotid endarterectomy can reveal technical defects that may lead to perioperative complications or recurrent carotid stenosis.

- Several methods have been used to examine the operated carotid artery, including angiography, angioscopy, transcranial Doppler, and carotid duplex scanning.

- Intraoperative carotid color-flow scanning is an easy method to use to ensure a satisfactory technical result.

- Major technical defects (e.g., flaps, clots, or high-grade stenosis) should be immediately revised. Minor defects can be safely observed.

REFERENCES

1. North American Symptomatic Carotid Endarterectomy Trial Collaborators: Beneficial effect of carotid endarterectomy in symptomatic patients with high-grade stenosis. N Engl J Med 325:445–453, 1991.
2. European Carotid Surgerty Trialists Collaborative Group: European Carotid Surgery Trial: Interim results for symptomatic patients with severe (70% to 99%) or with mild (0% to 29%) carotid stenosis. Lancet 337:1235–1243, 1991.
3. Executive Committee for the Asymptomatic Carotid Atherosclerosis Study: Endarterectomy for asymptomatic carotid stenosis. JAMA 273:1421–1428, 1995.
4. Moore WS, Quinones-Baldrich W, Krupski WC: Indications, Surgical Technique, and Results for Repair of Extracranial Occlusive Lesions. In Rutherford RB (ed): Vascular Surgery, 5th ed. Philadelphia, WB Saunders, 2000.
5. Kang SS, Labropoulos N, Baker WH: Intraoperative Assessment of Carotid Surgery. In Ernst CB, Stanley JC (eds): Current Therapy in Vascular Surgery, 4th ed. St. Louis: Mosby, 2001.
6. Blaisdell FW, Lin R, Hall AD: Technical results of carotid endarterectomy – arteriographic assessment. Am J Surg 106:239–246, 1967.
7. Roon AJ, Hoogerwerf D: Intraoperative arteriography and carotid surgery. J Vasc Surg 16:239–243, 1992.
8. Westerband A, Mills JL, Berman SS, et al: The influence of routine completion arteriography on outcome following carotid endarterectomy. Ann Vasc Surg 11:14–19, 1997.
9. Pross C, Shortsleeve CM, Baker JD, et al: Carotid endarterectomy with normal findings from a completion study: Is there need for early duplex scan? J Vasc Surg 33:963–967, 2001.
10. Branchereau A, Ede B, Magan PE, et al: Value of angioscopy for intraoperative assessment of carotid endarterectomy. Ann Vasc Surg 9:S67–S75, 1995.
11. Gaunt ME, Smith JL, Ratliff DA, et al: A comparison of quality control methods applied to carotid endarterectomy. Eur J Vasc Endovasc Surg 11:4–11, 1996.
12. Lennard N, Smith JL, Gaunt ME, et al: A policy of quality control assessment helps to reduce the risk of intraoperative stroke during carotid endarterectomy. Eur J Vasc Endovasc Surg 17:234–240, 1999.
13. Mueller DK, Haid SP, Painter TA, et al: Intraoperative assessment of carotid endarterectomy utilizing completion angioscopy. Vasc Surg 30:275–280, 1996.

14. Ackerstaff RGA, Moons KGM, van de Vlasakker CJW, et al: Association of intraoperative transcranial Doppler monitoring variables with stroke from carotid endarterectomy. Stroke 31:1817–1823, 2000.

15. Bandyk DF, Mills JL, Gahtan V, et al: Intraoperative duplex scanning: Fate of repaired and unrepaired defects. J Vasc Surg 20:426–433, 1994.

16. Zierler RE, Bandyk DF, Thiele BL: Intraoperative assessment of carotid endarterectomy. J Vasc Surg 1:73–83, 1984.

17. Baker WH, Koustas G, Burke K, et al: Intraoperative duplex scanning and late carotid artery stenosis. J Vasc Surg 19:829–833, 1994.

18. Mansour MA, Webb KM, Kang SS, et al: Timing and frequency of perioperative carotid color-flow duplex scanning: A preliminary report. J Vasc Surg 29:833–837, 1999.

19. Mays BW, Towne JB, Seabrook GR, et al: Intraoperative carotid evaluation. Arch Surg 135:525–529, 2000.

20. Mansour MA: Recurrent carotid stenosis: Prevention, surveillance, and management. Semin Vasc Surg 11:30–35, 1998.

21. Padayachee TS, Brooks MD, Modaresi KB, et al: Intraoperative high-resolution duplex imaging during carotid endarterectomy: Which abnormalities require surgical correction? Eur J Vasc Endovasc Surg 15:387–393, 1998.

22. Papanicolaou G, Toms C, Yellin AE, et al: Relationship between intraoperative color-flow duplex findings and early restenosis after carotid endarterectomy: A preliminary report. J Vasc Surg 24:588–596, 1996.

23. Sawchuk AP, Flanigan DP, Machi J, et al: The fate of unrepaired minor technical defects detected by intraoperative ultrasonography during carotid endarterectomy. J Vasc Surg 9:671–676, 1989.

24. Kinney EV, Seabrook GR, Kinney LY, et al: The importance of intraoperative detection of residual flow abnormalities after carotid endarterectomy. J Vasc Surg 17:912–923, 1993.

25. Golledge J, Cuming R, Ellis M, et al: Duplex imaging findings predict stenosis after carotid endarterectomy. J Vasc Surg 26:43–48, 1997.

26. Dykes JR, Bergamini TM, Lipski DA, et al: Intraoperative duplex scanning reduces both residual stenosis and postoperative morbidity of carotid endarterectomy. Am Surg 63:50–54, 1997.

27. AbuRahma AF, Robinson PA, Stickler DL: Analysis of regression of postoperative carotid stenosis from prospective randomized trial of carotid endarterectomy comparing primary closure versus patching. Ann Surg 229:767–773, 1999.

28. Krug RT, Calligaro KD, Dougherty MJ, et al: Comparison if intraoperative and postoperative duplex ultrasound for carotid endarterectomy. Ann Vasc Surg 15:666–668, 2001.

29. Panneton JM, Berger MW, Lewis BD, et al: Intraoperative duplex ultrasound during carotid endarterectomy. Vasc Surg 35:1–9, 2001.

30. Seelig MH, Oldenburg WA, Chowla A, et al: Use of intraoperative duplex ultrasonography and routine patch angioplasty in patients undergoing carotid endarterectomy. Mayo Clin Proc 74:870–876, 1999.

31. Walker RA, Fox AD, Magee TR, et al: Intraoperative duplex scanning as a means of quality control during carotid endarterectomy. Eur J Vasc Endovasc Surg 11:364–367, 1996.

32. Ascher E, Markevich N, Hingorani AP, et al: Internal carotid artery flow volume measurement and other intraoperative duplex scanning parameters as predictors of stroke after carotid endarterectomy. J Vasc Surg 35:439–433, 2002.

33. Karnik R, Ammerer HP, Winkler WB, et al: Initial experience with intravascular ultrasound imaging during carotid endarterectomy. Stroke 25:35–39, 1994.

Chapter 14

Noninvasive Screening and Utility of Carotid Intima-Media Thickness

LUIS R. LEON JR. • LUKE P. BREWSTER • NICOS LABROPOULOS

Introduction

Atherosclerosis is a progressive process that often begins in childhood.[1] Autopsy studies have correlated atherosclerotic plaques in young people with cardiovascular risk factors.[2] Ultrasound has shown increased intima-media thickening in children with risk factors but without atherosclerosis.[3] These risk factors persist longitudinally into adulthood[4,5] and may be predictive of coronary heart disease (CHD).[6,7] Hypercholesterolemia alone is associated with the development of cardiovascular disease (CVD: coronary and peripheral vascular disease) in later years.[8]

Carotid artery intima-media thickness (IMT) represents a marker of preclinical atherosclerosis because of its correlation with vascular risk factors.[9] It also correlates to the severity and extent of CHD and may be useful as a surrogate end-point to measure likelihood of disease or effectiveness of treatment modalities.[10-14] The benefit of IMT measurements may arise from an ability to treat or prevent atherosclerosis before the disease is symptomatic. However, the correlation is not absolute, and the presence of these risk factors in a youth does not always predict atherosclerosis in the same person as an adult.[15]

End-organ injury from atherosclerosis is a morbid and costly consequence of a variety of risk factors, genetics, and associations with other disease processes and results in 16.6 million deaths worldwide per year.[16] According to the American Heart Association, the cost in the United States alone for CVD and stroke is estimated to be $351.8 billion for 2003.[16] In the last several years clinicians and researchers have begun to understand the disease and address its horrific consequences. Better prevention will be the key to limiting this disease, and IMT may provide a role in this effort.

This chapter defines IMT, shows its correlation with various risk factors, and illustrates its potential utility in the treatment of patients with atherosclerosis.

Methods of Measuring IMT

IMT is defined as the width including lumen-intima and the media-adventitia interface (Fig. 14-1). Delineation of this distance is possible because of the clear interfaces between the anechoic vessel lumen and the echogenic intima, and between the hypoechoic media and the echogenic adventitia. The far arterial wall is used because of the proximal wall's dependence on the gain. The intima and media thickness cannot be measured on their own in vivo because they lack a definable border at their

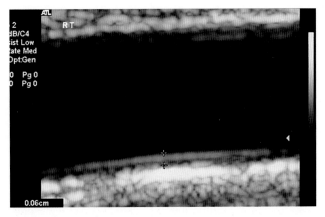

Figure 14-1. *Normal CCA IMT from a 50-year-old male without any risk factors. The measurement is performed in the far wall because the acoustic impedance enhancement allows better visualization compared with the near wall. The calipers are placed at the lumen-wall interface and at the adventitia-media border. This distance represents the intima plus media thickness.*

edges and the intima itself is exceedingly small.[17,18] The endothelium is the thickest part of the intima and it measures about 0.003 to 0.004 mm,[19] which is well beyond the resolution of ultrasound and other noninvasive methods. In addition to correlating directly with cardiovascular risk factors and atherosclerotic disease and its progression, IMT has been shown to correlate well with histologic findings.[20,21] Abnormal CCA and ICA IMT examples are shown in Figure 14-2.

B-Mode Ultrasonography

High-resolution ultrasound imaging can be used to measure IMT in major arteries within 4 cm from the skin. The common carotid artery (CCA) is ideal because it is close to the skin, homogenous, and often devoid of plaque. IMT is usually measured as an average continuous variable in arterial segments not involved by localized atherosclerotic plaques in the CCA.[22] In the authors' institution a high-resolution ultrasound is used to obtain longitudinal images from three different views (i.e., anterior, anterior-lateral, and posterior-lateral). The intra-operator and intraobserver variability of IMT measurements ranges from 3.7% to 7.8%.[23] This is consistent with the published variability (Table 14-1).[1,24-27]

High-resolution B-mode imaging repeated and averaged manual measurement is easy to perform[28,29]; however, it suffers from being operator-dependent and it can have poor reproducibility.[30] Modern computer-assisted measurements allow ease of measurement with improved reproducibility.[31,32] Computerized imaging can quantify the area of IMT and may be a more accurate way to follow IMT over time. This is done with horizontal visualization of the artery in a longitudinal view. The region of interest is defined and the IMT detection and measurement is then automated. Gray scale analysis is performed in each column of pixels perpendicular to the vessel wall. Through interpolation, a continuous curve is derived from the histogram of gray density values. The curve is then analyzed by a dedicated mathematical algorithm that defines the exact position of lumen-intima and media-adventitia interfaces. Because there are substantial systolic-diastolic differences in IMT, images are frozen in end-diastole where IMT changes are minimal.[30] The readings are recorded and the mean values are used. Other researchers have measured the CCA and internal carotid artery (ICA) (including or excluding the carotid bulb).[33,34] ARIC used images from CCA and ICA bilaterally[35] and found a greater correlation with atherosclerotic disease when the IMT for the CCA and ICA was combined.

Increased wall thickening has been assumed if the IMT exceeds a threshold, but this value is dependent on the number of risk factors present and on the patient's age and gender.[23,36]

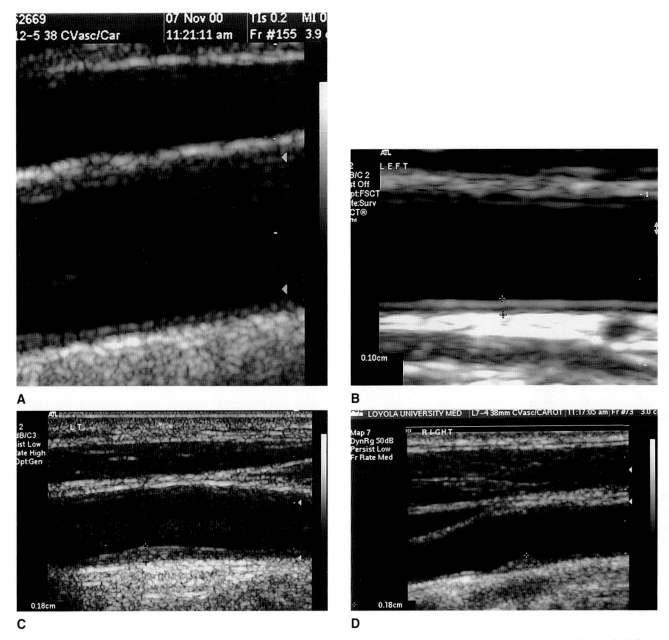

Figure 14-2. **A**, *Irregular CCA endothelial lining. This is one of the first atherosclerotic changes seen as the endothelium from smooth becomes irregular. The acoustic holes are caused by the concave surface that does not reflect sound waves from its center.* **B**, *Increased CCA IMT in a female patient with a recent stroke and absence of carotid stenosis.* **C**, *High IMT in the CCA of a female patient with hypertension, diabetes, hypercholesterolemia, and peripheral vascular disease.* **D**, *Increased IMT in the ICA. IMT measurements are performed in the ICA. These measurements can be used alone or in combination with the CCA.*

By defining a plaque as a localized irregularity of 1.5 mm or more protruding into the lumen,[37] IMT can be expressed as the maximal measured value including the thickness of a plaque, if present.[38] Physical forces alone can cause an increase in the IMT, and thus this process is not only associated with atherosclerotic disease.[37,39,40]

M-Mode Ultrasonography

M-mode ultrasonography utilizes discrete points along the CCA. Using a high-resolution probe, real-time images are generated on a standard monitor. The images are frozen, and three end-diastolic measurements are taken

TABLE 14-1. **Variability of Ultrasound Measurements of IMT**

Study	Number of Patients	Interobserver Variability	Intraobserver Variability	Within Subject Variation
Salonen 1991[24]	10	CV 10.5%	CV 5.4% to 5.8%	
Touboul 1992[25]	13	r = 0.71	r = 0.77	
KAPS 1995[26]	63		CIMT r = 0.89 Bulb IMT r = 0.79 Femoral IMT r = 0.9	r = 0.79–0.9
BRHS 1999[27]	NR	3% to 5%	3% to 5%	
Finns study 2003[1]	173	n = 60 5.2%	n = 113 6.4%	

KAPS, Kuopio Atherosclerosis Prevention Study; BRHS, British Regional Heart Study; EVA, Etude du Vieillissement Arteriel, aging vascular study; Finns study, Cardiovascular Risk in Young Finns Study.
IMT, intima-media thickness; CV, coefficient of variation; r, correlation coefficient; CIMT, carotid IMT; NR, not reported.

on the far wall 1 cm proximal to the carotid bulb.[41] It may also be used as M-mode-derived radio frequency signal.[41,42] The main drawback to this modality is the application of a single-point measurement to a diffuse and sometimes uneven parietal process.[30]

Transesophageal Echocardiography

This modality allows excellent visualization of the ascending and proximal descending aorta. It can be used to find aortic plaques and measure IMT. When the carotid IMT is greater than 2 mm, it correlates with complex aortic arch disease.[43] Aortic IMT less than 3 mm has been shown to be a predictor of the absence of CHD.[44] Carotid artery plaques have also been suggestive of aortic arch plaques.[45] The need for sedation, invasiveness, and the discomfort associated with swallowing the tube warrant its use as a secondary study and not as a screening modality.

Intravascular Ultrasound

Intravascular ultrasound (IVUS) can be utilized during arteriography. This is an accurate way of defining plaques and atheroma burden. There are studies promoting its utility in cardiac transplant patients, for stent deployment, and in certain patients with coronary artery disease. Arteriography and IVUS carry a small but real risk of major complications (up to 2% stroke/myocardial infarction [MI] risk). Briefly, the ultrasound probe is advanced over a guide wire to the artery of interest and the transducer is placed distal to a side branch. Then,

a motorized pullback apparatus is used to take serial images at a set velocity over a standardized distance.

Despite theoretical advantages of IVUS over B-mode ultrasound (e.g., shortest possible distance between points and improved acoustics from initiating the sound wave in a fluid medium to the wall) and studies showing IVUS's utility to measure coronary IMT, there are no studies comparing the measurement of carotid IMT between B-mode and IVUS.[46,47] IVUS is ideal for visualizing luminal irregularities, but it is more likely to help clinicians further evaluate this disease than prevent it. Given its size (i.e., larger introducing catheter and probe than a standard arteriography catheter) and invasiveness, it is plausible that IVUS denudes the endothelium of the targeted vessels. Thus, it is not an optimal screening modality.

Magnetic Resonance Imaging

Magnetic resonance imaging (MRI) has been used to identify and serially follow atherosclerotic plaques and to document regression of plaque volume following the use of a lipid-lowering agent.[48,49] The measurements have been shown to correlate in cadavers using fat-suppressed T1-weighted sequences with contrast enhancement.[50] There were no articles using MRI for IMT measurements only.

Risk Factors for IMT

IMT has shown to represent the sum of the risk factors that we carry; therefore, IMT reflects atherosclerotic changes and can be used to predict cardiovascular risk.

Some of the important risk factors associated with increased IMT are discussed in following:

- Age: Aging is the main determinant of IMT, except in subjects under 18 without cardiovascular risk factors.[51] This is supported in the Kuopio Atherosclerosis Prevention Study (KIHD) and Atherosclerosis Risk in Communities Study (ARIC).[28,33,52]

- Gender/ethnicity: Men have higher IMT readings and a quicker progression than women.[33,40,53] There are not a lot of data regarding ethnicity outside of populations predisposed to other risk factors, but D'Agostino found African Americans to be predisposed to higher CCA IMT but not ICA IMT.[54]

- Body habitus: Many studies show a correlation between body mass index and IMT.[55,56] The android body morphology has also been shown to correlate with increased IMT.[56] The reason may be the tendency to have concurrent hyperlipidemia, or that other characteristics shared by obese individuals contribute to the progress of atherosclerosis in an independent fashion. These factors have been postulated to include hyperinsulinemia with insulin resistance, inflammatory cytokines, and the perturbation of the renin-angiotensin system.[57–60]

- Blood pressure: Patients with established arterial hypertension have increased IMT.[53,61,62] It has also been correlated with isolated systolic hypertension[29] and pulse pressure.[63]

- Blood lipids: Hyperlipidemia leads to intimal atherosclerotic infiltration. This association is seen in familial forms of hypercholesterolemia.[64] There exists a linear correlation between plasma cholesterol and IMT,[28,63] and another between IMT and low-density lipoproteins (LDL) alone.[63,65] There is an inverse relationship between high-density lipoproteins (HDL) and IMT; this is especially important in diabetics.[65,66] Low HDL is associated with increased IMT.[67] Not surprisingly, IMT correlates directly with the LDL/HDL ratio.[68] The Monitored Atherosclerosis Regression Study (MARS) showed a positive relationship between IMT and triglycerides.[69]

- Smoking: Smoking is an independent risk factor for the development of IMT, and its cessation has been shown to slow or even regress IMT in patients in the KIHD, ARIC, and the European Lacidipine Study on Atherosclerosis (ELSA).[52,63,70] The association between IMT and smoking depends on lifelong smoking dose, with active smokers having thicker walls compared with former smokers.[71] Passive smoking is associated with increased IMT values.[70] Smoking correlates with the amount of thickening and progression of IMT in these patients.[52,72] MARS showed that stopping tobacco slows progression.[73]

- Diabetes: For diabetics, the highest IMT values are associated with end-organ dysfunction (e.g., microvascular complications[74] and microalbuminuria[75]). Diabetes-related IMT is linked to both duration of disease and quality of disease control.[66,76]

- Radiation: Radiotherapy for malignant diseases has been shown to promote atherosclerosis. Significant plaques and cardiovascular events usually develop 5 to 10 years after treatment. The acceleration in atherosclerosis was recently shown in a prospective study in which it was demonstrated that neck irradiation increased carotid IMT about 21 times more than in matched control volunteers from large epidemiologic studies.[77]

- Genetics: Current data do support the role of genetics in the development of increased IMT. It may exist, however, and operate through inflammatory mediators[78] or through various susceptibilities of certain genes to certain risk factors.[79] A study in 310 middle-aged women found that certain polymorphisms of the paraoxonase gene were an independent risk factor for increased IMT in both the CCA (odds ratio [OR] = 2.75; 95% confidence intervals [CI] 1.01 to 7.50) and carotid bulb (OR = 2.40; 95% CI 1.00 to 5.90).[80] Beilby and colleagues[81] have also shown that polymorphism of the apoE gene correlates with increased LDL-C levels and plaque formation in men but not with IMT in either sex.

Impact on Clinical Practice

A dynamic relationship between treatment of cardiovascular disease and IMT will likely develop; this can be used to study IMT in childhood and its prevention with diet and exercise modification. Its progression may also be slowed or halted with medication treating the underlying causes.[82] It may also be used to selectively screen patients with unknown atherosclerosis and streamline their evaluation. This has been endorsed by a recent statement of an American Heart Association working group on prevention of atherosclerosis. They state:

> . . . The severity of carotid IMT is an independent predictor of transient cerebral ischemia, stroke, and coronary events such as myocardial infarct (MI). Writing Group III concluded that in asymptomatic persons younger than 45 years old, carefully performed carotid ultrasound examination with IMT measurement can add incremental information to traditional risk factor assessment. In experienced laboratories, this test can now be considered for further clarification of CHD risk assessment at the request of a physician.[83]

The correlation between CVD risk factors and IMT progression has led the Food and Drug Administration

(FDA) to accept B-mode ultrasound as a valid technique in studying atherosclerosis.

Economics

The cost of CVD is consuming a major part of the health care budget, with sales of the cholesterol-lowering group of drugs, statins, reaching $12.5 billion in the United States in 2002. Nationalized health programs have had to create stringent criteria to exclude payment for medications that have been shown to benefit patients.[84] Certain studies support the cost-effectiveness of IMT measurement.[85] Undoubtedly, prevention is preferred to treatment and more effort is being made towards this direction.

IMT as a Predictor of Peripheral Vascular Disease

IMT has a strong association with peripheral vascular disease (PVD). Three prospective studies showed that an increased carotid IMT has been associated with a higher risk of PVD.[86] The Rotterdam study[87] enrolled 7983 people aged 55 years or older to identify determinants of PVD. The carotid IMT was measured and correlated with ankle-brachial index (ABI). Multiple linear regression was used adjusted for age, sex, and other cardiovascular risk factors. An increase of 0.1 mm in the CCA IMT was associated with a mean reduction of the ABI of 0.026 (95% CI = 0.018 to 0.034). To assess the association between PVD and ABI a logistical regression analysis was also used. The IMT values were divided in quintiles. PVD was increased in patients with IMT values in the upper quintiles (0.89 mm or greater; OR = 3.4; 95% CI = 2.2 to 5.2) when compared with values within the lower four. Among patients with claudication (n = 12) the IMT was 0.87 mm; it was 0.76 mm for those without claudication.

Three years later, the Edinburgh Artery Study[88] reported similar results. A cross-sectional survey was initially performed in 1988 including 1592 patients. A 5-year follow-up was later obtained including a new questionnaire, ABI, and IMT measurements. These investigators used the maximum IMT from both sides and not the mean, arguing that a more realistic indicator of atherosclerosis severity can thus be reached. Multiple regression analysis was used for the relation between IMT and ABI, univariately and after adjustment for age and sex. The study subjects included male and female participants 55 to 74 years old from a population that was geographically and socioeconomically spread across the city. Out of that cohort, 1156 subjects attended the 5-year follow-up examination; of those, 1106 had IMT readings recorded. After adjusting for age, men had higher mean IMT values in all age groups (p ≤ 0.01); but when stratified for age groups, significance was reached in the 65 to 69 year group (p ≤ 0.05). The age groups were stratified in quartiles, and continuously higher IMT values with increasing quartile in both sexes were found. Subjects with ABI less than 0.9 had significantly higher IMT readings than those without, even after adjusting for age and sex (p ≤ 0.01).

The SMART (Secondary Manifestations of Arterial Disease) study[89] analyzed carotid IMT in 570 patients with either high-risk factors or manifestations of CVD. Baseline survey, blood chemistry, and ultrasonography were performed. PVD was defined as ABI at rest of 0.9 or less; or ABI after treadmill testing decreasing 20% or more in 1 or both legs. Three risk scores were used to determine each patient's cardiovascular risk: (1) the authors developed a SMART risk score[90] to assess their vascular risk; (2) the Framingham score was used to assess their coronary risk; and (3) the Epidemiological Prevention study of Zoetermeer (EPOZ) score[91] was used to assess mortality risk. The association between IMT and the risk scores was assessed using a linear regression analysis. The risk scores increased nearly in a linear manner, with IMT increasing at a rate of 1.37 standard deviations (95% CI = 1.15 to 1.6) per each mm increase in IMT. Therefore, the predictive value of IMT was not only demonstrated for general populations but also for patients at risk or with extensive cardiovascular disease.

IMT and Other Vascular Territories

Carotid IMT and atherosclerosis have been evaluated in other vascular territories such as the abdominal aorta. The cardiovascular health study (CHS)[92] evaluated CHD and stroke in adults aged 65 years or older to identify factors related to their onset and course. It enrolled participants in each of four United States communities sampled from Medicare lists. The prevalence of abdominal aortic aneurysms (AAA) for the entire cohort was 9.5% (451/4741). After adjusting for age, sex, smoking, height, and weight, the presence of AAA was strongly related to ICA IMT (p < 0.0001) and an ABI of 0.9 or less (p < 0.0001).

A literature search was performed to investigate the correlation between IMT and visceral disease, and no studies were found. It is well known, however, that presence of plaque in carotid arteries, CHD, and an abnormal ABI are associated with visceral atherosclerotic disease. It would appear therefore that carotid IMT has an association with visceral artery disease, although is not studied yet.

IMT as Predictor of CHD

Several cohort and prospective studies have shown a strong association between CHD and increased IMT (Table 14-2).[12,14,27,28,93] This relationship remains strong even after adjusting for age, sex, and other risk factors. Often it was shown that a small increase in IMT significantly elevated the risk for CHD. Furthermore, subjects in the upper IMT quintile had the highest risk. Overall, the chance for developing CHD was higher in men, but after certain threshold it was significantly higher in women.

IMT as a Predictor of Stroke

A relationship between brain infarction and higher IMT readings has been shown using different methods such as ultrasound, computed tomography, and MRI. Several reports showed a clear relation of increasing IMT values and higher relative risk of stroke (Table 14-3).[12,14,27,94,101] In the CHS the occurrence of stroke was ascertained by yearly visits, phone interviews every 6 months, Medicare medical records, and reporting of events by subjects in the study. IMT was measured in CCA and ICA and the maximal value was used for analysis rather than the mean. A composite value that combined the maximal IMT in CCA and ICA was obtained by averaging both numbers after standardization. These values were divided in quintiles and they were also used as continuous variables. With a median follow-up of 6.2 years, 284 new strokes and 55 combined with MI were diagnosed. The relative risk of stroke increased with higher IMT (p < 0.001). After adjustment, the relative risk of stroke for those within the highest quintile was 3.9 times higher than the lowest (95% CI = 2.7 to 5.5). Therefore, a clear association between IMT measurements and the incidence

of new stroke in patients aged more than 65 years without a history of CVD was established.[14]

Cognitive function impairment was also shown to be related to IMT, based on application of neuropsychological testing in large populations with carotid atherosclerotic disease.[96]

Carotid IMT may help to reliably identify different subtypes of ischemic stroke patients.[100] Carotid IMT and atrial fibrillation were found to be the only independent factors capable of discriminating between lacunar and nonlacunar strokes in another study.[101]

IMT and the Femoral Artery

Limited information is produced by the use of ultrasound to assess atherosclerotic changes in the femoral artery in relation to femoral or carotid IMT. The mean femoral IMT was calculated in population-based studies on healthy subjects between the ages of 20 and 60 years; it was found to be 0.562 ± 0.074 mm for men and 0.543 ± 0.063 mm for women, with a growth rate of 0.0031 and 0.0012 mm per year, respectively.[86] Risk factors for its progression include cigarette smoking, hypercholesterolemia, familial hypercholesterolemia, high levels of plasma homocysteine, and fibrinogen.[86,102]

Suurkula and colleagues[103] examined morphologic changes in the common femoral artery wall and correlated them to ABIs and to symptoms of lower-extremity PVD. Their population was divided into two groups:

- A high-risk group (143) comprising hypertensive men 50 to 72 years old (at randomization) with 1 or more of the following: serum cholesterol level 6.5 mmol/L or greater, tobacco smoking 1 cigarette or moer per day, or diabetes mellitus

TABLE 14-2. **Correlation Between IMT and CHD**

Study	Number of Patients	Results
KIHD 1991[28]	1224	0.1-mm increase in IMT had a 4.4% increase in MI
ARIC 1997[93]	772	IMT >1 mm was associated with 5.07 (95% CI 3.08–8.36) ↑ in RR of CHD in women and 1.85 (95% CI 1.28–2.69) in men
ERGO 1997[12]	7983	MI risk ↑ 43% per SD increase in CIMT (OR = 1.43; 95% CI = 1.16–1.78)
BRHS 1999[27]	7735	CHD increased with ↑ IMT; OR = 2.8 (95% CI = 1.1–6.6)
CHS 1999[14]	4476	MI risk ↑ per SD increase in CCA-IMT (OR = 1.24; 95%CI = 1.12–1.36) ICA-IMT (OR = 1.34; 95% CI = 1.2–1.5) Combined (OR = 1.36; 95% CI = 1.23–1.52)

KIHD, Kuopio Ischemic Heart Disease Risk Factor Study; ARIC, Atherosclerosis Risk in Communities; ERGO Rotterdam, Association between the intima-media thickness of the common carotid and subsequent cardiovascular events in subjects, 55 years and older, in the Rotterdam study; BRHS, British Regional Heart Study; CHS, Cardiovascular Health Study.
RR, relative risk; IMT, intima-media thickness; CIMT, carotid intima-media thickness; CCA, common carotid artery; ICA, internal carotid artery; OR, odds ratio; CI, confidence intervals; SD, standard deviation; MI, myocardial infarct.

TABLE 14-3. IMT and the Risk of Stroke

Study	Number of Patients	Population	Measured Outcome	Results	Type of Study
Polak 1993[94]	5201	Older than 65 years	Plaque morphology, CIMT	Severity of ICA stenosis was associated with ↑ IMT (r = 0.37, p < 0.0001)	Prospective
Bots 1993[95]	111	Cohort from Rotterdam study[87] 65 to 85 years old	CIMT, brain MRI	Difference in IMT = 0.13 mm (95% CI 0.04–0.21)	Randomized
Auperin 1996[96]	1279	59- to 71-year-old people from the electoral rolls of Nantes (western France)	CIMT, MMSE, 7 neuropsychological tests	Slight association of ↑ CIMT and poor cognitive scores in men with plaques	Cross-sectional analysis
Chambless 1996[97]	12205	ARIC study subjects	Questionnaire on symptoms of TIA and stroke, CIMT	OR for TIA/stroke were significantly ↑ (p ≤ 0.01) for ↑ IMT (not in African Americans)	Cross-sectional analysis
Bots 1997[12]	7983	Cohort from Rotterdam study[87] >55 years old	CIMT images and determination of incident stroke based on discharge records	Stroke risk increased with increasing IMT OR per SD increase (0.163 mm) = 1.41 (95% CI = 1.25–1.82)	Nested case-control study
Yamakado 1998[98]	243	Normal and asymptomatic brain infarction	CIMT	Higher CIMT in asymptomatic brain infarction group	Cohort study
Kawamura 1998[99]	82	Diabetes >60 years old	CIMT	Higher CIMT with age; in patients with asymptomatic brain infarction; (+) correlation with sVCAM-1	Cohort study
Ebrahim 1999[27]	800	Males from the BRHS cohort; females an age-matched random sample	CIMT	Stroke risk with increased IMT OR 1.9 (95% CI = 0.4–10.2)	Cohort study
O'Leary 1999[14]	4476	>65 years old without CVD	Cardiovascular events (new MI or stroke) and CIMT	Relative risk of stroke increased with IMT (p < 0.001)	Prospective multicenter study
Touboul 2000[100]	470	MRI-proven brain infarction	CIMT	↑ IMT was associated with brain infarction	Cohort study
Cupini 2002[101]	292	Acute ischemic stroke	CIMT	IMT and AF discriminate independently stroke subtypes; IMT was significantly ↑ in nonlacunar vs. lacunar and controls	Cohort study

IMT, intima-media thickness; CIMT, carotid intima-media thickness; ICA, internal carotid stenosis; MRI, magnetic resonance imaging; sVCAM-1, vascular cell adhesion molecule-1; MMSE, Mini-Mental State Examination; ARIC, Atherosclerosis Risk in Communities Study; TIA, transient ischemic attack; OR, odds ratio; ICA, internal carotid artery; SD, standard deviation; AF, atrial fibrillation; CI, confidence intervals.

- An age-matched low-risk group (46) with the following criteria: diastolic blood pressure lower than 95 mmHg, no antihypertensive treatment, no smoking during the last 3 years, serum cholesterol 6.5 mmol/L or less, normal fasting blood glucose, and normal sinus rhythm on electrocardiogram

More and larger plaques were found in the high-risk group than in the low-risk group (p < 0.0001). Femoral IMT increased in proportion with the occurrence and severity of plaques in the common, superficial, or profunda femoral arteries. Femoral artery plaques were found in 28% of the patients in the low-risk group, indicating a prevalence of subclinical atherosclerosis higher than previously thought.

Veller and colleagues[104] correlated carotid IMT and atherosclerotic disease in the carotid and femoral bifurcations. They showed a mean IMT of 0.55 mm in subjects without a plaque in the mentioned bifurcations (0.36 to 0.81), and 0.77 in those with a plaque (0.56 to 1.07) (p < 0.001). If the mean IMT was less than 0.6 mm, a plaque was found in 5% of subjects; if it was between 0.6 and 0.8 mm, a plaque was found in 53%; and plaque was found in 96% if it was greater than 0.8 mm. The IMT increased at a rate of 0.009 mm/yr (r = 0.65) in subjects with a plaque in those locations, compared with 0.005 mm/yr (r = 0.64) in subjects without a plaque. The lifetime amount of smoking (0.003 mm/pack-year smoked; r = 0.39; p < 0.05) and the systolic blood pressure (0.004 mm/kPa; r = 0.51; p < 0.01). Sex, diameter of the vessel, mean and diastolic blood pressures did not have a significant effect on IMT.

Intravascular Ultrasound and IMT

IVUS has been extensively reported in clinical applications, mostly in relation to plaque morphology; its use for IMT assessment has been scarce. Wakeyama and colleagues[105] studied the extent and nature of 100 radial artery injuries after transradial approach for coronary angiography or intervention using IVUS and IMT measurements. The IMT values were higher in patients after repeated transradial interventions (p < 0.0001). Petronio and colleagues[46] used IVUS and IMT values to assess gender differences in patients that were referred for percutaneous coronary angioplasty. The left anterior coronary artery was smaller in women after correcting for body size, suggesting an intrinsic sex effect on the coronary anatomic dimensions.

IMT Effect on Treatment

IMT have been extensively studied in a broad field of applications including lipid-lowering agents, antihypertensive drugs and others (Tables 14-4, 14-5, and 14-6).[26,106–130]

TABLE 14-4. Impact of IMT Analysis on Treatment With Statins

Study	Number of Patients	Population	Treatment	Outcome	Results	Study
Byington 1994[106] (ACAPS study)	919	Asymptomatic with early carotid stenosis	Lovastatin 20–40 mg/d or placebo+ Coumadin 1 mg/d or placebo ± aspirin	3-year change in CIMT	Among patients with no coumadin, IMT ↓ significantly in statin group	Double-blind, randomized clinical trial
De Groot 1995[107] (REGRESS study)	255	Symptomatic CHD confirmed by angiography	Pravastatin	CIMT	↓ IMT progression	Double-blind, placebo-controlled, multicenter study
Crouse 1995[108] (PLAC-II study)	151	Men with CHD	Pravastatin	CIMT	Statistically significant 35% ↓ IMT progression	Randomized
Salonen 1995[26] (KAPS study)	447	Mostly asymptomatic	Pravastatin (40 mg/d) or placebo for 3 years	CIMT	↓ IMT progression, ↑ effect if ↑ baseline IMT values, smokers and ↓ plasma vitamin E levels	Randomized population-based trial

Continued

TABLE 14-4. Impact of IMT Analysis on Treatment With Statins—cont'd

Study	Number of Patients	Population	Treatment	Outcome	Results	Study
Mercuri 1996[109] (CAIUS study)	305	Asymptomatic Mediterranean patients with moderately ↑ cholesterol	Pravastatin (40 mg/d) or placebo for 3 years	CIMT	Stops IMT progression	Prospective, randomized, placebo-controlled study
Hodis 1996[110] (MARS study)	188	CHD confirmed by angiography	Lovastatin	CIMT	↓ IMT progression	Randomized, double-blind, placebo-controlled study
MacMahon 1998[111]	522	History of MI or unstable angina	Low-fat diet +pravastatin 40 mg/d or placebo	CIMT	IMT ↑ by 0.048-mm in placebo; ↓ by 0.014-mm with treatment	Randomized, double-blind, placebo-controlled study
Smilde 2001[112] (ASAP study)	325	Familial hypercholesterolemia	Atorvastatin 80 mg/d vs. simvastatin 40 mg/d	Lipoprotein, fibrinogen, IMT	Atorvastatin ↓ mean IMT by 0.031mm and simvastatin ↑ by 0.036mm ($p < 0.0001$)	Multicenter, randomized, double-blind clinical
Taylor 2002[113] (ARBITER study)	161	CHD	Atorvastatin 80 mg/d vs. pravastatin 40 mg/d	CIMT	Atorvastatin ↓ IMT while pravastatin was related to stable IMT (only significant after 1 year)	Single-center, randomized clinical trial
Youssef 2002[114]	25	Peripheral arterial disease	Atorvastatin 20 mg/d for 4 weeks	CIMT	Trend after 4 years to regress; after 8 weeks significant	Prospective, randomized, blinded
de Sauvage Nolting 2003[115]	153	Familial hypercholesterolemia	Simvastatin 80 mg/d for 2 years ± antihypertensive meds	CIMT, FIMT	↓Combined IMT in 69.8%; with antihypertensives more benefit	Prospective

ACAPS, Asymptomatic Carotid Artery Progression Study; REGRESS, Regression Growth Evaluation Statin Study; METEOR, Measuring Effects on Intima-Media Thickness: an Evaluation of Rosuvastatin; PLAC, Pravastatin, Lipids, and Atherosclerosis in the Carotid Arteries; KAPS, Kuopio Atherosclerosis Prevention Study; CAIUS, Carotid Atherosclerosis Italian Ultrasound Study; MARS, Monitored Atherosclerosis Regression Study; ASAP, Atorvastatin vs. Simvastatin on Atherosclerosis Progression; ARBITER, Arterial Biology for the Investigation of the Treatment Effects of Reducing Cholesterol. MI, myocardial infarct; CHD, coronary heart disease; IMT, intima-media thickness; CIMT, carotid intima-media thickness; FIMT, femoral intima-media thickness.

TABLE 14-5. Impact of IMT Analysis on Treatment With Antihypertensives

Study	Number of Patients	Population	Treatment	Outcome	Result	Type of Study
Pitt 2000[116] (PREVENT trial)	825	Angiographically documented CHD	Amlodipine 5 mg/d, increased to 10 mg/d after 2 weeks if tolerated	CIMT, clinical events, angiographic change in mean minimal diameter of segments with baseline diameter stenosis of 30%	IMT 0.033 mm ↑ with placebo; 0.0126-mm ↓ with amlodipine	Multicenter, randomized, placebo controlled, double masked trial

TABLE 14-5. Impact of IMT Analysis on Treatment With Antihypertensives—cont'd

Study	Number of Patients	Population	Treatment	Outcome	Results	Type of Study
Hedblad 2001[117] (BCAPS trial)	793	Asymptomatic subjects with carotid plaque	Metoprolol 25 mg/d for 1.5 to 3 years + fluvastatin 40 mg/d vs. placebo	CIMT	IMT progression at 18 and 36 months was ↓ by metoprolol (−0.058 mm/y; 95% CI, −0.094 to −0.023; p = 0.004; and −0.023 mm/y; 95% CI, −0.044 to −0.003; p = 0.014, respectively)	Randomized, double-blind, placebo-controlled, single-center trial
Simon 2001[118]	439	Hypertensive patients 55- to 80-years-old, with ≥1 cardiovascular risk factor	Nifedipine 30 mg or HCTZ + amiloride 25/2.5 mg with titration	CIMT	IMT ↑ on HCTZ + amiloride, not on nifedipine	Prospective, randomized, placebo-controlled trial
Hoogerbrugge 2002[119] (DAPHNE study)	80	Peripheral arterial disease, hypercholesterolemia	Doxazosin, HCTZ	CIMT, FIMT, fasting lipid profile	No differences after 3 years, but both ↓ significantly	Randomized, double-blind trial
Yamakado 2002[120]	20	HTN	Candesartan* vs. diuretics	BP, CIMT, superoxide dismutase activity, lipid peroxidase	ARB ↓ IMT significantly. Effects through antioxidation not only through BP control	Prospective
Bozec 2003[121]	98	Untreated with essential hypertension	Enalapril vs. celiprolol for 5 months	CIMT, M235T polymorphism for angiotensinogen gene	↑ IMT if homozygous for the T allele than MM patients; IMT was more significantly ↓ with treatment in TT than MM	Randomized, double-blind parallel group study
Terpstra 2003[122]	131	Newly diagnosed hypertension	Nifedipine 30–60 mg for 26 weeks	CIMT	IMT inhibition, more benefit in pretreatment ↑ IMT	Prospective, open-label study with blinded end-point analysis
Wiklund 2002[123] (ELVA trial)	129	Hypercholesterolemia	Metoprolol 100 mg/d for 1.5–3 years vs. placebo + concomitant statin therapy	CIMT	Metoprolol ↓ IMT at 1 (−0.08 vs −0.01 mm; p = 0.004) and 3 years (−0.06 vs +0.03 mm; p = 0.011)	Randomized, double-blind, placebo-controlled, single-center trial

*Candesartan is a angiotensin receptor blocker (ARB).

PREVENT, Prospective Randomized Evaluation of the Vascular Effects of Norvasc Trial; BICAPS, Beta-Blocker Cholesterol-Lowering Asymptomatic Plaque Study; ELVA, Effects of Long-Term Treatment of Metoprolol CR/XL on Surrogate Variables for Atherosclerotic Disease; DAPHNE, Doxazosin Atherosclerosis Progression Study in Hypertensives in the Netherlands.

IMT, intima-media thickness; CIMT, carotid intima-media thickness; FIMT, femoral intima-media thickness; CHD, coronary heart disease; HCTZ, hydrochlorotiazide; CI: confidence intervals.

TABLE 14-6. Impact of IMT Analysis on Treatment

Study	Number of Patients	Population	Treatment	Outcome	Results	Type of Study
Raal 1999[124]	15	Homozygous familial hypercholesterolemia	1g/d vitamin E for 2 years; then simvastatin started at 80–160 mg/d and subsequently atorvastatin 80 mg/d + diet	CIMT	↑ IMT rapidly with vitamin E. With statins mean ↓ of 28% in LDL cholesterol, no further IMT progression and regression	Prospective, blind trial
Drueke 2002[125]	60	ESRD	Iron	AOPP, iron, IMT and vessel diameter	↑ IMT with ↑ AOPP, ↑ IMT with ↑ iron and ferritin	Prospective
Moreau 2002[126]	104	Healthy postmenopausal	Sedentary vs. active; HRT and no-HRT within each group	CIMT, FIMT	No-HRT sedentaries had ↑ FIMT than rest; no differences for IMT; in >65, IMT is ↓ in HRT compared with no-HRT	Prospective
Chironi 2003[127]	36	Human immunodeficiency virus patients	Antiretroviral meds	CIMT, lipid panel, waist circumference	↓ HDL may be involved in early atherosclerosis in HIV patients	Prospective controlled
DCCT/EDIC 2003[128]	1229	IDDM and control group	Conventional (611) vs. intensive treatment (618)	CIMT	<IMT progression with intensive treatment	Observational follow-up
Erenus 2003[129]	20	Postmenopausal healthy females	Tibolone 2.5 mg/d for 12 weeks	CIMT, RI CCA/ICA/ ECA/VA	Significant ↓ in CIMT	Prospective
Salonen 2003[130]	440	Males, smokers and non-smokers, and postmenopausal females, 45–69 years old and cholesterol >193	136 IU vitamin E and 250 mg vitamin C BID	CIMT	Significant ↓ combined IMT in male and combined, not in females	Prospective

IMT, intima-media thickness; CIMT, carotid intima-media thickness; BP, blood pressure; ESRD, end-stage renal disease; AOPP, advanced oxidation protein products; CIMT, carotid IMT; FIMT, femoral IMT; HRT, hormone-replacement therapy; HCTZ, hydrochlorothiazide; BID, twice a day; RI, resistivity index; CCA, common carotid artery; ECA, external carotid artery; ICA, internal carotid artery; VA, vertebral artery; IDDM, insulin-dependent diabetes mellitus; DCCT, Diabetes Control and Complications Trial; EDIC, Epidemiology of Diabetes Interventions and Complications.

The subendothelial accumulation of inflammatory products in the arterial wall increases the IMT in atherosclerosis. Several randomized, multicenter, placebo-controlled trials showed conclusively that the use of statins slows the progression of atherosclerosis and decreases the IMT in several studies (see Table 14-4).[26,106–115]

Reported adverse outcomes included major cardiovascular events (e.g., death, stroke, nonfatal heart attacks) in both groups, significantly higher in the placebo group (p = 0.04).

Pitt and colleagues[116] studied in a multicenter, randomized, placebo-controlled trial the impact of amlodipine in 825 patients with angiographic-documented CHD. The primary goal was to determine if the drug would reduce early atherosclerosis progression as measured by a change in the mean minimal diameter using quantitative coronary angiography. A secondary goal was to test atherosclerosis progression through IMT estimation in 12 carotid segments (i.e., near and far walls of the CCA, bifurcation, and ICA bilaterally). At 3 years the average reduction in the mean minimal diameter was almost identical for both groups. The IMT increased by 0.033 mm in the placebo group and decreased by 0.013 mm with amlodipine (p = 0.007). Similar conclusions have been obtained in several other studies (see Table 14-5).[116–123] The use of amlodipine reduced the rates of combined nonfatal congestive heart failure and unstable angina (p = 0.01) and the need for coronary revascularization (p = 0.001).

Flow-Mediated Dilatation and IMT

Arteries of large caliber are capable to accommodate bloodflow changes by increasing their internal diameter; this is called flow-dependent dilatation (FMD), and it represents another surrogate marker for vascular disease. It opposes neurogenic and myogenic vasoconstriction, increases conductance on exertion, and maintains shear stress within physiologic range.[131] Experiments in isolated arteries or in animals suggest that FMD of conduit arteries is mediated through the release of endothelium-derived nitric oxide (NO) and/or prostacyclin.[132] FMD of large arteries in vivo has been used as an index of endothelial function in humans and is impaired in atherosclerosis.[131] Human studies have shown that NO is essential for FMD of human radial arteries in vivo.[131]

Few studies have addressed the relation between FMD and IMT. Ravikumar and colleagues[133] measured FMD in the brachial artery and correlated it with the carotid IMT in 50 diabetic and 50 age- and sex-matched nondiabetic control subjects. Overall, FMD had a significant inverse correlation with IMT (p = 0.001), and that finding was also true within the nondiabetic group. Lower FMD values were seen with an increase in quartiles of IMT both in diabetics and nondiabetics. Diabetic subjects had decreased FMD and increased arterial stiffness compared with nondiabetics.[133] Another study addressed the influence of apolipoprotein E (apoE) polymorphism on plasma lipoprotein levels and the development of cardiovascular disease. A negative correlation between brachial-FMD and carotid IMT was found in all subjects (r = −0.21, p < 0.05) being most clear in the E3E4 group (r = −0.53, p < 0.02).[134] A study of 122 patients with clinically suspected CHD before coronary angiography was performed analyzing carotid IMT and brachial FMD.[135] A negative correlation was shown between FMD and IMT (r = −0.317, p = 0.0004).

Receiver-operator characteristic curves showed that FMD was a better predictor of CHD, and IMT had a positive correlation with the extent of CHD.

Current Research and the Future

Other surrogate markers are being currently investigated. They include high-sensitivity C-reactive protein, soluble vascular cell adhesion molecule, soluble intercellular adhesion molecule, endothelial selectin, homocysteine, and von Willebrand factor (vWF).[136] Cell adhesion molecules are thought to have a key role in onset of atherosclerosis. They have been studied as possible predictive markers of presence and severity of atherosclerotic disease in patients with familial hypercholesterolemia, known to develop early severe coronary artery disease. Carotid IMT was also measured in this study. The use of individual levels of these molecules was found to be not predictive of atherosclerosis in this subgroup of patients.[137] Another paper that studied 42 subjects with familial hypercholesterolemia showed that after multivariate analysis, only LDL cholesterol and the cholesterol-years score were strong predictors of carotid IMT (multiple r = 0.82; r^2 = 0.68; p < 0.001).[138]

The coagulation profile of individuals with PVD and high IMT measurements was also studied. Cortellaro and colleagues[139] analyzed 64 patients with PVD. Some 24 patients had high IMT values, and the other 40 did not. Their coagulation profiles were compared; elevated plasma concentrations of factor VII and von Willebrand factor correlated with increasing IMT, and they were thought to possibly play a role in atherosclerosis progression.

REFERENCES

1. Raitakari OT, Juonala M, Kahonen M, et al: Cardiovascular risk factors in childhood and carotid artery intima-media thickness in adulthood: The cardiovascular risk in young Finns study. JAMA 290:2277–2283, 2003.
2. Berenson GS, Srinivasan SR, Bao W, et al: Association between multiple cardiovascular risk factors and atherosclerosis in children and young adults: The Bogalusa Heart Study. N Engl J Med 338:1650–1656, 1998.
3. Pauciullo P, Iannuzzi A, Sartorio R, et al: Increased intima-media thickness of the common carotid artery in hypercholesterolemic children. Arterioscler Thromb 14:1075–1079, 1994.
4. Mahoney LT, Lauer RM, Lee J, et al: Factors affecting tracking of coronary heart disease risk factors in children: The Muscatine Study. Ann N Y Acad Sci 623:120–132, 1991.
5. Porkka KV, Viikari JS, Taimela S, et al: Tracking and predictiveness of serum lipid and lipoprotein measurements in childhood: A 12-year follow-up: The cardiovascular risk in young Finns study. Am J Epidemiol 140:1096–1110, 1994.
6. Akerblom HK, Viikari J, Raitakari OT, et al: Cardiovascular risk in young Finns study: General outline and recent developments. Ann Med 31 (Suppl 1):45–54, 1999.
7. Berenson GS: Childhood risk factors predict adult risk associated with subclinical cardiovascular disease: The Bogalusa Heart Study. Am J Cardiol 90(Suppl):3L–7L, 2002.

8. Stamler J, Daviglus ML, Garside DB, et al: Relationship of baseline serum cholesterol levels in three large cohorts of younger men to long-term coronary, cardiovascular, and all cause mortality and to longevity. JAMA 284:311–318, 2000.

9. Poli A, Tremoli E, Colombo A, et al: Ultrasonographic measurement of the common carotid artery wall thickness in hypercholesterolemic patients: A new model for the quantitation and follow-up of preclinical atherosclerosis in living human subjects. Atherosclerosis 70:253–261, 1988.

10. Burke GL, Evans GW, Riley WA, et al: Arterial wall thickness is associated with prevalent cardiovascular disease in middle-aged adults: The Atherosclerosis Risk in Communities (ARIC) Study. Stroke 26:386–391, 1995.

11. Salonen JT, Salonen R: Ultrasonographically assessed carotid morphology and the risk of coronary heart disease. Arterioscler Thromb 11:1245–1249, 1991.

12. Bots ML, Hoes AW, Koudstaal PJ, et al: Common carotid intima-media thickness and risk of stroke and myocardial infarction: The Rotterdam Study. Circulation 96:1432–1437, 1997.

13. Hodis HN, Mack WJ, La Bree L, et al: The role of carotid arterial intima-media thickness in predicting clinical coronary events. Ann Intern Med 128:262–269, 1998.

14. O'Leary DH, Polak JF, Kronmal RA, et al: Cardiovascular Health Study Collaborative Research Group. Carotid-artery intima and media thickness as a risk factor for myocardial infarction and stroke in older adults. N Engl J Med 340:14–22, 1999.

15. Davis PH, Dawson JD, Riley WA, et al: Carotid intimal-medial thickness is related to cardiovascular risk factors measured from childhood through middle age: The Muscatine Study. Circulation 104:2815–2819, 2001.

16. www.americanheart.org/downloadable/heart/10590179711482 003HDSStatsBookREV7-03.pdf

17. Montauban van Swijndregt AD, The SH, Gussenhoven EJ, et al: An in vitro evaluation of the line pattern of the near and far walls of carotid arteries using B-mode Ultrasound. Ultrasound Med Biol 22:1007–1015, 1996.

18. Wendelhag I, Gustavsson T, Suurkula M, et al: Ultrasound measurement of wall thickness in the carotid artery: Fundamental principles and description of a computerized analyzing system. Clin Physiol 11:565–577, 1991.

19. Glagov S, Newman WP III, Schaffer SA (eds): Pathobiology of the Human Atherosclerotic Plaque. New York: Springer-Verlag, 1990.

20. Pignoli P, Tremoli E, Poli A, et al: Intimal plus medial thickness of the arterial wall: A direct measurement with ultrasound imaging. Circulation 74:1399–1406, 1986.

21. Gamble G, Beaumont B, Smith H, et al: B-mode ultrasound images of the carotid artery wall: Correlation of ultrasound with histological measurements. Atherosclerosis 102:163–173, 1993.

22. Linhart A, Gariepy J, Girai P, et al: Carotid artery and left ventricular relationship in asymptomatic men at risk for cardiovascular disease. Atherosclerosis 127:103–112, 1996.

23. Labropoulos N, Zarge J, Mansour MA, et al: Compensatory arterial enlargement is a common pathobiologic response in early atherosclerosis. Am J Surg 176:140–143, 1998.

24. Salonen JT, Korpela H, Salonen R, et al: Precision and reproducibility of ultrasonographic measurement of progression of common carotid artery atherosclerosis. Lancet 341:1158–1159, 1993.

25. Touboul PJ, Prati P, Scarabin PY, et al: Use of monitoring software to improve the measurement of carotid wall thickness by B-mode imaging. J Hypertens 10(Suppl):37–41, 1992.

26. Salonen R, Nyyssonen K, Porkkala E, et al: Kuopio Atherosclerosis Prevention Study (KAPS): A population-based primary preventive trial of the effect of LDL lowering on atherosclerotic progression in carotid and femoral arteries. Circulation 92:1758–1764, 1995.

27. Ebrahim S, Papacosta O, Whincup P, et al: Carotid plaque, intima media thickness, cardiovascular risk factors, and prevalent cardiovascular disease in men and women: The British Regional Heart Study. Stroke 30:841–850, 1999.

28. Salonen R, Salonen JT: Determinants of carotid intima-media thickness: A population-based ultrasonography study in eastern Finnish men. J Intern Med 229:225–231, 1991.

29. Ferrara LA, Mancini M, Celentano A, et al: Early changes of the arterial carotid wall in uncomplicated primary hypertensive patients. Study by ultrasound high-resolution B-mode imaging. Arterioscler Thromb 13:1290–1296, 1994.

30. Linhart A, Gariepy J, Massonneau M, et al: Carotid intima-media thickness: The ultimate surrogate end-point of cardiovascular involvement in atherosclerosis. Applied Radiology 29:25–39, 2000.

31. Wendelhag I, Liang Q, Gustavsson T, et al: A new automated computerized analyzing system simplifies readings and reduces the variability in ultrasound measurement of intima media thickness. Stroke 28:2195–2200, 1997.

32. Wikstrand J, Wendelhag I: Methodological considerations of ultrasound investigation of intima-media thickness and lumen diameter. J Intern Med 236:555–559, 1994.

33. Howard G, Sharrett AR, Heiss G, et al: Carotid artery intimal-medial thickness distribution in general populations as evaluated by B-mode ultrasound. ARIC Investigators. Stroke 24:1297–1304, 1993.

34. Riley WA, Barnes RW, Applegate WB, et al: Reproducibility of noninvasive ultrasonic measurement of carotid atherosclerosis. The asymptomatic carotid artery plaque study. Stroke 23:1062–1068, 1992.

35. Bond MG, Barnes RW, Rile WA, et al: High-resolution B-mode ultrasound reading methods in the Atherosclerosis Risk in Communities cohort: The ARIC study group. J Neuroimaging 1:168–172, 1991.

36. Bonithon-Kopp C, Touboul PJ, Berr C, et al: Factors of carotid arterial enlargement in a population aged 59 to 71 years: The EVA study. Stroke 27:654–660, 1996.

37. Labropoulos N, Mansour A, Kang SS, et al: Viscoelastic properties of normal and atherosclerotic carotid arteries. Eur J Vasc Endovasc Surg 19:221–225, 2000.

38. Tell GS, Howard G, McKinney WM: Risk factors for site-specific extracranial carotid artery plaque distributions measured by M-mode ultrasound. J Clin Epidemiol 42:551–559, 1989.

39. Glagov S, Zarins CK, Masawa N, et al: Mechanical functional role of non-atherosclerotic intimal thickening. Front Med Biol Eng 5:37–43, 1993.

40. Bonithon-Kopp C, Touboul PJ, Berr C, et al: Factors of carotid arterial enlargement in a population aged 59-71: The EVA study. Stroke 27:654–660, 1996.

41. Hoeks AP, Willekes C, Boutouyrie P, et al: Automated detection of local artery wall thickness based on M-line signal processing. Ultrasound Med Biol 23:1017–1023, 1997.

42. Tardy Y, Hayoz D, Mignot JP, et al: Dynamic noninvasive measurements of arterial diameter and wall thickness. J Hypertens 10(Suppl)6:105–109, 1992.

43. Fasseas P, Brilakis ES, Leybishkis B, et al: Association of carotid artery intima-media thickness with complex aortic atherosclerosis in patients with recent stroke. Angiology 53:185–189, 2002.

44. Belhassen L, Carville C, Pelle G, et al: Evaluation of carotid artery and aortic intima-media thickness measurements for exclusion of significant coronary atherosclerosis in patients scheduled for heart valve surgery. J Am Coll Cardiol 39:1139–1144, 2002.

45. Kallikazaros IE, Tsioufis CP, Stefanadis CI, et al: Closed relation between carotid and ascending aortic atherosclerosis in cardiac patients. Circulation 102(19 Suppl 3):263–268, 2000.

46. Petronio AS, Musumeci G, Limbruno U, et al: Coronary angioplasty in women: Risk factors and sex-related differences in coronary anatomy evaluated with intravascular ultrasonography.

Italian Heart Journal: Official Journal of the Italian Federation of Cardiology 3(1 Suppl):71–77, 2002.

47. Anderson TJ, Meredith IT, Uehata A, et al: Functional significance of intimal thickening as detected by intravascular ultrasound early and late after cardiac transplantation. Circulation 88:1093–1100, 1993.

48. Corti R, Fuster V, Fayad ZA, et al: Lipid lowering by simvastatin induces regression of human atherosclerotic lesions: 2 years' follow-up by high-resolution noninvasive magnetic resonance imaging. Circulation 106:2884–2887, 2002.

49. Helft G, Worthley SG, Fuster V, et al: Progression and regression of atherosclerotic lesions: Monitoring with serial noninvasive magnetic resonance imaging. Circulation 105:993–998, 2002.

50. Abolmaali N, Langenfeld M, Krahforst R, et al: Vessel wall MRI of the thoracic aorta: Correlation to histology and transesophageal ultrasound. Preliminary results. Rofo Fortschr Geb Rontgenstr Neuen Bildgeb Verfahr 174:568–572, 2002.

51. Sass C, Herbeth B, Chapet O, et al: Intima-media thickness and diameter of carotid and femoral arteries in children, adolescents, and adults from the Stanislaus cohort: Effect of age, sex, anthropometry, and blood pressure. J Hypertens 16:1593–1602, 1998.

52. Salonen R, Salonen JT: Progression of carotid atherosclerosis and its determinants: A population-based ultrasonography study. Atherosclerosis 81:33–40, 1990.

53. Paivansalo M, Rantala A, Kauma H, et al: Prevalence of carotid atherosclerosis in middle-aged hypertensive and control subjects. A cross-sectional systematic study with duplex ultrasound. J Hypertens 14:1433–1439, 1996.

54. D'Agostino RB Jr, Burke G, O'Leary D, et al: Ethnic differences in carotid wall thickness. The insulin resistance atherosclerosis study. Stroke 27:1744–1749, 1996.

55. Stevens J, Tyroler HA, Cai J, et al: Body weight changes and carotid artery wall thickness. The Atherosclerosis Risk in Communities Study. Am J Epidemiol 147:563–573, 1998.

56. Folsom AR, Eckfeldt JH, Witzman S, et al: Atherosclerosis risk in communities. Relation of carotid artery wall thickness to diabetes mellitus, fasting glucose and insulin, body size, and physical activity. Stroke 5:66–73, 1994.

57. Reaven GM: Banting lecture 1988: Role of insulin resistance in human disease. Diabetes 37:1595–1607, 1988.

58. Yudkin JS, Stehouwer CD, Emeis JJ, et al: C-reactive protein in healthy subjects: Associations with obesity, insulin resistance, and endothelial dysfunction: A potential role for cytokines originating from adipose tissue? Arterioscler Thromb Vasc Biol 19:972–978, 1999.

59. Hotamisligil GS, Arner P, Caro JF, et al: Increased adipose tissue expression of tumor necrosis factor-alpha in human obesity and insulin resistance. J Clin Invest 95:2409–2415, 1995.

60. Engeli S, Negrel R, Sharma AM: Physiology and pathophysiology of the adipose tissue rennin-angiotensin system. Hypertension 35:120–177, 2000.

61. Cuspidi C, Marabini M, Lonati L, et al: Cardiac and carotid structure in patients with established hypertension and white-coat hypertension. J Hypertens 13:1707–1711, 1995.

62. Muisan ML, Pasini G, Salvetti M, et al: cardiac and vascular structural changes. Prevalence and relation to ambulatory blood pressure in a middle-aged general population in northern Italy: The Vobarno study. Hypertension 27:1046–1052, 1996.

63. Zanchetti A, Crepaldi G, Bond MG, et al: Systolic and pulse blood pressures (but not diastolic blood pressure and serum cholesterol) are associated with alterations in carotid intima-media thickness in the moderately hypercholesterolaemic hypertensive patients of the Plaque Hypertension Lipid Lowering Italian Study. PHYLLIS study group. J Hypertens 19:79–88, 2001.

64. Wendelhag I, Wiklund O, Wikstrand J: Arterial wall thickness in familial hypercholesterolemia. Ultrasound measurement of intima-media thickness in the common carotid artery. Arterioscler Thromb 12:70–77, 1992.

65. Sharrett AR, Patsch W, Sorlie PD, et al: Associations of lipoprotein cholesterols, apolipoproteins A-I and B, and triglycerides with carotid atherosclerosis and coronary heart disease. The atherosclerosis risk in communities study. Arterioscler Thromb 14:1098–1104, 1994.

66. Pujia A, Gnasso A, Irace C, et al: Common carotid arterial wall thickness in NIDDM subjects. Diabetes Care 17:1330–1336, 1994.

67. Wilt TJ, Rubins HB, Robins SJ, et al: Carotid atherosclerosis in men with low levels of HDL cholesterol. Stroke 28:1919–1925, 1997.

68. Mowbray PI, Lee AJ, Fowkes GR, et al: Cardiovascular risk factors for early carotid atherosclerosis in the general population: The Edinburgh artery study. J Cardiovasc Risk 4:357–362, 1997.

69. Hodis HN, Mack WJ, Dunn M, et al: Intermediate-density lipoproteins and progression of carotid arterial wall intima-media thickness. Circulation 95:2022–2026, 1997.

70. Howard G, Burke GL, Szklo M, et al: Active and passive smoking are associated with increased carotid wall thickness. The atherosclerosis risk in communities study. Arch Intern Med 154:1277–1282, 1994.

71. Tell GS, Polka JF, Ward BJ, et al: Relation of smoking with carotid artery wall thickness and stenosis in older adults. The cardiovascular health study collaborative research group. Circulation 90:2905–2908, 1994.

72. Diez-Roux AV, Nieto FJ, Comstock GW, et al: The relationship of active and passive smoking to carotid atherosclerosis 12–14 years later. Prev Med 24:48–55, 1995.

73. Markus RA, Mack WJ, Azen SP, et al: Influence of lifestyle modification on atherosclerotic progression determined by ultrasonographic change in the common carotid intima-media thickness. Am J Clin Nutr 65:1000–1004, 1997.

74. Visona A, Lusiani L, Bonanome A, et al: Wall thickening of common carotid arteries in patients affected by noninsulin-dependent diabetes mellitus: Relationship to microvascular complications. Angiology 46:793–799, 1995.

75. Mykka Nen L, Zaccaro DJ, O'Leary DH, et al: Microalbuminuria and carotid artery intima-media thickness in nondiabetic and NIDDM subjects. The Insulin Resistance Atherosclerosis Study. Stroke 28:1710–1716, 1997.

76. Wagenknecht LE, D'Agostino R, Savage PJ, et al: Duration of diabetes and carotid wall thickness. The Insulin Resistance Atherosclerosis Study. Stroke 28:999–1005, 1997.

77. Muzaffar K, Collins SL, Labropoulos N, et al: A prospective study of the effects of irradiation on the carotid artery. Laryngoscope 110:1811–1814, 2000.

78. Chapman CM, Beilby JP, Humphries SE, et al: Association of an allelic variant of interleukin-6 with subclinical carotid atherosclerosis in an Australian community population. Eur Heart J 24:1494–1499, 2003.

79. Inamoto N, Katsuya T, Kokubo Y, et al: Association of methyl-enetetrahydrofolate reductase gene polymorphism with carotid atherosclerosis depending on smoking status in a Japanese general population. Stroke 34:1628–1633, 2003.

80. Fortunato G, Rubba P, Panico S, et al: A paraoxonase gene polymorphism, PON 1 (55), as an independent risk factor for increased carotid intima-media thickness in middle-aged women. Atherosclerosis 167:141–148, 2003.

81. Beilby JP, Hunt CC, Palmer LJ, et al: Apolipoprotein E gene polymorphisms are associated with carotid plaque formation but not with intima-media wall thickening: Results from the Perth Carotid Ultrasound Disease Assessment Study (CUDAS). Stroke 34:869–874, 2003.

82. Ludwig M, von Petzinger-Kruthoff A, von Buquoy M, et al: Intima-media thickness of the carotid arteries: Early pointer to arteriosclerosis and therapeutic endpoint. Ultraschall Med 24:162–174, 2003.

83. Smith SC, Greenland P, Grundy SM: Prevention Conference V. Beyond secondary prevention: Identifying the high-risk patient for primary prevention: Executive summary citation AHA. Circulation. 101:111(e16–e22), 2000.

84. Mika M: Expanding statin use to help more at-risk patients is causing financial heartburn. JAMA 290:2243–2245, 2003.

85. Blankenhorn DH, Hodis HN: George Lyman Duff Memorial Lecture. Arterial imaging and atherosclerosis reversal. Arterioscler Thromb 14:177–192, 1994.

86. Cheng KS, Mikhailidis DP, Hamilton G, et al: A review of the carotid and femoral intima-media thickness as an indicator of the presence of peripheral vascular disease and cardiovascular risk factors. Cardiovasc Res 54:528–538, 2002.

87. Bots ML, Hofman A, Grobbee DE: Common carotid intima-media thickness and lower extremity arterial atherosclerosis. The Rotterdam Study. Arterioscler Thromb 14:1885–1891, 1994.

88. Allan PL, Mowbray PI, Lee AJ, et al: Relationship between carotid intima-media thickness and symptomatic and asymptomatic peripheral arterial disease. The Edinburgh Artery Study. Stroke 28:348–353, 1997.

89. Simons PC, Algra A, Bots ML, et al: Common carotid intima-media thickness in patients with peripheral arterial disease or abdominal aortic aneurysm: The SMART study. Second Manifestations of ARTerial disease. Atherosclerosis 146:243–248, 1999.

90. Anderson KM, Wilson PW, Odell PM, et al: An updated coronary risk profile. A statement for health professionals. Circulation 83:356–362, 1991.

91. Hoes AW, Grobbee DE, Valkenburg HA, et al: Cardiovascular risk and all-cause mortality: A 12-year follow-up study in The Netherlands. Eur J Epidemiol 9:285–292, 1993.

92. Alcorn HG, Wolfson SK, Sutton-Tyrrell K, et al: Risk factors for abdominal aortic aneurysms in older adults enrolled in the Cardiovascular Health Study. Arterioscler Thromb Vasc Biol 16:963–970, 1996.

93. Chambless LE, Heiss G, Folsom AR, et al: Association of coronary heart disease incidence with carotid arterial wall thickness and major risk factors: The Atherosclerosis Risk in Communities (ARIC) Study, 1987–1993. Am J Epidemiol 146:483–494, 1997.

94. Polak JF, O'Leary DH, Kronmal RA, et al: Sonographic evaluation of carotid artery atherosclerosis in the elderly: Relationship of disease severity to stroke and transient ischemic attack. Radiology 188:363–370, 1993.

95. Bots ML, van Swieten JC, Breteler MM, et al: Cerebral white matter lesions and atherosclerosis in the Rotterdam Study. Lancet 341:1232–1237, 1993.

96. Auperin A, Berr C, Bonithon-Kopp C, et al: Ultrasonographic assessment of carotid wall characteristics and cognitive functions in a community sample of 59- to 71-year-olds. The EVA Study Group. Stroke 27:1290–1295, 1996.

97. Chambless LE, Shahar E, Sharrett AR, et al: Association of transient ischemic attack/stroke symptoms assessed by standardized questionnaire and algorithm with cerebrovascular risk factors and carotid artery wall thickness. The ARIC Study, 1987–1989. Am J Epidemiol 144:857–866, 1996.

98. Yamakado M, Fukuda I, Kiyose H: Ultrasonographically assessed carotid intima-media thickness and risk for asymptomatic cerebral infarction. J Med Syst 22:15–18, 1998.

99. Kawamura T, Umemura T, Kanai A, et al: The incidence and characteristics of silent cerebral infarction in elderly diabetic patients: Association with serum-soluble adhesion molecules. Diabetologia 41:911–917, 1998.

100. Touboul PJ, Elbaz A, Koller C, et al: Common carotid artery intima-media thickness and brain infarction: The Etude du Profil Genetique de l'Infarctus Cerebral (GENIC) case-control study. The GENIC Investigators. Circulation 102:313–318, 2000.

101. Cupini LM, Pasqualetti P, Diomedi M, et al: Carotid artery intima-media thickness and lacunar versus nonlacunar infarcts. Stroke 33:689–694, 2002.

102. Joensuu T, Salonen R, Winbland I, et al: Determinants of femoral and carotid atherosclerosis. J Intern Med 236:79–84, 1994.

103. Suurkula M, Fagerberg B, Wendelhag I, et al: Atherosclerotic disease in the femoral artery in hypertensive patients at high cardiovascular risk. The value of ultrasonographic assessment of intima-media thickness and plaque occurrence. Risk Intervention Study (RIS) Group. Arterioscler Thromb Vasc Biol 16:971–977, 1996.

104. Veller MG, Fisher CM, Nicolaides AN, et al: Measurement of the ultrasonic intima-media complex thickness in normal subjects. J Vasc Surg 4:719–725, 1993.

105. Wakeyama T, Ogawa H, Iida H, et al: Intima-media thickening of the radial artery after transradial intervention. An intravascular ultrasound study. J Am Coll Cardiol 41:1109–1114, 2003.

106. Byington RP, Evans GW, Espeland MA, et al: Effects of lovastatin and warfarin on early carotid atherosclerosis: Sex-specific analyses. Asymptomatic Carotid Artery Progression Study (ACAPS) research group. Circulation 100:e14–e17, 1999.

107. de Groot E, Jukema JW, van Boven AJ, et al: Effect of pravastatin on progression and regression of coronary atherosclerosis and vessel wall changes in carotid and femoral arteries: A report from the Regression Growth Evaluation Statin Study. Am J Cardiol 76:40C–46C, 1995.

108. Crouse JR III, Byington RP, Bond MG, et al: Pravastatin, lipids, and atherosclerosis in the carotid arteries (PLAC-II). Am J Cardiol 75:455–459, 1995.

109. Mercuri M, Bond MG, Sirtori CR, et al: Pravastatin reduces carotid intima-media thickness progression in an asymptomatic hypercholesterolemic Mediterranean population: The Carotid Atherosclerosis Italian Ultrasound Study. Am J Med 101:627–634, 1996.

110. Hodis HN, Mack WJ, LaBree L, et al: Reduction in carotid arterial wall thickness using lovastatin and dietary therapy: A randomized controlled clinical trial. Ann Intern Med 124:548–556, 1996.

111. MacMahon S, Sharpe N, Gamble G, et al: Effects of lowering average of below-average cholesterol levels on the progression of carotid atherosclerosis: Results of the LIPID Atherosclerosis Substudy. LIPID Trial Research Group. Circulation 97:1784–1790, 1998.

112. Smilde TJ, van Wissen S, Wollersheim H, et al: Effect of aggressive versus conventional lipid lowering on atherosclerosis progression in familial hypercholesterolaemia (ASAP): A prospective, randomised, double-blind trial. Lancet 357:577–581, 2001.

113. Taylor AJ, Kent SM, Flaherty PJ, et al: ARBITER: Arterial biology for the investigation of the treatment effects of reducing cholesterol: A randomized trial comparing the effects of atorvastatin and pravastatin on carotid intima-medial thickness. Circulation 106:2055–2060, 2002.

114. Youssef F, Seifalian AM, Jagroop IA, et al: The early effect of lipid-lowering treatment on carotid and femoral intima-media thickness (IMT). Eur J Vasc Endovasc Surg 23:358–364, 2002.

115. Nolting PR, de Groot E, Zwinderman AH, et al: Regression of carotid and femoral artery intima-media thickness in familial hypercholesterolemia: Treatment with simvastatin. Arch Intern Med 163:1837–1841, 2003.

116. Pitt B, Byington RP, Furberg CD, et al: Effect of amlodipine on the progression of atherosclerosis and the occurrence of clinical events. PREVENT Investigators. Circulation 102:1503–1510, 2000.

117. Hedblad B, Wikstrand J, Janzon L, et al: Low-dose metoprolol CR/XL and fluvastatin slow progression of carotid intima-media thickness: Main results from the Beta-Blocker Cholesterol-Lowering Asymptomatic Plaque Study (BCAPS). Circulation 103:1721–1726, 2001.

118. Simon A, Gariepy J, Moyse D, et al: Differential effects of nifedipine and co-amilozide on the progression of early carotid wall changes. Circulation 103:2949–2954, 2001.

119. Hoogerbrugge N, de Groot E, de Heide LH, et al: Doxazosin and hydrochlorothiazide equally affect arterial wall thickness in hypertensive males with hypercholesterolaemia (the DAPHNE study). Doxazosin Atherosclerosis Progression Study in Hypertensives in the Netherlands. Neth J Med 60:354–361, 2002.

120. Yamakado M: Protective vascular effect of angiotensin receptor blocker (ARB). Nippon Rinsho 60:2020–2027, 2002.

121. Bozec E, Fassot C, Tropeano AI, et al: Angiotensinogen gene M235T polymorphism and reduction in wall thickness in response to antihypertensive treatment. Clin Sci (Lond) 105:637–644, 2003.

122. Terpstra WF, May JF, Smit AJ, et al: Effects of nifedipine on carotid and femoral arterial wall thickness in previously untreated hypertensive patients. Blood Press Suppl (Suppl 1):22–29, 2003.

123. Wiklund O, Hulthe J, Wikstrand J, et al: Effect of controlled release/extended release metoprolol on carotid intima-media thickness in patients with hypercholesterolemia: A 3-year randomized study. Stroke 33:572–577, 2002.

124. Raal FJ, Pilcher GJ, Veller MG, et al: Efficacy of vitamin E compared with either simvastatin or atorvastatin in preventing the progression of atherosclerosis in homozygous familial hypercholesterolemia. Am J Cardiol 84:1344–1346, 1999.

125. Drueke T, Witko-Sarsat V, Massy Z, et al: Iron therapy, advanced oxidation protein products, and carotid artery intima-media thickness in end-stage renal disease. Circulation 106:2212–2217, 2002.

126. Moreau KL, Donato AJ, Seals DR, et al: Arterial intima-media thickness: Site-specific associations with HRT and habitual exercise. Am J Physiol Heart Circ Physiol 283:H1409–H1417, 2002.

127. Chironi G, Escaut L, Gariepy J, et al: Brief report: Carotid intima-media thickness in heavily pretreated HIV-infected patients. J Acquir Immune Defic Syndr 32:490–493, 2003.

128. Nathan DM, Lachin J, Cleary P, et al: Diabetes Control and Complications Trial; Epidemiology of diabetes interventions and complications research group. Intensive diabetes therapy and carotid intima-media thickness in type 1 diabetes mellitus. N Engl J Med 348:2294–2303, 2003.

129. Erenus M, Ilhan AH, Elter K: Effect of tibolone treatment on intima-media thickness and the resistive indices of the carotid arteries. Fertil Steril 79:268–273, 2003.

130. Salonen RM, Nyyssonen K, Kaikkonen J, et al: Antioxidant supplementation in atherosclerosis prevention study. Six-year effect of combined vitamin C and E supplementation on atherosclerotic progression: The Antioxidant Supplementation in Atherosclerosis Prevention (ASAP) Study. Circulation 107:947–953, 2003.

131. Joannides R, Haefeli WE, Linder L, et al: Nitric oxide is responsible for flow-dependent dilatation of human peripheral conduit arteries in vivo. Circulation 91:1314–1319, 1995.

132. Joannides R, Haefeli WE, Linder L, et al: Role of nitric oxide in flow-dependent vasodilation of human peripheral arteries in vivo. Arch Mal Coeur Vaiss 87:983–985, 1994.

133. Ravikumar R, Deepa R, Shantirani C, et al: Comparison of carotid intima-media thickness, arterial stiffness, and brachial artery flow mediated dilatation in diabetic and nondiabetic subjects (The Chennai Urban Population Study [CUPS-9]). Am J Cardiol 90:702–707, 2002.

134. Haraki T, Takegoshi T, Kitoh C, et al: Carotid artery intima-media thickness and brachial artery flow-mediated vasodilation in asymptomatic Japanese male subjects amongst apolipoprotein E phenotypes. J Intern Med 252:114–120, 2002.

135. Enderle MD, Schroeder S, Ossen R, et al: Comparison of peripheral endothelial dysfunction and intimal media thickness in patients with suspected coronary artery disease. Heart 80:349–354, 1998.

136. Grewal J, Chan S, Frohlich J, et al: Assessment of novel risk factors in patients at low risk for cardiovascular events based on Framingham risk stratification. Clin Invest Med 26:158–165, 2003.

137. Paiker JE, Raal FJ, Veller M, et al: Cell adhesion molecules: Can they be used to predict coronary artery disease in patients with familial hypercholesterolaemia? Clin Chim Acta 293:105–113, 2000.

138. Raal FJ, Pilcher GJ, Waisberg R, et al: Low-density lipoprotein cholesterol bulk is the pivotal determinant of atherosclerosis in familial hypercholesterolemia. Am J Cardiol 83:1330–1333, 1999.

139. Cortellaro M, Baldassarre D, Cofrancesco E, et al: Relation between hemostatic variables and increase of common carotid intima-media thickness in patients with peripheral arterial disease. Stroke 27:450–454, 1996.

Chapter 15

Surveillance and Follow-Up After Carotid Endarterectomy

ALI F. ABURAHMA

Introduction

Restenosis is a known entity that occurs after carotid endarterectomy (CEA), but the frequency of restenosis varies, depending on the diagnostic method used and the frequency of follow-up examinations.[1-12] Several studies have reported on the value of postoperative carotid duplex surveillance, but no consensus has been reached.[1-12] The advantages cited are detection of significant restenosis befor the onset of neurologic events, which aids in the prevention of potential strokes, and follow-up on the contralateral carotid artery, to document the development of surgically correctable stenosis. Opponents of routine postoperative carotid duplex sur-veillance claim that restenosis is benign in nature, and therefore a large number of strokes may not be prevented by this surveillance.[5,6,8,9,12] Some of these studies have reported restenoses of more than 50% in 12% to 36% of the endarterectomized arteries.[1] Despite the high rate of restenosis, symptoms attributed to restenoses are rare; therefore several authorities have suggested that routine surveillance of patients after CEA is not efficacious.[4-6,9]

Mattos and colleagues[6] described their experience with postoperative carotid duplex surveillance and found an equal stroke-free survival at 5 years between patients with or without > 50% restenosis. In addition, only 1 of 380 patients suffered a stroke in their study, suggesting a benign clinical significance of recurrent carotid artery stenosis. Based on these results, the authors suggest an initial 6-month duplex examination and subsequent yearly duplex surveillance examinations. Mackey and colleagues claim a low rate of clinically significant restenosis.[5] Their retrospective series of 258 patients (348 arteries) show a potential 4% incidence of late strokes, but this included all patients who underwent repeat CEA for asymptomatic restenosis. They also note that the majority of restenoses (53%) remained asymptomatic and did not progress to occlusion through-out follow-up. Of 10 documented late occlusions, 8 did not result in stroke. Eight patients with operable resteno-sis had transient ischemic attacks (TIAs) and under-went reoperation. The authors found that even patients with 75% to 99% restenosis most often remained asymptomatic (37%) or had TIAs (32%). Only 2 of 19 patients (11%) with 75% to 99% restenosis had an unheralded stroke. The authors feel that postoperative carotid duplex surveillance is not justified because of the low incidence of symptomatic restenosis.

In spite of these findings, investigators have been reluctant to advise that postoperative carotid duplex surveillance be abandoned because the cost-effectiveness of this surveillance has not been formally investigated. Others have reported that high-grade stenosis (>75%), whether caused by myointimal hyperplasia of the CEA site or by progressive atherosclerosis of the contralateral carotid artery, is associated with an increased risk of late stroke.[12,13]

Ouriel and Green reported an 11% incidence of restenotic lesions greater than 80%. Although the incidence of symptoms with restenotic lesions was low (12%), the onset of symptoms at the time of occlusion was significant.[7] Some 42% of patients became symptomatic at the time of occlusion, with 33% resulting in a stroke. This led to the observation that critical restenoses are precursors to stroke, even if asymptomatic, and therefore the detection of greater than 80% restenosis allows future stroke prevention if operative intervention is undertaken.[7] Mattos and colleagues also described the outcome for greater than 80% restenosis. In their group of three patients with greater than 80% restenosis, one suffered a stroke, one had a TIA, and one remained asymptomatic. This suggests a more serious course once restenosis reaches greater than 80%.[6,7]

So far, a consensus has not yet been reached in the surgical literature regarding the usefulness, cost-effectiveness, or timing of postoperative carotid duplex surveillance.

Timing of Postoperative Carotid Duplex Surveillance

Several authors have recommended an initial surveillance duplex on the operative carotid system within the first 6 months[3,6–8,12] to detect residual stenosis from the operative procedure or early restenosis.[7] For example, Roth and colleagues recently recommended an initial duplex ultrasound to ensure a technically successful CEA, with subsequent postoperative carotid duplex surveillance at 1 to 2 years as long as restenosis and contralateral stenoses remain less than 50%. More frequent follow-up (every 6 months) is warranted if greater than 50% stenosis is noted, or with the onset of symptomatic disease.[12]

Several studies have reported that the majority of restenoses occur during the first 1 to 2 years after CEA. Zierler and colleagues[1] noted that 91% of restenoses occur during the first year. Mattos and colleagues[3] also noted that 70% of restenoses were detected within 1 year after the CEA, and 96% developed within 15 months. Thomas and colleagues[2] reported that 70% of restenoses in their study occurred within 1 year of the CEA. Similar observations were noted previously by the author.[10]

Cost-Effectiveness of Postoperative Carotid Duplex Surveillance

There have been reports that postoperative carotid duplex surveillance is not cost-effective because there is such a low incidence of symptomatic restenosis. Patel and colleagues evaluated the cost-effectiveness of postoperative carotid duplex surveillance[11] and concluded that postoperative carotid duplex surveillance after CEA has an unfavorable cost-effectiveness ratio. In the process of their analysis, they identified a subset of patients in whom postoperative carotid duplex surveillance may be cost-effective. These included patients in whom the rate of progression to greater than 80% stenosis exceeded 6% per year. In their analysis, they felt that some groups of patients could potentially have a rate of disease progression that approaches or exceeds the level at which postoperative carotid duplex surveillance becomes cost-effective. Some of these include patients with multiple risk factors (e.g., smoking, hypertension, hyperlipidemia, diabetes mellitus, coronary artery disease, female gender, and a young age). In addition, they concluded that with postoperative carotid duplex surveillance, the rate of carotid artery occlusion could be reduced by 15% per year. The author's evaluation of the cost of postoperative carotid duplex surveillance agrees with these conclusions (see the following).

The Author's Clinical Experience

Three hundred and ninety-nine CEAs were randomized into 135 with primary closure, 134 with polytetrafluoroethylene (PTFE) patch closures, and 130 with vein patch closures; these patients were followed for a mean of 47 months. Postoperative carotid duplex surveillance was done at 1, 6, and 12 months, and every year thereafter (a mean of 4.0 studies/artery). A Kaplan-Meier analysis was used to estimate the rate of 80% or greater restenosis over time and the time frame of progression from less than 50%, to 50% to 79%, and to 80% or greater stenosis.

Restenoses of 80% or greater developed in 24 (21%) with primary closure, and 9 (4%) with patching. A Kaplan-Meier estimate of freedom from 50% to 79% restenosis at 1, 2, 3, 4, and 5 years was 92%, 83%, 72%, 72%, and 63%, respectively, for primary closure, and 99%, 98%, 97%, 97%, and 97%, respectively, for patching (Table 15-1 and Fig. 15-1). A Kaplan-Meier estimate of freedom from 80% or greater restenosis at 1, 2, 3, 4, and 5 years was 92%, 83%, 80%, 76%, and 68%, respectively, for primary closure; and 100%, 99%, 98%, 98%, and 91%, respectively, for patching (p < 0.01; Table 15-2 and Fig. 15-2).

Out of 56 arteries with 20% to 50% restenosis, 2/28 patch closures and 10/28 primary closures progressed to 50% to less than 80% restenosis (p = 0.02), and 0/28 patch closures and 6/28 primary closures pro-gressed to 80% or greater restenosis (p = 0.03). In primary closures, the median time to progression from less than 50% to 50% to 79%, from less than 50% to 80% or greater, and from 50% to 79% to 80% or greater was 42, 46, and 7 months, respectively. Of the 24 arteries with 80% or greater restenosis in primary closures, 10 were symptomatic (Table 15-3). Thus assuming that symptomatic restenosis would have undergone duplex examinations anyway, there were 14 asymptomatic arteries (12%) that could have been detected only by postoperative carotid duplex surveillance (at an estimated

TABLE 15-1. **Lifetable Analysis of Time to 50% to 79% Restenosis According to CEA Closure**

Time Interval (Months)	Number At Risk At Start	Number Failed	Cumulative (%)	Standard Error (%)
Patch				
0	222	0	100	0
6	220	0	100	0
12	201	2	99.04	0.68
18	173	1	98.48	0.92
24	157	0	98.48	0.97
30	131	2	97.12	1.44
36	114	0	97.12	1.54
42	93	0	97.12	1.71
48	71	0	97.12	1.96
54	46	0	97.12	2.43
60	34	0	97.12	2.83
Primary				
0	116	0	100	0
6	109	3	97.37	1.51
12	93	6	91.77	0.68
18	75	5	86.46	3.09
24	63	3	82.73	4.33
30	49	6	74.08	5.39
36	41	1	72.47	5.94
42	35	0	72.47	6.43
48	26	0	72.47	7.46
54	18	1	68.66	9.06
60	10	1	62.94	12.12

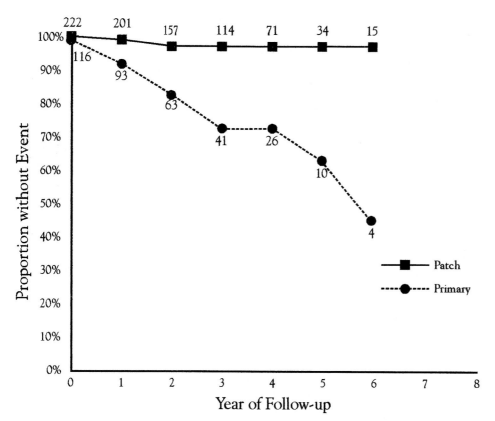

Figure 15-1: Kaplan-Meier estimate of time to 50% to 79% restenosis according to closure. (From AbuRahma AF, Robinson PA, Hannay RS, et al: Frequency of postoperative carotid duplex surveillance and type of closure: Results from a randomized trial. J Vasc Surg 32:1043–1051, 2000.)

cost of $139,200) and would have been candidates for redo CEA. Of the nine arteries with patch closures (three PTFE and six vein patch closures) with 80% or greater restenosis, six asymptomatic arteries (four vein patch closure and two PTFE, or 3%) could have been detected by postoperative carotid duplex surveillance. In patients with a normal duplex at the first 6 months, only 4/222 (2%) patched arteries (two asymptomatic) developed 80% or greater restenosis versus 5/13 (38%) in patients with abnormal duplex examinations (p < 0.001).

Assuming a 5% stroke rate for the 14 repeat CEAs for asymptomatic 80% or greater restenosis in the primary closure group in our series,[14] 0.7 strokes would be associated with the 14 repeat CEAs and approximately 4.7 strokes would have been prevented through surgical intervention before occlusion (assuming a similar outcome of 80% or greater restenosis as described by Mattos and colleagues[6]). A net reduction of four strokes in patients with primary closure would have an approximate cost of $56,150 per stroke prevented.

Also, assuming a similar outcome of greater than 80% restenosis as described by Ouriel and Green,[7] and if one half of these greater than 80% restenoses would progress to total occlusion (7 patients), and assuming one third of patients with total occlusion would suffer a stroke; then approximately 2.3 strokes would be prevented by doing the 14 redo CEAs. Because 0.7 strokes would result from repeating 14 CEAs,[14] the net

effect would be prevention of 1.6 strokes at a cost of $224,600 (i.e., $140,250 per stroke prevented). This analysis does not take into consideration the value of duplex screening of the contralateral nonoperated side.

The justification for this cost is unclear without a definite estimate of the economic burden of caring for these stroke victims. Considering the low incidence of greater than 80% restenosis in patients with patch angioplasty closure, the cost-effectiveness of postoperative carotid duplex surveillance appears to be unfavorable. and therefore should be limited to a single duplex ultrasound to detect residual stenosis. Subsequent follow-up should be dictated by the results found on the initial scan and the onset of neurologic symptoms.

Natural History of Carotid Artery Stenosis Contralateral to CEA

A few nonrandomized studies have reported on the natural history of carotid artery stenosis contralateral to CEA. Recently, the author analyzed the natural history of carotid artery stenosis contralateral to CEA from two randomized prospective trials.[10,15]

The contralateral carotid arteries of 534 patients who participated in two randomized trials comparing CEA with primary closure versus patching were followed

TABLE 15-2. Lifetable Analysis of Time to 80% or Greater Restenosis According to CEA Closure

Time Interval (Months)	Number At Risk At Start	Number Failed	Cumulative (%)	Standard Error (%)
Patch				
0	222	0	100	0
6	220	0	100	0
12	202	0	100	0
18	174	1	99.50	0.53
24	158	1	98.89	0.83
30	134	2	97.51	1.33
36	116	0	97.51	1.43
42	95	0	97.51	1.58
48	73	0	97.51	1.80
54	47	2	93.79	3.41
60	35	1	91.19	4.58
Primary				
0	116	0	100	0
6	111	4	96.51	1.71
12	97	5	91.96	2.65
18	79	5	86.77	3.55
24	68	3	83.19	4.14
30	55	2	80.48	4.79
36	49	0	80.48	5.08
42	41	0	80.48	5.55
48	30	2	76.18	6.68
54	22	1	72.72	8.10
60	13	1	67.52	10.67

clinically and had duplex ultrasounds at 1 month and every 6 months. Carotid artery stenoses were classified into less than 50%, 50% to less than 80%, 80% to 99%, and occlusion. Late contralateral CEAs were done for significant carotid artery stenoses. Progression of carotid artery stenosis was defined as progress to a higher category of stenosis. A Kaplan-Meier lifetable analysis was used to estimate freedom from progression of carotid artery stenosis. The correlation of risk factors and carotid artery stenosis progression was also analyzed.

Out of 534 patients, 61 had initial contralateral CEAs within 30 days of the ipsilateral CEA, and 53 had contralateral occlusions. Overall, 109/420 (26%) progressed at a mean follow-up of 41 months (range, 1 to 116 months). Progression of contralateral carotid artery stenosis was noted in 5/162 (3%) patients who had baseline normal carotids. Some 56/157 (36%) patients with less than 50% carotid artery stenosis progressed, vs. 45/95 (47%) patients with 50 to less than 80% carotid artery stenosis ($p = 0.003$). The median time for progression was 24 months for less

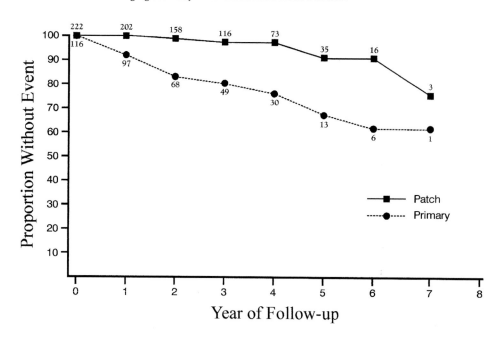

Figure 15-2: *Kaplan-Meier estimate of time to 80% or greater restenosis according to closure. (From AbuRahma AF, Robinson PA, Hannay RS, et al: Frequency of postoperative carotid duplex surveillance and type of closure: Results from a randomized trial. J Vasc Surg 32:1043–1051, 2000.)*

TABLE 15-3. Correlation Between 80% or Greater Restenosis and Neurologic Events (TIA/Stroke)

Neurologic Events	Patients Without 80% or Greater Restenosis	Patients With 80% or Greater Restenosis	Total
Whole Series			
No neurologic events	281 (92%)	20 (61%)	301 (89%)
Neurologic events	24 (8%)*	13 (39%)*	37 (11%)
Total	305 (100%)	33 (100%)	338 (100%)
Patients with Patch Closure			
No neurologic events	198 (93%)	6 (67%)	204 (92%)
Neurologic events	15 (7%)†	3 (33%)†	18 (8%)
Total	213 (100%)	9 (100%)	222 (100%)
Patients with Primary Closure			
No neurologic events	83 (90%)	14 (58%)	97 (84%)
Neurologic events	9 (10%)‡	10 (42%)‡	19 (16%)
Total	92 (100%)	24 (100%)	116 (100%)

*$p < 0.0001$; †$p = 0.027$; ‡$p < 0.001$.

than 50% carotid artery stenosis and 12 months for 50% to less than 80% carotid artery stenosis ($p = 0.035$). Freedom from progression for patients with baseline less than 50% and 50% to less than 80% carotid artery stenosis at 1, 2, 3, 4, and 5 years was, respectively, 95%, 78%, 69%, 61%, and 48%, and 75%, 61%, 51%, 43%, and 33% ($p = 0.003$). Freedom from progression in patients with baseline normal carotid arteries at 1, 2, 3, 4, and 5 years was, respectively, 99%, 98%, 96%, 96%,

and 94%. Late neurologic events referable to the contralateral carotid artery were infrequent in the whole series (28/420, or 6.7%) and included 10 strokes (2.4%) and 18 TIAs (4.3%) (28/258, or 10.9% in patients with contralateral carotid artery stenosis); however, late contralateral CEAs were done in 62 patients (62/420, or 15%; in the whole series, 62/258, or 24%). The survival rates were 96%, 92%, 90%, 87%, and 82% at 1, 2, 3, 4, and 5 years, respectively.

Conclusions

Our randomized prospective studies confirm that carotid restenosis is a known entity that follows a percentage of patients who undergo carotid surgery. In the past, the clinical significance of carotid restenosis has led some investigators to conclude that postoperative carotid duplex surveillance is not warranted. The author showed that, based on the incidence of greater than 80% restenosis, postoperative carotid duplex surveillance may be beneficial in patients with primary closure, with examinations at 6 months and at 1- to 2-year intervals for several years. For patients with patching, a 6-month postoperative duplex examination, if normal, is adequate.

The author also found that progression of contralateral carotid artery stenosis was noted in a significant number of patients with baseline contralateral carotid artery stenosis. Serial carotid duplex ultrasounds every 6 to 12 months for patients with 50% to less than 80% carotid artery stenosis, and every 12 to 24 months for 50% or less carotid artery stenosis, is adequate.

REFERENCES

1. Zierler RE, Bandyk DF, Thiele BR, et al: Carotid artery stenosis following endarterectomy. Arch Surg 117:1408–1414, 1982.
2. Thomas M, Otis S, Rush M, et al: Recurrent carotid artery stenosis following endarterectomy. Ann Surg 200:74–79, 1984.
3. Mattos MA, Shamma AR, Rossi N, et al: Is duplex follow-up cost-effective in the first year after carotid endarterectomy? Am J Surg 156:91–95, 1988.
4. Cook JM, Thompson BW, Barnes RW: Is routine duplex examination after carotid endarterectomy justified? J Vasc Surg 12:334–340, 1990.
5. Mackey WC, Belkin M, Sindhi R, et al: Routine postendarterectomy duplex surveillance: Does it prevent late stroke? J Vasc Surg 16:934–940, 1992.
6. Mattos MA, van Bemmelen PS, Barkmeier LD, et al: Routine surveillance after carotid endarterectomy: Does it affect clinical management? J Vasc Surg 17:819–831, 1993.
7. Ouriel K, Green RM: Appropriate frequency of carotid duplex testing following carotid endarterectomy. Am J Surg 170:144–147, 1995.
8. Ricotta JJ, DeWeese JA: Is routine carotid ultrasound surveillance after carotid endarterectomy worthwhile? Am J Surg 172:140–143, 1996.
9. Golledge J, Cuming R, Ellis M, et al: Clinical follow-up rather than duplex surveillance after carotid endarterectomy. J Vasc Surg 25:55–63, 1997.
10. AbuRahma AF, Robinson PA, Saiedy S, et al: Prospective randomized trial of carotid endarterectomy with primary closure and patch angioplasty with saphenous vein, jugular vein, and polytetrafluoroethylene: Long-term follow-up. J Vasc Surg 27:222–234, 1998.
11. Patel ST, Kuntz KM, Kent KC: Is routine duplex ultrasound surveillance after carotid endarterectomy cost-effective? Surgery 124:343–353, 1998.
12. Roth SM, Back MR, Bandyk DF, et al: A rational algorithm for duplex scan surveillance after carotid endarterectomy. J Vasc Surg 30:453–460, 1999.
13. Kinney EV, Seabrook GR, Kinney LY, et al: The importance of intraoperative detection of residual flow abnormalities after carotid artery endarterectomy. J Vasc Surg 17:912–923, 1993.
14. AbuRahma AF, Snodgrass KR, Robinson PA, et al: Safety and durability of redo carotid endarterectomy for recurrent carotid artery stenosis. Am J Surg 168:175–178, 1994.
15. AbuRahma AF, Hannay RS, Khan JH, et al: Prospective randomized study of carotid endarterectomy with polytetrafluoroethylene versus collagen impregnated Dacron (Hemashield) patching: Perioperative (30-day) results. J Vasc Surg 35:125–130, 2002.

Chapter 16

Surveillance and Follow-Up After Carotid Angioplasty and Stenting

TIMOTHY M. SULLIVAN

Introduction

Surgical endarterectomy of high-grade carotid lesions, both symptomatic and asymptomatic, has been identified as the treatment of choice for stroke prophylaxis in most patients when compared with "best medical therapy" (i.e., risk factor reduction and antiplatelet agents), as shown in the NASCET and ACAS studies.[1,2] Subsequently, carotid endarterectomy (CEA) has been performed in increasing numbers of patients, and now represents the most common operation performed by vascular surgeons. The results of this procedure have continued to improve, as exemplified by a report from Hertzer and colleagues[3] at the Cleveland Clinic Foundation. In a series of 2228 consecutive isolated CEA procedures, they documented an overall stroke rate of 1.8% (1.3% for asymptomatic patients) and a mortality rate of 0.5%, for a combined stroke-mortality rate of 2.3%. Despite the proven efficacy of CEA in the prevention of ischemic stroke, great interest has been generated in carotid angioplasty/stenting (CAS) as an alternative to surgical therapy.

Given the exemplary results of CEA, many vascular surgeons have reserved angioplasty/stenting for patients considered to be at high-risk for surgical therapy. Ouriel and colleagues[4] reviewed 3061 CEA procedures performed over a 10-year period; patients were stratified into high-risk and low-risk groups based on the presence or absence of the following comorbid conditions:

1. Severe coronary artery disease

2. Chronic obstructive pulmonary disease

3. Renal disease

The composite end-point of stroke/myocardial infarction/death was 3.8% for the entire cohort. Among the high-risk group, however, the result was 7.4%, significantly higher than those without these comorbidities (2.9%, $p < 0.005$). The authors suggest that initial clinical evaluation of CAS might best be performed in the group in whom CEA carries significant risk. A list of other potentially high-risk conditions are listed in Table 16-1. Table 16-2 lists limitations and contraindications to the technique.

TABLE 16-1. Indications for Carotid Angioplasty in High-Risk Patients

Severe Cardiac Disease
Requiring coronary PTA or CABG
Congestive heart failure (estimated ejection fraction <30%)
Severe chronic obstructive pulmonary disease
Requiring home oxygen
FEV-1 <20% predicted
Severe Chronic Renal Insufficiency
Serum creatinine >3.0 mg%
Dialysis-dependent
Prior Carotid Endarterectomy (Restenosis)
Contralateral vocal cord paralysis
Surgically inaccessible lesions
Radiation-induced carotid stenosis
Prior ipsilateral radical neck dissection

TABLE 16-2. Limitations of and Contraindications to Carotid Angioplasty/Stenting

Inability to obtain femoral artery access
Unfavorable aortic arch anatomy
Severe tortuosity of the common carotid artery
Severely calcified/undilatable stenoses
Lesions containing fresh thrombus
Extensive stenoses (longer than 2 cm)
Critical (99+%) stenoses ("string sign")
Lesions adjacent to carotid artery aneurysms

Carotid Angioplasty/Stenting

An insight into the technique involved in CAS may be useful to the clinician/sonographer caring for these patients and may aid in the interpretation of follow-up duplex ultrasound studies. As with any other surgical or interventional technique, careful preprocedural evaluation and planning is essential to success. All patients should have a carotid duplex ultrasound from an accredited vascular laboratory confirming both the presence of a high-grade stenosis and its location with respect to the carotid bifurcation. Careful attention should be paid to the presence of mobile atheroma or thrombus that could embolize during catheter/guidewire manipulation. Subsequently, all patients should have an arch/carotid/intracranial angiogram, either as a separate study before the procedure or at the time of the proposed intervention. Specific details to be gained from this complete study (which may not be evident on the preprocedure duplex ultrasound) include tortuosity of the brachiocephalic trunks (which impacts catheter/sheath access to the target lesion); location; character and extent of the stenosis; the presence of tandem common carotid/internal carotid lesions; the presence or absence of thrombus; and the presence of intracranial disease (e.g., occlusions, stenoses, or aneurysms). It is imperative to document the status of the intracranial circulation before intervention so that potential procedure-related embolic lesions can be identified when compared with the preangioplasty study.

At the time of the diagnostic study, measurements of lesion length and diameter of the arteries proximal and distal to the lesion can be made; this will aid in the selection of an appropriate stent and protection device. Potential candidates should have a thorough cardiopulmonary evaluation. Informed consent regarding the risks and potential benefits of the procedure, especially as they relate to alternative therapies (e.g., medical therapy or CEA) is imperative. Ideally, a team of physicians (e.g., surgeon, neurologist, and interventionist) should review all case summaries and radiographic studies, and reach a consensus regarding the most appropriate therapy for the individual patient. All patients are pretreated with aspirin and clopidogrel for several days before their procedures. In addition, most study protocols require both a pre- and postprocedural brain scan (computed tomography [CT] or magnetic resonance imaging [MRI]) and a thorough, documented neurologic evaluation by a certified neurologist.

Arterial access for carotid intervention is typically gained through a retrograde femoral approach using local anesthesia and mild intravenous sedation. A 7 Fr, 90-cm sheath is advanced over a guidewire into the distal common carotid artery under fluoroscopic guidance. The lesion is then crossed with a steerable guidewire (typically 0.014-inch) and a cerebral protection device (either a basket filter or an occlusion balloon) is deployed. Predilation of the carotid lesion is performed with a noncompliant balloon to facilitate advancing the stent across the lesion. The stent is deployed across the target lesion, and postdilation is performed with an appropriately sized balloon, typically 5 mm in diameter. A completion angiogram is then performed, and the procedure terminated. Following a brief stay in a monitored setting, patients are returned to a regular nursing floor. They are allowed to ambulate according to the status of their access site, and are typically discharged the next morning following completion of laboratory studies, carotid duplex ultrasound, and a neurologic evaluation. Medical therapy includes aspirin (81 mg) and clopidogrel (75 mg) daily for 1 month, followed by lifetime aspirin. Follow-up duplex studies are performed at 1 month, 3 months, 6 months, and every 6 to 12 months thereafter.

It is important to note the substantial differences between CEA and CAS with respect to management of carotid plaque; with CEA, the plaque is removed entirely, and the vessel often enlarged by means of patch angioplasty. With CAS, the plaque is simply displaced (and not compressed) and the adventitia stretched; the stent serves as a "scaffold" to prevent elastic recoil following angioplasty. Not infrequently, modest residual stenosis remains following CAS. In addition, displacement of plaque at the origin of the internal carotid artery (ICA) may impinge on the origin of the external carotid artery

(ECA), causing iatrogenic ECA stenosis (which is typically of no clinical consequence) (Fig. 16-1). Several studies have documented, on completion angiography, residual in-stent stenosis of 4% to 20% immediately following CAS.[5,6] Berkefeld and colleagues,[7] in a series of 40 consecutive carotid stent procedures using the Wallstent (Boston Scientific Corp), documented optimal widening of the carotid lumen and complete apposition of the stent to the vessel wall in only 28% of cases. Residual stenosis (40%), free stent filaments not attached to the vessel wall (53%), and stent-induced kinking of the internal carotid artery (15%) were identified in substantial numbers of patients. These differences between CEA and CAS have significant implications for the accurate interpretation of subsequent duplex studies.

The majority of CAS procedures are currently performed with the use of stents, all of which are metallic and are easily identified on duplex ultrasound. Most opera-

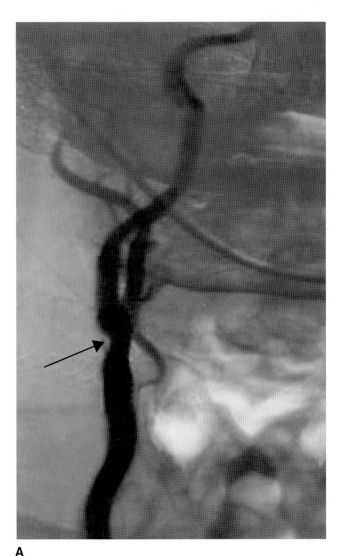
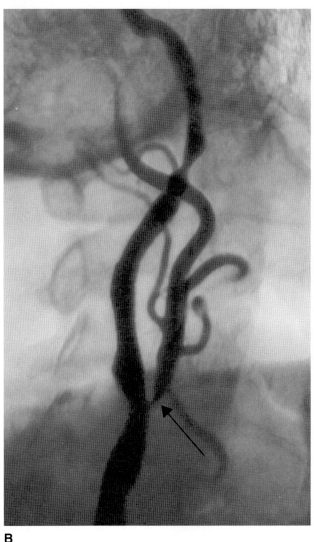

A   **B**

Figure 16-1. **A**, *Residual narrowing of distal CCA following successful PTA/stent.* **B**, *Induced ECA stenosis caused by compression of ECA origin from stent and displacement of ICA plaque.*

tors use either nitinol stents, which are self-expanding and shorten minimally upon deployment; or Wallstents (Boston Scientific Corporation), which are self-expanding and can foreshorten considerably following deployment in the carotid position. It is important, on follow-up duplex studies, to document the position of the stent struts with respect to the carotid bifurcation and the internal carotid artery. Figure 16-2 shows an example where a Wallstent shortened and extruded itself from the internal carotid artery over a 3-month period. The stent can easily be identified in the dilated common carotid artery, which measures 8 to 10 mm in diameter. Balloon-expandable stents were utilized early on for CAS, quite simply because they were some of the only stents available for use in medium-sized arteries. The use of these stents has been abandoned, in part because of a small but definite

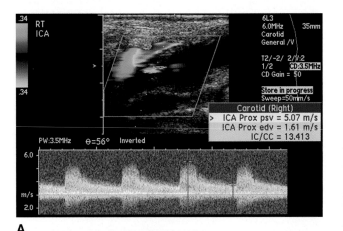

A

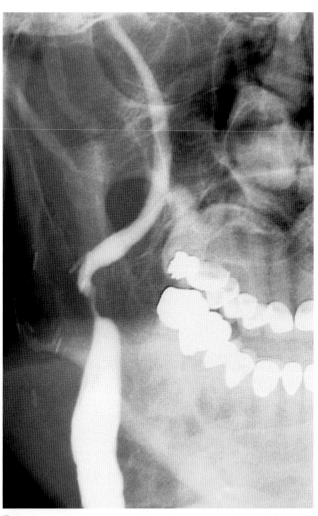

B

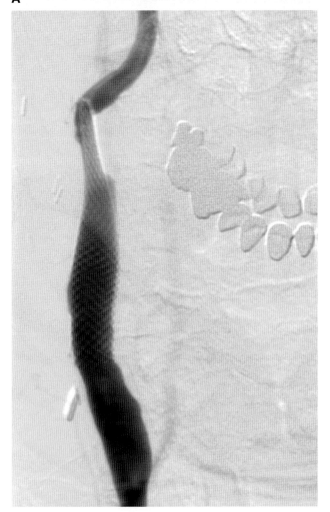

C

Figure 16-2. **A,** *Duplex ultrasound. Recurrent, high-grade symptomatic right internal carotid stenosis following two prior carotid endarterectomies. ICA:CCA ratio 13.4.* **B,** *Selective carotid arteriogram identifies high-grade lesion. Note large CCA and absence of ECA.* **C,** *Following PTA/stenting with Wallstent. Note incomplete apposition of stent to internal carotid artery.*

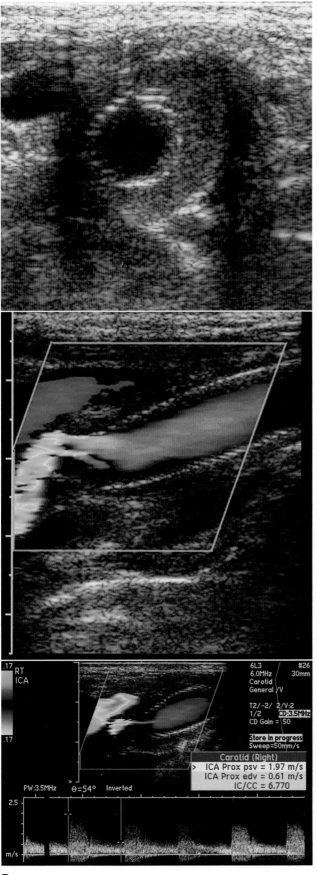

D

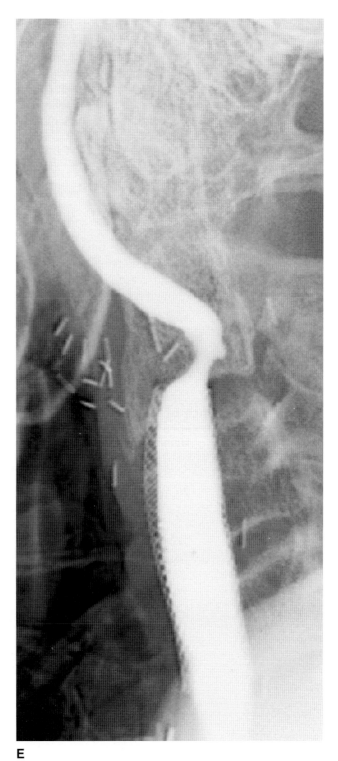

E

Figure 16-2, cont'd. **D**, *Follow-up duplex 3 months following index procedure. Metallic stent easily visualized; appears to have migrated into CCA. Suspected restenosis, with ICA:CCA ratio 6.77.* **E**, *Arteriogram confirms stent migration. Maximum stenosis 50%.*

incidence of stent deformation or "crushing" in the carotid position.[8,9] When evaluating patients who may have these types of stents, documentation of proper stent expansion is mandatory. Confirmation of stent deformation can then be confirmed by plain-film radiography in multiplanar views. When performing a follow-up duplex study, it is useful to identify which type of stent was used for the intervention.

Restenosis Following Carotid Angioplasty/Stenting

The rationale for routine surveillance following either CEA or CAS is to identify asymptomatic patients who have high-grade recurrent stenosis that, presumably, puts them at risk of stroke. Although it is not the purpose of this chapter to debate the pros and cons of this philosophy, most vascular specialists closely follow their patients who have had surgical or percutaneous carotid intervention.

Carotid endarterectomy has been proven both safe and durable in the treatment of patients with carotid stenosis. Although percutaneous therapy is certainly attractive, the risk of periprocedural stroke and the rate of recurrence currently exceed those of CEA for most patients. Table 16-3 highlights the risk of recurrent stenosis with CAS; only studies that have appeared in peer-reviewed journals within the last 5 years are included. Although the types of stents and periods of follow-up are quite variable, most authors report rates of significant restenosis between 5% and 15% at 6 to 12 months, with a range of 2% to 75% at 6 to 37 months follow-up. The vast majority of these restenoses are secondary to intimal hyperplasia.

Before the use of stents in conjunction with angioplasty (percutaneous transluminal angioplasty [PTA]) was routine, Crawley and colleagues[10] followed 12 patients with symptomatic carotid stenosis treated with PTA alone. The immediate angioplasty result decreased the mean percent stenosis from 82% to 51%. Six of the 12 showed further improvement in lumen diameter of more than 14% at 1 year, from a mean stenosis immediately post-

TABLE 16-3. **Incidence of Restenosis Following Carotid Angioplasty/Stenting**

Author/Year	Number of Patients (n)	Follow-Up (Mos)	Restenosis/Occlusion
Wholey 1998	2048	6	4.80%
Teitelbaum 1998	26	6	14.3%
Malek 2000	28	14	25%
Shawl 2000	170	19	2%
Cremonesi 2000	119	6-36	5.04%
Ahmadi 2001	320	12	10%
D'Audiffret 2001	83	16	7.2%
Chakhtoura 2001	50	18	8%
Leger 2001	8	20	75%
Paniagua 2001	62	17	5.7%
Dietz 2001	43	20	2.3%
Baudier 2001	54	34	28%
Pappada 2001	27	6-37	3.7%
Criado 2002	135	16	3%
Bonaldi 2002	71	12	8%
Willfort 2002	279	12	3%
Stankovic 2002	100	12	3.4%
Shawl 2002	343	26	2.7%
Gable 2003	31	28	6%

PTA of 47% to 28% at follow-up angiography. Obviously, there is substantial arterial remodeling that occurs following carotid PTA.

Schillinger and colleagues,[11] in a prospective study of 108 patients having CAS (with stenting), found restenosis of more than 50% in 6 patients (14%). Elevated levels of C-reactive protein (CRP) at 48 hours postintervention, indicative of a systemic inflammatory response, correlate strongly with restenosis at 6 months (p = 0.01). Both residual stenosis of 10% to 30% and restenosis

following prior stent implantation were independent predictors of restenosis in this study.

Carotid Duplex Ultrasound Following CAS

Due to the nature of CAS—the plaque is not removed, simply displaced, as described previously—the duplex

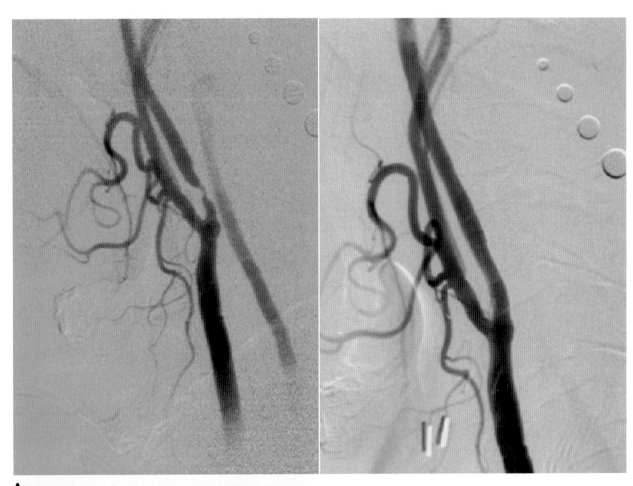

A

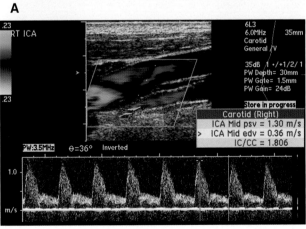

B

Figure 16-3. **A**, *Successful PTA/stent of high-grade, symptomatic right internal carotid stenosis. No residual stenosis on completion angiogram.* **B**, *Postprocedure duplex ultrasound suggests 40% residual stenosis.*

criteria used to follow patients post-CEA may not apply. Figure 16-2 is an illustrative case in point. This particular patient left the hospital before having a "baseline" duplex the day following his CAS procedure. As such, a direct correlation could not be made between the final angiographic appearance and the duplex velocities. In short-term follow-up, elevated velocities and a high ICA:CCA ratio suggested an early restenosis. A large, patulous CCA following two prior surgical repairs and an occluded ECA

likely falsely lowered the CCA velocities, compounding the problem. Subsequent angiography confirmed modest restenosis (50%) that did not require reintervention.

Robbin and colleagues,[12] reporting on patients treated at the University of Alabama at Birmingham by Yadav and his colleagues, prospectively studied 170 stented carotid arteries. Prospective duplex criteria for stenosis included peak systolic velocity greater than 125 cm/sec, ICA:CCA ratio greater than 3, and intrastent doubling

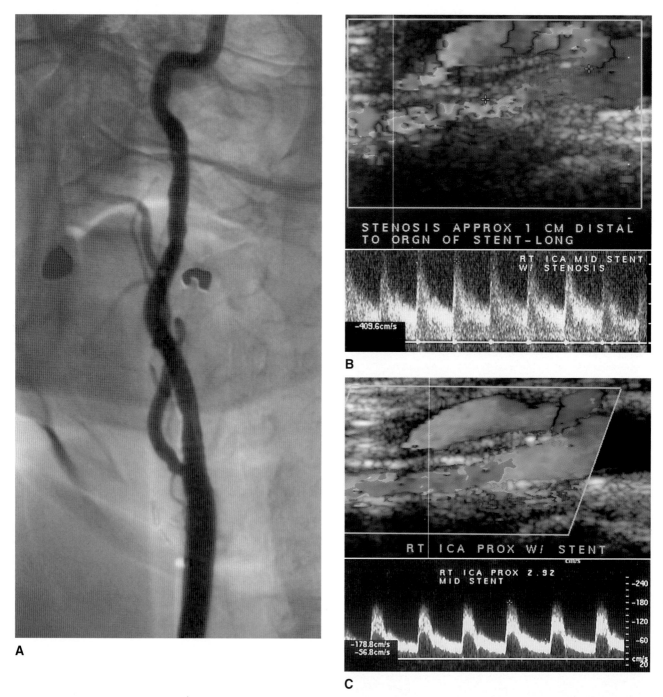

Figure 16-4. A, *Selective right carotid arteriogram following successful PTA/stent (nitinol stent).* **B,** *Two hours following procedure, patient has a right hemispheric transient ischemic attack (TIA) lasting 4 minutes. Duplex identifies high-grade stenosis (PSV >400 cps); stent is lined with thrombus.* **C,** *Follow-up duplex following 8-hour infusion of abciximab, shows resolution of thrombus and normalization of velocities.*

of velocity. Although very few stents showed significant restenosis, duplex was able to accurately identify restenosis, and correlated with angiographic findings at 1 year.

In a study that included blinded comparison of carotid angiograms at completion of CAS and 24-hour duplex ultrasound studies in 114 patients, Ringer and colleagues[13] found little correlation between the two modalities. Utilizing two standard criteria for high-grade stenosis (A, peak in-stent velocity > 125 cm/sec; B, ICA:CCA ratio > 3) and two customized criteria (C, peak in-stent velocity > 170 cm/sec; D, ICA:CCA ratio > 2), they found 61 patients who met one of these criteria for high-grade stenosis immediately following CAS. None of these 61 had more than 50% residual stenosis by angiography at the completion of their procedure. Most strikingly, in those patients found to have recurrent stenosis in follow-up, in-stent peak systolic velocities and ICA:CCA ratios had increased by more than 80% when compared with their immediate postprocedure study. These authors conclude that strict velocity criteria for restenosis is less reliable than are changes in velocity over time. Clearly, based on this data, a baseline duplex following CAS, which can be correlated with the completion angiogram and followed over time, is imperative. This policy will lead to fewer false-positive duplex studies (Fig. 16-3).

Lal and colleagues,[14] from Hobson's group in New Jersey, found that, among several duplex criteria, post-CAS peak systolic velocity correlated best with angiography in 90 stented arteries. A mean residual angiographic stenosis of 4.2% +/- 9.7% correlated with an internal carotid peak systolic velocity of 123 +/- 30 cm/sec. They concluded that a peak systolic velocity of 150 cm/sec or less correlates with a normal lumen (0% to 19% stenosis) follwing CAS. Contrast-enhanced color-coded duplex ultrasound using an ultrasound contrast agent, administered intravenously, that produces air-filled microbubbles may be a promising technique on the horizon for imaging post-CAS arteries, producing images comparable to contrast angiography.[15]

Carotid duplex ultrasound may also be a useful tool in evaluating the rare patient with postprocedure neurologic symptoms, as illustrated in Figure 16-4.

Conclusions

1. Duplex ultrasound follow-up of stented carotid arteries is an important tool to identify patients with restenosis. The current risk of restenosis is 5% to 15% at 6 to 12 months. Early restenosis is typically secondary to myointimal hyperplasia.

2. Because follow-up duplex ultrasound studies may be difficult to interpret based on traditional velocity criteria, a baseline study is imperative; this must be correlated with the degree of residual stenosis at the completion of the CAS procedure. Subsequent studies are performed at 3, 6, and 12 months, and at 6- to 12-month intervals thereafter.

3. Current evidence suggests that a peak systolic velocity of 150 cm/sec or less in the internal carotid artery correlates with a normal vessel (0% to 19% stenosis). Elevation of the peak systolic velocity and the ICA:CCA ratio (>80% increase) may be even more important criteria in determining significant restenosis following CAS. Identification of high-grade restenosis typically warrants futher evaluation with contrast angiography.

REFERENCES

1. North American Symptomatic Carotid Endarterectomy Trial Collaborators: Beneficial effect of carotid endarterectomy in symptomatic patients with high-grade carotid stenosis. N Engl J Med 325:445–453, 1991.
2. Executive Committee for the Asymptomatic Carotid Atherosclerosis Study. Endarterectomy for asymptomatic carotid artery stenosis. JAMA 273:1421–1428, 1995.
3. Hertzer NR, O'Hara PJ, Mascha EJ, et al: Early outcome assessment for 2228 consecutive carotid endarterectomy procedures: The Cleveland Clinic experience from 1989 to 1995. J Vasc Surg 26:1–10, 1997.
4. Ouriel K, Hertzer NR, Beven EG, et al: Preprocedural risk stratification: Identifying an appropriate population for carotid stenting. J Vasc Surg 33:728–732, 2001.
5. New G, Roubin GS, Iyer SS, et al: Safety, efficacy, and durability of carotid artery stenting for restenosis following carotid endarterectomy: A multicenter study. J Endovasc Ther 7:345–352, 2000.
6. Criado FJ, Lingelbach JM, Ledesma DF, et al: Carotid stenting in a vascular surgery practice. J Vasc Surg 35:430–434, 2002.
7. Berkefeld J, Turowski B, Dietz A, et al: Recanalization results after carotid stent placement. Am J Neuroradiol 23:113–120, 2002.
8. Calvey TA, Gough MJ: A late complication of internal carotid stenting. J Vasc Surg 27:753–735, 1998.
9. Johnson SP, Fujitani RM, Leyendecker JR, et al: Stent deformation and intimal hyperplasia complicating treatment of a post-carotid endarterectomy intimal flap with a Palmaz stent. J Vasc Surg 25:764–768, 1997.
10. Crawley F, Clifton A, Markus H, et al: Delayed improvement in carotid artery diameter after carotid angioplasty. Stroke 28:574–579, 1997.
11. Schillinger M, Exner M, Mlekusch W, et al: Acute-phase response after stent implantation in the carotid artery: Association with 6-month in-stent restenosis. Radiology 227:516–521, 2003.
12. Robbin ML, Lockhart ME, Weber TM, et al: Carotid artery stents: Early and intermediate follow-up with Doppler US. Radiology 205:749–756, 1997.
13. Ringer AJ, German JW, Guterman LR, et al: Follow-up of stented carotid arteries by Doppler ultrasound. Neurosurgery 51:639–643, 2002.
14. Lal BK, Hobson RW, Goldstein J, et al: Carotid artery stenting: A need to revise ultrasound velocity criteria for stenosis? Presented at the Vascular Annual Meeting 2003. Chicago, IL, June 8–11, 2003.
15. Yoshida K, Nozaki K, Kikuta K, et al: Contrast-enhanced carotid color-coded duplex sonography for carotid stenting follow-up assessment. Am J Neurorad 24:992–995, 2003.

Chapter 17

Vertebrobasilar Insufficiency: Technique and Clinical Applications

MARK D. MORASCH

- Diagnosis
- Surgical Reconstruction
- Results

Brain stem ischemia, most often the result of disease involving the vertebrobasilar arteries, remains poorly understood, and misdiagnosis is common. In contrast to the clear focal symptoms of anterior circulation ischemia, the symptoms associated with brain stem ischemia can be multiple, varied, and vague. There appears to be reluctance on the part of clinicians to aggressively pursue diagnosis or to recommend treatment for many of the surgically correctable lesions that may be responsible for these syndromes. In addition, there are a number of other medical conditions that mimic vertebrobasilar ischemia and that may confound proper diagnosis.

One reason the pathophysiology of vertebrobasilar ischemia is less well understood than carotid/hemispheric ischemia is that the peculiar anatomy of the vertebral artery makes it less accessible to surgical reconstruction and to postmortem examination. The surgical anatomy of the paired vertebral arteries has traditionally been divided into four segments: (1) V1, the origin of the vertebral artery arising from the subclavian artery to the point at which it enters the C6 transverse process; (2) V2, the segment of the artery buried deep within the intertransverse muscle and the cervical transverse processes of C6 to C2; (3) V3, the extracranial segment between the transverse process of the C2 and the base of the skull before it enters the foramen magnum; and (4) V4, the intracranial portion beginning at the atlanto-occipital membrane and terminating as the two vertebrals converge to form the basilar artery.

Ischemia affecting the temporo-occipital areas of the cerebral hemispheres or segments of the brain stem and cerebellum characteristically produces bilateral symptoms. The classic symptoms of vertebrobasilar ischemia are dizziness, vertigo, drop attacks, diplopia, perioral numbness, alternating paresthesias, tinnitus, dysphasia, dysarthria, and imbalance.

In general, the ischemic mechanisms can be broken down into those that are hemodynamic and those that are embolic. Hemodynamic symptoms occur as a result of brain stem hypoperfusion and can be precipitated by postural changes or transient reduction in cardiac output. For hemodynamic symptoms to occur, pathology must be present in both of the paired vertebral arteries and compensatory contribution from the carotid circulation must be incomplete. Alternatively, ischemic symptoms may follow proximal subclavian artery occlusion and the syndrome of subclavian/vertebral artery steal. Ischemia from hemodynamic mechanisms rarely results in infarction; rather, symptoms are short-lived, repetitive, and more of a nuisance than a danger.

Most infarctions in the vertebrobasilar distribution (one third of vertebrobasilar ischemic syndromes) result from embolization. Cerebellar, brain stem, and posterior hemispheric strokes follow microembolization from the heart and aortic arch or from the subclavian, vertebral, and basilar arteries. Arterial to arterial emboli can arise from atherosclerotic lesions; from intimal defects caused by extrinsic compression or repetitive trauma; and, rarely, from fibromuscular dysplasia, aneurysms (Fig. 17-1), or dissections. Compared to hemodynamic mechanisms of ischemia, emboli are more likely to cause fatal infarcts or to leave patients with permanent and debilitating strokes.

Diagnosis

A precise diagnosis of vertebrobasilar ischemia begins with an accurate assessment of the presenting symptom complex. This must be followed by efforts to exclude other causes for patient symptoms. Certain prescription medications can mimic vertebrobasilar ischemia; therefore, patient medications require thorough review. Investigation must be undertaken to exclude inner ear pathology including rare cerebellar-pontine angle tumors. A cardiac source may be the most common cause of brain stem ischemia, especially in the elderly. Because patients often present with a combination of cerebral hemispheric and posterior symptoms, investigation of the carotid circulation is usually warranted.

Duplex ultrasound is an excellent tool to detect lesions at the carotid bifurcation. In addition, ultrasound imaging can diagnose great vessel pathology, confirm subclavian steal, and detect reversed flow down a vertebral. Duplex ultrasound is also becoming a useful tool for identifying flow velocity changes and stenosis in the vertebral artery. As such, duplex ultrasound has become an invaluable screening tool for patients with vertebrobasilar symptomatology (for technique, see Chapter 9).

Recent developments in magnetic resonance imaging (MRI) show great promise for safe, noninvasive, detailed evaluation of both the extracranial and intracranial vasculature. New contrast-enhanced magnetic resonance angiography techniques provide full imaging coverage of the supra-aortic trunks and the carotid and vertebral arteries (Fig. 17-2). In contrast to traditional computed tomography (CT) scans, transaxial MRI can readily diagnose both acute and chronic posterior fossa infarcts.

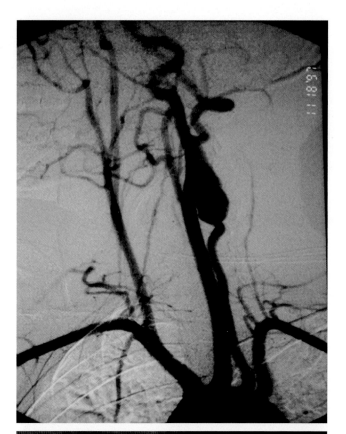

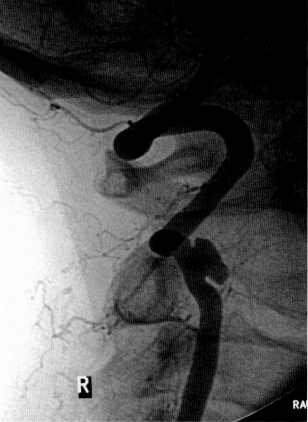

Figure 17-1. Angiograms showing aneurysms of the vertebral artery.

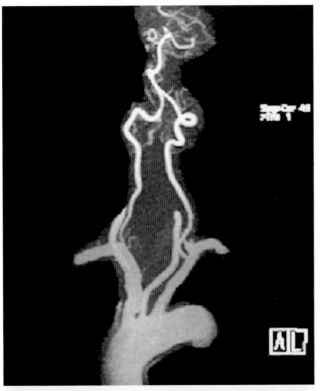

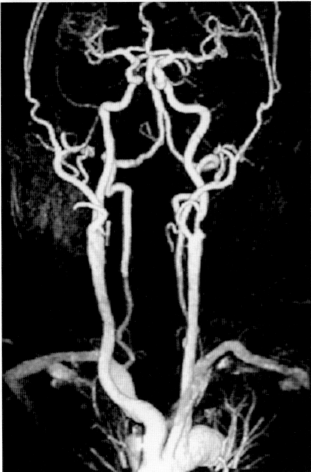

Figure 17-2. Contrast-enhanced magnetic resonance angiography showing the supra-aortic trunks and the carotid and vertebral arteries.

Transaxial MRI should be obtained routinely in all patients suspected to have suffered embolic infarction in the distribution of the posterior circulation.

Selective subclavian and vertebral angiography remains the gold standard for preoperative evaluation of patients with vertebrobasilar ischemia. Some surgeons still consider angiography mandatory before surgical reconstruction. The most common site of disease, the VA origin, may not be well imaged with ultrasound or magnetic resonance angiography (MRA) and, in fact, often can only be displayed with oblique projections that are not part of standard arch evaluation. Patients with VA compression syndromes who suffer from positional symptoms should undergo dynamic angiography, which incorporates provocative positioning. Delayed images may demonstrate reconstitution of an occluded extracranial vertebral artery through existing cervical connections (Fig. 17-3).

Surgical Reconstruction

Accumulated experience has shown that, with appropriate surgical intervention, predictable resolution of hemodynamic symptoms and cessation of embolic events can occur. Furthermore, vertebral artery reconstruction is attended by fewer ischemic complications and has better long-term results than carotid surgery.

A number of operations have been described to treat stenosing ostial lesions in V1. Transposition of the proximal vertebral artery onto the common carotid artery is the most common reconstruction. Endarterectomy and bypass are used less commonly.

The second segment of the VA, the portion that ascends within the foramina of the cervical vertebrae, is the site of a variety of pathology. Because this segment is relatively inaccessible, elective surgical reconstruction of the intravertebral segment is rarely undertaken. Disease in the first or second segments of the VA can result in extracranial occlusion, whereas stenotic lesions in the intraforaminal segment commonly give rise to emboli. Patency of the distal extracranial segment is often maintained via collaterals from the external carotid or subclavian artery. This patent segment (V3) can be exposed for bypass reconstruction.

Reconstruction of the distal vertebral artery is usually performed at the C1–C2 level. For more distal pathology, the VA can also be accessed surgically above the level of the transverse process of C1. The technique most often used to reconstruct the distal vertebral artery includes saphenous vein bypass from the common carotid, subclavian, or proximal vertebral artery. Transposition of the external carotid or hypertrophied occipital artery into the distal VA, as well as transposition of the distal VA into the side of the internal carotid artery, have also been described.

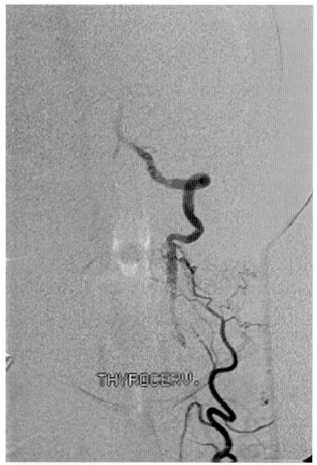

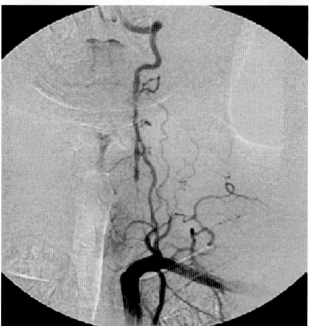

Figure 17-3. Delayed images showing reconstitution of an occluded extracranial vertebral artery through existing cervical connections.

Intraoperative completion imaging using digital angiography is necessary for all types of VA reconstruction. A significant number of reparable technical flaws may be identified, and repair can prevent reconstruction failure.

Results

Results following both proximal and distal VA reconstructions generally equal or exceed those reported in series reviewing other forms of extracranial cerebrovascular reconstruction. Reviews of VA reconstruction have demonstrated combined stroke and death rates of 4% or less, and long-term patency is excellent with greater than 80% cured or significantly improved.[1]

REFERENCES

1. Berguer R, Morasch MD, Kline RA: A review of 100 consecutive reconstructions of the distal vertebral artery for embolic and hemodynamic disease. J Vasc Surg 27:852–859, 1998.

PERIPHERAL ATHEROSCLEROTIC OCCLUSIVE DISEASE

Chapter 18

Vascular Diagnosis of Lower Extremity Occlusive Disease: An Overview

REESE A. WAIN • GEORGE BERDEJO • FRANK VEITH

- Introduction
- Patient Presentation
- Vascular Diagnostic Studies

Introduction

The presence of lower extremity arterial occlusive disease is usually suspected on the basis of a patient's risk factors for atherosclerotic disease and the history of present illness. Evidence supporting the diagnosis of peripheral occlusive disease is gathered on physical examination and confirmed with the appropriate diagnostic tests. Management of peripheral vascular disease may be noninvasive, consisting of risk factor and behavioral modification or medical therapy. Alternatively, invasive management via an endovascular or open operative approach may also be required. The decision on whether intervention is warranted is almost always based on history and examination findings alone; however, diagnostic testing is usually required to decide on what type of intervention is needed. This chapter provides an overview on the initial evaluation of patients with suspected lower extremity occlusive disease and how different diagnostic modalities can be used to confirm the diagnosis and develop an appropriate treatment plan.

Patient Presentation

Patients with lower extremity occlusive disease typically seek consultation for symptoms that may be acute or chronic in nature. Acute limb ischemia is generally a surgical emergency and must be diagnosed correctly and treated as quickly as possible to avoid limb loss. Symptoms of chronic occlusive disease may have been present for years or may worsen quickly over a subacute interval. Although the signs and symptoms of chronic occlusive disease may suggest a limb-threatening scenario, management decisions usually do not need to be made over a period of minutes to hours.[1]

The cornerstone of the physical examination in a patient with suspected peripheral occlusive disease is the pulse examination. Pulses should be palpated over the femoral, popliteal, posterior tibial, and dorsalis pedis arteries, and the quality of these pulses documented. We grade pulses as either being absent, 1+ (diminished), or 2+ (normal). The presence and quality of pulses at a particular location should be corroborated with the patient's history regarding the location and severity of symptoms. Bruits over the femoral artery in the groin may signify a hemodynamically significant stenosis.

Acute lower extremity arterial occlusions may be caused by embolization from a proximal source in the arterial tree or the heart; or they may be caused by thrombus at the site of pre-existing arterial stenoses. Most emboli originate within the heart; in the past, rheumatic heart disease and concomitant mitral valvular stenosis was the most common cause of cardiac emboli. Presently, atrial fibrillation is responsible for the majority of symptomatic peripheral emboli. Alternative cardiac sources of embolization include ventricular thrombus; and prosthetic valves, which are more prone to produce emboli when the patient is not properly anticoagulated. Finally, cardiac tumors and vegetations associated with endocarditis can also cause emboli. Other potential sources of emboli include cancer that has invaded the pulmonary veins; and "paradoxical" emboli, occurring when a venous thrombus passes through a patent foramen ovale in the heart into the arterial circulation.

Patients with acute lower extremity emboli usually present with some or all of the so-called five Ps: pain, pulselessness, palor, paralysis, and paresthesias. Typically, the symptoms occur abruptly and cause pain that is severe and unrelenting. Emboli tend to lodge at branch points within the lower extremity vasculature including the femoral and popliteal artery bifurcations. The pain and the majority of symptoms occur in the muscle groups distal to the level of obstruction. In addition to pain, the involved extremity may appear cyanotic, be cool to the touch, and develop neurologic changes including diminished proprioception and motor function. Calf tenderness upon palpation is a sign of advanced and potentially irreversible ischemia.

In situ thrombosis occurs at the site of a chronically diseased and stenotic artery. Rupture of a pre-existing arterial plaque has been implicated as the cause of these acute occlusive events. It is especially important to distinguish between acute embolic disease and acute arterial thrombosis because appropriate treatments are significantly different. Patients with acute embolic disease can be treated by removing the offending emboli; however, patients with acute arterial thrombosis superimposed upon chronic occlusive disease typically require definitive management via endarterectomy, patch angioplasty, or bypass surgery. The history and physical examination may be especially important in distinguishing between these two entities. Patients with embolic disease may have an obvious source of emboli such as atrial fibrillation or a recent myocardial infarction. Such patients may not have had any prior symptoms of arterial occlusive disease such as intermittent claudication or rest pain. Contrarily, patients with in situ thrombosis may not have an identifiable source of emboli and are more likely to have experienced claudication or other sequelae of chronic lower extremity occlusive disease in the past.

Physical findings more suggestive of embolic disease include a normal contralateral pulse examination and an obvious lack of pulses on the affected side. Patients with chronic atherosclerotic disease tend to have similar disease patterns in both extremities and may have an abnormal pulse examination on the contralateral side as well. Finally, patients with in situ thrombosis may have a less pronounced presentation secondary to collateral circulation that has developed in the face of chronic disease.

Although the diagnosis of acute ischemia is largely clinical and based on the patient's known risk factors, presentation, and physical examination, the appropriate diagnostic work-up and management varies significantly between embolic and thrombotic disease. Patients with obvious acute embolic disease and normal contralateral pulse examinations are often brought to the operating room for surgical embolectomy without additional diagnostic testing. If readily available, the authors obtain a duplex arterial scan of the involved extremity to help in operative planning (Fig. 18-1). Emboli at the femoral bifurcation without significant extension into the superficial femoral artery are most easily managed via a groin incision and femoral arteriotomy. More extensive emboli or emboli originating in the popliteal or crural vessels are managed by an infrapopliteal approach and exposure of the popliteal, anterior and posterior tibial, and peroneal arteries.

Patients with in situ thrombosis and chronic lower extremity occlusive disease are usually subjected to an imaging study in the preoperative period to help guide

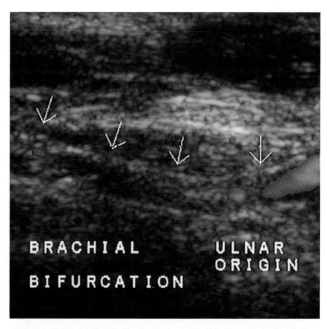

Figure 18-1. *Duplex study of a patient with atrial fibrillation who experienced the acute onset of a painful, cool hand. The examination revealed thrombus within the brachial artery* (arrows) *that ends at the brachial bifurcation.*

the operative procedure. In these cases, embolectomy alone may be unsuccessful and represents a prelude to the definitive procedure rather than the definitive procedure itself. In these cases, an imaging study capable of revealing distal vasculature suitable for potential bypass surgery is necessary. In addition, visualization of the contralateral lower extremity vasculature is often helpful in predicting which vessels and what pattern of disease might be present in the involved extremity. Angiography has typically been the most useful study in this regard; however, alternative imaging modalities such as magnetic resonance angiography (MRA), computed tomography (CT) angiography, and duplex mapping are assuming an increasingly important role.

Chronic occlusive disease represents a longstanding process that manifests itself clinically over weeks, months, and years rather than minutes to hours. Patients with chronic lower extremity occlusive disease have the typical risk factors for systemic atherosclerosis including cigarette smoking, hypertension, diabetes, and increased cholesterol. Similar to atherosclerotic coronary artery disease, lower extremity occlusive disease is usually present for years before becoming clinically significant. Many patients can have considerable lower extremity occlusive disease yet remain asymptomatic. Symptomatic patients present with intermittent claudication, rest pain, or tissue loss characterized by ulceration and/or gangrene.

The management of patients with chronic occlusive disease depends primarily on the severity of the symptoms and the findings on physical examination supplemented by the appropriate diagnostic testing. Patients with asymptomatic disease discovered on the basis of an abnormal pulse examination or via a diagnostic study performed to seek an alternative diagnosis do not require vascular reconstruction. Instead, medication and risk factor and behavioral modification constitute the cornerstone of their care. Counseling regarding the appropriateness of stopping cigarette smoking, maintaining a low-fat diet, keeping the blood pressure under control, and maintaining an exercise regimen should be stressed.

The earliest manifestation of lower extremity occlusive disease is often intermittent claudication. Claudication is a pain that occurs in a muscle group receiving inadequate blood supply when the increased metabolic demands of exercise are placed on it. Patients with claudication commonly describe pain in a particular muscle group that occurs exclusively when ambulating a certain distance. The pain is described either as a cramping sensation or as tiredness. The pain reliably disappears when the physical exertion is halted and is reproducible insofar as it returns when walking the exact same distance again. Careful patient questioning should be able to support a diagnosis of intermittent claudication fairly readily. Patients whose predominant disease is in the aortoiliac distribution will commonly describe pain in the buttocks and thighs when ambulating. Contrarily, patients with combined aortoiliac and infrainguinal disease or patients with predominantly infrainguinal disease typically have calf claudication.

Most patients with intermittent claudication do not develop limb-threatening symptoms or ultimately require amputation. Less than 10% of patients will ultimately experience complications related to lower extremity ischemia. In fact, those who do have complications most commonly include cigarette smokers who do not stop smoking and patients with diabetes. The risks of treating claudicants with lower extremity revascularization or balloon angioplasty must be carefully weighed against the patient's medical comorbidities and his or her lifestyle expectations. In general, the authors pursue lower extremity revascularization if the claudication is lifestyle limiting. Patients with severe cardiac or other major comorbidities or whose lifestyle is not limited by the claudication are managed medically.

Patients with intermittent claudication who are at acceptable surgical risk for revascularization require further diagnostic studies to decide what type of intervention will be required. Duplex arterial mapping, CT, MRA, and conventional contrast arteriography have all been used in this regard.

Rest pain is the next level of disease severity in patients with lower extremity occlusive disease. Rest pain occurs when resting metabolic requirements are not met by the blood reaching a muscle group secondary to proximal occlusive disease; it therefore characteristically occurs in the forefoot and toes. Patients with rest pain describe a constant pain affecting the involved region. Dependent rubor as well as cyanosis may be present, and the involved extremity may be cool. On physical examination, pulses are missing at one or more levels. The pulses that are present often indicate the anatomic level of disease and predict what type of treatment will be required. For example, patients with no femoral or distal pulses harbor aortoiliac occlusive disease. Patients with femoral and popliteal pulses but no pedal pulses have crural disease.

Rest pain is typically considered a limb-threatening condition and demands prompt attention in all but the sickest of patients. Diagnostic confirmation of a depressed circulatory status is mandatory, and imaging studies are required to help plan the most appropriate management. Patients who have severe medical comorbidities or unreconstructible disease on the basis of preoperative studies may be offered an amputation for pain control. Similarly, patients who have ischemic ulceration or gangrene are also considered to have threatened limbs and require imaging studies and prompt intervention.

Vascular Diagnostic Studies

A multitude of studies are available to the surgeon or interventionalist treating patients with lower extremity occlusive disease. Physiologic and anatomic information regarding the location and severity of a patient's disease may be obtained and imaging can occur via invasive or noninvasive means. The mainstay of the vascular non-invasive laboratory is the pulse volume recording (PVR). This noninvasive test is quickly performed, has reasonable reproducibility, and is inexpensive. PVRs are most often used to corroborate findings on physical examination and the patient's history. Information regarding the level and severity of disease may be gleaned as well. However, deciding what type of intervention is most appropriate requires additional imaging modalities such as contrast, MR and CT arteriography, and duplex arterial mapping.

Over the past 30 years, contrast arteriography has been the mainstay of vascular diagnostic imaging. The advantages of conventional arteriography include the ability to image the relevant vascular tree in its entirety, to readily delineate the site of arterial stenoses and occlusions, and to plan what type of intervention is most appropriate for the patient. Arteriography provides a view of the circulatory tree that is easily interpreted by the surgeon familiar with this format (Fig. 18-2). In addition to providing valuable anatomic information, pressure measurements across arterial stenoses can be used to gauge the homodynamic severity of a lesion, and intervention can be undertaken via concurrent balloon angioplasty and/or stenting. The disadvantages of arteriography are well documented and include procedure-related complications, patient discomfort, and high costs. Periprocedural complications can include hematoma, pseudoaneurysm or arteriovenous fistula formation, embolization, and dissection, to name a few. In addition, patients may experience temporary or permanent renal failure caused by the contrast infusion. Arteriography is uncomfortable for patients and requires them to undergo preprocedural bloodwork and to spend the better part of a day in the interventional suite. Finally, arteriography is an expensive undertaking that will be increasingly frowned upon by third-party payers as pressure increases to curtail skyrocketing medical care costs.

Technologic improvements in the 1980s through today have made possible noninvasive techniques for imaging the vascular tree. Several such modalities exist and will increasingly compete with contrast arteriography as the vascular diagnostic imaging study of choice. To date, duplex arterial mapping, MR, and CT angiography have proven capable of imaging the vascular system.

Duplex arterial mapping holds significant promise for replacing contrast arteriography before peripheral interventions. The major advantage of duplex ultrasound scanning is that it is a noninvasive study that is very well tolerated by patients and can be repeated as necessary without incurring the additional risk, cost, and inconvenience of angiography. In addition, it is significantly less expensive than contrast arteriography.

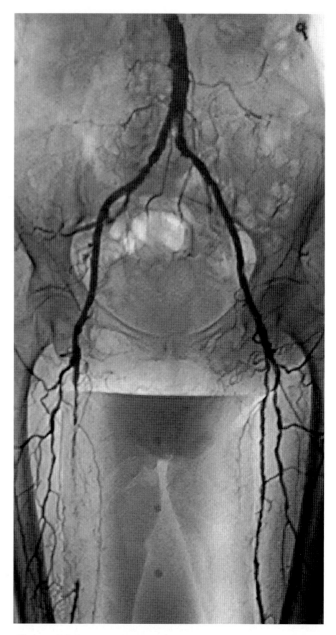

Figure 18-2. A conventional contrast arteriogram demonstrating patency of the aortoiliac segment and considerable bilateral superficial femoral artery disease.

Duplex mapping can provide important not only anatomic information but physiologic information as well. In the past, duplex ultrasound scanning has been employed more as a screening modality in patients with vascular disease than as a diagnostic study to help plan the necessary intervention. However, patients with vascular disease such as carotid artery lesions are now being safely treated using duplex scanning results alone without undergoing preoperative carotid angiograms.[2] Similarly, duplex scanning has also been applied to the evaluation of the lower extremity vasculature. Numerous studies have shown that duplex scanning can reliably distinguish between normal, disease-free vasculature;

mild (less than 50%) stenoses; severe (greater than 50%) stenoses; and arterial occlusions[3] (Fig. 18-3). The final step in duplex mapping's ascendancy as a rival to angiography has been a demonstration that lower extremity bypass procedures can safely be performed based on the results of this study alone. Findings from studies in the authors' laboratory, as well as those of others, have confirmed that lower extremity revascularization can safely be performed based on the results.

In order to evaluate whether duplex arterial mapping could replace angiography before lower extremity revascularization, the authors studied whether bypasses could be performed based on duplex ultrasound studies alone without relying on preoperative contrast arteriography. In the study, 41 patients who required lower extremity bypasses for claudication, rest pain, and foot lesions underwent preoperative contrast arteriography as well as duplex arterial mapping. An observer blinded to the results of the operation performed predicted what type of lower extremity bypass would be necessary based on each of the studies performed. In addition, the observer predicted where the anastomotic sites would be placed given the contrast study findings and the duplex findings. Finally, the predictions made by the blinded observer were compared to the actual procedure and anastomotic sites chosen by the operating surgeon.

The results indicated that duplex arterial mapping could decide whether a femoral-popliteal vs. a distal bypass graft was required in 90% of the patients studied. Both the proximal and distal anastomotic sites were correctly predicted in 90% of the patients who underwent femoral popliteal bypass grafts and in only 24% of the patients who had infrapopliteal revascularizations. Based on the results, the authors concluded that duplex arterial mapping was a reliable study to predict whether a patient required femoral popliteal or distal bypasses. Moreover, when a patient required a femoral popliteal bypass, the actual locations of the anastomotic sites could be predicted as well.[4] When a patient was found to require an infrapopliteal bypass, duplex arterial mapping was not sensitive enough to decide on the anastomotic sites. The primary problem with duplex mapping in this regard was that the technologist was unable to distinguish between the qualities of multiple patent, yet highly diseased, vessels. Other groups have met with more success by utilizing schemes whereby the operating surgeon's preference vessel of choice is evaluated for patency. If this vessel is patent it receives the terminus of the bypass graft. However, alternative vessels that are patent are not evaluated to see whether they might represent a preferable bypass target.[5,6]

Disadvantages of duplex arterial mapping include difficulty imaging patients with morbid obesity, circumferential and diffuse vascular calcification, and open wounds obscuring visualization of the underlying vasculature. In addition, some of the infragenicular vasculature (e.g., the terminal branches of the peroneal artery or the segment of anterior tibial artery that traverses the interosseous membrane) may be difficult to image. Moreover, there is no agreed-upon standard for grading the severity of stenoses within the lower extremity vasculature, and there is considerable subjectivity involved with duplex mapping such that interobserver reproducibility may be lacking. Finally, duplex arterial mapping is labor- and time-intensive, and the results may vary significantly depending on the technician performing the scanning and his or her level of training. Certainly, one must have confidence in the technician performing the study before proceeding with lower extremity revascularization based on duplex results alone. Physician comfort with contrast arteriography has centered on the ease with which the images can be interpreted. Until surgeons are comfortable with duplex technology and their own vascular technicians, the results of these studies might not be received with confidence or the study might not be requested at all.

Other alternatives for imaging the lower extremity vascular tree include magnetic resonance angiography and CT angiography.[7,8] Magnetic resonance angiography, unlike conventional arteriography, is a noninvasive study that does not require the administration of iodinated intravenous contrast. Therefore the potential for complications is negated. Numerous studies have been performed demonstrating the high sensitivity of MRA for adequately visualizing the infrainguinal vasculature in a complimentary fashion to contrast arteriography. In addition, there have been several studies documenting the ability of MRA to supplant contrast arteriography in planning infrainguinal revascularizations. Similar to duplex ultrasonography, the technique is operator depen-

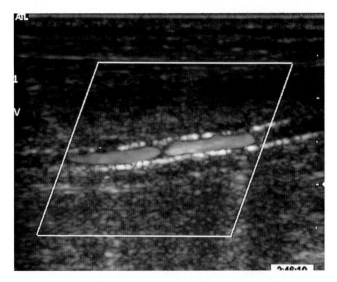

Figure 18-3. A duplex arteriogram of an anterior tibial artery. The artery is noted to be calcified, yet widely patent with uniform color flow in the lumen. This vessel could therefore serve as the terminus of a distal bypass graft in this patient with limb-threatening ischemia.

dant, and there appears to be a significant learning curve. In addition, there is variability among equipment in different institutions that may alter the usefulness of the procedure in a particular location. The authors have seen MRAs of the central and peripheral vasculature that have better resolution than conventional angiograms (Figs. 18-4 and 18-5) and MRs of such poor qualtity that identification of the imaged vessels is not possible.

Another potential disadvantage of magnetic resonance imaging is that only anatomic information is provided: There is no physiologic means to grade the degree of stenosis or the significance of a lesion, once discovered. Finally, MRA does not possess widespread applicability to all patient populations. Patients who have indwelling cardiac pacemakers, metallic clips from cerebral aneurysm surgery, or other metallic objects implanted in their bodies cannot be placed in the scanner. In addition, many patients may not be able to tolerate the claustrophobic conditions and the time required for MRA scanning. Critically ill patients with ventilator support, or those who require hemodynamic monitoring may be denied access to this study.

CT angiography is an alternative imaging study that is also undergoing considerable investigation as an alternative to contrast arteriography. In the past, CT scans were much better at imaging the central vasculature (e.g., the aorta and iliac arteries) than the infrainguinal

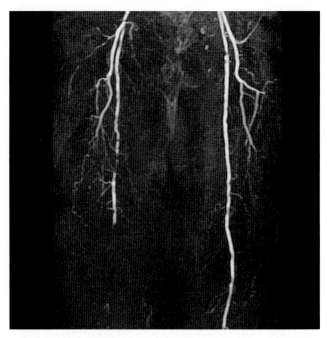

Figure 18-5. *MRA of the femoropopliteal vessels in the same patient seen in Figure 18-4 demonstrates an occlusion of the superficial femoral artery in the adductor canal on the right and widespread stenoses within the same vessel on the left. (From Dr. Joseph Divito, Assistant Professor of Radiology, Weiler Hospital of the Albert Einstein Hospital.)*

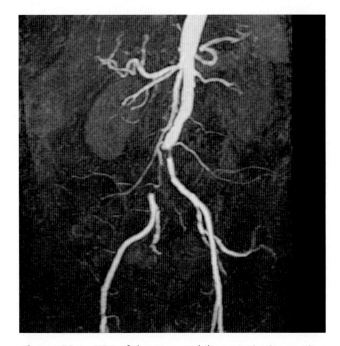

Figure 18-4. *MRA of the aorta and iliac arteries in a patient with severe bilateral claudication. The study reveals a long segment occlusion of the right common iliac artery and a high-grade stenosis of the left common iliac artery. Note that the quality of the study is equivalent to a conventional angiogram. (From Dr. Joseph Divito, Assistant Professor of Radiology, Weiler Hospital of the Albert Einstein Hospital.)*

vessels. However, technologic improvements are allowing the peripheral vessels to be imaged in an improved fashion. Similar to MRA, CT angiography is dependant on the software and the technician performing the studies for optimal image acquisition and interpretation. In addition, anatomic information regarding the location of stenosis may be obtained; however, the hemodynamic significance of these lesions is difficult to quantify. Improvements in software design and imaging technology should continue to improve the quality and the ease of acquisition of MRA and CT angiographic studies and to increase their applicability in the future.

REFERENCES

1. Mazzariol F, Ascher E, Salles-Cunha SX, et al: Values and limitations of duplex ultrasonography as the sole imaging method of preoperative evaluation for popliteal and infrapopliteal bypasses. Ann Vasc Surg 13:1–10, 1998.
2. Mazzariol F, Ascher E, Hingorani A, et al: Lower-extremity revascularization without preoperative contrast arteriography in 185 cases: Lessons learned with duplex ultrasound arterial mapping. Eur J Vasc Endovasc Surg 19:509–515, 2000.
3. Moneta G, Yeager R, Antonovic R, et al: Accuracy of lower extremity arterial duplex mapping. J Vasc Surg 15:275–284, 1992.
4. Wain RA, Berdejo GL, Delvalle W, et al: Can duplex scan arteriography replace contrast arteriography as the test of choice before infrainguinal revascularization? J Vasc Surg 29:100–109, 1999.

5. Wain RA, Lyon RT, Veith FJ, et al: Accuracy of duplex ultrasound in evaluating carotid artery anatomy before endarterectomy. J Vasc Surg 27:235–244, 1998.

6. Gambria RP, Kaufman JA, L'Italien GJ, et al: Magnetic resonance angiography in the management of lower extremity arterial occlusive disease: A prospective study. J Vasc Surg 25(2):380–389, 1997.

7. Koelemay MJ, Lijmer J, Stoker J, et al: Magnetic resonance angiography for the evaluation of lower extremity arterial disease: A Meta-analysis. JAMA 285(10):1338–1345, 2001.

8. Stoffers H, Kester A, Kaiser V, et al: The diagnostic value of signs and symptoms associated with peripheral arterial occlusive disease in general practice. A multivariate approach. Med Decis Making 17:61–70, 1997.

Chapter 19

Evaluation of Claudication

PAUL J. NORDNESS • SAMUEL R. MONEY

Claudication as a Manifestation of Peripheral Arterial Disease

*C*laudication may be the first recognizable symptom of peripheral arterial occlusive disease (PAOD). The term is derived from the Latin verb *claudico* meaning "to limp." The terms *claudication* or *intermittent claudication* (IC) are used almost exclusively to describe ischemic muscular pain induced by exercise and relieved by rest.

Lower extremity claudication and other manifestations of PAOD in the lower extremities are typically related to atherosclerosis and the progressive narrowing of large and intermediate size arteries. Narrowed vessels have a reduced capacity to deliver oxygenated blood and a reduced ability to compensate for increased oxygen demand in the extremity. During times of increased work (exercise) in an affected limb, the metabolic demands exceed the maximum oxygen delivery capacity. Muscular fatigue and cramping pain develop in the temporarily ischemic muscles, until the limb is rested and the pain resolves.

Claudication may also be used to describe ischemic fatigue of the upper extremities, though this is less common. Upper extremity claudication accounts for a small percentage of patients with symptomatic PAOD. However, claudication of the upper extremities may be a more complex diagnostic dilemma because of the higher frequency of nonatherosclerotic diseases (e.g., Beurger's disease and thoracic outlet syndrome).

As the vascular disease progresses, and the arteries become highly stenotic or occluded, the signs and symptoms of PAOD become more apparent and more severe (Table 19-1). The claudication can become lifestyle limiting, making the person unable to work or to easily undertake the activities of daily life. At some point the baseline metabolic needs of the muscle may exceed the maximum oxygen supply through the diseased arteries. The depressed cardiac output as seen with sleep, coupled with postural changes that deprive the limb of gravity's influence, may lead to "rest pain." Rest pain typically awakens the patient with cramping pains across the foot. These pains are relieved as the patient increases his or

TABLE 19-1. Classification of PAOD: Rutherford Categories

Grade	Category	Clinical Description
0	0	Asymptomatic
	1	Mild claudication
I	2	Moderate claudication
	3	Severe claudication
II	4	Ischemic rest pain
III	5	Minor tissue loss
	6	Major tissue loss

Adapted from Rutherford RB, Baker JD, Ernst C, et al: Recommended standards for reports dealing with lower extremity ischemia: Revised version. J Vasc Surg 26:517–538, 1997.

her cardiac output and augments the perfusion pressure by lowering the limb. Eventually the vascular disease may limit perfusion to such an extent that even the baseline metabolic needs cannot be met. At this point the generalized atrophy of the skin and muscles progresses, leading to ulceration and tissue necrosis.

The classic presentation of IC involves the calf muscles with cramping pain that is rapidly relieved by brief periods of rest; however, this is found in a distinct minority of patients with identifiable PAOD.[1,2] Atypical claudication may still be related to PAOD, but symptoms may present in other muscle groups such as the upper extremity, thigh, or gluteal regions. Claudication in the foot is uncommon but may suggest involvement of smaller vessels as a result of thromboangiitis obliterans (Beurger's disease), which is a form of vascular disease distinct from atherosclerotic arterial disease.

It is important, however, to emphasize that the absence of claudication does not preclude the existence of PAOD. Patients, especially the elderly, may not be active enough to induce claudication during their daily routine. Their sedentary lifestyle may or may not be caused by their compromised vascular supply. Coexisting arthritis, cognitive impairment, coronary heart disease, depression, previous strokes, visual problems, or other medical or social problems may severely affect the lifestyle of many elderly persons. Despite progressive PAOD these patients may not be identified unless the clinician is attentive and thorough in the history and examination. Approximately 25% to 50% of patients with PAOD will present with claudication.

Prevalence

Vascular disease is common in Western societies. Peripheral vascular disease may affect up to 12% of the population over age 65,[3] and studies suggest that primary care physicians could identify PAOD in approximately 20% of their patients over 55 years old.[2]

Intermittent claudication is strongly related to age. A consensus study recently reviewed seven large studies on the prevalence of IC[4] (Table 19-2). The weighted mean prevalence of IC was roughly 2% among those 50 to 54 years old, 3% among those 60 to 64 years old, and over 7% in those over 70 years old. Therefore, as the life expectancy and median age of Western countries increase over the foreseeable future, clinicians can expect that PAOD and IC will be increasingly common within their practices. In addition, claudication will be of even further importance as the baby boomer generation has expectations for increased activity and independence in their later years.

Using slightly different diagnostic criteria, two studies, one by Meijer and colleagues from Rotterdam[5] and one by Criqui and colleagues from San Diego,[6] studied the prevalence of PAOD. These population studies demonstrate a clear association between PAOD and age, with

TABLE 19-2. Prevalence of Intermittent Claudication by Age

Study	Population Size	Age (yrs)	Prevalence (%)
Hughson (1978)	1716	45–69	2.2
De Backer (1979)	8252	40–49	0.8
		50–59	2.9
Reunanen (1982)	5738	30–39	0.6
		40–49	1.9
		50–59	4.6
Fowkes (1991)	1592	55–74	4.5
Stoffers (1991)	3654	45–54	0.6
		55–64	2.5
		65–74	8.8
Smith (1991)	10,042	40–59	1.1
Novo (1992)	1558	40–49	4.7
		50–59	9.2

Adapted from Dormandy JA, Rutherford RB: Management of peripheral arterial disease (PAD). TASC Working Group. J Vasc Surg 31(1 pt 2):S1–S296, 2000.

noninvasive diagnostic studies identifying PAOD in 2.5% of people 40 to 59 years old but in 18.8% of subjects 70 to 79 years old.[4] The prevalence of PAOD is also higher in men than women (1.4:1.0), and this becomes more prominent when severe disease is considered.[4,6] Recent data suggest that as the rate of smoking increases among women, the difference in prevalence between the genders may be reduced.

Risk Factors

Risk factors for IC are similar to those noted for PAOD and for other atherosclerotic diseases, with the notable exception that a family history of the disease has not been clearly identified as a risk factor for PAOD or IC (although it has been noted for coronary artery disease [CAD] and stroke).[4] Beyond age and gender, four risk factors are implicated in the development of IC: diabetes mellitus, tobacco use, hypertension, and hematologic disorders[4] (Fig. 19-1).

Of great significance, diabetes mellitus is a risk factor associated with accelerated atherosclerosis and claudication.[7] Indeed, claudication appears to be two to four times as common in diabetics compared with nondiabetic controls.[4] Much of the association between diabetes and atherosclerosis is related to the "metabolic syndrome" (i.e., concurrent obesity, type 2 diabetes, hyperinsulinemia, hyperlipidemia, hyperuricemia, and hypertension) that is just recently being appreciated as having a close association with PAOD and IC.[8]

Tobacco use is another well-known risk factor for IC[5,7,9,10-12] and may play a more dramatic role among males.[11] Depending on the severity of the habit, the odds ratio for developing IC may be between 1 and 4.[4] Although tobacco cessation has been central to vascular therapeutic programs for many years, at this time it is controversial to speculate as to how long a person must quit smoking before he or she reverses the effects of prolonged tobacco use.[12-14]

The causative relationship between hypertension and IC is less clear than that for IC and diabetes or tobacco use. Hypertension is thought to be both a cause and a symptom of atherosclerosis, and therefore its association with PAOD and IC is complex. Nevertheless, hypertension is a risk factor for IC,[7,9] and this is more apparent in women.[15]

Hematologic factors thought to be associated with IC include elevated cholesterol, elevated plasma fibrinogen, hyperhomocysteinemia, and any functional hypercoaguability. Elevated cholesterol has been the most thoroughly studied. Although not consistently shown to be an independent risk factor, an elevated total cholesterol (or an elevated ratio of total lipids to high density lipids) seems to be associated with IC.[16] In addition, pharmacotherapy can lower cholesterol levels and reduce the incidence of IC.[17] Other hematologic factors (e.g., fibrinogen,[18] homocysteine,[19-21] and hypercoaguability[22]) have not been as rigorously studied, although some association with PAOD and IC likely exists.

Natural History of Claudication

Among patients with IC, progression to a more severe state of PAOD (i.e., rest pain or tissue loss) is uncommon. By far the most common outcome of untreated IC is that the disease and the disability associated with the disease will remain stable. Based on studies that used objective means to evaluate vascular occlusions in patients with IC, over 50% to 70% of patients will have stable disease.[23-26] These studies demonstrate that progressive occlusion is noted in 22% to 60% of these patients over a period of 2.5 to 8 years. Of clinical importance, roughly 20% to 30% will require an intervention during this same period,[27] but less than 12% of patients with IC will require amputation in the next 10 years.[28] Although the diagnosis of PAOD and IC has been associated with early death, this is primarily because of their association with concurrent coronary and carotid artery occlusions.

Concurrent Vascular Disease

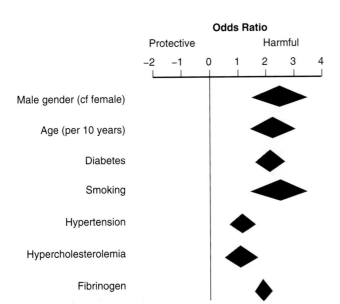

Figure 19-1. Range of odds ratios for developing IC. (Adapted from Dormandy JA, Rutherford RB: Management of peripheral arterial disease (PAD). TASC Working Group. J Vasc Surg 31(1 pt 2):S1–S296, 2000.)

Given that atherosclerotic vascular disease plays a central role in coronary, carotid, and peripheral disease, it is not surprising that patients presenting with symptoms of PAOD are at greater risk of also having cardiac or cerebral vascular disease (CVD). Peripheral symptoms have been associated with a markedly increased risk of CAD, including both symptomatic and asymptomatic heart disease. When compared with other patients, it can be expected that patients presenting with PAOD will have a three- or fourfold increase in their incidence of CAD.[29] The true prevalence of CAD among patients presenting with PAOD is dependent on the diagnostic technique used and the definitions applied to those studies. Using routine coronary angiography in patients with claudication, CAD was identified in 90% of patients and severe CAD was identified in 28% of patients.[30] However, such routine evaluation by coronary arteriography cannot be justified for patients without cardiac symptoms. In contrast, using only clinical history and electrocardiograms (ECGs) may identify CAD in up to 62% of PAOD patients, which is not markedly different from the number found by treadmill or dipyridamole-thallium stress evaluations.[31] At present, appropriate indications and techniques for selective cardiac evaluation in patients presenting with IC have not been standardized.

The importance of identifying CAD in a patient with claudication revolves around the profound impact heart disease has on that patient's health. The Framingham Study highlighted the impact of CAD on patients with IC. In this study, CAD accounted for 50% of all deaths among patients with IC, whereas deaths caused by progressive PAOD were much less common.[16,32]

Similarly, patients with symptomatic PAOD are at high risk for having clinically important carotid artery disease. This can be identified by clinical history alone (15%) or by duplex examination in about 25% of patients with claudication, rest pain, or tissue loss.[31] In addition, the Framingham Study demonstrated a 10% risk of fatal stroke in patients with claudication,[16,32] and patients with PAOD have a 25% to 30% 5-year mortality rate from cardiac and cerebrovascular events.

Undiagnosed Disease

Despite the high prevalence of PAOD in our aging society, and the expanding range of therapies now available for patients with all forms of vascular disease, there is an increasing suspicion that both patients and clinicians often overlook PAOD and claudication. In contrast to CAD or CVD, the public remains largely unaware of the symptoms of progressive limb ischemia. Primary care providers may not routinely screen patients for claudication symptoms or recognize claudication when the symptoms are atypical. Hirsch and colleagues[1] studied nearly 7000 high-risk individuals and found that, among patients with previously documented peripheral artery occlusions, less than half of their physicians had recognized or documented this diagnosis. Failure to recognize this diagnosis could mean clinicians are overlooking

clues to asymptomatic coronary or cerebral disease. It would also delay the implementation of therapies (e.g., exercise, glucose control, tobacco cessation, antiplatelet drugs, phosphodiesterase inhibitors, or beta-adrenergic blockade) that could benefit the patient by slowing the progression of PAOD, CAD, and CVD.

Clinical Evaluation

Though classic claudication symptoms may not be obvious, a thorough history can usually discriminate between peripheral arterial disease and other nonvascular diagnoses. Special attention should be given to cardiac and cerebrovascular symptoms; or a history of diabetes, tobacco use, and other atherosclerosis risk factors. When given a complaint suggestive of IC the clinician must allow the patient to fully describe the symptoms. The character and location of the pain are important. Calf pain is often reported with infrainguinal disease, whereas gluteal or thigh claudication may result from lesions in the aortoiliac region. Foot claudication is rare but can be seen with severe infrapopliteal disease.

Claudication is not strongly suggested by joint pain or pain that is inconsistent in its presentation. With further questioning, the patient can usually describe a specific walking distance or activity level required to bring about the cramping pain. Claudication is not relieved by anti-inflammatory medications but improves after brief periods of inactivity. The clinician must also assess whether a patient is active and is developing limitations that strongly affect his or her work (lifestyle), or whether a patient is primarily sedentary and minimally troubled by this pain.

Further inquiry into the presence of ischemic rest pain should be explored, even if not initially noted by the patient. Especially in the relatively inactive patient, claudication can present as a late symptom, with the patient already having signs and symptoms of severe limb-threatening ischemia (e.g., rest pain or nonhealing skin lesions) in the extremity.

The initial history and physical examination should go a long way toward suggesting vascular claudication or suggesting one of many nonischemic limb pain syndromes, generally referred to as "pseudoclaudication" (Table 19-3). Herniated spinal disks with nerve root compression may masquerade as IC; however, the pain is more commonly sharp and radiates down the posterior or lateral leg. The pain may occur while at rest or soon after initiating activities. Neurospinal root compression is another neurologic symptom that may be mistaken for ischemic claudication. These symptoms are most severe in the buttocks or thigh, and weakness is often more prominent than pain. With neurospinal root compression, symptoms may develop during periods of inactivity and resolve reliably with any flexing of the spine.

TABLE 19-3. **Differential Diagnosis of Intermittent Claudication**

	Location	Character	Effect of Exercise	Effect of Rest	Effect of Body Position	Other Characteristics
Intermittent claudication	Calf, thigh, gluteal	Cramp	Predictable	Rapid relief	None	Reproducible
Chronic compartment syndrome	Calf	Tightness	After prolonged exercise	Slow relief	Elevation helps	Athletes
Venous claudication	Entire leg	Tightness	Less predictable	Slow relief	Elevation helps	History of venous disease
Nerve root compression	Radiates posteriorly	Sharp pain	Rapid onset	May present at rest	Back position affects pain	History of back pain/injury
Hip arthritis	Hip, thigh	Aching	Variable	May present at rest	Relief with sitting	Highly variable
Spinal cord compression	Dermatomal	Weakness	Predictable	Variable, based on back position	Relief with lumbar flexion	History of back problems

Adapted from Dormandy JA, Rutherford RB: Management of peripheral arterial disease (PAD). TASC Working Group. J Vasc Surg 31(1 pt 2):S1–S296, 2000.

Pseudoclaudication may also have arthritic etiologies affecting the hip or foot. This pain is usually associated with one or many joints and may be worse after periods of inactivity. Often the pain is relieved by over-the-counter anti-inflammatory medications. Patients will often emphasize the variability in the severity of the pain, which contrasts with the typically uniform pain seen with IC.

Venous pseudoclaudication may be differentiated from arterial claudication by the history of deep venous thrombosis (or by a history placing the patient at risk for venous thrombosis). This pain is less localized and may involve the whole extremity with a painful sensation that is relieved by elevation of the affected limb.

After taking a thorough history, the patient should be examined completely, paying particular attention to cardiac auscultation, abdominal auscultation, and palpation of peripheral pulses. Pulses that are difficult to palpate should not be ignored or attributed to obesity or edema. In these situations, a handheld Doppler ultrasound device is an invaluable aid in identifying and characterizing peripheral bloodflow. Of note, aplasia of the anterior tibial artery results in a congenital absence of the dorsalis pedis pulse in about 10% of humans without specific clinical significance, whereas the posterior tibial artery is congenitally absent in up to 5% of the population.[33]

Upon initial examination, arterial bruits should be identified. In the neck these may be suggestive of carotid or cardiac disease, whereas abdominal bruits are usually related to aortic or renal artery lesions. Pulsatile masses along the arterial system can result from aneurysms or pseudoaneurysms that compress or obstruct flow to an extremity.

Examining the skin along the affected extremity is also critically important. Hairless legs with cool, scaly, and fragile skin may suggest ischemia. The skin may also demonstrate pallor on elevation, dependent rubor, or delayed (greater than 3 seconds) capillary refill. Neuropathy, either ischemic or diabetic, should be noted and the entire extremity should be evaluated for ulceration and subclinical infections (bacterial or fungal). The examination of a patient with claudication (and all diabetic patients) must also look for evidence of poor foot hygiene (e.g., long nails, ingrown nails, or abrasions from ill-fitting shoes) because these problems may rapidly develop into nonhealing lesions in the presence of ischemia.

Ankle-Brachial Index

During the initial evaluation of a patient with claudication, the ankle-brachial index (ABI) should be obtained in order to aid in the diagnosis of IC and to serve as an objective measurement that can be followed on subsequent examinations. Recent clinical studies have demonstrated a strong and independent association between lower ABI and poor lower extremity function as measured by 6-minute walking distance, balance, 4-meter walking velocity, and physical activity assessment.[34] In addition, a low ABI is a strong independent predictor of increased cardiovascular morbidity and mortality.[35,36]

This technique may be performed in a medical office and requires only a blood pressure cuff and a handheld

Doppler. Bilateral supine upper extremity systolic blood pressures are determined using the Doppler device for detection of vascular flow. The higher of the two measurements is used to calculate the ABI (eliminating possible error because of subclinical arterial stenosis in either extremity). Similarly, the systolic pressures in both ankle arteries are determined using the Doppler. ABI is calculated as the highest ankle Doppler pressure divided by the highest brachial Doppler pressure (Fig. 19-2).

Persons without vascular disease will typically have an ABI between 1.05 and 1.15. An ABI greater than 1.30 must be questioned because it is likely an aberrant value caused by medial calcification of the lower extremity vasculature from longstanding diabetes. PAOD is suspected when the ABI is below 0.90. The mean ABI of a patient presenting with claudication has been shown to be 0.59 (standard deviation 0.15), whereas those presenting with rest pain or tissue loss have mean ABIs even lower at 0.26 +/− 0.13 and 0.05 +/− 0.08, respectively.[37]

Toe Systolic Pressure Index

As noted above, ABI measurement in patients with heavily calcified vessels will be falsely elevated. Given the prevalence of IC among diabetics this is a significant limitation of the ABI examination. For these patients, special cuffs may be applied to the great toes to obtain a toe systolic measurement, and then a toe-brachial index (TBI) can be calculated. The small arteries of the toes are not heavily involved by medial calcification and therefore are less susceptible to this artifact. A normal TBI is greater than 0.60 and some degree of PAOD may be inferred from any value below 0.50. The toe's systolic pressure is often used to assess the likelihood that a diabetic foot ulcer will heal because ulcers associated with a systolic pressures less than 30 mmHg are unlikely to heal without intervention.[38]

Treadmill Testing

Despite the high sensitivity (95%) and specificity (99%) of ABI when combined with an appropriate clinical history,[33] some patients with claudication could be overlooked with ABI alone. Challenging the painful extremity with exercise may, however, increase the sensitivity of the ABI. Though this test usually requires a vascular laboratory, the clinician should be aware of the principles behind performing post-treadmill ABIs. In standard treadmill testing, the patient walks at a constant rate of 2 miles per hour on a 12% grade. The walking continues until the point of claudication (maximum walking distance) or 5 minutes. The patient is then immediately placed in a supine position and ankle pressures are

$$\text{Ankle brachial index (ABI)} = \frac{\text{Doppler determined systolic pressure using the higher of either the dorsalis pedis or posterior tibial artery}}{\text{Doppler determined systolic pressure using the higher of either the left or right brachial artery}}$$

Figure 19-2. *Calculation of ankle brachial index.*

obtained every minute until they return to baseline. The resting arm pressure is used when calculating the post-treadmill ABI.

With exercise, the peripheral vasculature is maximally dilated for increased bloodflow; however, proximal lesions limit the effect of distal arterial dilation, and blood is therefore shunted to other dilated arterial regions. As a result, the ABI will be lower after the affected limb is stressed than it was in the resting state. A test is considered abnormal if the value drops by 20% and remains low for longer than 3 minutes. In practice, patients with true ischemic claudication will often have ankle pressures that fall dramatically and may be difficult to measure for several minutes. Also, if the post-treadmill ABI returns to baseline within 5 minutes, then a single lesion is suggested, whereas delays over 10 minutes suggest multi-level disease. In contrast, after this modest activity level, a healthy person should see an ABI value very close to normal or have rapid normalization of any modestly decreased ABI. Recently, many vascular laboratories have been substituting toe raises (up to 50 repetitions) for treadmill walking with good results, and this can even be performed in the office setting.

Further Evaluation

As discussed in full detail in subsequent chapters, a variety of tests may be performed in the vascular laboratory to more accurately assess vascular insufficiency and provide some insight into the anatomic location of the significant lesions. Segmental limb pressures (SLPs), segmental pulse volume recordings (PVRs), and Doppler velocity waveform analysis (VWF) are all noninvasive tests used during the initial evaluation of claudication. These are particularly useful for patients with significantly disabling claudication. The decision to proceed with invasive diagnostic tests and possible intervention, or to continue with conservative management (e.g., pharmacotherapies, smoking cessation, and a formal exercise regimen) can be influenced by these noninvasive tests. Tests suggesting aortoiliac disease with preserved vasculature below the inguinal ligament may, in appropriate patients, be referred for arteriography in hopes that other minimally invasive endovascular angioplasty and stenting techniques or surgery may provide relief. On the other hand, a patient with similar disability but

TABLE 19-4. Suggested Tests for Evaluation of Patient With New Claudication Symptoms

Test	When Used
Ankle-brachial index (ABI)	
ABI with toe raises or treadmill	Indicated when clinical suspicion exists with normal ABI
Toe brachial pressure index (TBI)	Indicated when ABI falsely elevated
Further anatomic or physiologic studies	Ordered only when indicated
Electrocardiography	
Complete blood count	
Diabetic screening test	
Serum creatinine	
Fasting lipid profile	
Hypercoagulability studies or homocysteine levels	Ordered only when indicated

with noninvasive tests suggesting multilevel disease or significant infrageniculate disease may tolerate further conservative therapy before opting to undergo diagnostic arteriography and open bypass procedure.

Routine Tests During Initial Evaluation of Claudication

Several laboratory tests may provide valuable information to help evaluate claudication or coexisting disease. Recently, an American and European consensus conference[4] has provided the following recommendations regarding initial routine laboratory testing. Physicians should consider ordering these tests on a patient with new claudication symptoms if they have not been recently studied. These recommended tests are: ECG, complete blood count (CBC), diabetic screening, renal function screening, and a lipid profile. An ECG is an accurate and inexpensive means to evaluate for silent myocardial ischemia. A CBC may identify polycythemia or anemia, either of which can induce claudication. A screening evaluation for glucose intolerance (e.g., urine glucose test, fasting blood glucose level, or hemoglobin A1c) should be obtained because of the close association between PAOD and glucose intolerance. Renal function can be tested with a serum creatinine level and urine protein measurement. Finally, as discussed earlier, a fasting lipid profile should be considered to help identify cholesterol disorders that are associated with CAD as well as PAOD. Further testing may be considered by the clinician to address specific concerns regarding an individual patient. In general, hypercoaguability studies and homocysteine levels are not routinely indicated, although they may be helpful in selected patients where family or personal medical history is suggestive (Table 19-4).

REFERENCES

1. Hirsch AT, Criqui MH, Treat-Jacobson D, et al: Peripheral arterial disease detection, awareness, and treatment in primary care. JAMA 286(11):1317–1324, 2001.
2. Fowkes FG, Housley E, Cawood EH, et al: Edinburgh Artery Study: Prevalence of asymptomatic and symptomatic peripheral arterial disease in the general population. Int J Epidemiol 20:384–392, 1991.
3. Newman AB, Siscovick DS, Manolio TA, et al: Ankle-arm index as a marker of atherosclerosis in the Cardiovascular Health Study. Cardiovascular Heart Study (CHS) Collaborative Research Group. Circulation 88:837–845, 1993.
4. Dormandy JA, Rutherford RB: Management of peripheral arterial disease (PAD). TASC Working Group. J Vasc Surg 31(1 pt 2):S1–S296, 2000.
5. Meijer WT, Hoes AW, Rutgers D, et al: Peripheral arterial disease in the elderly: The Rotterdam Study. Arterioscler Thromb Vasc Biol 18:185–192, 1998.
6. Criqui M, Fronek A, Barrett-Connor E, et al: The prevalence of peripheral arterial disease in a defined population. Circulation 71:510–515, 1985.
7. Murabito JM, D'Agostino RB, Silbershatz H, et al: Intermittent claudication: A risk profile from the Framingham Heart Study. Circulation 96:44–49, 1997.
8. Reaven GM: Banting Lecture: Role of insulin resistance in human disease. Diabetes 37:1595–1607, 1988.
9. Kannel WB: Risk factors for atherosclerotic cardiovascular outcomes in different arterial territories. J Cardiovasc Risk 1:333–339, 1994.
10. Criqui MH, Browner D, Fronek A, et al: Peripheral arterial disease in large vessels is epidemiologically distinct from small vessel disease: An analysis of risk factors. Am J Epidemiol 129:1110–1119, 1989.
11. Bowlin SJ, Medalie JH, Flocke SA, et al: Epidemiology of intermittent claudication in middle-aged men. Am J Epidemiol 140(5):418–430, 1994.

12. Ingolfsson IO, Sigurdsson G, Sigvaldason H, et al: A marked decline in the prevalence and incidence of intermittent claudication in Icelandic men 1968-1986: A strong relationship to smoking and serum cholesterol. The Reykjavik Study. J Clin Epidemiol 47(11):1237–1243, 1994.

13. Fowkes GR, Housley E, Riemersma RA, et al: Smoking, lipids, glucose intolerance, and blood pressure as risk factors for peripheral atherosclerosis compared with ischemic heart disease in the Edinburgh Artery Study. Am J Epidemiol 135:331–340, 1992.

14. Dagenais GR, Maurice S, Robitaille NM, et al: Intermittent claudication in Quebec men from 1974-1986: The Quebec Cardiovascular Study. Clin Invest Med 14:93–100, 1991.

15. Kannel WB, McGee DL: Update on some epidemiological features of intermittent claudication. J Am Geriatr Soc 33:13–18, 1985.

16. Kannel WB, Skinner JJ Jr, Schwartz MJ, et al: Intermittent claudication: Incidence in the Framingham study. Circulation 41:875–883, 1970.

17. Duffield RGM, Lewis B, Miller NE, et al: Treatment of hyperlipidaemia retards progression of symptomatic femoral atherosclerosis: A randomized controlled trial. Lancet 2:639–642, 1983.

18. Kannel WB, D'Agostino RB, Belanger AJ: Update on fibrinogen as a cardiovascular risk factor. Ann Epidemiol 2:457–466, 1992.

19. Kang SS, Wong PW, Malinow MR: Hyperhomocysteinaemia as a risk factor for occlusive vascular disease. Annu Rev Nutr 12:279–298, 1992.

20. Fermo I, d'Angelo V, Paroni R, et al: Prevalence of moderate hyperhomocysteinemia in patients with early onset venous and arterial occlusive disease. Ann Intern Med 123(32):747–753, 1995.

21. Caldwell S, McCarthy M, Martin SC, et al: Hyperhomocysteinaemia, peripheral vascular disease and neointimal hyperplasia in elderly patients. Br J Surg 85:685–715, 1998.

22. Ray SA, Rowley MR, Loh A, et al: Hypercoagulable states in patients with leg ischaemia. Br J Surg 81:811–814, 1994.

23. Cronenwett JL, Warner KG, Zelenock GB, et al: Intermittent claudication: Current results of nonoperative management. Arch Surg 119:430, 1984.

24. Rosenbloom MS, Flanigan DP, Schuler JJ, et al: Risk factors affecting the natural history of claudication. Arch Surg 123:867, 1988.

25. Jonason T, Ringqvist I: Factors of prognostic importance for subsequent rest pain in patients with intermittent claudication. Acta Med Scand 218:27, 1985.

26. Walsh DB, Gilbertson JJ, Zwolak RM: The natural history of superficial femoral artery stenosis. J Vasc Surg 14:299, 1991.

27. Weitz JI, Byrne J, Clagett GP, et al: Diagnosis and treatment of chronic arterial insufficiency of the lower extremities: A critical review. Circulation 94:3026–3049, 1996.

28. Boyd AM: The natural course of arteriosclerosis of the lower extremities. Angiology 11:10, 1960.

29. Stoffers HE, Rinkens PE, Kester AD, et al: The prevalence of asymptomatic and unrecognized peripheral arterial occlusive disease. Int J Epidemiol 25:282–290, 1996.

30. Hertzer NP, Beven EG, Young JR, et al: Coronary artery disease in peripheral vascular patients: A classification of 1000 coronary angiograms and results of surgical management. Ann Surg 199:223–233, 1984.

31. Golomb B, Criqui MH, Bundens W: Epidemiology. In Creager MA (ed): Management of Peripheral Arterial Disease. London: Remedica Publishing, 2000.

32. Dormandy J, Mahir M, Ascada G, et al: Fate of the patient with chronic leg ischemia. J Cardiovasc Surg 30:50–57, 1989.

33. Keck GM, Zwiebel WJ: Arterial Anatomy of the Extremities. In Zwiebel WJ (ed): Introduction to Vascular Ultrasonography, 4th ed. Philiadelphia: WB Saunders, 2000.

34. McDermott MM, Greenland P, Liu K, et al: The ankle brachial index is associated with leg function and physical activity: The walking and leg circulation study. Ann Intern Med 136(12):873–883, 2002.

35. Newman AB, Tyrrell KS, Kuller LH: Mortality over 4 years in SHEP participants with a low ankle-brachial index. J Am Geriatr Soc 45:1472–1478, 1997.

36. McKenna M, Wolfson S, Kuller LH: The ratio of ankle and arm arterial pressure as an independent predictor of mortality. Atherosclerosis 87:119–128, 1991.

37. Yao JST: Hemodynamic studies in peripheral arterial disease. Br J Surg 57:761–766, 1970.

38. Orchard TJ, Strandness DE: Assessment of peripheral vascular disease in diabetics: Reports and recommendations of an international workshop sponsored by the American Diabetes Association and the American Heart Association. September 18–20, 1992, New Orleans, Louisiana. Circulation 88:819–828, 1993.

Chapter 20

Physiologic Testing of Lower Extremity Arterial Disease: Segmental Pressures, Plethysmography, and Velocity Waveforms

TERRY NEEDHAM

- Plethysmography
- Doppler
- Systolic Pressures
- Stress Testing

Physiologic modalities for the noninvasive detection and assessment of peripheral arterial occlusive disease (PAOD) are indirect, nonimaging modalities that use plethysmography and Doppler ultrasound. These modalities do not generate images of the arteries; therefore, the status of the arterial circulation must be inferred from systolic pressure gradients, pressure indices, and pulse waveforms. Despite this limitation, plethysmographic and Doppler-based modalities are well established and remain appropriate for the initial assessment of persons with signs and symptoms of PAOD, in addition to the follow-up of those patients on medical therapy.

Systolic pressures and Doppler/plethysmographic waveform recordings can indicate when PAOD has caused a detectable loss in flow energy through a segment of narrowed artery and/or any collateral channels. These energy losses are identified from significant changes in the pulse or blood velocity waveforms and from abnormally large reductions in systolic pressures along a particular arterial segment. Plethysmographic waveforms represent the changes in limb volume throughout the cardiac cycle (i.e., the difference between the arterial flow into a limb segment and its venous outflow). These waveforms are a combination of the pulsatility of all the vasculature under the sensing cuff, whereas Doppler waveforms are recorded from specific blood vessels.

At rest, arterial pulse waveforms in a normal lower extremity are characterized by a rapid upstroke during systole followed by a transient net reversal of flow at the end of systole/beginning of diastole. Forward flow resumes throughout the remainder of diastole, although this may not be obvious if the extremity is cold or the patient is vasoconstricted. Hemodynamically significant narrowing in an artery will alter the waveform, and it is these changes that are used to indicate the presence and the severity of the disease.

Digit pressures can be measured using photoplethysmography (PPG); however, systolic pressures at other levels in an extremity most commonly are measured with Doppler, followed by air and, rarely, straingauge plethysmography. The same normal/abnormal systolic pressure criteria are used whatever modality is employed. Some volume plethysmographs use only one large cuff above the knee, whereas two cuffs are used most commonly with Doppler.

As stated, plethysmographs are integrating instruments, so they indicate only the highest pressure at the level of the cuff and not the pressure from a specific artery. Doppler systolic pressures are measured from individual arteries and, as such, these techniques demand more from the operator than when using plethysmography. A limitation of measuring ankle systolic pressures occurs when an arterial wall becomes calcified or stiffened to the point where a blood pressure cuff cannot compress it—even when inflated to 300 mmHg. This situation is commonly encountered with patients having long-term diabetes or those with renal failures. This should be suspected if an ABI is greater than 1.4 or if the measured ankle pressures exceed the higher brachial pressure by more than 60 mmHg. Pulse volume recordings are particularly valuable when this is the case, especially when they are combined with pressures measured from the toes.

Plethysmographic waveforms, at any level in an extremity, are less affected by calcification than are Doppler signals because extremity Doppler systolic pressures are measured from moderate- to small-sized arteries, whereas plethysmography includes perfusion through smaller (but less affected) vessels. Measurements of digit pressure are valuable when proximal pressures are artifactually elevated because digit arteries are less affected by stiffening of their walls. In these cases, the plethysmographic waveform provides diagnostic information about the presence of PAOD superior to that provided by Doppler. Digit pressures are more valid than ankle pressures in this situation because the walls of digital arteries are affected less by calcification than are those of larger vessels. That being the case, toe pressures should be measured routinely when testing a diabetic patient, and a case can be made for measuring these pressures on all patients.

It should be remembered that an apparently normal resting systolic pressure gradient of less than 20 mmHg can exist across a segment with PAOD when a lesion in a more proximal artery has already reduced significantly the pressure energy entering that segment. Under these circumstances, it is unreliable to use only systolic pressure gradients to detect the presence/site/severity of PAOD; they should be combined with information from the pulse waveform.

Plethysmography

Waveforms

Volume plethysmography (VP) and PPG are common plethysmographic modalities for recording arterial pulse waveforms. Although PPG is regarded as experimental by federal agencies, it is used widely to record digit waveforms and systolic pressures. VP can be used also to record digit pulse waveforms, in addition to all other limb segments.

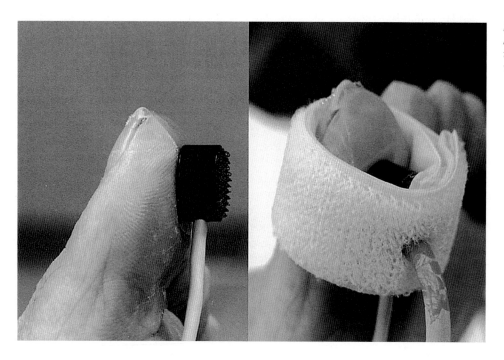

Figure 20-1. Photoplethysmography transducer applied to digit for recording pulse waveforms.

PPG transducers are applied with double-sided tape (Fig. 20-1). This helps to prevent it moving during cuff inflation when measuring digit pressures, making it unnecessary to apply the cuff firmly (which can cause blanching of the skin). VP waveforms are reproducible, provided that the sensing cuffs are wrapped around the limb segment at a moderate tension and are inflated to 50 to 60 mmHg (Fig. 20-2). Because VP and PPG waveforms do not indicate flow direction, neither modality will exhibit the flow reversal at the end of systole (as seen in normal arterial Doppler signals). However, a normal plethysmographic waveform will have a notching in its dicrotic portion; this corresponds to the flow reversal (Figs. 20-3 and 20-4). Hemodynamically significant PAOD proximal to the limb segment being examined will cause first a loss of the dicrotic notch (see Fig. 20-4, *B*) in mild/moderate disease. More severe PAOD results in a dampened flow pulsality, causing waveform amplitude to be reduced and prolongation of the upstroke (Fig. 20-5; see Fig. 20-4, *C*).

Systolic Pressures

Using plethysmography, segmental systolic pressures are measured using a sensing cuff (inflated to 50 to 60 mmHg) distal to the inflation cuff. Waveforms are recorded from the sensing cuff during deflation of the proximal pressure cuff from a superior systolic pressure, the systolic pressure at the level of the pressure cuff being the pressure at which the pulses reappear (Fig. 20-6).

Doppler

Waveforms

Directional Doppler instruments are able to demonstrate the transient reversal of flow occurring at the end of systole and the beginning of diastole in normal lower extremity arteries (Fig. 20-4, *D*). PAOD changes the normal triphasic waveform to biphasic signals in mild/moderate disease (Fig. 20-4, *E*), which progresses to monophasic signals where PAOD is severe (Fig. 20-4, *F*). Severe proximal PAOD can cause Doppler signals distally to be continuous or absent. The greater the degree of PAOD, the more similar the plethysmographic and Doppler waveforms become. Blood velocity waveforms from the common femoral artery can characterize significant PAOD proximal or distal to the probe. When PAOD is at more than one level in a lower extremity, the comparison of waveforms from adjacent segments can indicate the areas of greatest disease.

Systolic Pressures

Ankle-Brachial Systolic Pressure Indices (ABIs)

A well-established method for assessing the status of peripheral arteries in the lower extremity is to compare systolic pressures at ankle level with that in the arms

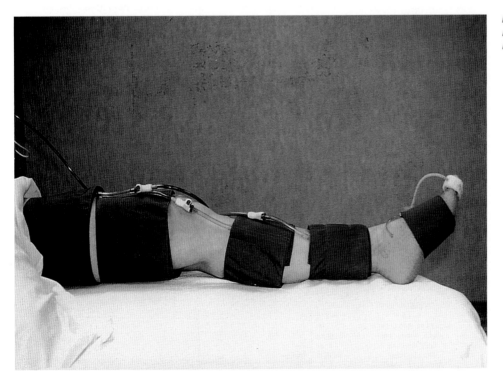

Figure 20-2. Volume plethysmography cuffs applied on a lower extremity.

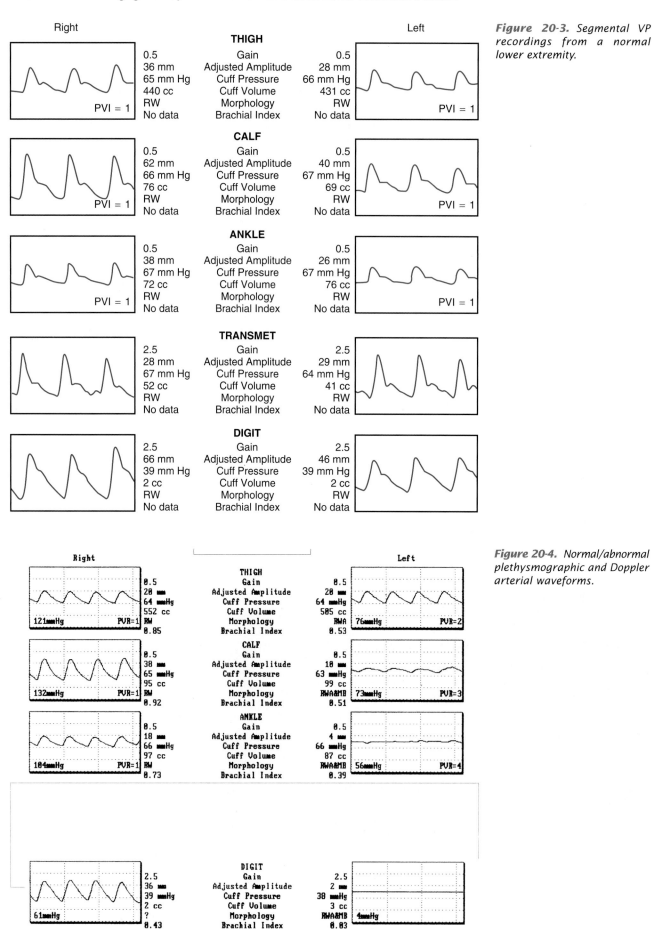

Figure 20-3. Segmental VP recordings from a normal lower extremity.

Figure 20-4. Normal/abnormal plethysmographic and Doppler arterial waveforms.

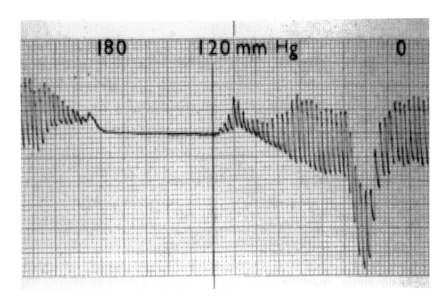

Figure 20-5. Segmental volume pressure recordings from an extremity with peripheral arterial occlusive disease affecting inflow to both lower extremities plus disease more distally in the left lower extremity.

Chapter

Arteria
Throml

LUIS R. LEON JR. •

Plethysmography

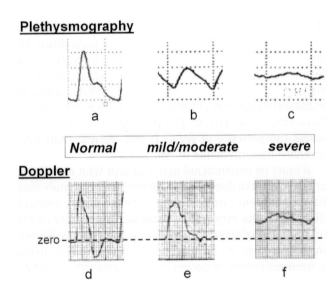

a	b	c

Normal	mild/moderate	severe

Doppler

zero

d	e	f

Figure 20-6. Systolic pressures measured using plethysmography. The systolic pressure is where the pulse reappears during deflation of a cuff from a super systolic pressure (120 mmHg in this example).

signals from the anterior tibial artery are absent or difficult to hear.

$$\text{Ankle-brachial index (ABI)} = \frac{\text{Highest pressure at ankle level}}{\text{Higher brachial pressure}}$$

Using a 10- or 12-cm wide cuff at the ankle, a normal ABI is 0.92 or greater (Table 20-1). When the ABI is in the abnormal range, pressures should be measured more proximally to localize where the pressure drop is occurring; these are called segmental pressure measurements.

Segmental Systolic Pressures

It is normal for some pressure energy to be lost as blood moves along an artery; a small amount of flow energy is converted into heat, which is conducted through the artery wall into the surrounding tissue. However, any drop in systolic pressures between adjacent segments of the extremity (e.g., from upper thigh to above knee, from

while the patient is supine. Pressures are measured from the posterior tibial and anterior tibial/dorsalis pedis arteries. Although arterial collateralization in the presence of significant PAOD may maintain systolic pressures to be normal at rest, functional impairment can be assessed from measurements of postexercise pressures. Although nonimaging, measurements of ankle-brachial indices are an important complement to duplex ultrasound imaging for assessing lower extremity arteries.

ABIs are calculated by dividing the highest systolic pressure at ankle level (from the anterior tibial, posterior tibial, or dorsalis pedis arteries) by the higher of the two brachial systolic pressures. Systolic pressures from the dorsalis pedis artery can be measured when

TABLE 20-1. Ankle-Brachial Indices and Category of Peripheral Arterial Occlusive Disease

ABI	PAOD category
0.92–1.4	Normal
0.75–0.91	Mild
0.50–0.74	Moderate
0.35–0.49	Severe
< 0.35	Ischemic

ABI, ankle-brachial index; PAOD, peripheral arterial occlusive disease.

Thigh systolic pressu
systolic pressure or l
Maximum difference
cent segments equal:

- 20 to 30 mmHg i
- Greater than 30
  proximal PAOD

is present. This balance is influenced by many factors. First, different tissues can tolerate ischemia in different degrees. For example, brain cells show signs of irreversible cell damage after only 4 to 6 minutes of total ischemia. Peripheral nerves demonstrate signs of prolonged functional deficits after 3 hours of ischemia. Skeletal muscle is relatively tolerant, with histologic changes occurring after 4 to 6 hours of ischemia. Second, even within the same tissue, the temperature and the metabolic activity of the cells determine their tolerance of decreased flow states. Kidneys can only tolerate less than an hour of warm ischemia; however, if stored at low temperatures and flushed with iced solutions, they can tolerate ischemic times up to hours. Third, the time over which the arterial occlusion develops may allow for the formation of collateral channels that will continue to perfuse the tissues even when the main arterial source is occluded. Even more, there is evidence that chronically ischemic tissue is more tolerant to total ischemia than is normally perfused tissue.

Reperfusion

An acutely ischemic limb needs to be revascularized in order to avoid limb loss and to preserve as much limb function as possible. Revascularization, when performed in the inappropriate patient or at an inappropriate time, can be harmful. Following revascularization, oxygenated blood reaches the ischemic area. The bloodflow to the ischemic extremity is much higher than in a normal condition because there is significant vasodilatation caused by ischemia (Fig. 21-1). The complement system is activated and adhesion molecules are expressed on the endothelial surface, recruiting neutrophils. With oxygen now available, neutrophils produce oxygen radicals that cause membrane lipid peroxidation and tissue damage.[6] This entity is known as reperfusion syndrome and it comprises a local and a systemic response.[7] The local response is caused by an increased permeability in the damaged capillaries, leading to significant swelling (most often in the anterior compartment). The intramuscular pressure is usually less than 8 mmHg. When the pressure is elevated to greater than 30 mmHg, it is higher than the perfusion pressure and results in compartment syndrome by compromising the intramuscular flow (Fig. 21-2).[8] It can lead to tissue necrosis, infection, and sepsis if not treated in a timely fashion.[9] The systemic response occurs as a consequence of leakage of metabolic products from damaged cells, causing acidosis and hyperkalemia. Cardiac arrhythmias and myoglobinemia may follow; these can result in acute tubular necrosis, multiple organ failure, and death. Acute respiratory distress syndrome and bowel edema with associated increased vascular permeability may occur, leading to endotoxic shock.[7] If the ischemic process involves the bulk of the lower extremity, amputation rather than revascularization may be the procedure of choice to avoid the entrance of toxic products from the damaged limb into the systemic circulation.[7] Although the development of the compartment syndrome after reperfusion is most common in the calf, it can also occur in the foot, thigh, gluteal muscles, and upper extremity.

Etiology

Total flow arrest in an artery can be the result of three things: (1) an embolism; (2) local thrombosis; and (3) traumatic transection. This last cause will not be included in this discussion.

Embolism

Embolic phenomena are the most common cause of acute arterial ischemia, accounting for approximately 80% of the cases seen in clinical practice. Sources of embolism include the heart; aortoiliac, femoral, and popliteal aneurysms; and proximally located lesions responsible for artery-to-artery emboli (e.g., carotid bifurcation atherosclerotic lesions causing stroke). Of all these, the heart is the most common source. Cardiac thrombi more commonly form after anterior myocardial transmural infarcts, but also occur because of ventricular aneurysms, valvular lesions, and arrhythmias. In 75% of patients with lower extremity embolic occlusion, a history of acute myocar-

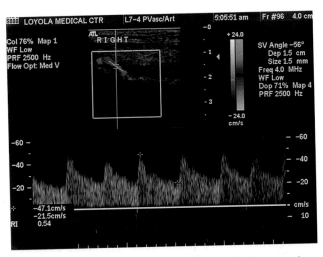

Figure 21-1. *High flow in the anterior tibial artery in a patient with acute thrombosis of the popliteal artery. The anterior tibial fills through the recurrent anterior tibial artery. There is absence of reverse flow and a very high end-diastolic velocity indicating the drop in the peripheral resistance from the vasodilatation of the ischemic tissues beyond the level of occlusion.*

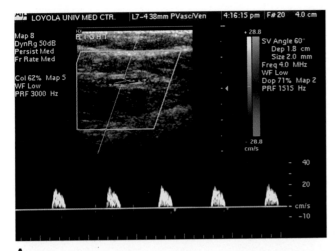

A

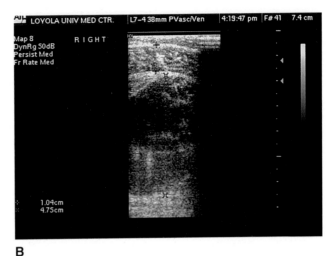

B

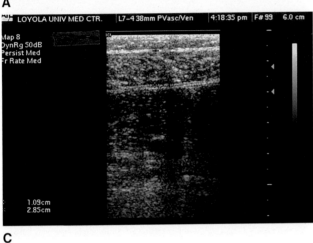

C

Figure 21-2. **A**, *Very resistant intramuscular flow in a patient with compartment syndrome. The reversed flow is negligible and there is absence of forward flow in the end-diastole.* **B**, *The soleus muscle is swollen and almost twice the size of the soleus muscle in the contralateral normal limb at the same anatomic level (**C**).*

dial infarction or atrial fibrillation is present during the preceding weeks. Emboli originating in the heart lodge in the lower extremities in 60% to 70% of patients, in the cerebral circulation in 20% of patients, in the upper extremities in 14% of patients, and in the visceral circulation in 7% to 10% of patients.[9] These emboli tend to locate at bifurcation points. In the mesenteric circulation, they lodge beyond the first few branches of the superior mesenteric artery. In the legs, they locate at the bifurcation of the common femoral artery or at the popliteal trifurcation.

Abdominal Aortic Aneurysms

Regarding artery-to-artery embolism, almost every artery has been found to be the source of emboli, but the abdominal aorta is the most common source. Both atherosclerotic disease and aneurysms are known to cause embolization of distal arteries (Fig. 21-3). It is of interest that neither large abdominal aneurysms nor

iliac artery aneurysms are common sources of emboli. Instead, abdominal aortic aneurysms (AAAs) smaller than 5.0 cm are associated with embolism (see Fig. 21-3).[10] Data from Northwestern University have shown that 5% (15/302) of patients there presented with distal emboli. This resulted in critical limb ischemia in 3 patients, digital in 11, and necrosis of calf muscles in 1. All but 1 of these patients had a CT scan; it showed luminal thrombus within the AAA and a size of less than 5 cm in 12 patients.[10]

Iliac Artery Aneurysms

An isolated iliac aneurysm is an uncommon entity with a relative incidence of 0.9 (compared with 4.7% for abdominal aortic aneurysms); however, these aneurysms have a rupture rate of 37.5%, higher than that reported for abdominal aortic aneurysms.[11] Almost half of iliac artery aneurysms are bilateral.[12] These patients most commonly present with rupture or local compression

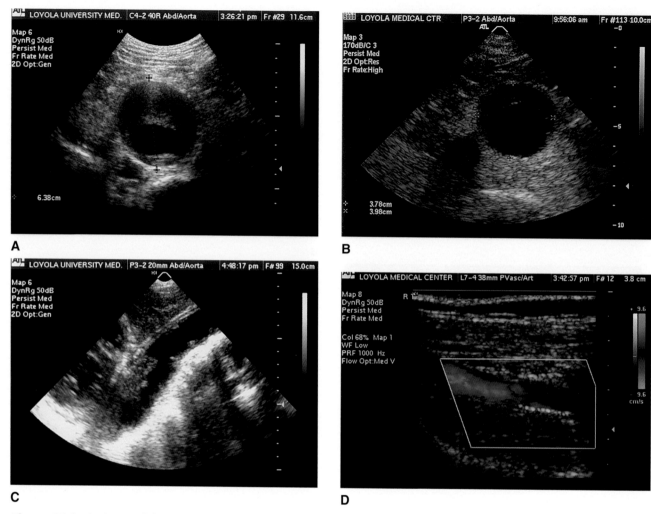

Figure 21-3. **A,** *Large abdominal aortic aneurysm with thrombus. This aneurysm was repaired because of its large size.* **B,** *Small abdominal aortic aneurysm containing thrombus. Aneurysms like this are more prone to distal embolization. When distal embolization occurs they are fixed regardless of their size.* **C,** *Shaggy aorta with a large mobile atheroma on the suprarenal segment. The patient had many emboli in three extremities and a larger embolus in the right popliteal artery (**D**).*

of neighboring structures (e.g., ureter, bowel, or iliac veins).[13-16] Iliac artery aneurysm can be associated with acute limb ischemia after spontaneous dissection because of cystic medial necrosis[17] or fibromuscular dysplasia.[18]

Popliteal Artery Aneurysms

Popliteal artery aneurysms represent over 70% of peripheral aneurysms. This can be a life-threatening condition because of constant embolization to the distal arterial tree, and have been associated with subacute ischemia in 20% to 40% of patients following thrombotic occlusion. Approximately half of patients with these aneurysms will need extremity amputation as an emergency treatment because of distal artery occlusion not suitable to surgical thrombectomy.[19] Therefore, sur-

gical repair is indicated for all symptomatic or complicated cases, with some clinicians recommending surgery also for asymptomatic aneurysms, except in high-risk patients.

Paradoxical Embolism

Paradoxical embolism of a venous thrombosis through a right-to-left shunt is an important cause of acute limb ischemia. This commonly occurs through a patent foramen ovale,[20] which has a prevalence thought to be as high as 35% in the general population.[21] Given that the presence of deep vein thrombosis or pulmonary embolus may be clinically silent, a high degree of suspicion for paradoxical embolism is needed in cases of unexplained arterial occlusion.

Artery-to-Artery Embolism

Another kind of arterial occlusion arises when dislodged emboli from a proximal source are trapped distally at an arterial bifurcation. Sites of predilection for emboli are acutely angled branching points of arteries (primarily in the lower extremities).[22] The most common site of embolism in the lower extremity is the common femoral and popliteal arteries; in the upper extremity, it is the brachial and ulnar arteries. The most common source is cardiac; atrial fibrillation accounts for about 70% of patients, followed by myocardial infarcts in about 20%.[23] Noncardiac sources include aortic[24] and peripheral aneurysms; persistent sciatic artery[25]; arterial dissection, either spontaneous or iatrogenic[26]; foreign bodies[27]; tumor cells[28]; aortoiliac stent placement[29]; primary aortic mural thrombus[30,31]; hematologic conditions[32]; thoracic outlet syndrome[33]; and, in about 10% of cases, the source remains unidentified.[9]

Hematologic conditions deserve a separate mention as an etiologic factor: these include deficiencies of natural anticoagulants, fibrinolytic system disorders, presence of antiphospholipid antibody, and platelet abnormalities. Vascular reconstructions may have catastrophic results in in patients with unrecognized and untreated hypercoagulable states. The most effective screening tool is a meticulous history related to thrombosis. If a positive history is found, determination of platelet count, antithrombin III, protein C, free protein S and total protein S levels, along with platelet aggregometry, is imperative.[34] Factor V Leiden mutation, present in 4% of whites, is one of the leading abnormalities resulting in an increased risk for deep leg vein thrombosis.[35] Arterial thromboembolism caused by factor V Leiden mutation is rare and, to date, it has only been described in the supraaortic, coronary, and upper extremity circulation.[36] Other disorders include protein S deficiency; protein C deficiency; proteins C and S deficiency; and hyperaggregable platelet conditions (e.g., inherited thrombophilia with a G20210A prothrombin gene mutation).[34,36]

Thrombosis

Local thrombosis of an artery is the consequence of one or a combination of several predisposing factors (e.g., atherosclerotic stenosis, hypercoagulable conditions, low flow states, and outflow venous occlusion).

Acute limb ischemia secondary to peripheral arterial thrombosis is an ominous event, although the clinical course associated with thrombosis is less dramatic than that associated with embolic episodes. In the large arteries of the legs, stenosis of greater than 70% diameter is needed to impair normal exercise capacity; it can be assumed that even substantial vascular changes may be present in an asymptomatic patient.[37] Select inherited and acquired hypercoagulable states appear to contribute to an initial arterial thrombosis and, more importantly, recurrent thrombotic events.[38] Popliteal artery entrapment syndrome causes repeated arterial compression and trauma to its wall, leading to localized atherosclerosis. It is a progressive disease, with arterial thrombosis occurring in some as part of its natural history.[39] Persistent sciatic artery can present as a pulsatile mass in the buttocks, caused by aneurismal dilatation; or as chronic or acute limb ischemia.[40] Thrombosis can also occur on an atherosclerotic plaque or as a complication of surgical reconstructions. The latter can derive from the occlusion of a previously placed arterial bypass graft[41] or as a complication related to an endovascularly placed device.[42]

The risk of emergent interventions for acute thrombosis is thought to be usually less than that associated with embolectomy, although limb preservation is often less satisfactory.[43]

A detailed history and a careful physical examination performed by an experienced practitioner will provide clues to the etiology. Claudication is a symptom often lacking with acute embolic episode, and examination of the contralateral limb does not reveal any evidence of atherosclerotic changes. Patients with background occlusive disease have a better-developed collateral system, and therefore the level of temperature change in the affected limb is not as well demarcated as in embolic cases.[9] A detailed cardiac history and a careful cardiac evaluation should be performed in order to identify possible embolic sources. Aortic pathology can be suggested as a cause of both emboli and thrombosis, especially in patients with Marfanoid body habitus and/or a history of hypertension.[9] Blue-toe syndrome causes acute digital ischemia by microembolization from a proximal source via a patent arterial tree in an otherwise well-perfused foot. The prompt delineation of the embolic source is paramount to prevent further deterioration through continuous embolization.[24]

Catastrophic events in the venous system (e.g., phlegmasia cerulea dolens, neurologic entities, and low output states) can also be missed or confused with acute arterial occlusion.[9]

Clinical Presentation

Acute ischemia in the extremities is classically described with the six "Ps": pallor, pain, poikilothermia, pulselessness, paresthesias, and paralysis. In general, acute ischemia caused by embolism presents in a more dramatic form: the onset is acute, and because no time for the development of collateral circulation has elapsed, the ischemic symptoms are severe. In cases of thrombotic ischemia, the presence of an underlying arterial lesion has allowed for the formation of collaterals. This may make the presentation more insidious and the symptoms less pronounced. This is not always true, however, and the differentiation between an embolic and a thrombotic event on the basis of clinical presentation may be difficult. In any case, one cannot overemphasize the value of a conscientious yet expeditious history and physical examination. Special attention should always be paid to the neurologic status of the limb. Any sensory or motor deficit should be clearly documented; this will alert the practitioner about the imminent threat of permanent sequelae and limb loss.

Pain is the most common symptom and is typically located in the foremost part of the arterial tree. It is commonly of sudden onset, with or without preceding claudication symptoms depending on the etiology.[44] It is also severe and constant, and often at the level of the major muscle group below the occlusion level. The pain may be masked by sensory disturbances that result from nerve ischemia.[9] A careful pulse examination can often lead to the clinical diagnosis of the level of occlusion. This examination must be done with the aid of a Doppler device for an accurate analysis.[44] A sudden loss of a previously palpable pulse is a key clue in the differential diagnosis. The pulse quality is also helpful. The augmentation of the pulse at the site of the occlusion represents the pulse waves encountering the thrombus.[9] Coolness, often associated with pallor in the affected extremity, is an important finding, and is more so if relative to the contralateral unaffected limb. The capillary refill time and the presence of venous return must be addressed as well. Sensory deficits can involve paresthesias or numbness. Those symptoms can be confounded by the neuropathy of diabetic patients. With more pronounced ischemia, motor deficits are evident.[44]

Noninvasive Evaluation

Unidirectional Doppler

Insonation of the arteries is performed to determine the following: presence or absence of flow; characteristics of the flow signal (e.g., monophasic, biphasic, or triphasic); and determination of ankle-brachial indexes (ABIs). The combination of physical examination findings and bedside, handheld, Doppler insonation of the distal arteries provides the necessary information to determine the severity of ischemia and to formulate an initial plan. The Society for Vascular Surgery/International Society for Cardiovascular Surgery (SVS/ISCVS) revised reporting standards[45] stratify acute limb ischemia into four classes:

- Class I: Doppler signals clearly audible; no motor or sensory deficits

- Class IIa: No Doppler signal audible; paresthesias and limited (toes) sensory loss

- Class IIb: Persisting pain, greater sensory loss, any motor deficit

- Class III Early: Complete anesthesia and paralysis

- Late: Muscle rigor, marbling of the skin; no detectable venous flow, even with compressive maneuvers

This classification has important prognostic and therapeutic value. Class I and IIa limbs are viable or only marginally threatened. Further diagnostic studies can be pursued. Class IIb and early Class III limbs are immediately threatened and require immediate revascularization in the operating room. Late Class III limbs are nonsalvageable.

Duplex Ultrasound

In patients with acutely ischemic but viable limbs (Class I, Class IIa) the use of duplex ultrasound (DUS) can provide valuable information about the cause of the ischemia. It can determine the distribution and extent of thrombosis, and the source of emboli from artery-to-artery embolism, by detecting aneurysms or plaques proximal to affected arteries. Aneurysms in the abdominal aorta containing thrombus (see Fig. 21-3), or aneurysms in the femoral (Fig. 21-4) and popliteal arteries (see Fig. 21-4) are common findings. Complete thrombosis of the aneurysm can be determined as well (see Fig. 21-4). Thrombosis of an artery at an atherosclerotic lesion may be also seen (Fig. 21-5). Patients with both acute arterial and venous symptoms may be accurately diagnosed (Fig. 21-6). DUS is often used to determine the absence or presence of flow in bypass grafts thought to be thrombosed (Fig. 21-7). In most instances, the whole graft is occluded unless there is an in situ graft being patent through a fistula or partial thrombosis near the anastomosis (see Fig. 21-7). An acutely thrombosed arterial segment is characterized by DUS in the absence of atherosclerotic disease from the smooth interface of the arterial wall and the thrombus. In this scenario, no significant collateral vessels are seen. The outer layer of the thrombus appears bright because it contains fibrin (Fig. 21-8). In the presence of atherosclerotic plaque, arterial segments not affected by it appear as described above except that collateral vessels are often found. Thrombosis over an atherosclerotic plaque can be recognized by the segmental calcification of the arterial wall. If the plaque is echogenic, material that is brighter than the thrombus is seen (see Fig. 21-5). The flow characteristics before, at, and after the occlusion are seen in Figure 21-9. The severity of the occlusion and the levels of pre-existing disease determine the patterns of the Doppler waveforms

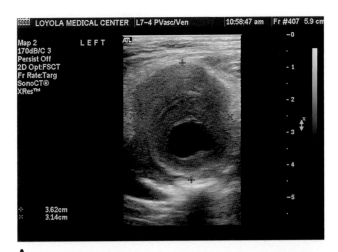

A

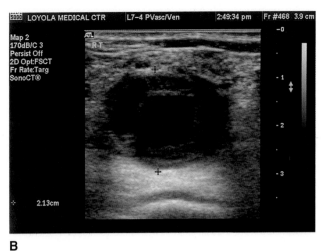

B

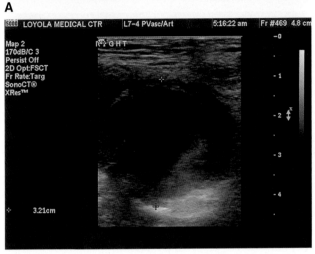

C

Figure 21-4. **A**, *Large common femoral artery aneurysm with thrombus. The patient had occlusion of his superficial femoral artery, but it is not known if the aneurysm was the cause because it was diagnosed later.* **B**, *Popliteal artery aneurysm containing thrombus. The aneurysm had occluded two of the runoff vessels and was repaired.* **C**, *Complete thrombosis of a popliteal artery aneurysm in a patient who presented with acute ischemia.*

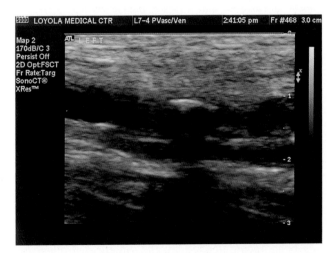

Figure 21-5. *Acute thrombosis of the superficial femoral artery over an atherosclerotic plaque. The patient presented with stable limb ischemia and no other reason was found for the thrombosis during the work-up other than the local plaque. The calcification with the acoustic shadow is seen over the thromboses segment. No flow or Doppler signal was detected. The popliteal artery was filled through the deep femoral artery branches.*

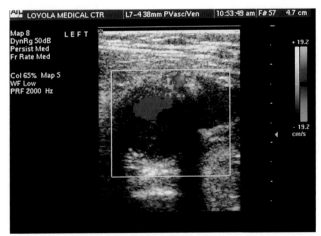

Figure 21-6. *Significant compression of the popliteal vein (blue) from a popliteal artery aneurysm containing thrombus. The patient had swelling and was sent to the vascular lab to rule out venous thrombosis. He had a previous documented episode of deep vein thrombosis and pulmonary embolism; however, during the clinical examination, the affected limb was colder. The aneurysm had embolized to segments of all three runoff vessels. The compression of the vein by the aneurysm can explain the swelling. The aneurysm was repaired and the patient did well.*

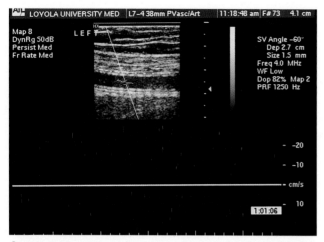

A

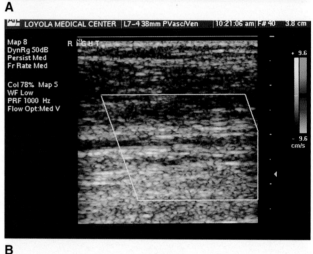

A

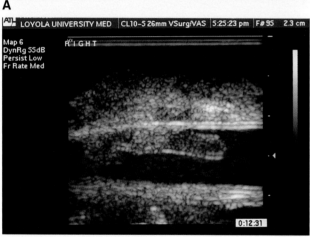

B

B

Figure 21-7. **A,** *Acute thrombosis of a femoropopliteal bypass graft with an externally supported polytetrafluoroethylene (PTFE) graft as shown by the acoustic shadows created by the rings. There is no Doppler signal, and thrombus is seen within the graft. The patient presented with acute ischemia and no apparent reason was found for the graft thrombosis.* **B,** *Acute partial thrombosis of a common femoral artery to superficial femoral artery PTFE graft. The patient had a small drop in the ankle brachial index from 0.9 to 0.8 and was placed on heparin. A week later the thrombus resolved and there was no other complication.*

Figure 21-8. **A,** *Acute thrombosis of the popliteal artery after aortocoronary bypass graft. The patient presented with a cool extremity, absence of pedal pulses, and nonthreatening limb ischemia. Echogenic material can be seen within the arterial lumen. The arterial wall is free of plaque and has a smooth interface with the thrombus. The outer layer of the thrombus appears bright because it contains fibrin.* **B,** *Acute thrombosis of the anterior tibial artery in a patient with atrial fibrillation and no peripheral arterial disease. There is absence of color filling within the artery despite the pulse repetition frequency being at 1000 Hz and the color gain at 78%. The arterial wall has no irregularities or calcification.*

Echocardiography to Determine the Source of Embolism

Once an embolic etiology is determined, investigation about the source of the emboli is indicated. The role of transesophageal echocardiography (TEE) in patients with or suspected to have peripheral arterial emboli has not been determined. It is well known that the heart is the most common source of emboli. These are of variable sizes, and include the emboli that usually occlude larger arteries. A few studies have shown that the prevalence

of embolization from the heart is estimated to be 80% to 90%; however, these studies had a small sample size and did not evaluate patients with multiplanar TEE, which can image better pathology in the thoracic aorta.[46] It has been recommended by the American College of Cardiology and the American Heart Association that TEE should be used in patients with major peripheral or visceral vessel acute occlusions.[47]

Because heart and peripheral vascular disease often coexist it is difficult to differentiate embolism from thrombosis. TEE has the best resolution for imaging pathologies of the heart and the aorta and therefore

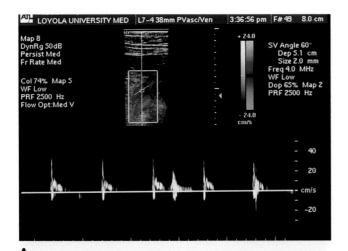

A

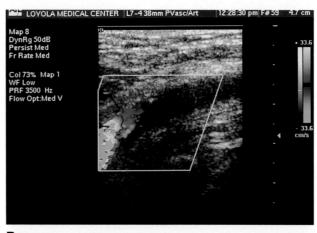

B

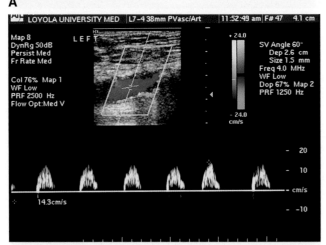

C

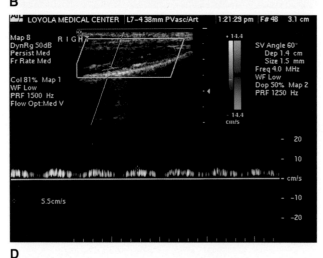

D

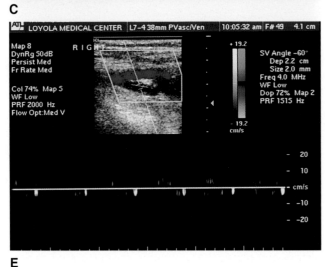

E

Figure 21-9. Very resistive low amplitude flow in the external iliac artery (**A**) of a patient with acute thrombosis of the common femoral artery and (**B**) after cardiac catheterization. The characteristic "blue cup" is seen at the site of the occlusion (**C**). Very low amplitude flow with monophasic waveform in the common femoral artery of a patient with acute iliac artery thrombosis. The first patient had a strong femoral pulse, whereas the pulse was absent in the second patient. **D**, Very low flow with venous-like signal in the dorsalis pedis artery of a patient with multiple levels of acute thrombosis from a cardiac source. **E**, No Doppler signal and absence of color flow in the deep femoral artery of a patient who presented with acute onset of thigh pain. The source of emboli was never identified.

provides a greater yield in defining cardiovascular emboli (Fig. 21-10).[48] Transthoracic echo is often used, but it has a low sensitivity in identifying a cardiac source of emboli, and its use is limited. When transthoracic echo is positive, no further testing is required; when it is negative, either TEE or MRI is usually performed.[49,50]

Invasive Evaluation

Arteriography

An arteriogram offers several advantages in the evaluation of an acutely ischemic limb. Besides helping to determine the cause of thrombosis, it provides informa-

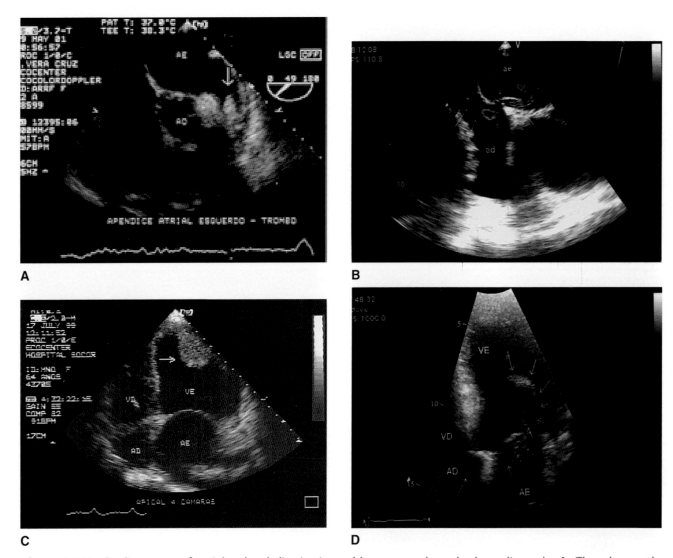

Figure 21-10. *Cardiac source of peripheral embolization imaged by transesophageal echocardiography.* **A,** *Thrombus on the left atrial appendage.* **B,** *Thrombus in both atria.* **C,** *Large thrombus in the left ventricle.* **D,** *Thrombus in the left atrium and the left ventricle. (A and C courtesy of Dr. Marcia Barbosa, Belo Horizonte, Brasil; B and D courtesy of Dr. Salomon Israel do Amaral, Rio De Janeiro, Brasil.)*

tion regarding the circulation proximal and distal to the obstruction that will be vital in planning the revascularization procedure. Also, it allows for the use of catheter-directed thrombolysis, which is especially useful in cases of graft failure and thrombosed popliteal aneurysms. Today most centers possess high-quality angiographic capabilities in the operating room. This eliminates any potential delays that could increase the revascularization time and allows for the prompt performance of an angiogram even in acutely threatened limbs that require immediate intervention.

Management

The primary goal in the management of an ischemic limb is prompt revascularization. Other objectives are the deter-

mination of the causes of the ischemic event; the prevention of recurrent ischemic episodes; and the management of sequelae caused by the ischemic insult (e.g., fasciotomy for compartment syndrome, acute renal failure for myoglobinuria, or management of hyperkalemia).

An algorithm on the evaluation and management of acute limb ischemia is shown in Figure 21-11. Detailed history and physical examination are performed as previously described. As soon as the diagnosis is suspected, full systemic anticoagulation with intravenous heparin should be administered to prevent further thrombi formation. The adequacy of anticoagulation must be monitored using the activated partial thromboplastin time (aPTT). This is a common practice, although a randomized study advised against preoperative and early postoperative anticoagulation: researchers found that these efforts failed to improve the short-term results of thrombectomy and increased bleeding complications.[51]

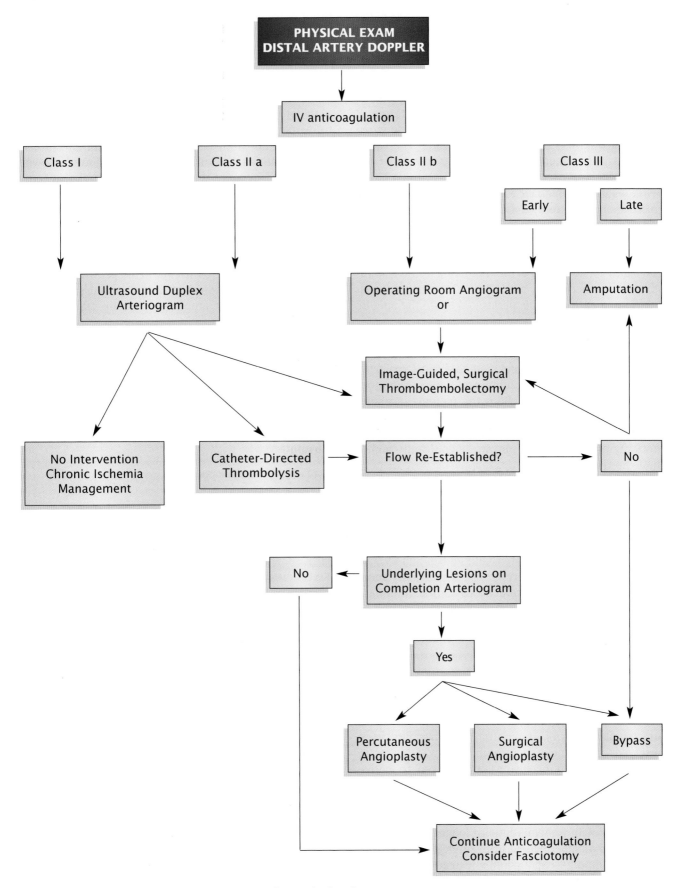

Figure 21-11. *Algorithm for the management of acute limb ischemia.*

The next step is to classify the patient into one of the four SVS/ISCVS clinical classes to direct therapy. Intervention is tailored to the particular patient as described previously.

With a viable limb, there is enough time to obtain further diagnostic testing or to consider thrombolytic therapy if there are no contraindications for its use. It has been shown that high-risk patients do worse when revascularization is performed emergently.[5] The viable limb has to be diagnosed as such and remain in the same category under close scrutiny. On the other hand, better results are obtained when stabilization and revascularization are performed as soon as possible. Judgment and common sense are mainstay elements of this algorithm.[52] When time permits, catheter-directed thrombolysis is the treatment of choice. It can restore perfusion, may allow identification of an underlying lesion responsible for the occlusion, and often allows an endovascular intervention to be performed with therapeutic purposes.[3]

Three clinical trials addressed the comparison between thrombolysis and surgery for acute limb ischemia. The Rochester study compared urokinase to surgery, analyzing 114 patients with class IIb limbs and a mean symptom duration of about 2 days. Both the patients receiving urokinas and those undergoing surgery achieved identical limb salvage rates after a follow-up of 1 year, but the mortality of the surgical group was significantly higher than the thrombolysis group, mainly because of perioperative cardiopulmonary complications.

The TOPAS (Thrombolysis or Peripheral Arterial Surgery) trial also studied 544 patients in two groups: urokinase or surgery. Amputation-free survival rates in the thrombolysis group were 71.8% at 6 months and 65.0% at 1 year, as compared with 74.8% and 69.9%, respectively, for the surgery group. Significantly more bleeding complications were noted in the urokinase group.[53] Even though no improvement in survival or limb salvage with thrombolysis was demonstrated, the success was comparable to surgery.[3]

The STILE (Surgery or Thrombolysis for the Ischemic Lower Extremity) trial[54] randomized 393 patients to three groups: urokinase, recombinant tissue plasminogen activator (rt-PA), or surgery. When surgery was compared with the combined data obtained from the thrombolysis arm, similar rates of amputation and mortality were observed. The benefit of thrombolysis was higher in patients with graft occlusions as opposed to native occluded arteries. It was found that patients with acute ischemia (0 to 14 days) in the thrombolysis group had better amputation-free survival rates and shorter hospital stays; those with ischemia time of longer than 14 days experienced a higher benefit from surgical intervention.

For profoundly ischemic limbs (category IIb or early class III), immediate treatment should be instituted in the operating room. Surgical interventions include thrombectomy, embolectomy, or bypass grafting. Intraoperative thrombolysis is often used as an adjunctive measure by direct injection. Surgery is also needed when contraindications to thrombolysis (Table 21-1) are found.[4]

Early decompression with fasciotomy may avoid ischemic complications, permanent disability, or amputation. Fasciotomy is associated with an increased risk of minor wound morbidity, but limb loss and death result from persistent ischemia and underlying systemic processes, not from fasciotomy wound complications. Owen described the double-incision technique for lower extremity fasciotomy, which is the technique most commonly used.[55] In the upper extremity, the curvilinear volar and volar-ulnar techniques are used. The curved incision allows better exposure to nerves and vessels and is preferred.[56]

Limbs classified in late class III groups generally have permanent neuromuscular damage; they result in poor outcomes regardless of the promptness or nature of therapy. Primary amputation is the treatment of choice.

TABLE 21-1. Contraindications to Thrombolysis

Absolute
Active or recent bleeding
Recent stroke
Recent intracranial or spinal interventions or trauma
Relative
Recent major or eye surgery, trauma, or cardiopulmonary resuscitation
Uncontrolled hypertension
Recent puncture of uncompressible vessel like the subclavian artery
Intracranial tumor
Mitral valve disease and intracardiac thrombus
Intracranial aneurysm or vascular malformation
Minor
Renal or liver failure (especially if coagulopathy is present)
Bacterial endocarditis
Pregnancy
Diabetic hemorrhagic retinopathy
Antiplatelet therapy

Modified from Costantini V, Lenti M: Treatment of acute occlusion of peripheral arteries. Thromb Res 106:V285–V294, 2002.

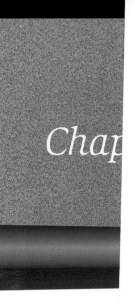

REFERENCES

1. Davies B, Braithwaite BD, Birch PA, et al: Acute leg ischemia in Gloucestershire. Br J Surg 84:504–508, 1997.
2. Bergqvist D, Troeng T, Elfstrom J, et al: Auditing surgical outcome: Ten years with the Swedish Vascular Registry-Swedvasc. The Steering Committee of Swedvasc. Eur J Vasc Endovasc Surg 164(Suppl 581):3–8, 1998.
3. Ouriel K: Current status of thrombolysis for peripheral arterial occlusive disease. Ann Vasc Surg 16:797–804, 2002.
4. Costantini V, Lenti M: Treatment of acute occlusion of peripheral arteries. Thromb Res 106:V285–V294, 2002.
5. Blaisdell FW, Steele M, Allen RE: Management of acute lower extremity arterial ischemia due to embolism and thrombosis. Surgery 84:822–834, 1978.
6. Novelli GP, Adembri C, Gandini E, et al: Vitamin E protects human skeletal muscle from damage during surgical ischemia-reperfusion. Am J Surg 173:206–209, 1997.
7. Blaisdell FW: The pathophysiology of skeletal muscle ischemia and the reperfusion syndrome: A review. Cardiovasc Surg 10:620–630, 2002.
8. Mubarak SJ, Owen CA, Hargens AR, et al: Acute compartment syndromes: Diagnosis and treatment with the aid of the wick catheter. J Bone Joint Surg Am 60:1091–1095, 1978.
9. Greenberg RK, Ouriel K: Arterial thromboembolism. In Rutherford RB (ed): Vascular Surgery. Philadelphia: WB Saunders, 2000.
10. Baxter BT, McGee GS, Flinn WR, et al: Distal embolization as a presenting symptom of aortic aneurysms. Am J Surg 160:197–201, 1990.
11. Sato O, Tada Y, Akimoto S, et al: Isolated iliac aneurysms. Nippon Geka Gakkai Zasshi 85:1370–1375, 1984.
12. Krupski WC, Selzman CH, Floridia R, et al: Contemporary management of isolated iliac aneurysms. J Vasc Surg 28:1–11, 1998.
13. Marino R, Mooppan UM, Zein TA, et al: Urological manifestations of isolated iliac artery aneurysms. J Urol 137:232–234, 1987.
14. Nelson RP: Isolated internal iliac artery aneurysms and their urological manifestations. J Urol 124:300–303, 1980.
15. Ozergin U, Vatansev C, Durgut K, et al: An internal iliac artery aneurysm causing a colonic obstruction: Report of a case. Surg Today 31:839–841, 2001.
16. Rosenthal D, Matsuura JH, Jerius H, et al: Iliofemoral venous thrombosis caused by compression of an internal iliac artery aneurysm: A minimally invasive treatment. J Endovasc Surg 5:142–145, 1998.
17. Sogaro F, Toffon A, Galeazzi E, et al: Spontaneous limited dissection of the external iliac artery. Case report after 14-year follow-up. VASA 23:370–372, 1994.
18. Patel KS, Wolfe JH, Mathias C: Left external iliac artery dissection and bilateral renal artery aneurysms secondary to fibromuscular dysplasia: a case report. Neth J Surg 42:118–120, 1990.
19. Steinmetz E, Bouchot O, Faroy F, et al: Preoperative intraarterial thrombolysis before surgical revascularization for popliteal artery aneurysm with acute ischemia. Ann Vasc Surg 14:360–364, 2000.
20. Ahmed S, Sadiq A, Siddiqui AK, et al: Paradoxical arterial emboli causing acute limb ischemia in a patient with essential thrombocytosis. Am J Med Sci 326:156–158, 2003.
21. Ward R, Jones D, Haponik EF: Paradoxical embolism: An under-recognized problem. Chest 108:549–558, 1995.
22. Morl H: Anatomic and functional diagnosis in arterial occlusive disease. Herz 13:351–357, 1988.
23. Vrtik L, Zernovicky F, Kubis J, et al: Arterial embolisms in the extremities. Rozhl Chir 80:465–469, 2001.
24. Karmody AM, Powers SR, Monaco VJ, et al: "Blue toe" syndrome. An indication for limb salvage surgery. Arch Surg 111:1263–1268, 1976.
25. Tomczak R, Gorich J, Pamler R, et al: Ischemia of the lower extremity due to a persistent a. ischiadica—a possible interventional therapeutic approach. Radiologe 40:745–747, 2000.
26. Rahmani O, Gallagher JJ: Spontaneous superficial femoral artery dissection with distal embolization. Ann Vasc Surg 16:358–362, 2002.
27. Roubal P, Korger J, Ondruskova O, et al: An unusual embolization of a projectile in the superficial femoral artery. Rozhl Chir 76:557–559, 1997.
28. Fernandez BB, Grove M, Carman TL: An unusual presentation of simultaneous bilateral popliteal artery embolism: A case report. Angiology 49:573, 1998.
29. Lin PH, Bush RL, Conklin BS, et al: Late complication of aortoiliac stent placement- atheroembolization of the lower extremities. J Surg Res 103:153–159, 2002.
30. Stadler P, Sebesta P, Hoffmann R, et al: An unusual extensive thrombus in the abdominal aorta of a young female patient after recurrent embolisms in the pelvis and lower extremity. Rozhl Chir 80:294–296, 2001.
31. Hahn TL, Dalsing MC, Sawchuk AP, et al: Primary aortic mural thrombus: Presentation and treatment. Ann Vasc Surg 13:52–59, 1999.
32. Dorweiler B, Neufang A, Kasper-Koenig W, et al: Arterial embolism to the upper extremity in a patient with factor V Leiden mutation (APC resistance): A case report and review of the literature. Angiology 54:125–130, 2003.
33. Davidovic LB, Kostic DM, Jakovljevic NS, et al: Vascular thoracic outlet syndrome. World J Surg 27:545–550, 2003.
34. Eason JD, Mills JL, Beckett WC: Hypercoagulable states in arterial thromboembolism. Surg Gynecol Obstet 174:211–215, 1992.
35. Wilcken DE: Overview of inherited metabolic disorders causing cardiovascular disease. J Inherit Metab Dis 26:245–257, 2003.
36. Nanas JN, Gougoulakis A, Kanakakis J: Acute coronary and peripheral arterial thrombosis following percutaneous coronary intervention in a patient with previously undiagnosed inherited thrombophilia. Can J Cardiol 19:1063–1065, 2003.
37. Morl H: Anatomic and functional diagnosis in arterial occlusive disease. Herz 13:351–357, 1988.
38. Deitcher SR, Carman TL, Sheikh MA, et al: Hypercoagulable syndromes: Evaluation and management strategies for acute limb ischemia. Semin Vasc Surg 14:74–85, 2001.
39. Stager A, Clement D: Popliteal artery entrapment syndrome. Sports Med 28:61–70, 1999.
40. Ito H, Okadome K, Odashiro T, et al: Persistent sciatic artery: Two case reports and a review of the literature. Cardiovasc Surg 2:275–280, 1994.
41. O'Donnell TF Jr: Arterial diagnosis and management of acute thrombosis of the lower extremity. Can J Surg 36:349–353, 1993.
42. Carroccio A, Faries PL, Morrissey NJ, et al: Predicting iliac limb occlusions after bifurcated aortic stent grafting: Anatomic and device-related causes. J Vasc Surg 36:679–684, 2002.
43. Brewster DC: Acute peripheral arterial occlusion. Cardiol Clin 9:497–513, 1991.
44. Katzen BT: Clinical diagnosis and prognosis of acute limb ischemia. Rev Cardiovasc Med 3(Suppl 2):S2–S6, 2002.
45. Rutherford RB, Baker JD, Ernst C, et al: Recommended standards for reports dealing with lower extremity ischemia. J Vasc Surg 26:517–538, 1997.
46. Vongpatanasin W, Brickner ME, Willett DL, et al: Usefulness of transesophageal echocardiography in determining the source of emboli in patients with acute limb ischemia. Am J Cardiol 8:253–255, 1998.
47. Cheitlin MD, Alpert JS, Armstrong WF, et al: ACC/AHA guidelines for the clinical application of echocardiography: executive summary. A report of the American College of Cardiology/American Heart Association Task Force on Practice Guidelines (Committee on Clinical Applications of Echocardiography). J Am Coll Cardiol 29:862–879, 1997.
48. Hoffmann M, Talaszka A, Liesse A, et al: Difficulties in diagnosing an aortic arch thrombus. Rev Med Interne 23:943–947, 2002.

49. Barkhausen
    characteriza
    Roentgenol
50. Mariano M(
    esophageal
    embolizatio
51. Jivegard L,
    Failure of a
    arterial thr(
    centre stud
52. Rutherford
    J (eds): De
    Saunders,

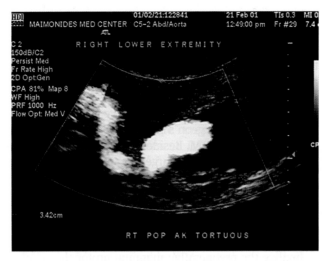

Figure 22-2. *A thrombosed large popliteal aneurysm (3.4 cm) that was missed by contrast arteriography.*

of concomitant veins may avoid misinterpretation of main trunk or collateral arteries. Flow velocities and run-off viability may be estimated quantitatively. Diameters are accurately measured. Nonvascular anatomic landmarks are noticeable as needed.

Another major benefit is the evaluation of the arterial wall at the site of the intended anastomosis. Wall thickness can be observed and measured. Calcification can be ruled out and quantitated. A skin mark at the site of anastomosis facilitates and minimizes surgical dissection.

US Limitations

Deep vessels must be imaged with low-frequency transducers. The tradeoff to accomplish penetration is

deterioration of image resolution. Gas and edema produce US imaging artifacts. Arterial wall calcifications create acoustic shadows. Potential stenosis or occlusion may be masked within this shadow.

Transmission of information is impaired by the small field of view inherent to US. The ultrasonographer draws an arterial map to rely the information that is obtained segment by segment (Fig. 22-4). This process creates a significant dependency on who performs the test. The possibility of a second, independent opinion of the data collected is limited.

Patient lack of cooperation has hampered a few US studies. Some patients cannot adapt to the positioning required for appropriate insonation. Others are not patient enough if the US test is prolonged. US cannot be performed over casts and bandages. It may be performed over ulcers and wounds with a protecting sheet.

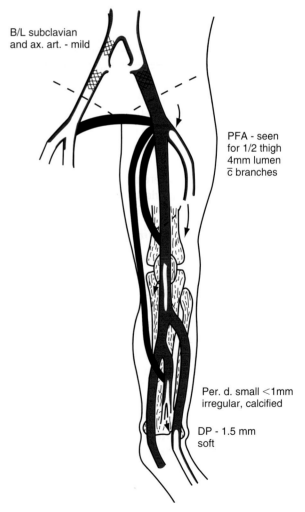

Figure 22-4. *An arterial map of a patient with multiple failed PTFE bypasses.*

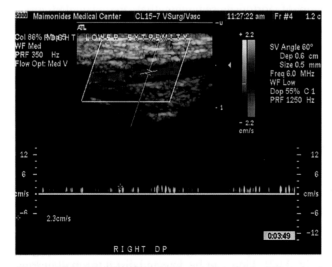

Figure 22-3. *Very low flow (peak systolic velocity 2.3 cm/sec) registered by duplex in the dorsalis pedis artery (appeared occluded on contrast arteriogram).*

Chapter 22

Duplex Ultrasound Arterial Mapping Before Infrainguinal Revascularization

ENRICO ASCHER • SERGIO X. SALLES-CUNHA
• ANIL HINGORANI • NATALIA MARKEVICH

Introduction

Many years of experience with duplex ultrasound (US) as the primary imaging modality before infrainguinal revascularization have been well-described.[1-9] Bypass surgeries based on US imaging were performed not only to the popliteal artery but also to the infrapopliteal, para-malleolar, and foot arteries.[5,7] This chapter describes basic protocols emphasizing the advantages and limitations of the US method. Additional standby and/or complementary intraoperative techniques are also mentioned. Knowledge of US-based protocols, however, is not enough to gain the confidence necessary to shift away from the traditional protocol based on preoperative x-ray arteriography (XRA). Therefore, various approaches have been investigated to document the feasibility of preoperative US mapping of the arteries feeding the lower extremity.

US images of arterial segments have been compared to XRA and to magnetic resonance arteriography (MRA).[3,10-31] Aortoiliac XRA can be avoided based on US findings.[15] Decision-making studies compared virtual bypasses that would be implanted based on US and XRA images.[8,32-36]

Decision to revascularize the lower extremity has been made based on US.[1,5-8,37-41] Intraoperative XRA has been performed for two reasons: (1) as part of preprocedure to confirm US findings[28,29]; or (2) post-bypass to demonstrate a viable revascularization. Successful revascularizations have been accomplished based on US despite failure of XRA to demonstrate viable target vessels.[42] Intraoperative iliofemoral pressure measurements have been performed to complement US findings after a bypass graft implantation.[1,5-8]

The Maimonides Medical Center experience includes several of the issues mentioned above; it has shown that the majority of infrainguinal revascularizations can be performed based on preoperative US mapping and intraoperative completion US arteriography without the need for preoperative XRA or other imaging modality. This experience can be subdivided in four phases: (1) training of an US/vascular surgery expert team; (2) virtual decision making focused on XRA acceptance/rejection of US selected bypasses; (3) US proposed bypass surgery with complementary intraoperative pressure measurements and post-bypass completion XRA; and (4) replacement of XRA for US completion arteriography.

This chapter summarizes these topics and includes a brief literature review of investigations related to US diagnosis, preoperative mapping, and decision making leading to US-based infrainguinal revascularizations.

Duplex Ultrasound Arterial Mapping (DUAM)

This section describes and expands on the four phases of the Maimonides Medical Center experience. Long and short US protocols for arterial mapping are summarized (phase 1 and subsequent modifications). US advantages and limitations are listed. A section on avoiding pitfalls emphasizes the lessons learned during this continuing education process. Results of the virtual decision-making comparison based on the first 55 cases are briefly reported (phase 2). Complementary techniques employed in the operating room are also briefly described (phases 3 and 4). Finally, the results obtained are summarized.

Long DUAM Protocol

The primary objective of US protocols before an infrainguinal bypass is to select arterial segments for placement of proximal and distal anastomoses. Such locations should be marked on the patient's skin to facilitate the surgical approach. Ideally, such anastomotic sites are nondiseased

arteries without calcifications (clearly, above and below the segments that need to be bypassed) consistent with available length of a venous or prosthetic conduit and easily assessed during surgery. In the process of selecting anastomotic sites, clinical suspicion of arterial obstruction, location, extent of occlusions, and stenoses are confirmed and quantitated.

Long US protocol includes imaging of the aorta, iliac, common femoral, superficial femoral, deep femoral, popliteal, crural, and pedal arteries. This protocol may last from 40 to 90 minutes and was initially designed to mimic XRA. Nowadays it is rarely performed because detailed imaging of all arterial segments is not always necessary and it is time-consuming.

The US scan is performed with patient in supine position with legs slightly dependent to fill the venous side of the circulation. Imaging concomitant veins may help in the identification of chronic occluded or barely opened main arterial trunks.

Patient Preparation

Aortoiliac imaging requires patient preparation to avoid artifacts caused by bowel interposition in the abdomen and pelvis. Ideally, the test is performed in the morning after 10 hours of abstinence from food, drinks, and smoking. Antigas medication helps and should be administered if not contraindicated.

Imaging of distal arteries requires a comfortable (warm) room temperature. Maneuvers to vasodilate the peripheral arteries and veins facilitate US imaging.

US Technology

Color-flow US scans facilitate identification of arteries and concomitant veins. Power Doppler imaging improves sensitivity in low-flow conditions. Color-flow gain, scale, sensitivity, persistence, and other adjustable parameters improve visualization under abnormal conditions. B-mode colorization may increase contrast and facilitate identification of vessel walls and obstructing plaques.

Doppler spectrum analysis is used to confirm occlusion or to grade stenosis. Hemodynamically significant stenosis greater than 50% usually doubles the peak-systolic velocity in comparison with velocities adjacent to the obstruction. A severe (greater than 70%) stenosis triples the peak-systolic velocity. A critical stenosis may be associated with low velocities.

A triphasic Doppler waveform with an acceleration time less than 100 ms usually rules out a significant proximal stenosis. A monophasic waveform is associated with occlusion or high-grade stenosis proximal to the site of measurement (Fig. 22-1). Analysis of a biphasic waveform is not very specific. Cardiac function and stenosis proximal or distal to the site of recording stenosis may alter spectral waveform.

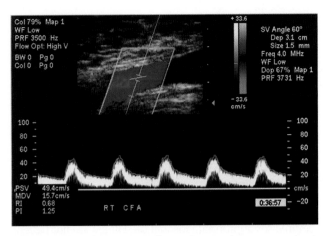

Figure 22-1. *This common femoral artery has a monophasic waveform because of common iliac artery occlusion.*

Aortoiliac US Imaging

The US scan is performed with a 3- to 5-MHz transducer for adequate penetration to permit imaging of deep vessels. A higher frequency probe may be used to scan thinner patients. Anterior and anterolateral approaches are used to visualize the aorta. Various angles of insonation and varying degrees of probe pressure are employed according to the shape of the patient's body. Arteries are imaged in transverse and longitudinal sections. The iliac veins and the inferior vena cava may serve as landmarks, particularly in the presence of occlusions. A complete scan includes the observation of several flow waveforms at the suprarenal and infrarenal aorta and proximal, mid-, and distal common and external iliac arteries.

The use of reactive hyperemia may be considered to challenge and evaluate a mild-to-moderate iliac stenosis.

Femorodistal US Imaging

The US scan is performed with a 5- to 10-MHz transducer. On occasion, a sector probe with a wide angle and lower frequencies is employed to improve visualization of deeper vessels. Such probes may facilitate identification of the superficial femoral artery at the adductor canal, the tibioperoneal trunk, and the proximal anterior tibial artery. Extremity rotation and repositioning often help improve imaging of femoral, popliteal, and tibial arteries. Leg dependence may help in imaging of diseased or occluded arteries by filling the adjacent veins. The traditional imaging approaches are anteromedial for the superficial femoral, posterior for the popliteal, medial for the posterior tibial, lateral for the anterior tibial, and posterolateral for the peroneal artery. The ultrasonographer should be adept in identifying collaterals or anomalous anatomy. Enlarged collaterals are often detected proximal to severe stenosis or occlusion. Collaterals that reconstitute a main arterial trunk are landmarks to

determine extent of occlusions. The anterior and posterior terminal branches of the peroneal artery may be identified in connection with reconstitution of the distal tibial arteries. Anatomic variances of the dorsal, pedal, and tarsal arteries; and the common and lateral plantar arteries need to be recognized in cases when pedal bypasses are planned.

Knowledge of surgeon's preferences is fundamental for infrainguinal DUAM. Besides a preference for a tibial or a peroneal bypass, the surgeon may elect to perform a distal anastomosis over the most distal stenosis, with concomitant endarterectomy. This alternative may increase flow significantly in both directions of the anastomosis.

Saphenous and/or arm vein mapping may be required to finalize the preoperative mapping protocol.

Short DUAM Protocol

Short protocols may vary according to the objective of treatment. Such procedures may be different for limb salvage, claudication, or emergency situations. A simple protocol includes five items:

1. Evaluation of the common femoral artery waveform to exclude significant aortoiliac disease
2. Scanning distally from the common femoral down until the origin of a superficial femoral artery occlusion or severe stenosis
3. Imaging of the proximal deep femoral artery
4. Imaging of the popliteal artery
5. Scanning from the pedal arteries up the tibial and peroneal arteries until the location of the distal end of respective occlusions or severe stenosis

With this approach, time is saved by avoiding evaluation of aortoiliac segments that are evaluated intraoperatively, diseased or occluded superficial femoral at the adductor canal, and/or scanning of diseased tibioperoneal arteries in the upper calf. If a distal bypass is not being considered, initial scanning could be limited to the femoropopliteal segment.

US Advantages

US is often contemplated to avoid the risks and complications of XRA. US is noninvasive, can be repeated at will, and has significant cost advantages. Once experience is acquired with US mapping, several other benefits become evident. US combines lumen and arterial wall imaging (Fig. 22-2). Flow can be detected distal to small or long occlusions. Blood movement can be forced and detected in arteries with minimal or no flow (Fig. 22-3). Imaging

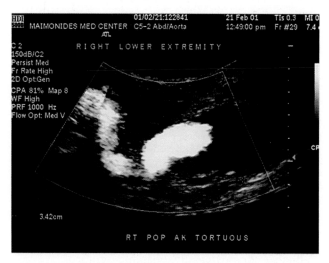

Figure 22-2. *A thrombosed large popliteal aneurysm (3.4 cm) that was missed by contrast arteriography.*

of concomitant veins may avoid misinterpretation of main trunk or collateral arteries. Flow velocities and run-off viability may be estimated quantitatively. Diameters are accurately measured. Nonvascular anatomic landmarks are noticeable as needed.

Another major benefit is the evaluation of the arterial wall at the site of the intended anastomosis. Wall thickness can be observed and measured. Calcification can be ruled out and quantitated. A skin mark at the site of anastomosis facilitates and minimizes surgical dissection.

US Limitations

Deep vessels must be imaged with low-frequency transducers. The tradeoff to accomplish penetration is

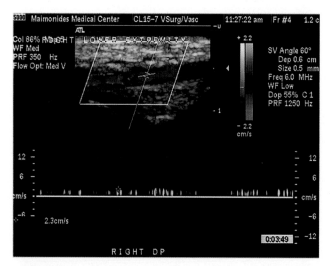

Figure 22-3. *Very low flow (peak systolic velocity 2.3 cm/sec) registered by duplex in the dorsalis pedis artery (appeared occluded on contrast arteriogram).*

deterioration of image resolution. Gas and edema produce US imaging artifacts. Arterial wall calcifications create acoustic shadows. Potential stenosis or occlusion may be masked within this shadow.

Transmission of information is impaired by the small field of view inherent to US. The ultrasonographer draws an arterial map to rely the information that is obtained segment by segment (Fig. 22-4). This process creates a significant dependency on who performs the test. The possibility of a second, independent opinion of the data collected is limited.

Patient lack of cooperation has hampered a few US studies. Some patients cannot adapt to the positioning required for appropriate insonation. Others are not patient enough if the US test is prolonged. US cannot be performed over casts and bandages. It may be performed over ulcers and wounds with a protecting sheet.

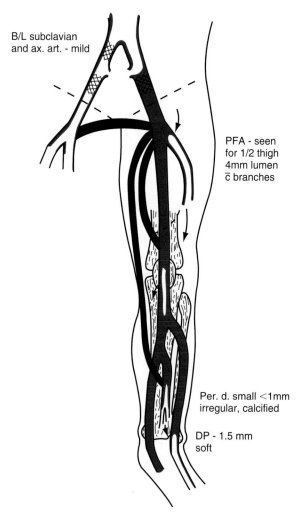

Figure 22-4. *An arterial map of a patient with multiple failed PTFE bypasses.*

Avoiding Pitfalls

Several potential problems facing US mapping can be avoided or minimized. This section includes a discussion of pitfalls related to velocity measurements, color-flow, B-mode imaging, and specific training.

Velocity criteria used for a single, isolated stenosis may not be applied to serial stenoses. The energy lost in the first major stenosis affects velocity increases in distal stenoses. Modern US, using B-mode and color-flow imaging besides velocity criteria, however, allows for high predictive values in assessing normalcy, significant stenoses, and occlusions.[43] A meta-analysis of papers published between 1984 and 1994 demonstrated the superiority of color-flow, duplex ultrasound imaging over duplex scanning alone.[44] Color-flow shortens imaging time by readily identifying patent arteries, the location of stenosis, or the collaterals that feed the reconstituted channels of the main infrainguinal occluded arteries.

Lack of sensitivity to low flow states may be addressed with echo-enhancing agents.[45,46] US contrast agents improve sensitivity of medium-quality US scanners and speed up examinations performed with high-quality scanners. Because flow detection increases, collateral flow is also significantly enhanced. A pitfall to avoid is in the distinction between main arterial trunks and their collaterals. Identification of the main veins can help in this differentiation.

Interobserver variation exists in the measurement of velocities and in the estimation of stenosis or occlusion.[47] This variability increases from popliteal to pedal arteries. Uniform training and interaction with the surgical team is a requirement for large vascular laboratories employing many sonographers. With appropriate training, US interobserver agreement can become similar to that of XRA.[48]

The specialist performing US of the peripheral arteries must have knowledge not only of vascular diseases but also about the preferences of the vascular surgeon treating the patient. Vascular surgeons have performed US mapping, and fast, short protocols have been described.[49] Ultrasound training of vascular surgeons has been recommended.[50]

Virtual Decision Making

Although valuable to document proficiency and increase reliance on the noninvasive method, comparison between US and XRA is a secondary objective. The main purpose of US preoperative arterial mapping is not to mimic XRA but to provide information for successful revascularization. XRA is not essential for this primary goal. Therefore, the authors' learning curve focused not on a comparison with arteriography segment by segment, but on decision making analyzing virtual bypass grafts selected based on US imaging.

Furthermore, the authors were aware of potential variability or inconsistency associated with treatment selection by surgeons. Kohler and colleagues provided evidence indicating that treatment variability was larger than differences between the imaging methods.[51] Therefore, direct comparison of bypasses based on US vs. XRA was avoided. The method selected was acceptance/rejection of US-selected bypasses based on the reading of arteriographic films by an independent observer.[8] A series of 55 studies were included in this virtual decision-making phase. This process revealed a learning curve of 15 cases with an acceptance ratio of 60%. In the last 40 cases, the acceptance ratio increased to 88%. The five rejections highlighted potential pitfalls in iliac imaging, alternative surgical philosophies, and misidentification of distal vessels in uncooperative patients with edema and/or obesity. The example illustrating surgical decision was a case of selecting a popliteal-distal bypass and balloon angioplasty of a superficial femoral stenosis vs. performing a proximal superficial femoral-distal bypass. These observations confirmed the need for intraoperative pressure measurements, further training of the ultrasonographer in the surgical preferences of the surgeon, and specific description of segments poorly visualized by US.

Intraoperative Pressure Measurements

Intraoperative pressure measurements complement and confirm US findings regarding aortoiliac disease. At first, inflow pressures were measured before and after infrainguinal bypass revascularization. If a gradient between inflow and radial pressures was found, then intraoperative arteriography was performed with intent to dilate potential stenosis. Lately, pressure measurements have been performed after revascularization. The increased iliac flow caused by improved outflow exacerbates the hemodynamic effects of a potentially significant iliac stenosis.

Intraoperative Arteriography

Initially, completion XRA was performed to demonstrate adequacy of the distal anastomosis and run-off. As the surgical team gained experience with intraoperative US imaging, XRA has been replaced by US completion arteriography. US permits visualization of vessel walls, flaps, displaced plaques, vein webs, graft torsions, graft constrictions, and other anomalies not necessarily detected by XRA lumenography (Fig. 22-5).

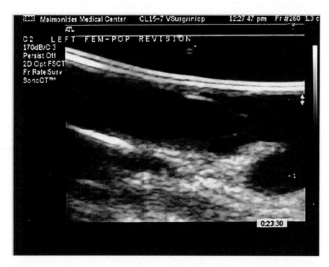

Figure 22-5. Intraoperative image of a "frozen" valve in the femoral-popliteal bypass with reversed greater saphenous vein missed on the completion contrast arteriogram.

Surgical Experience

The authors have reported experience with 485 lower extremity revascularizations performed between January 1998 and May 2001.[1,5] Revascularizations caused by acute arterial occlusions or bypass graft thrombosis totaled 87. It is estimated that over 700 revascularizations have been performed based on preoperative DUAM thus far. Indications for surgery were severe claudication (about 20%); tissue loss (about 40%); rest pain (about 20%); and other conditions (e.g., acute ischemia, popliteal aneurysm, and failing grafts) (about 20%). The average age of patients was 72 years. Cardiovascular risk factors such as diabetes, hypertension, smoking, coronary artery disease, and end-stage renal disease were noted in 45%, 45%, 44%, 44%, and 13% of the patients, respectively. The ratio of infrapopliteal to popliteal bypasses was approximately 3 to 2. Overall, 6-, 12-, and 24-month secondary patency rates were 86%, 80%, and 66%, respectively.

Literature Review

Several reviewed articles concluded that DUAM was feasible, avoided XRA complications, was competitive with XRA in diagnosis, could help select patients for a bypass or an endovascular procedure, was a reasonable replacement for preoperative arteriography if intraoperative arteriography was performed, or was good enough to limit the role of arteriography to interventional procedures.[9, 52-55] This section presents several study approaches used in the investigation of potential applications for US arterial mapping.

US-XRA Imaging Comparison

Jager and colleagues,[10] working with DE Strandness Jr. group at the University of Washington, reported in 1985 that noninvasive duplex ultrasonography was not only suitable for clinical use but was as good as arteriography in defining the location and extent of iliac, femoral, and/or popliteal arterial disease. Different results have been reported regarding diagnostic or preoperative mapping role for US mapping.[11-13] Moneta and colleagues[11] reported that sensitivity to detect stenosis was better in the aortoiliac than in the femoropopliteal segment (89% vs. 67%), with occlusion successfully distinguished from stenosis in 98% of the cases. Koelemay's meta-analysis[12] reported specificity of 97% and 96% and sensitivity of 86% and 80% in the aortoiliac and femoropopliteal tracts, respectively.

In 1986, Sherman and colleagues[14] showed that the level of a leg bypass could be predicted correctly in 88% of the cases by using clinical and Doppler US data. Schneider and Ogawa[15] suggested that short acceleration time of the common femoral velocity waveform (less than 140 ms) and normal duplex US studies were sufficient to limit arteriography to the infrainguinal arteries without the need for an aortoiliac angiogram.

Comparisons between US and XRA imaging findings in the infrapopliteal arteries have also produced mixed results. Katsamouris and colleagues[16] reported that US diagnostic agreement and decision making was excellent at the femoropopliteal level, good at the aortoiliac segment, and moderate for infrapopliteal arteries. In their study, US detected tibial arteries and above-the-knee popliteal stenosis not opacified or perceived by XRA. Alexander and colleagues[17] reported an accuracy of 96% for US-XRA comparison of femoral, popliteal, and tibial arteries. In contrast, Bostrom Ardin and colleagues[18] reported retrospectively that US could correctly select a superficial femoral, popliteal, or crural artery in 85%, 66%, and 32% of cases, respectively. US contrast may significantly improve assessment of infrapopliteal arteries.[46]

Imaging of tibial arteries has been more successful than peroneal artery imaging. In patients with femoropopliteal obstructions, Larch and colleagues[19] reported similar judgments between US and XRA to select the dominant infrapopliteal artery; but despite good sensitivity to detect severe stenosis or occlusion, agreement between US and XRA findings was poor, particularly for the peroneal artery. Accuracy of 80% for detection of tibioperoneal trunk, crural, and pedal artery obstructions has been reported,[20] with poor specificity for detection of normal or minimally diseased peroneal arteries. US selection of patients for transluminal angioplasty has been inferior in the popliteal and crural arteries as compared with the femoral segment.[21]

Incomplete infrapopliteal imaging was more common with XRA (36%) than with the expanded field of view

US technique (15%), and it was more common during imaging of the peroneal artery.[22,23] Although agreement was high among studies with complete images (92%), comparison could only be performed in about two thirds of the infrapopliteal arteries.

Multiple lesions may lead to inadequate predictions of stenosis based on Doppler spectra.[24,25] Sensitivity may drop in low-flow segments distal to total occlusions in patients with severe iliac and distal femoropopliteal lesions.[26] Better results can be achieved if all facets of color-flow US duplex imaging are employed.[27,30]

US Comparison With Intraoperative XRA

Significant differences may be observed if the standard of comparison shifts from preoperative to intraoperative arteriography. Lujan and colleagues[28] showed that US correlated with preoperative arteriography diverging only in 6% of 52 cases. Decisions based on the two preoperative imaging techniques, however, were modified after intraoperative arteriography in about 20% of the cases. McCarthy and colleagues[29] demonstrated that color-flow and dependent Doppler US could predict very well an optimal cruropedal run-off (kappa = 1.0), the site of distal anastomosis (kappa = 0.85), and the patency of the pedal arch and the predominant feeding artery (kappa = 1.0).

Comparison With Final Surgical Decision

Most modern-day surgical decisions in infrainguinal reconstruction rely on a complex set of data. Surgeons, in most cases, rely on data confirmed by more than one source of information. However, in exceptional cases, such decision must favor one source over another. For example, Aly and colleagues[30] determined that US had positive and negative predictive values of 91% and 100% in comparison with XRA. Length of the XRA arterial lesion was also predicted correctly by US in more than 90% of the cases. However, the accuracy of both techniques, when compared with the final decision, was inferior, being 84% and 85% for US and XRA, respectively. This work emphasized that neither US nor XRA imaging per se completely influences surgical decisions.

Validation of Arterial Mapping

Comparisons of decisions to perform virtual bypasses based on US and XRA face a double source of variability: (1) differences in imaging information and (2) alternative preferences by different surgeons. Even the same surgeon may be inconsistent in treatment selection, given similar information.[51] These observations played an important role in the modified design of the authors' own virtual decision-making study described above and

should be taken into consideration in the analysis of data with variable results.

Wain and colleagues[32] demonstrated that preoperative US mapping could select patients for a femoropopliteal or infrapopliteal bypass and show a 90% agreement with arteriography. Agreement in selection of the actual anastomotic site for infrapopliteal grafts, however, was poor at 24%. Koelemay and colleagues[33] reported similar results, with agreement in 79% of femoropopliteal and 41% in crural bypasses. These data emphasize the inconsistencies of infrapopliteal imaging. Although XRA may be traditionally favored in comparison with US, inadequacies of infrapopliteal XRA have been documented.[16,22,23] Avenarius and colleagues reported that about 10% of 112 limbs could not be properly analyzed, and that US and XRA offered the same strategy in 90% of the remainder.[34] These authors observed that if severe calcification prevented visualization of crural vessels, or if no patent anterior or posterior tibial artery were noted by US, then XRA should be performed.

In a comparison with intraoperative clinical findings and completion flow studies/arteriograms, for a sample of 44 consecutive femorocrural reconstructions, dependent Doppler, XRA, and US correctly predicted a suitable run-off in 21 (48%), 32 (73%), and 44 (100%) limbs, respectively.[35] The proportion of correctly assessed run-offs was significantly higher with US than with XRA (p < 0.001).

A recent report from Dartmouth Medical Center validated selection of tibial or peroneal distal anastomotic sites by US and XRA.[36] The study was performed on a blinded fashion, and actual bypasses performed served as the standard of comparison. US-predicted artery sites were actually used in 88% of the cases, XRA were used in 93%, and agreement between the two selections occurred in 85%. Arteries used for bypass grafting had higher peak-systolic and end-diastolic velocities and larger diameters. The authors concluded that if US identifies a target artery and visualizes the peroneal artery well, then US-based decision making should rarely be altered by XRA findings.

In a specific study of pedal artery imaging, Hofmann and colleagues[31] reported moderate agreement accomplished between two radiologists interpreting XRA and MRA (respective Kappa scores of 0.63 and 0.60). US and MRA were superior to XRA in predicting distal outflow. This study underscores the inadequacy of relying solely on XRA as a comparison standard.

Actual Decision Making

The Maimonides Medical Center experience has been described above. Others have examined imaging methods available for planning leg revascularization. Walsh and LaBombard[37] pointed out deficiencies of XRA in iliac and infrainguinal arterial occlusive disease. They noted that US can be performed successfully and can contribute in a variety of situations. Isolated stenosis or short occlusions can be identified by US, and percutaneous endovascular treatment can be performed. Patients with severe disease can be taken to the operating room, where inflow can be evaluated with pressure measurements. For the outflow, if US fails to demonstrate a distal site for bypass, XRA should be performed as a preoperative or intraoperative study before considering amputation. Pemberton and London[38] concluded that arteriography should no longer be the standard of imaging peripheral arteries, and that future studies should concentrate on the efficacy of US in guiding clinical decisions.

Intraoperative X-ray Arteriography

Decision to operate has been performed based on US. Patients have been taken to the operating room without preoperative arteriography. US findings have been corroborated by intraoperative arteriography. Bostrom and colleagues[39] have performed close to half of their interventions without preoperative arteriography. In cases of femoral endarterectomy, US correctly diagnosed the extent of stenosis and the status of the deep femoral artery in all but one patient. The US selection of a distal anastomosis for an infrainguinal bypass was confirmed by intraoperative arteriography in 98% of the cases, and agreement of run-off status was 90%. In 1996, Pemberton and colleagues[40] reported 29 cases of infragenicular reconstruction based on preoperative US findings. With one exception, the US information was confirmed by prereconstruction intraoperative arteriography.

No X-ray Arteriography

Most surgeons who have performed infrainguinal revascularizations based on US imaging focused their initial experience in the femoropopliteal level. Pemberton and colleagues[40] described a wide range of femoropopliteal revascularizations performed with color Doppler alone. Schneider and colleagues evaluated prospectively 24 femoropopliteal bypasses and femoral endarterectomies performed based on US mapping.[41] This selected group represented 15% of their revascularizations. Assisted primary patency was 100% at 18 months.

US: Intraoperative

As an extension of intraoperative carotid endarterectomy evaluation, B-mode imaging was employed as a complement or replacement for preoperative arteriography to define placement of an anastomosis or to guide in the design of additional reconstruction.[56]

US: Completion Arteriography

Several authors employed either B-mode or color-flow duplex US to perform completion arteriography in the operating room.[56,57] Sawaqed and colleagues[57] correlated duplex scanning to cut-film angiography and real-time fluoroscopy as techniques for intraoperative bypass graft assessment. Duplex scanning obtained a 100% correlation with XRA findings, was performed in about half of the time (10 minutes vs. 22 and 17 minutes for cut-film and fluoro, respectively), and for half of the cost ($350 vs. $650).

Conclusions

Significant evidence was gathered to justify infrainguinal arterial revascularization based primarily on duplex ultrasound arterial mapping. US can be the technique of choice for prereconstruction mapping and for intraoperative postimplantation completion angiography. Implementation of such a program requires special training of an ultrasound/surgery team with focus on arterial US mapping and surgical preferences. Inadequate US studies must be clearly identified. US findings should be complemented by intraoperative manometry. Intraoperative arteriography should be available for special circumstances. A single imaging modality, either US, XRA, or MRA, may not be the basis for leg amputation. Routine, standard bypass graft is recommended.

REFERENCES

1. Ascher E, Hingorani A, Markevich N, et al: Acute lower limb ischemia: The value of duplex ultrasound arterial mapping (DUAM) as the sole preoperative imaging technique. Ann Vasc Surg 17:284–289, 2003.
2. Ascher E, Markevich N, Schutzer RW, et al: Small popliteal aneurysms: Are they clinically significant? J Vasc Surg 37:755–760, 2003.
3. Soule B, Hingorani A, Ascher E, et al: Comparison of magnetic resonance angiography (MRA) and duplex ultrasound arterial mapping (DUAM) prior to infrainguinal arterial reconstruction. Eur J Vasc Endovasc Surg 25:139–146, 2003.
4. Hingorani A, Ascher E: Dyeless vascular surgery. Cardiovasc Surg 11:12–18, 2003.
5. Ascher E, Hingorani A, Markevich N, et al: Lower extremity revascularization without preoperative contrast arteriography: Experience with duplex ultrasound arterial mapping in 485 cases. Ann Vasc Surg 16:108–114, 2002.
6. Mazzariol F, Asher E, Hingorani A, et al: Lower-extremity revascularization without preoperative contrast arteriography in 185 cases: Lessons learned with duplex ultrasound arterial mapping. Eur J Vasc Endovasc Surg 19:509–515, 2000.
7. Ascher E, Mazzariol F, Hingorani A, et al: The use of duplex ultrasound arterial mapping as an alternative to conventional arteriography for primary and secondary infrapopliteal bypasses. Am J Surg 178:162–165, 1999.
8. Mazzariol F, Ascher E, Salles-Cunha SX, et al: Values and limitations of duplex ultrasonography as the sole imaging method of preoperative evaluation for popliteal and infrapopliteal bypasses. Ann Vasc Surg 13:1–10, 1999.
9. Salles-Cunha SX, Andros G: Preoperative duplex scanning prior to infrainguinal revascularization. Surg Clin North Am 70:41–59, 1990.
10. Jager KA, Phillips DJ, Martin RL, et al: Noninvasive mapping of lower limb arterial lesions. Ultrasound Med Biol 11:515–521, 1985.
11. Moneta GL, Yeager RA, Antonovic R, et al: Accuracy of lower extremity arterial duplex imaging. J Vasc Surg 15:275–283, 1992.

12. Koelemay MJ, den Hartog D, Prins MH, et al: Diagnosis of arterial disease of the lower extremities with duplex ultrasonography. Br J Surg 83:404–409, 1996.
13. Ramaswami G, Al-Kutoubi A, Nicolaides AN, et al: The role of duplex scanning in the diagnosis of lower limb arterial disease. Ann Vasc Surg 13:494–500, 1999.
14. Sherman CP, Gwynn BR, Curran F, et al: Noninvasive femoropopliteal assessment: Is that angiogram really necessary? BMJ (Clin Res Ed) 293:1086–1089, 1986.
15. Schneider PA, Ogawa DY: Is routine preoperative aortoiliac arteriography necessary in the treatment of lower extremity ischemia? J Vasc Surg 28:28–34, 1998.
16. Katsamouris AN, Giannoukas AD, Tsetis D, et al: Can ultrasound replace arteriography in the management of chronic arterial occlusive disease of the lower limb? Eur J Vasc Endovasc Surg 21:155–159, 2001.
17. Alexander JQ, Leos SM, Katz SG: Is duplex ultrasonography an effective single modality for the preoperative evaluation of peripheral vascular disease? Am Surg 68:1107–1110, 2002.
18. Bostrom Ardin A, Lofberg AM, Hellberg A, et al: Selection of patients with infrainguinal arterial occlusive disease for percutaneous transluminal angioplasty with duplex scanning. Acta Radiol 43:391–395, 2002.
19. Larch E, Minar E, Ahmadi R, et al: Value of color duplex sonography for evaluation of tibioperoneal arteries in patients with femoropopliteal obstruction: A prospective comparison with antegrade intraarterial digital subtraction angiography. J Vasc Surg 25:629–636, 1997.
20. Karacagil S, Lofbert AM, Granbo A, et al: Value of duplex scanning in evaluation of crural and foot arteries in limbs with severe lower limb ischaemia: A prospective comparison with arteriography. Eur J Vasc Endovasc Surg 12:300–303, 1996.
21. Lofberg AM, Karacagil S, Hellberg A, et al: The role of duplex scanning in the selection of patients with critical lower-limb ischemia for infrainguinal percutaneous transluminal angioplasty. Cardiovasc Intervent Radiol 24:229–232, 2001.
22. Engelhorn CA: Comparison of expanded field-of-view ultrasound imaging and arteriography in the diagnosis of infrainguinal arterial obstructions. Doctoral dissertation. Universidade Federal de Sao Paulo, Escola Paulista de Medicina, 2001.
23. Salles-Cunha S, Engelhorn C, Miranda F Jr, et al: Distal revascularization: Comparison of incomplete images of infrapopliteal images in severely ischemic lower extremities. J Vasc Bras 2(Supp 1):S34, 2003.
24. Allard L, Cloutier G, Durand LG, et al: Limitations of ultrasonic duplex scanning for diagnosing lower limb arterial stenosis in the presence of adjacent segment disease. J Vasc Surg 19:650–657, 1994.
25. Bergamini TM, Tatum CM Jr, Marshall C, et al: Effect of multilevel sequential stenosis on lower extremity arterial duplex scanning. Am J Surg 169:564–566, 1995.
26. Karacagil S, Lofberg AM, Almgren B, et al: Duplex ultrasound scanning for diagnosis of aortoiliac and femoropopliteal arterial disease. Vasa 23:325–329, 1994.
27. Sensier Y, Hartshorne T, Thrush A, et al: The effect of adjacent segment disease on the accuracy of colour duplex scanning for the diagnosis of lower limb arterial disease. Eur J Vasc Endovasc Surg 12:238–242, 1996.
28. Lujan S, Criado E, Puras E, et al: Duplex scanning or arteriography for preoperative planning of lower limb revascularization. Eur J Vasc Endovasc Surg 24:31–36, 2002.
29. McCarthy MJ, Nydahl S, Hartshorne T, et al: Colour-coded duplex imaging and dependent Doppler ultrasonography in the assessment of cruropedal vessels. Br J Surg 86:33–37, 1999.
30. Aly S, Sommerville K, Adiseshiah M, et al: Comparison of duplex imaging and arteriography in the evaluation of lower limb arteries. Br J Surg 85:1099–1102, 1998.
31. Hofmann WJ, Forstner R, Kofler B, et al: Pedal artery imaging: A comparison of selective digital subtraction angiography, contrast enhanced magnetic resonance angiography, and duplex ultrasound. Eur J Vasc Endovasc Surg 24:287–292, 2002;
32. Wain RA, Berdejo GL, Delvalle WN, et al: Can duplex scan arterial mapping replace contrast arteriography as the test of choice before infrainguinal revascularization? J Vasc Surg 29:100–107, 1999.
33. Koelemay MJ, Legemate DA, de Vos H, et al: Can cruropedal colour duplex scanning and pulse-generated run-off replace angiography in candidates for distal bypass surgery? Eur J Vasc Endovasc Surg 16:13–18, 1998.
34. Avenarius JK, Breek JC, Lampman LE, et al: The additional value of angiography after colour-coded duplex on decision making inn patients with critical limb ischemia. A prospective study. Eur J Vasc Endovasc Surg 23:393–397, 2002.
35. Wilson YG, George JK, Wilkins DC, et al: Duplex assessment of run-off before femorocrural reconstruction. Br J Surg 84:1360–1363, 1977.
36. Grassbaugh JA, Nelson PR, Rzucidlo EM, et al: Blinded comparison of preoperative duplex ultrasound scanning and contrast arteriography for planning revascularization at the level of the tibia. J Vasc Surg 37:1186–1190, 2003.
37. Walsh DB, LaBombard E: Lower extremity bypass using only duplex ultrasonography: Is the time now? Semin Vasc Surg 12:247–251, 1999.
38. Pemberton M, London NJ: Colour flow duplex imaging of occlusive arterial disease of the lower limb. Br J Surg 84:912–919, 1997.
39. Bostrom A, Ljungman C, Helberg A, et al: Duplex scanning as the sole preoperative mapping method for infrainguinal arterial surgery. Eur J Vasc Endovasc Surg 23:140–145, 2002.
40. Pemberton M, Nydahl S, Hartshorne T, et al: Can lower limb vascular reconstruction be based on colour duplex imaging alone? Eur J Vasc Endovasc Surg 12:452–454, 1966.
41. Schneider PA, Ogawa DY, Rush MP: Lower extremity revascularization without contrast arteriography: A prospective study of operation based upon duplex mapping. Cardiovasc Surg 7:699–703, 1999.
42. Felizzola LR, Camargo O Jr, Guillaumon AT, et al: Limb salvage surgery based on color-flow ultrasonography with contrast. J Vasc Br 2(Supp 1):S51, 2003.
43. Aly S, Jenkins MP, Zaidi FH, et al: Duplex scanning and effect of multisegmental arterial disease on its accuracy in lower limb arteries. Eur J Vasc Endovasc Surg 16:345–349, 1998.
44. De Vries SO, Hunink MG, Polak JF: Summary receiver operating characteristic curves as a technique for meta-analysis of the diagnostic performance of duplex ultrasonography in peripheral arterial disease. Acad Radiol 3:361–369, 1996.
45. Ubbink DT, Legemate DA, Llull JB: Color-flow duplex scanning of the leg arteries by use of a new echo-enhancing agent. J Vasc Surg 35:395–396, 2002.
46. Eiberg JP, Hansen MA, Jensen F, et al: Ultrasound contrast-agent improves imaging of lower limb occlusive disease. Eur J Vasc Endovasc Surg 25:23–28, 2003.
47. Koelemay MJ, Legemate DA, van Gurp JA, et al: Interobserver variation of colour duplex scanning of the popliteal, tibial and pedal arteries. Eur J Vasc Endovasc Surg 21:160–164, 2001.
48. Eiberg JP, Madycki G, Hansen MA, et al: Ultrasound imaging of infrainguinal arterial disease has a high interobserver agreement. Eur J Vasc Endovasc Surg 24:293–299, 2002.
49. Elsharawy M, Elzayat E: A fast arterial duplex ultrasound performed by vascular surgeons. Is the time now? Int Angiol 21:374–378, 2002.
50. Ascher E: Presidential address: The modern vascular specialist-surgeon, clinician, and interventionist. J Vasc Surg 38(4):633–638, 2003.
51. Kohler TR, Andros G, Porter JM, et al: Can duplex scanning replace arteriography of lower extremity arterial disease? Ann Vasc Surg 4:280–287, 1990.
52. Pellerito JS, Taylor KJ: Doppler color imaging: Peripheral arteries. Clin Diagn Ultrasound 27:97–112, 1992.
53. London NJ, Sensier Y, Hartshorne T: Can lower limb ultrasonography replace arteriography? Vasc Med 1:115–119, 1996.

54. Zierler RE: Vascular surgery without arteriography: Use of duplex ultrasound. Cardiovasc Surg 7:74–82, 1999.

55. Eiberg JP, Schroeder TV: Can ultrasonography replace arteriography in arteriosclerosis of the lower limb? Ugeskr Laeger 163:278–281, 2001.

56. Kresowik TF, Hoballah JJ, Sharp WJ, et al: Intraoperative B-mode ultrasonography is a useful adjunct to peripheral arterial reconstruction. Ann Vasc Surg 7:33–38, 1993.

57. Sawaqed RS, Podbielski FJ, Rodriguez HE, et al: Prospective comparison of intraoperative angiography with duplex scanning in evaluating lower-extremity bypass grafts in a community hospital. Am Surg 67:601–604, 2001.

Chapter 23

The Role of Skin Perfusion Pressure and Transcutaneous Partial Pressure Oxygen Measurements in Chronic Critical Limb Ischemia

JOHN J. CASTRONUOVO, JR.

- Critical Limb Ischemia
- Skin Perfusion Pressures
- Methodology and Limitations of SPP
- Transcutaneous Oxygen Partial Pressures
- Methodology and Limitations of $TcPO_2$
- Conclusions

Individuals with peripheral arterial disease (PAD) comprise a wide spectrum of patients whose clinical management varies considerably.[1] Many of these patients have widespread arterial disease and may eventually require treatment for conditions other than PAD. For a substantial proportion of PAD patients, the disease has progressed to such severity that the survival of the affected limb is in question. *Critical limb ischemia* (CLI) is the term commonly used to describe this condition.

Patients with CLI present with skin lesions, rest pain, or both. In any case, physiologic arterial examination of the leg (i.e., segmental arterial pressures and plethysmography or Doppler waveforms) should be done immediately to document the presence of PAD. A shortcoming of these tests, however, is that the pressure measurements may be falsely elevated. McDermott and colleagues reported that the ankle-brachial index (ABI) was unable to gauge arterial perfusion accurately in 136 of 460 (29.5%) patients with PAD.[2]

Skin is the tissue most seriously affected in CLI. Although the pathophysiology of CLI is not well understood, there is a consensus that it causes alterations to the microcirculation in skin and other tissues. These should not be understood simplistically as events secondary to the macrocirculatory occlusions in PAD, even though PAD may be the underlying cause. In fact, current treatments are often focused on the correction of microcirculatory deficiencies, particularly in patients for whom revascularization is not an option.

For CLI patients, it is imperative that appropriate diagnostic testing be performed to provide data for clinical decision making. In addition to conventional vascular diagnostic testing of the arteries, CLI requires an evaluation of microcirculatory conditions.

Various types of investigations proposed for this purpose include skin perfusion pressure (SPP),[3-6] radionuclide perfusion scans,[7] transcutaneous oxygen partial pressure (TcPO$_2$),[8-10] laser Doppler flowmetry (LDF),[6,11-12] and capillary microscopy.[13] Two of these measurement types, SPP and TcPO$_2$, afford a relatively simple and inexpensive noninvasive test method that measures the effect of microcirculatory lesions of PAD on the microcirculation. This chapter reviews the methodology, principles, relative advantages, and limitations of SPP and TcPO$_2$ testing, and provides criteria that can be helpful in choosing the method best suited to particular patients and clinical decisions.

Critical Limb Ischemia

The TransAtlantic Inter-Society Consensus Working Group (TASC) has defined the term *CLI* to include patients with chronic ischemic rest pain, ulcers, or gangrene attributable to proven PAD.[1] Inherent in this definition is the assumption that arterial occlusive disease is not acute and is at least partly responsible for the symptoms and findings in the limbs of CLI patients. Also implied by the definition is that the absence of PAD, as determined by conventional vascular testing (e.g., segmental arterial pressures, plethysmography, and Doppler waveforms), should be used as evidence to exclude a diagnosis of CLI.

The clinical decision-making process varies considerably from one situation to the next, especially if arterial reconstruction is not possible. For example, in one case a decision may be made concerning the optimum level of amputation. In a patient with a diabetic foot ulcer, it may be whether hyperbaric oxygen (HBO) therapy should be attempted or if a reconstructive surgery procedure should be performed. In yet another case it may be whether to try systemic treatments, perform debridement with local wound care, or proceed to amputation. Sometimes the decision is summarized as being a choice between conservative therapy and surgical intervention.

It is helpful, in light of the above, to determine as precisely as possible the question being asked of the physiologic investigation. If the goal is to make a positive diagnosis of CLI, for example, it would not be prudent

to apply a test which only does well at excluding the presence of the condition. If one is looking for arterial blockage or other macrovascular abnormalities, an arterial examination is indicated; but if there is evidence of vessel calcification, or if one is looking for more localized microvascular abnormalities, a test assessing the skin microcirculation should be employed. When the question relates to a particular therapeutic decision (e.g., whether a patient will benefit from HBO therapy), then the choice of test should be consistent with the type of physiologic changes that are expected.

In statistical terms, the ideal test of CLI is both sensitive and specific, and also has both a strong *positive predictive value* (PPV) and a strong *negative predictive value* (NPV). These terms can be explained using the test result (i.e., either normal vs. abnormal, or predicting healing vs. failure in the case of a lesion) and the actual patient condition or outcome.

If a positive test indicates that the outcome will be failure to heal (i.e., CLI), for example, then let:

- a = % of patients with healing failure, for which the test predicted failure (i.e., true positives)
- b = % of patients healed, for which the test predicted failure (i.e., false positives)
- c = % of patients with healing failure, for which the test predicted healing (i.e., false negatives)
- d = % of patients healed, for which the test predicted healing (i.e., true negatives)

The definitions pertinent to our discussion are as follows[14]:

$$\text{Sensitivity} = a / (a + c)$$
$$\text{Specificity} = d / (d + b)$$
$$\text{PPV} = a / (a + b)$$
$$\text{NPV} = d / (d + c)$$

Clearly it is preferable to have all four of these parameters as close to 1.00 as possible for the test method in use and with respect to the clinical question to be resolved. To accomplish this, it is necessary to minimize the occurrence of false positives and false negatives (i.e., b and c above).

In patients with symptoms of CLI, it is unfortunately quite common to perform arterial testing without follow-up microvascular investigations, and where microvascular tests are actually done, they may not provide relevant information. This can result in misguided clinical decision making.

For example, conventional arterial testing usually includes segmental systolic pressures, or at least an ankle systolic pressure (ASP). This testing is not considered sensitive when it is used to detect the presence of CLI because of the high number of false-negative test results. This can be a result of falsely elevated systolic pressure measurements caused by arterial calcification,[15] by the absence of disease in just one of the infrageniculate arteries,[16] or even by the aging process.[17] The PPV is much better for ASP because there are few false-positive test results. However, because the NPV is poor, the measurement of ankle pressure does not conclusively rule out CLI.[18] Conventional testing should therefore be followed by appropriate microvascular testing when it is necessary to rule out CLI because accurate measurement of the perfusion of the microcirculation is not affected by incompressible arteries at the macrocirculatory level.

A corollary problem often occurs when $TcPO_2$ tests are performed to determine if CLI is present. This testing is considered relatively sensitive when it is used to diagnose the presence of CLI (i.e., yielding few false-negative test results). However, as will be discussed later, $TcPO_2$ results are not very specific for CLI because they can be falsely lowered when skin bloodflow is depressed,[17] resulting in an unacceptable number of false-positive tests. The NPV is quite high, but the PPV and specificity are both poor. The reporting of normal $TcPO_2$ values is more or less conclusive for demonstrating the absence of CLI, but an abnormal $TcPO_2$ value is not a reliable indicator of its presence, and should be followed by a more specific test.

It should be emphasized that there is no single test that is optimal for all situations; however, as the preceding demonstrates, the correct choice of physiologic test, and its proper interpretation, is vitally important.

Skin Perfusion Pressures

SPP is defined as the external pressure threshold required for skin blanching. Ordinarily the skin perfusion is measured at the location of applied pressure using a microcirculatory sensing technique. The pressure is first elevated to a level sufficient to completely arrest the skin bloodflow, and then is slowly decreased. The definition of SPP then translates into the external pressure at which the sensor registers the first reappearance of perfusion.

In this respect the SPP measurement is performed much like arterial pressure measurements, in which the external pressure (usually applied with a cuff encircling the limb or digit) is first elevated and then slowly decreased. The appearance of bloodflow is registered with a sensor distal to the cuff, and the systolic pressure is taken as that external cuff pressure at which the first indication of bloodflow occurs. For SPP measurements, the appearance of flow is sensed directly beneath the externally applied pressure cuff (Fig. 23-1).

SPP investigations were reported as early as 1973 by Nielsen and colleagues[19] and Holstein,[20] using a photoelectric surface probe as the perfusion sensor. Subsequently, Holstein and colleagues,[21] Faris and Duncan,[5] and Dwars and colleagues[22] substituted the use of radioisotope washout in place of the photoelectric probe to improve the sensitivity of the bloodflow detection.

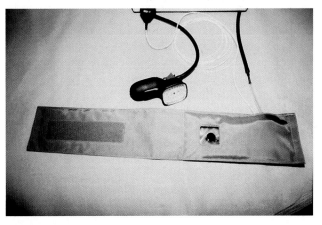

Figure 23-1. The fenestrated cuff used to measure skin perfusion pressure.

The radioisotope washout method (RI-SPP) improved the reproducibility of the technique such that it could reliably predict clinical outcomes in ischemic limbs. Its use nevertheless did not become popular because it required the involvement of nuclear medicine, was cumbersome to perform, and was uncomfortable for patients because of the length of time of cuff inflation required for measurement of SPP using washout of the isotope.

A later development reported by Malvezzi and colleagues[23] was the substitution of laser Doppler (LD) sensing in place of the radioisotope washout technique. With the LD sensor placed inside the cuff used to apply external pressure, this new method correlated very well with RI-SPP (Fig. 23-2). Because the LD sensor is real-time and exceptionally sensitive, SPP testing could be done much faster and with less discomfort to the patient.

Recent studies have been reported in which SPP, using a LD sensor, is used to identify patients with CLI who require vascular reconstruction or surgical intervention,[6] and also to predict amputation wound healing.[24] The critical SPP level in these studies, below which wound healing is unlikely to occur with conservative therapy, is consistent with previously reported values.

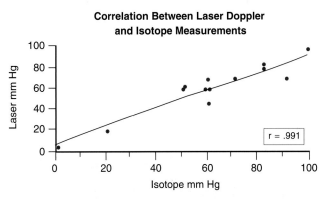

Correlation Between Laser Doppler and Isotope Measurements

r = .991

Figure 23-2. A good correlation has been shown between the radioisotope method of skin perfusion pressure determination and the laser Doppler method of measuring skin perfusion pressure.

Table 23-1 sets forth a summary of the clinical findings on the use of SPP in amputation wound healing in critical limb ischemia. With reference to the preceding remarks, it should be noted that the clinical question asked of SPP investigation should be whether a patient's skin circulation is insufficient for healing. SPP testing (as well as other physiologic testing) does not evaluate other noncirculatory causes of healing failure (e.g., infection). Therefore, the sufficiency of perfusion does not, by itself, predict healing, unless noncirculatory pathology can be fully ruled out. On the other hand, a low SPP does, by itself, predict healing failure, whether or not other pathology is present, because there is not enough perfusion to support healing. In light of this, a "positive" test outcome in Table 23-1 is a low SPP indicative of the presence of CLI and predictive of healing failure.

The comparison of SPP and toe systolic pressure values is of interest because both measurements are made in the distal circulation. Tsai and colleagues[25] have reported a good correlation between SPP measurements at the foot dorsum and toe systolic pressures on both healthy and diseased patients, with toe pressure values approximately 20% higher than foot SPP (Fig. 23-3).

Toe pressure measurements are recommended when CLI is suspected,[1,26–28] especially for diabetic patients whose ankle pressures may be falsely elevated. Values of 30 to 40 mmHg are considered to be positive indications for this diagnosis. The measurement of toe pressure is sometimes problematic, as when the large toe is missing or ulcerated, when the pulsatile signals (PPG or Doppler) are very faint, or when the toes are disfigured. In those cases the measurement of SPP at the dorsum of the foot is a good substitute. An abnormal SPP in a limb with a normal ABI is certain evidence of the spurious nature of the ankle systolic pressure.

Methodology and Limitations of SPP

In current practice, SPP measurements are performed much the same way as are arterial segmental pressure measurements in the lower extremities. The patient first

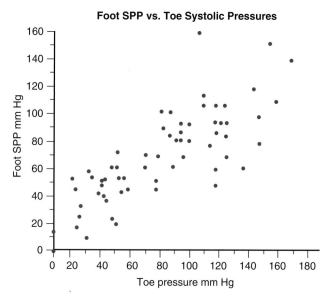

Figure 23-3. *In patients in whom toe pressures cannot be measured, SPP measured on the dorsum of the foot is a good substitute measurement and has been shown to correlate well with pressure measurements in the great toe using either photoplethysmograhy or strain gauge techniques.*

should be acclimatized, and the limb of interest should be kept as warm as possible. The patient should be supine, as with any lower extremity vascular test.

A specialized blood pressure cuff that incorporates a LD sensing device inside the pressurized bladder is wrapped around the limb, foot, or digit. A cuff size is chosen to fit the anatomic dimensions. The cuff should not be tightly applied because capillary blanching may result.

The use of a perfusion sensing device external and underneath the cuff is not recommended because the sensor will create a high pressure point, and the actual counterpressure on the skin at that location will be higher than the air pressure in the bladder. As a result, the SPP measurement will be falsely lowered.

The cuff is then inflated to a pressure sufficient to arrest capillary perfusion. On patients with suspected CLI, a pressure of 50 mmHg is probably high enough, whereas a pressure in excess of 120 mmHg may be necessary for patients with normal SPP. The disappear-

TABLE 23-1. SPP Predictions of Nonhealing of Foot Lesions and Lower Extremity Amputations (Excluding Toes)

Author	Criteria	Sensitivity (%)	Specificity (%)	PPV (%)	NPV (%)
Faris[5]	40 mmHg	80	97	94	90
Dwars[22]	20 mmHg	89	99	89	99
Adera[24]	30 mmHg	100	97	83	100
Castronuovo[6]	30 mmHg	85	73	75	85

PPV, positive predictive value; NPV, negative predictive value.

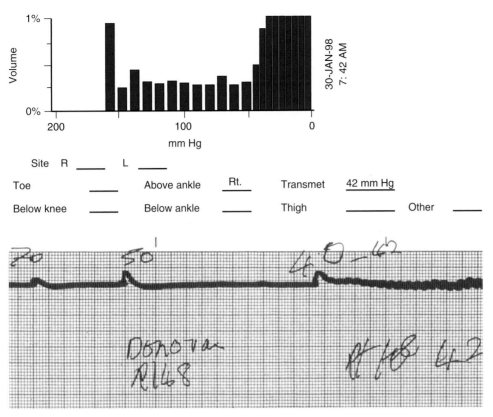

Site R _____ L _____

Toe _____   Above ankle Rt.   Transmet 42 mm Hg

Below knee _____   Below ankle _____   Thigh _____   Other _____

Figure 23-4. Simultaneous toe pressure measurement (bottom tracing) with a photoptheysmograph and SPP measurement (top tracing). Note the initiation of a pulsatile waveform occurs at the same pressure as the pressure at which initiation of capillary bloodflow in the skin causes the LD sensor in the SPP cuff to register flux. The baseline LD flux level is well above 0 even at high inflation pressure (left side of top tracing). Nevertheless, an SPP measurement is possible because of the distinct increase in LD flux that occurs as cuff pressure is lowered to 40 mmHg. Reasons for inter-individual variation in baseline LD flux values include skin pigmentation and the sensitivity of the LD instrument. Minimizing the baseline value will make the detection of the initiation of capillary flow, which is essential to SPP measurement, easier; this can be accomplished by elevating the leg before the application of the SPP cuff and inflation to suprasystolic levels.

ance of capillary flow, as detected by the LD sensor, does not occur immediately because the blood is gradually eliminated by the cuff counterpressure, which may take 30 to 45 seconds or more. However, it is imperative that the perfusion indication of the LD sensor be allowed to reach a 0 or low baseline condition, or else it will not clearly indicate the restarting of perfusion when the cuff pressure reaches the SPP level (Fig. 23-4).

The deflation of the cuff pressure may proceed either in a stepwise or continuous fashion, provided that the rate is not too rapid. Above cuff pressures of 50 mmHg, the deflation rate should be about 2 mmHg per second. Below 50 mmHg, the optimum deflation rate has been found to be 5 mmHg per 15 seconds.[25] This slower cuff deflation allows for the fact that capillary refilling is a slower process than arterial reflow.

The resumption of capillary perfusion is reported graphically on a display that shows the perfusion magnitude as a function of cuff pressure. It is easy to determine the SPP from this graph, and a paper report can be generated for record keeping (Fig. 23-5).

SPP measurements do not require the technologist to locate an artery or identify a pulse, making them easier to perform than arterial pressures on patients with faint pulses. The test is also somewhat more comfortable for the patient, in view of the lower maximum cuff pressure that must be applied. Most significantly, SPP values are

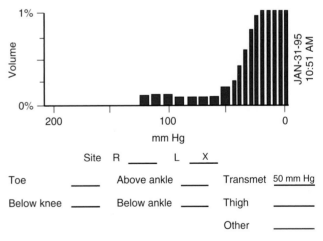

Site R _____ L X

Toe _____   Above ankle _____   Transmet 50 mm Hg

Below knee _____   Below ankle _____   Thigh _____

Other _____

Figure 23-5. This patient demonstrates a low baseline with the result that the pressure at which capillary skin bloodflow resumes is easy to detect. In this instance the SPP is 50 mmHg. The narrow bars on the right of the perfusion-pressure readout denote the fact that below 50 mmHg the instrument is designed to measure SPP at 5-mmHg intervals.

not falsely elevated on patients with medial calcification because this process does not affect the microvessels in the skin. Another advantage is that SPP measurements can be done on the foot, where the bone structure precludes arterial measurements.

SPP investigations are inhibited by motion artifacts on patients who cannot remain still for the duration of the test. The presence of edema does not cause a problem with SPP measurements, and the authors' experience has demonstrated that nearly all patients with suspected CLI can be reliably evaluated with this test.[24]

Transcutaneous Oxygen Partial Pressures

The availability of oxygen in tissues is important for nutritional needs and wound healing. Although oxygen levels in the blood may be sufficiently high, skin tissue may still suffer if perfusion rates are not high enough to deliver the needed oxygen. Therefore, $TcPO_2$ is often measured in patients with suspected CLI to determine whether this is the case. $TcPO_2$ is defined as the partial pressure of oxygen gas at the skin surface, and is usually reported in units of mmHg or kPa.

Devices for $TcPO_2$ measurements incorporate a modified Clark-type oxygen electrode, which has a silver anode and a platinum cathode. When the electrode is exposed to oxygen, an electrochemical reaction occurs, causing the flow of electric current proportional to the oxygen pressure. This current is measured and reported as the local $TcPO_2$ value.

Other device components include a disposable permeable membrane covering the electrode, a means of sealing the electrode to eliminate room air, and a heating coil that maintains an elevated skin temperature (typically 42 to 44 °C) to maximize blood perfusion in the capillaries. The last feature is essential particularly in ischemic skin, because 0 readings are likely when the skin is not vasodilated.[18]

This technique was first described by Huch and colleagues,[28] who found it useful for pulmonary function monitoring in neonates. Their relatively thin skin enables the $TcPO_2$ to accurately reflect the arterial oxygenation level. Others later investigated its use in adults with PAD.[9,29-31] Although $TcPO_2$ was not found to be reliable for separation of PAD patients from individuals with normal calculations, it has commonly been used in CLI patients to evaluate skin viability.

Franzeck and colleagues[9] and Byrne colleagues[10] demonstrated that $TcPO_2$ levels decreased as peripheral arterial flow was lowered, and also that patients with ischemic rest pain tended to have low $TcPO_2$ measurements. Byrne and colleagues[10] showed that $TcPO_2$ levels in claudicants decreased during exercise. Increases in $TcPO_2$ following revascularization procedures have also been documented,[30-32] suggesting that an improvement in cellular oxygenation may be related to an increase in arterial inflow. These studies lend support for the idea that limb viability and wound healing may be correlated with $TcPO_2$ in patients with CLI.

A prospective study of lower extremity amputations by Malone and colleagues[33] found that a $TcPO_2$ measurement greater than 20 mmHg was predictive of healing. Wutschert and Bounameaux[34] more recently reported primary healing in 80% of cases with a value greater than 20 mmHg. Burgess and colleagues[35] found that $TcPO_2$ measurements above 40 mmHg always predicted stump healing in below-knee amputations, but measurements from 0 to 40 mmHg were not predictive. Ray and colleagues[36] studied a series of patients undergoing vascular reconstruction, and found that $TcPO_2$ measurements above 33.5 mmHg were predictive of symptomatic improvement, whereas measurements below 19 mmHg were predictive of a lack of improvement or the need for a subsequent amputation. Ubbink and colleagues[37] reported that CLI patients with $TcPO_2$ measurements at or below 10 mmHg would require an amputation within 18 months.

The prediction of healing outcome with $TcPO_2$ values ranging from 10 to 40 mmHg suffers from the same limitations as healing prediction with SPP. Some of the discrepancy is caused by differing sensitivity and calibration of the instruments from various manufacturers, but the wide range of values is also related to the way the clinical question is analyzed: a prediction of healing is different than a prediction of nonhealing. As will be discussed in the following, $TcPO_2$ measurements tend to be reliable when they are in the normal range but are not reliable when they are low. High $TcPO_2$ levels may reliably predict healing success, but low readings are not predictive.[38]

Therefore, $TcPO_2$ as a test of CLI appears to generate an unacceptable number of false-positive test results (i.e., $TcPO_2$ falsely indicates the presence of CLI). Numerous attempts to improve the predictive value of this test have been made. For example, studies have shown that patients with low $TcPO_2$ measurements (less than 10 mmHg) at the level of amputation would nevertheless heal provided that the $TcPO_2$ value would increase by at least 10 mmHg after oxygen inhalation.[39-41] A study by McCollum and colleagues[42] showed that the rate of change of $TcPO_2$ during oxygen inhalation was more predictive, and that at least 9 mmHg/min was needed for healing to occur. The use of an oxygen challenge in some form may be beneficial for improving the diagnostic accuracy of $TcPO_2$ for CLI.

Another method proposed to improve the usefulness of $TcPO_2$ measurements is to perform testing with differing elevations of the patient's leg. Supine, sitting, and leg elevated positions have been recommended.[43-45] Unfortunately, these maneuvers require serial testing with instrument and patient stabilization for each position, which further extends the time required for testing.

The measurement of $TcPO_2$ to select patients for HBO therapy is commonly done. $TcPO_2$ is particularly well suited to determine whether HBO therapy will increase oxygenation of the affected extremity. Patients with CLI are not usually good candidates for HBO therapy. $TcPO_2$ should be measured after breathing oxygen for the patient in the HBO chamber in order to confirm that elevating arterial PO_2 will result in greater oxygen delivery to the skin.[38]

In spite of numerous clinical studies on $TcPO_2$ there remains skepticism about whether it is reliable as a test of perfusion in the diagnosis of CLI. A recent study to compare the relative reproducibility of $TcPO_2$ vs. blood pressure measurements concluded that it is only moderately reproducible, in contrast to blood pressure measurements, which were found to be well reproducible.[43] In a review of the clinical literature, Fronek[39] found it "difficult to explain the relatively wide range of critical $TcPO_2$ values."

Methodology and Limitations of $TcPO_2$

Measurement of $TcPO_2$ with commercially available instruments requires first the setup of a calibration device, which may include a gas cylinder to provide a known concentration of oxygen (room air is commonly used instead). The sensor, with its heater, must be allowed to reach the desired operating temperature (typically 42 to 44 °C), after which it is placed in the calibration device for a few minutes. Calibration adjustments are then made to the system as needed.

The skin site must be cleaned and degreased, and also shaved if necessary to ensure an airtight seal between the sensor and the skin. A small amount of contact gel is applied to the sensor face, and then adhesive tape is attached; this acts to seal out room air and fix the sensor to the skin. Once the sensor is in place and the heater is turned on, the instrument takes about 30 minutes to give a measurement. This is the time required for the heater to elevate the skin temperature and then for the oxygen diffusion to reach a steady-state condition (Fig. 23-6).

A membrane and electrolyte fluid, which cover the Clark-type electrode, must also be replaced every 1 to 3 days, depending on usage.

The skin site selection is very important because of the requirement for good capillary bloodflow and also for an airtight seal around the sensor. Bony prominences, fatty tissue, areas with edema, hairy skin, and callused or thickened skin must all be avoided. Toe measurements are generally not feasible because the sensor needs a larger flat surface to achieve an airtight seal. Measurements of $TcPO_2$ are typically done where the skin thickness is minimal (e.g., the foot dorsum and the lateral or medial aspects of the lower leg). A reference measurement on the chest area is often taken; this allows for the calculation of an index.

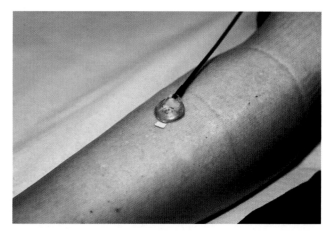

Figure 23-6. *The $TcPO_2$ electrode in some instruments consists of a sensor in a heated probe that is placed in a contact gel solution. Other $TcPO_2$ instruments do not require a holder for the probe to contain a gel solution and are easier to apply to skin sites.*

Conclusions

Both SPP and $TcPO_2$ measurements have been suggested for diagnostic testing of the microcirculation of patients with CLI. Neither is a substitute for conventional vascular examinations to identify occlusive arterial disease, but if such investigations indicate the possibility of CLI, then these methods can be employed to provide additional needed information for determining the best clinical treatment.

SPP investigations are easy to perform and interpret and can be used to determine if segmental systolic pressures measured with noninvasive conventional lower extremity arterial examination are falsely elevated. Reported studies show good agreement regarding the measurement threshold below which CLI is likely to be present. The sensitivity and specificity for determining the presence of CLI are both very high. These tests can be beneficially performed on all types of patients regardless of their skin conditions, provided some area of intact skin is available at the area of interest. Further, SPP can be used to test the reliability of standard noninvasive arterial examination in patients with diabetes and suspected arterial calcification.

$TcPO_2$ tests are also easy to interpret, but performance of the test is often problematic. Patients with abnormal skin conditions, which are very common among the CLI population, generally cannot be measured reliably because of the effects of low perfusion levels and the oxygen diffusion impairment in thickened and edemic skin. Published reports show a wide range of $TcPO_2$ values in CLI, and as a result the specificity and predictive value are decreased. Most errors with this method cause an underestimation of the actual $TcPO_2$ level.

The utility of $TcPO_2$ measurements is better for evaluating patients who could benefit from HBO treatment.

Patients with normal TcPO$_2$ levels, or who demonstrate a response to an oxygen challenge, are more likely to respond to HBO treatment. Low TcPO$_2$ levels after O$_2$ challenge, while not predictive of CLI, may nevertheless be predictive of a failure to benefit from HBO therapy.

When microcirculatory investigations are required for clinical treatment decisions, the predictive value of the method should be considered. For determining whether the presence of CLI will cause wound healing failure in chronic ulcers or at an amputation site, SPP measurements give more specific and reliable information. If the TcPO$_2$ is high, CLI can probably be ruled out, but low TcPO$_2$ readings are not predictive. SPP can also be used to identify unreliable ankle systolic pressures.

REFERENCES

1. Dormandy JA, Rutherford RB: Management of peripheral arterial disease (PAD). TransAtlantic Inter-Society Consensus (TASC). J Vasc Surg 31:1(2), 2000.
2. McDermott MM, et al: Leg symptoms in peripheral artery disease. JAMA 386:1599–1606, 2001.
3. Holstein P, Sager P, Lassen NA: Wound healing in below-knee amputations in relation to skin perfusion pressure. Acta Orthop Scand 50:49–58, 1979.
4. Holstein P, Lassen NA: Healing of ulcers of the feet correlation with distal blood pressure measurements in occlusive arterial disease. Acta Orthop Scand 51:995–1006, 1980.
5. Faris I, Duncan H: Skin perfusion pressure in the prediction of healing in diabetic patients with ulcers or gangrene of the foot. J Vasc Surg 2:536–540, 1985.
6. Castronuovo JJ Jr, Adera HM, Smiell JM, Price RM: Skin perfusion pressure measurement is valuable in the diagnosis of critical limb ischemia. J Vasc Surg 26:629–637, 1997.
7. Ohta T: Noninvasive technique using thallium-201 for predicting ischemic ulcer healing of the foot. Br J Surg 72:892–895, 1985.
8. Matsen FA III, Wyss CR, Pedegana LR, et al: Transcutaneous oxygen tension measurement in peripheral vascular disease. Surg Gynecol Obstet 150:525, 1980.
9. Franzeck UK, Talke P, Bernstein EF: Transcutaneous PO$_2$ measurements in health and peripheral arterial occlusive disease. Surg 91:156–163, 1982.
10. Byrne P, Provan JL, Ameli FM, Jones DP: The use of transcutaneous oxygen tension measurements in the diagnosis of peripheral vascular insufficiency, Ann Surg 200:159–165, 1984.
11. Winsor T, Haumschild DJ, Winsor DW, et al: Clinical application of laser Doppler flowmetry for measurement of cutaneous circulation in health and disease. J Angiol 38(10):727–736, 1987.
12. Belcaro G, Vasdekis S, Rulo A, Nicolaides AN: Evaluation of skin blood flow and venoarteriolar response in patients with diabetes and peripheral vascular disease by laser Doppler flowmetry. Angiol 40(11):953–957, 1989.
13. Fagrell B, Lindberg G: A simplified evaluation of vital capillary microscopy for predicting skin viability in patients with severe arterial insufficiency. Clin Physiol 4:403–411, 1984.
14. Dwars BJ, van den Broeck TAA, Rauwerda JA, Bakker FC: Criteria for reliable selection of the lowest level of amputation in peripheral vascular disease. J Vasc Surg 15:536–542, 1992.
15. Carter SA: The relationship of distal systolic pressures to healing of skin lesions in limbs with arterial occlusive disease, with special reference to diabetes mellitus. Scand J Clin Lab Invest 31(Suppl 128):239, 1973.
16. Carter SA: Indirect systolic pressures and pulse waves in arterial occlusive disease of the lower extremities. Circulation 37:624, 1968.
17. Carter SA: Response of ankle systolic pressure to leg exercise in mild or questionable arterial disease. N Engl J Med 287:578, 1972.
18. Burgess EM, Romano RL, Zettl JH, Schrock RD: Amputations of the leg for peripheral vascular insufficiency. J Bone Joint Surg 53A:874–890, 1971.
19. Nielsen PE, Poulsen HL, Gyntelberg F, et al: Arterial blood pressure in the skin measured by a photoelectric probe and external counterpressure. VASA 2:65–75, 1973.
20. Holstein P: Distal blood pressure as guidance in choice of amputation level. Scand J Clin Lab Invest (Suppl)128:245–248, 1973.
21. Holstein P, Lund P, Larsen B, Schomacker T: Skin perfusion pressure measured as the external pressure required to stop isotope washout. Scand J Clin Lab Invest 37:649–659, 1977.
22. Dwars BJ, Rauwerda JA, van den Broeck TA, et al: A modified scintigrafic technique for amputation level selection in diabetics. Eur J Nucl Med 15:38–41, 1989.
23. Malvezzi L, Castronuovo JJ, Swayne LC, et al: The correlation between three methods of skin perfusion pressure measurement: Radionuclide washout, laser Doppler flow, and photoplethysmography. J Vasc Surg 15:823–830, 1992.
24. Adera HM, James K, Castronuovo JJ, et al: Prediction of amputation wound healing with skin perfusion pressure. J Vasc Surg 21:823–829, 1995.
25. Tsai FW, Tulsyan N, Jones DN, et al: Skin perfusion pressure of the foot is a good substitute for toe pressure in the assessment of limb ischemia. J Vasc Surg 32:32–36, 2000.
26. Rutherford RB, Baker JD, Ernst C, et al: Recommended standards for reports dealing with lower extremity ischemia: Revised version. J Vasc Surg 26:517–538, 1997.
27. Carter SA: Role of Pressure Measurements. In Bernstein EF (ed): Vascular Diagnosis, ed 4. St. Louis: Mosby, 1993.
28. Huch A, Huch R, Lubbers DW: Quantitative polarographische Sauerstoff-druckmessung auf der Kopfhaut des Neugeborenen. Arch Gynakol 207:443–448, 1969.
29. Clyne CAC, Ryan J, Webster JH, Chant AD: Oxygen tension on the skin of ischemic legs. Am J Surg 143:315–318, 1982.
30. White RA, Nolan L, Harley D, et al: Noninvasive evaluation of peripheral vascular disease using transcutaneous oxygen tension. Am J Surg 144:68–72, 1982.
31. Moosa HH, Peitzman AB, Makaroun MS, et al: Transcutaneous oxygen measurements in lower extremity ischemia: Effects of position, oxygen inhalation, and arterial reconstruction. Surgery 103:193–198, 1988.
32. Ubbink DT, Tulevski II, de Graaf JC, et al: Optimisation of the noninvasive assessment of critical limb ischemia requiring invasive treatment. Eur J Vasc Endovasc Surg 19:131–137, 2000.
33. Malone JM, Anderson GG, Lalka SG, et al: Prospective comparison of noninvasive techniques for amputation level selection. Am J Surg 154:179–184, 1987.
34. Wutschert R, Bounameaux H: Determination of amputation level in ischemic limbs: Reappraisal of the measurement of TcPO$_2$. Diabetes Care 20:1315–1318, 1997.
35. Burgess EM, Matsen FA, Wyss CR, Simmons CW: Segmental transcutaneous measurements of PO$_2$ in patients requiring BK amputation for peripheral vascular insufficiency. J Bone Joint Surg 64A:378–382, 1982.
36. Ray SA, Buckenham TM, Belli AM, et al: The predictive value of laser Doppler fluxmetry and transcutaneous oximetry for clinical outcome in patients undergoing revascularization for severe leg ischaemia. Eur J Vasc Endovasc Surg 13:54–59, 1997.
37. Ubbink DT, Spincemaille GH, Reneman RS, Jacobs MJ: Prediction of imminent amputation in patients with nonreconstructable leg ischaemia by means of microcirculatory investigations. J Vasc Surg 30:114–121, 1999.

38. Grolman RE, Wilkerson DK, Taylor J: Transcutaneous oxygen measurements predict a beneficial response to hyperbaric oxygen therapy in patients with nonhealing wounds and critical limb ischemia. Am Surg 67:1072–1079, 2001.

39. Fronek A: Clinical Experience With Transcutaneous P_{O_2} and P_{CO_2} Measurements. In Bernstein EF (ed): Vascular Diagnosis, ed 4. St. Louis: Mosby, 1993.

40. Harward TRS, Volny J, Golbranson F, et al: Oxygen inhalation-induced transcutaneous P_{O_2} changes as a predictor of amputation level. J Vasc Surg 2:220–227, 1985.

41. Oishi C, Fronek A, Golbranson FL: The role of noninvasive vascular studies in determining levels of amputation. Am J Bone Joint Surg 70:1520–1530, 1988.

42. McCollum PT, Spence VA, Walker WF: Oxygen inhalation induced changes in the skin as measured by transcutaneous oximetry. Br J Surg 73:882–885, 1986.

43. de Graff JC, Ubbink DT, Legemate DA, et al: Interobserver and intraobserver reproducibility of peripheral blood and oxygen pressure measurements in the assessment of lower extremity arterial disease. J Vasc Surg 33:1033–1040, 2001.

44. Scheffler A, Rieger H: A comparative analysis of transcutaneous oximetry (TcPO$_2$) during oxygen inhalation and leg dependency in severe peripheral arterial occlusive disease. J Vasc Surg 16:218–224, 1992.

45. Bacharach JM, Rooke TW, Osmundson PJ, Gloviczki P: Predictive value of transcutaneous oxygen pressure and amputation success by use of supine and elevation measurements. J Vasc Surg 15:558–563, 1992.

Chapter 24

Vascular Trauma: The Role of Noninvasive Testing

DOUGLAS B. HOOD • FRED A. WEAVER

Introduction

As with all areas of vascular disease, the diagnosis of peripheral vascular trauma has undergone significant evolution as the technology for noninvasive imaging has improved. A minority of patients with arterial trauma present with classic findings such as hemorrhage or frank limb ischemia, and in these patients the diagnosis is obvious. However, the identification of occult arterial injuries is more challenging, and it is for this group that the diagnostic algorithm has changed most significantly. Because of the low yield of routine operative exploration and of routine arteriography for the evaluation of penetrating wounds in proximity to major vessels, many authors now recommend the selective application of diagnostic imaging techniques based on the results of clinical examination and noninvasive pressure determinations. This chapter will review the authors' approach to the diagnosis of peripheral arterial injuries.

The management of vascular injuries since the time of the Korean War has taught that not all arterial injuries require operative intervention. Diagnostic emphasis has shifted from identification of all arterial injuries, no matter how minor, to identifying only those injuries that are clinically significant and require therapeutic intervention. The goal is to design a diagnostic algorithm for arterial trauma with maximum sensitivity and specificity while minimizing the use of invasive and costly angiography. Achievement of this goal requires a thorough understanding of the strengths and limitations of each of the diagnostic modalities and acceptance of the premise that some small, nonocclusive arterial injuries ("minimal injuries") will heal without intervention and therefore need not be identified and treated.

Doppler Indices

Two studies performed at the authors' institution have addressed these concerns. The first was performed to determine the diagnostic and therapeutic yield of arteriography when routinely performed for proximity alone, as well as for other signs more directly suggestive of arterial injury.[1] Over an 18-month period, 373 patients with a unilateral penetrating injury to an upper or lower extremity were studied prospectively. Patients with a penetrating injury distal to the deltopectoral groove or inguinal ligament underwent arteriography if a distal pulse deficit, neurologic deficit, hematoma, history of hemorrhage or hypotension, bruit, fracture, major soft-tissue injury, or delayed capillary refill was present. Arteriography was also performed in the absence of these findings if the path of the penetrating object was judged by the admitting surgeon to be in proximity to a major neurovascular bundle. Patients with bilateral penetrating injuries, injuries outside the defined anatomic boundaries, or arterial injuries that required immediate operation because of severe limb ischemia or active hemorrhage were excluded from study. Before arteriography, the wounding agent (e.g., stab wound, gunshot wound, or shotgun wound) was noted. Physical findings including bruit; pulse deficit; hematoma; associated fracture; major soft-tissue destruction; neurologic deficit (e.g., sensory, motor, combined, or glove distribution); or decreased capillary refill were assessed in all patients. In 210 of the 373 patients, the posterior tibial/dorsalis pedis or radial/ulnar Doppler pressures of the injured and contralateral uninjured extremity were obtained and indexed using the brachial Doppler pressure of an uninjured arm as a reference (ankle-arm/brachial index [ABI]). The minimum ABI (MABI), defined as the lower of the two ABIs at the ankle or wrist, was recorded.

Arteriograms were interpreted as "normal" or "injured." If an injury was seen, the affected arterial segment was identified. All arterial injuries were then classified as "major" or "minor." Major injuries were injuries to arterial segments that, if interrupted, would likely result in clinically significant limb ischemia (e.g., the superficial femoral artery). All other arterial injuries were termed minor. The arterial injuries were further classified as an intimal defect, intimal flap, pseudoaneurysm, arteriovenous fistula, stenosis, or occlusion. Therapy was based on the clinical and arteriographic findings and included observation, arteriographic embolization, arterial ligation, or repair.

Of the 373 patients enrolled in this study, 216 presented with one or more of the abnormal physical findings listed above. Arterial injuries were identified arteriographically in 65 (30%) of these 216 patients. Proximity alone was the indication for arteriography in the remaining 157 patients, with arterial injuries identified in 17 (11%). Data analysis revealed that a pulse deficit or neurologic deficit noted on physical examination and injury with a shotgun correlated significantly ($p < 0.05$) with arteriographic evidence of arterial injury, major or minor. The presence of one or more of these variables identified a high-risk group of 104 patients with 40 injuries (38%). Of those 40 injuries, 15 required repair or embolization and 25 were observed. An intermediate-risk group was identified with a 20% (33/165) incidence of arterial injury. The intermediate-risk group consisted of those patients with an MABI less than 1.00 or with "soft" signs of arterial injury (e.g., fracture, hematoma, bruit, decreased capillary refill, history of hemorrhage, hypotension, or soft-tissue injury). Five of 33 injuries in the intermediate-risk group required intervention. A low-risk group of 104 patients with none of the above findings remained. Nine injuries (9%) were identified in this low-risk group, none of which required intervention.

A policy of performing arteriography exclusively for intermediate- and high-risk groups and eliminating proximity alone as an indication would have identified 89% of all injuries in this study and 100% of injuries that required intervention. Nearly one third of the arteriograms performed in this study could have been eliminated without significant risk to a single patient. This study confirmed that by relying on a careful clinical examination and readily available, simple, noninvasive ABI testing, arteriography for the evaluation of penetrating extremity trauma could be more precisely applied.

To confirm the reliability of this risk classification scheme and to further investigate the role of the Doppler index in detecting clinically occult arterial injuries, a subsequent prospective study was performed with another consecutive cohort of patients with unilateral, isolated. penetrating extremity trauma.[2] Arteriography was performed for all patients in the previously identified high-risk group (i.e., with pulse deficit, neurologic deficit, or shotgun injury) and in the intermediate-risk group (i.e., one or more "soft" signs or an MABI < 1.00). Arteriography was not performed for those patients in the low-risk group (no "hard" or "soft" signs with an MABI (1.00). Low-risk patients were observed in the hospital for 24 hours and then were monitored as outpatients.

Some 514 consecutive patients were initially assessed. Excluded from this analysis were 22 (4%) patients with obvious limb-threatening ischemia who required immediate operation and 23 (4%) patients who refused arteriography. Of the remaining 469 patients, 276 (59%) had lower extremity injuries and 193 (41%) had upper extremity injuries. Some 213 patients (45%) were determined to be at low risk, 151 (32%) at intermediate risk, and 105 (23%) at high risk for arterial injury.

No clinical findings indicative of arterial injury developed in any of the patients in the low-risk group during the 24-hour observation period. In addition, no clinical signs were apparent during follow-up visits in 78 (37%) of these patients from 1 to 8 weeks (median 2.5 weeks) after discharge. Arteriography identified injuries in 39 of 151 patients (26%) in the intermediate-risk group and 38 of 105 patients (36%) in the high-risk group. A total of 24 major and 53 minor injuries were found. Multivariate analysis showed that only pulse deficit and an MABI less than 1.00 were found to significantly ($p < 0.05$) correlate with all (major and minor) injuries and with major injuries alone. All major injuries except one had an MABI less than 1.00 (sensitivity 23 of 24 or 96%). Five major injuries that required therapeutic intervention (i.e., surgical repair or transcatheter embolization) had an MABI of 0.90 or greater. For the identification of major injuries, an MABI less than 1.00 had a sensitivity of 96%, specificity of 30%, positive predictive value of 12%, negative predictive value of 99%, and overall accuracy of 36%. Compared to lower cutoff values, an MABI less than 1.00 was the most sensitive indicator of injury with the highest negative predictive value; however, it was also the least specific as a result of a large number of false-positive readings. Because it is critical to identify these injuries, which may cause significant morbidity, the authors feel it is best to select the cutoff value with the highest sensitivity and tacitly accept the trade-off in specificity.

The findings of this second study further strengthened the argument that a careful physical examination and the judicious use of Doppler indices can accurately select those patients with penetrating extremity trauma who should be subjected to arteriography. On the basis of these findings, the following diagnostic algorithm can be constructed. Patients with penetrating extremity injuries who have a normal pulse examination and an MABI of 1.00 or greater do not require diagnostic arteriography. A brief period of observation is all that is necessary. Because all significant, clinically occult arterial injuries are found in extremities that have a distal pulse deficit, an MABI less than 1.00, or both, it is in this group of patients that diagnostic arteriography is indicated and will have its greatest yield.

These indications for arteriography for penetrating trauma are equally applicable to blunt extremity trauma. Another prospective study from the authors' institution analyzed the results of arteriography in 53 patients with unilateral blunt lower extremity trauma.[3] Thirty-one patients presented with physical findings suggestive of arterial injury; in 22 patients, the presence of a fracture, knee dislocation, or significant soft-tissue injury without other suggestive findings was the indication for arteriography. Arterial injuries were demonstrated in 15 patients. A pulse deficit or decreased capillary refill was shown to significantly correlate ($p < 0.05$) with arteriographic evidence of injury. Arterial injuries were found in 12 of 31 patients (39%) with one or both of these findings; 4 of those injuries required repair. In the 22 patients with neither a pulse deficit nor decreased capillary refill, 3 minor injuries were found, none of which required repair. ABIs were determined in 27 of the 53 patients. An ABI less than 1.00 identified arterial injuries with a sensitivity of 100% and a specificity of 26% in this series.

Similar evidence for the reliability of the clinical examination combined with noninvasive pressure determination has been provided by other authors. Johansen and colleagues reported a series of 100 limbs that had sustained blunt or penetrating trauma.[4,5] All patients underwent ABI determination and arteriography. Arterial injuries requiring intervention were discovered in 14 cases. An ABI less than 0.90 predicted arteriographic evidence of injury with 87% sensitivity and 97% specificity.

Minimal Injuries

Although careful physical examination and pressure measurements will appropriately select which patients have a higher likelihood of significant arterial injury and should therefore undergo further diagnostic testing (usually with arteriography), there are some minor injuries that will be missed by adhering to such a policy of selective arteriography. Injuries that may be missed are generally not clinically important and include injuries to minor branch vessels and some nonocclusive injuries of major vessels. Many of these nonocclusive injuries will heal without specific intervention. The healing power of these minimal, nonocclusive injuries has been likened to that of the puncture site for percutaneous vascular catheterization and to the extensive intimal disruption that occurs with balloon angioplasty. In the authors' experience, the following "minimal" injuries may be safely observed, provided that the wounding agent is low velocity, the distal circulation is intact, and no active hemorrhage is present: intimal defects or pseudoaneurysms of less than 5 mm, and intimal flaps that are adherent or protrude downstream.

The authors' initial experience with selective management of 50 patients with 61 minimal injuries has been previously reported.[6] Included in that report were 44 injuries of major arteries: 12 in the cerebrovascular system, 11 in the upper extremities, and 20 in the lower extremities. Some 17 injuries occurred in minor arteries. All patients were initially managed nonoperatively. Repeat arteriography was performed from 1 to 3 weeks after the injury in 40 patients; 21 patients were observed clinically without repeat study. Percutaneous transcatheter embolization of noncritical branch arteries was performed at the time of repeat arteriography for the treatment of 5 pseudoaneurysms and 5 arteriovenous fistulae. Of the 24 injuries to major arteries that were evaluated with serial arteriography, 21 (88%) had healed or were stable and asymptomatic and 3 had progressed. Those that progressed were all small pseudoaneurysms that enlarged and were then treated. None of these injuries resulted in delayed hemorrhage or thrombosis. Although this study documented that the majority of "minimal" injuries will heal on their own, careful follow-up with repeat clinical examination, arteriography, and/or color-flow duplex scanning is essential. Nonoperative management is a reasonable option only in carefully selected patients. During the past 10 years, the authors have continued a policy of nonoperative management of minimal injuries without any evidence of delayed complications. Similar results for the nonoperative management of "minimal" injuries have been reported by Frykberg and colleagues.[7,8]

Color-Flow Duplex

Color-flow duplex ultrasonography (CFD) has been evaluated as a potential alternative to arteriography for the diagnosis of occult arterial trauma. There are several potential advantages of CFD: It is noninvasive; the patient morbidity rate is virtually 0%; the necessary equipment is portable and can be brought to the bedside, emergency room, or operating room; it is easily repeatable; and it is relatively inexpensive. However, there is some controversy regarding the ability of CFD to detect all arterial injuries. Bynoe and colleagues reported a sensitivity of 95%, specificity of 99%, and accuracy of 98% for CFD when used to evaluate blunt and penetrating injuries of the neck or extremities.[9] However, because confirmatory arteriography was not performed in this study when results of CFD were normal, false-negative results of CFD may have been underestimated and the sensitivity may have been overestimated. A report by Fry and colleagues reporting 100% sensitivity and 97.3% specificity of CFD suffered from a similar flaw; arteriography for confirmation of CFD results was performed for only 50 of 200 patients with 225 extremity injuries.[10] Bergstein and colleagues published a series of 67 patients with 75 penetrating injuries to the extremities without obvious arterial injury.[11] All patients underwent both CFD and arteriography. Compared with arteriography, there were 2 false-negative and 1 false-positive results of CFD, resulting in a sensitivity of 50% and specificity of 99%. The authors of that report stated that CFD is most likely to be of value in the evaluation of injuries to the thigh and arm, followed by the forearm and then the calf. The accuracy of CFD in the thoracic outlet, axilla, and calf was considered questionable. Gagne and colleagues published a small series of 37 patients with proximity injuries in 43 extremities.[12] Arteriography identified 3 injuries, 1 each in the profunda femoris, superficial femoral, and posterior tibial arteries. None of these 3 injuries was identified with CFD. CFD did detect an intimal flap in the superficial femoral artery that was not identified with arteriography. Hence, in that study, CFD and arteriography were complementary in their ability to detect arterial injuries. Interestingly, in this last study, 22% of extremities were found to have isolated occult venous injuries that would not be detected arteriographically. Despite some uncertainty regarding the ability of CFD to detect all vascular injuries, it seems that nearly all major injuries that require therapeutic intervention can be identified, and this modality continues to be advocated by a number of authors for the evaluation of potential peripheral vascular injuries.[13,14]

Perhaps the least controversial application of CFD to the management of vascular trauma is the use of this modality for the serial examination of "minimal" injuries that do not require immediate intervention but do require repeat imaging to document healing. The authors' experience with CFD in the evaluation of extremity trauma is that this is a highly operator-dependent examination that requires the immediate availability of both experienced technologists and experienced interpreters to be reliable.[15] Because trauma commonly occurs outside of the hours of the usual business day, these personnel are not always present, and CFD has not been widely adopted as a primary modality for the diagnosis of vascular injury.

Conclusions

In summary, the evaluation of occult extremity arterial trauma has evolved from routine operative exploration to the selective use of ancillary diagnostic testing based on risk stratification criteria. The criteria that are most useful at present are an abnormal pulse examination and reduction of the Doppler-derived pressure index. Patients with either of these findings are most reliably evaluated with arteriography, although noninvasive color-flow duplex scanning has proven reliable enough in centers experienced with this technique to supplant arteriography.

REFERENCES

1. Weaver FA, Yellin AE, Bauer M, et al: Is arterial proximity a valid indication for arteriography in penetrating extremity trauma? Arch Surg 125:1256–1260, 1990.
2. Schwartz MR, Weaver FA, Bauer M, et al: Refining the indications for arteriography in penetrating extremity trauma: A prospective analysis. J Vasc Surg 17:116–124, 1993.
3. Applebaum R, Yellin AE, Weaver FA, et al: Role of routine arteriography in blunt lower-extremity trauma. Am J Surg 160:221–225, 1990.
4. Johansen K, Lynch K, Paun M, et al: Noninvasive vascular tests reliably exclude occult arterial trauma in injured extremities. J Trauma 31:515–522, 1991.
5. Lynch K, Johansen K: Can Doppler pressure measurement replace "exclusion" arteriography in the diagnosis of occult extremity arterial trauma? Ann Surg 214:737–741, 1991.
6. Stain SC, Yellin AE, Weaver FA, et al: Selective management of nonocclusive arterial injuries. Arch Surg 124:1136–1141, 1989.
7. Frykberg ER, Crump JM, Dennis JW, et al: Nonoperative observation of clinically occult arterial injuries: A prospective evaluation. Surgery 109:85–96, 1991.
8. Dennis JW, Frykberg ER, Vendenz HC, et al: Validation of nonoperative management of occult vascular injuries and accuracy of physical examination in penetrating extremity trauma: 5- to 10-year follow-up. J Trauma 44:243–253, 1998.
9. Bynoe RP, Miles WS, Bell RM, et al: Noninvasive diagnosis of vascular trauma by duplex ultrasonography. J Vasc Surg 14:346–352, 1991.
10. Fry WR, Smith RS, Sayers DV, et al: The success of duplex ultrasonographic scanning in diagnosis of extremity vascular proximity trauma. Arch Surg 128:1368–1372, 1993.
11. Bergstein JM, Blair J, Edwards J, et al: Pitfalls in the use of color-flow duplex ultrasound for screening of suspected arterial injuries in penetrated extremities. J Trauma 33:395–402, 1992.

12. Gagne PJ, Cone JB, McFarland D, et al: Proximity penetrating extremity trauma: The role of duplex ultrasound in the detection of occult venous injuries. J Trauma 39:1157–1163, 1995.

13. Knudson MM, Lewis FR, Atkinson K, et al: The role of duplex ultrasound arterial imaging in patients with penetrating extremity trauma. Arch Surg 128:1033–1038, 1993.

14. Meissner M, Paun M, Johansen K: Duplex scanning for arterial trauma. Am J Surg 161:552–555, 1991.

15. Schwartz M, Weaver F, Yellin A, et al: The utility of color-flow Doppler examination in penetrating extremity arterial trauma. Am Surg 59:375–378, 1993.

Chapter 25

Guiding Endovascular Interventions with Color-Flow Scanning

KENNETH K. KAO • SAMUEL S. AHN

- Background
- Validation Studies
- Benefits
- Limitations
- What Information Does It Give You?
- How Does This Information Influence Your Treatment?
- Conclusions

Background

B-mode ultrasonography is a noninvasive diagnostic tool that generates images from differential tissue reflection of high-frequency sound waves (2 to 10 MHz). In addition to anatomic representations, hemodynamic images can be derived using the principle of Doppler shift. This principle mathematically describes the change in the detected frequency of a sound wave originating from a moving source. In the case of bloodflow, red blood cells act as a reflective interface for sound waves. Cells moving towards a detector will increase the frequency of the reflected wave, whereas their motion away will decrease it. When the angle of incidence is known, these changes in frequency can then be used to calculate bloodflow velocity.

Continuous-wave Doppler ultrasound provides hemo-dynamic information by simultaneously transmitting and detecting sound waves and then generating an audio waveform from the data. This method provides an average measurement of all fluid motion within the path of the sound waves. Thus rather than processing data from specific regions within a given vessel, it provides a single velocity reading for the entire cross-section being scanned. Conversely, pulsed Doppler alternately transmits and detects sound waves. By varying transmission and detection times, a sample area can be defined. This method permits more definite localization within the scanned region, thereby providing more detailed information (e.g., bloodflow pattern within the vessel) that can be examined by spectral waveform analysis.

Normal arterial Doppler waveforms are pulsatile with a triphasic flow pattern. The initial forward-flow component is of greatest magnitude and represents systolic flow. The ensuing reverse-flow component occurs during diastole, and the final forward-flow component represents bloodflow secondary to arterial resistance. Proximal to a stenotic lesion, a pattern of high-resistance flow is illustrated by an increase in the reverse-flow component. Distal to a region of stenosis the spectral waveform is dampened, with reduced amplitude, delayed peaks, and attenuated reverse-flow. Regions with biphasic flow are considered normal unless proximal patterns were already characterized as triphasic. If monophasic waveforms are seen, some proximal occlusive disease should be suspected.

The continuity equation for steady one-dimensional flow states that with a constant volume flow through a vessel, any reduction in the cross-sectional area would result in a compensatory increase in fluid velocity after the point of constriction. Thus stenotic lesions may be identified by a relative velocity increase across the site in question. In order to determine the percent stenosis, peak systolic flow velocity is recorded at the nearest proximal point of normal bloodflow and at that of maximal velocity; the ratio of peak systolic velocity (PSV) between these two readings, in turn, correlates with a percent vessel stenosis.

PSV Ratio = Intrastenotic PSV / Prestenotic PSV

Ratios of 2.0 and 4.0 are interpreted as at least 50% or 75% reduction in lumen diameter, respectively.[1-5] Typically, a ratio of 2.5 indicates a hemodynamically significant stenosis of at least 50%.[6]

Doppler spectral waveforms are limited in that the reading alone does not provide any information applicable to plaque characterization. Furthermore, sampling volumes cannot be targeted to specific regions within the vessel without anatomic visual guidance. Duplex scanning overcomes this limitation by combining pulsed Doppler detection with B-mode ultrasonography. The B-mode image may be used to identify anatomic variations, plaque structure, and vessel wall thickening or calcification. Furthermore, the gray scale image can be used to localize a Doppler sample volume within the target vessel, whereas the local flow pattern is assessed by spectral waveform analysis.

Color-coded scanning may be used in place of spectral waveform analysis to obtain qualitative flow information. This system, rather than presenting velocity data as a waveform, generates a pictorial representation of flow velocity and direction within the gray scale B-mode image. Flow toward the scanning head may be denoted with red, whereas flow away may be indicated with blue. The velocity magnitude is signified by changes in hue; high-flow and low-flow areas are shaded more lightly and darkly, respectively. Thus color-velocity hemodynamic information is superimposed in real-time on stationary gray scale B-mode images of lesions and vessels (Figs. 25-1 through 25-7). This visual inter-

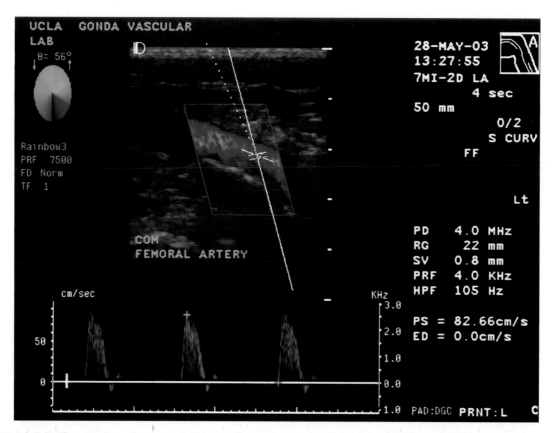

Figure 25-1. Color-flow duplex of a normal common femoral artery with triphasic Doppler signal and normal peak systolic velocity (PSV) for this segment.

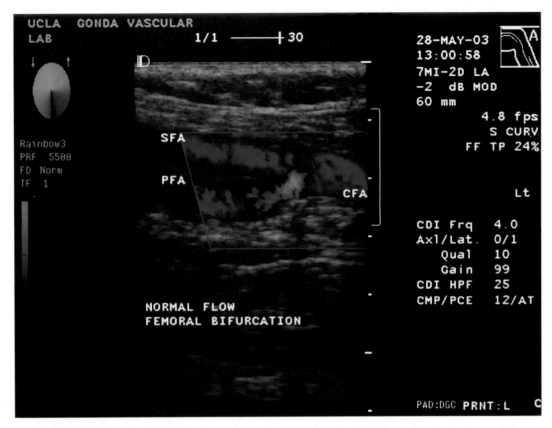

Figure 25-2. *Color-flow duplex of a normal common femoral artery showing the bifurcation with origins of the superficial and profunda femoral artery (PFA).*

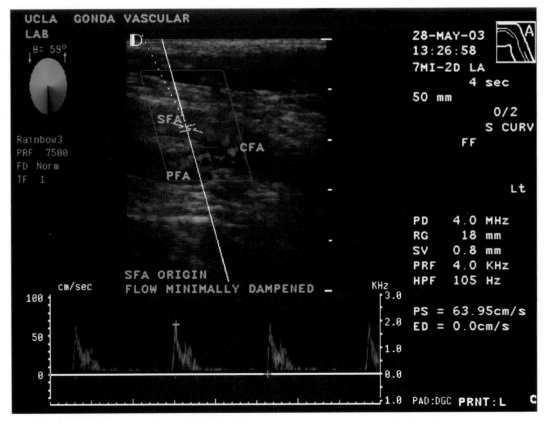

Figure 25-3. *Color-flow image of some dampening of flow in proximal superficial femoral artery.*

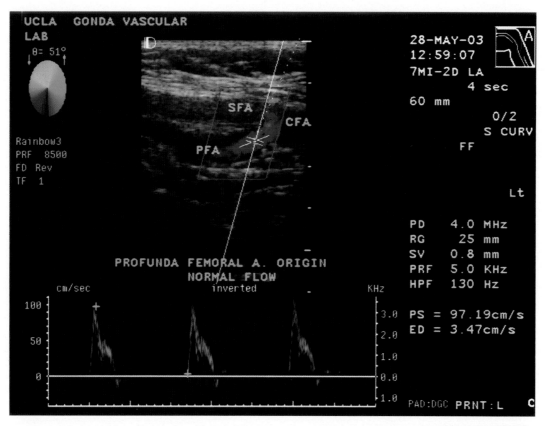

Figure 25-4. Color-flow image of a femoral bifurcartion showing complete occlusion of the superficial femoral artery (SFA) with no color within the artery, and normal flow in the profunda.

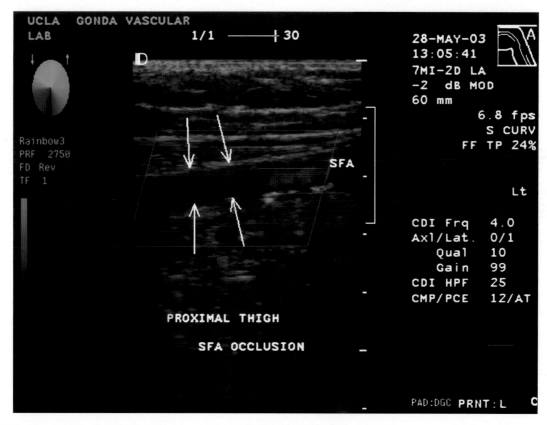

Figure 25-5. Image of occluded superficial femoral artery (SFA) in mid-thigh.

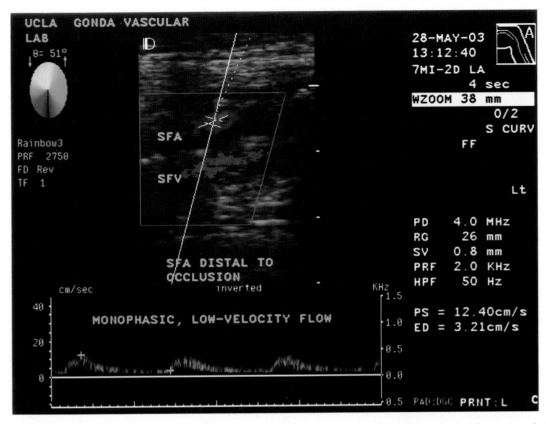

Figure 25-6. *Monophasic flow with low velocity (peak systolic velocity = 12 cm/sec) provide a clue to distal superficial femoral artery (SFA) occlusion just beyond the segment being imaged. Compare normal SFA flow in Figure 25-2.*

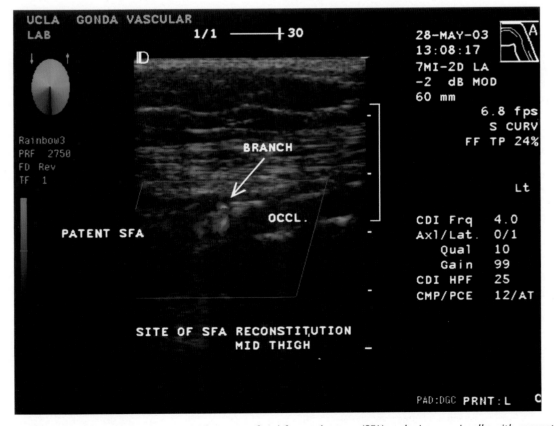

Figure 25-7. *This color-flow image shows complete superficial femoral artery (SFA) occlusion proximally with reconstitution of the distal SFA via a patent collateral.*

pretation permits more rapid localization of normal arterial flow, thus reducing examination time. However, because of the limitations of semiquantitative visual representation, more accurate flow data are provided by waveform analysis.[7,8]

Validation Studies

Traditionally, the gold standard of arterial diagnostic examination has been contrast angiography; however, good correlations have been reported between angiography and duplex scanning. Jager and colleagues compared spectral waveform analysis and angiographic data from 338 arterial segments. Sensitivity and specificity for detecting a 50% or greater diameter reduction for duplex scanning were 77% and 98%, respectively, whereas the rates for arteriography were 87% and 94%, respectively.[9] Koelemay and colleagues performed a meta-analysis of 71 studies and found that the sensitivity and specificity of duplex scanning has been excellent.

Scanning of aortoiliac segments revealed a sensitivity of 86% and specificity of 97%, respectively; that of femoropopliteal tracts resulted in a sensitivity of 80% and specificity of 96%, respectively; and that of infrapopliteal segments had a sensitivity of 83% and specificity of 84%, respectively. Other studies have revealed sensitivities and specificities for infrainguinal vessels as a whole ranging from 83% to 100% and 89% to 99%, respectively.[10–13] Agreement between duplex scan and angiography findings in infrainguinal arterial segments have kappa values ranging from 0.59 to 0.94[3–5,7,14,15] (Table 25-1). Kohler and colleagues further examined these correlations by calculating the agreement between surgeons planning lower extremity intervention. A very high intraobserver agreement was found between decisions based on angiogram versus those based on duplex scan (kappa = 0.70), and a significantly smaller interobserver agreement was found (kappa = 0.56). These results concur with previous findings; furthermore, they suggest that variations in operative planning are the consequence of individual decision-making processes rather than differences in duplex or angiogram interpretation.[16]

TABLE 25-1. Summary of Duplex Ultrasound Performance

Author	Year	Modality	*n*	Sensitivity	Specificity	PPV	NPV	Accuracy	Kappa
Overall									
‡Löfberg and colleagues[11]	2001	Duplex vs. Angio	486	86	84	87	86	86	N/A
Ramaswami and colleagues[17]	1999	Duplex vs. Angio	216	91	98	80	99	97	0.92
‡Lai and colleagues[55]	1996	Duplex vs. Angio	38	75	90	77	89	N/A	0.57
‡Bergamini and colleagues[39]	1995	Duplex vs. Angio	80	80	95	88	92	91	N/A
‡Allard and colleagues[40]	1994	Duplex vs. Angio	110	74	96	N/A	N/A	93	N/A
Aortoiliac									
‡Katsamouris and colleagues[14]	2001	Duplex vs. Angio	80	86	90	88	90	88	0.69
*Schneider and colleagues[56]	1998	Duplex vs. Angio	85	100	76	78	100	87	N/A
*Aly and colleagues[13]	1998	Duplex vs. Angio	177	89	99	92	99	N/A	0.81
‡Sensier and colleagues[2]	1996	Duplex vs. Angio	148	65	96				0.59
Common Iliac									
‡Lai and colleagues[55]	1996	Duplex vs. Angio	49	79	80	61	90	N/A	0.46

Continued

TABLE 25-1. Summary of Duplex Ultrasound Performance—cont'd

Author	Year	Modality	n	Sensitivity	Specificity	PPV	NPV	Accuracy	Kappa
‡Allard and colleagues[40]	1994	Duplex vs. Angio	110	84	97	N/A	N/A	93	N/A
External Iliac									
‡Lai and colleagues[55]	1996	Duplex vs. Angio	49	71	83	63	88	N/A	0.48
‡Allard and colleagues[40]	1994	Duplex vs. Angio	110	60	96	N/A	N/A	92	N/A
Femoropopliteal									
‖Boström Ardin and colleagues[10]	2002	Duplex vs. Angio	952	83	92	94	78	89	N/A
‡Katsamouris and colleagues[14]	2001	Duplex vs. Angio	80	99	94	97	99	96	0.89
‡Aly and colleagues[13]	1998	Duplex vs. Angio	177	95	99	94	99	N/A	0.92
‖Lai and colleagues[52]	1995	Duplex vs. Angio	86	61	88	61	86	N/A	N/A
‡Sensier and colleagues[2]	1996	Duplex vs. Angio	148	86	97	N/A	N/A	N/A	0.80
Common Femoral									
‡Mazzariol and colleagues[12]	2000	Duplex vs. Angio	214	100	93	100	100	N/A	N/A
‡Lai and colleagues[55]	1996	Duplex vs. Angio	89	61	99	92	91	N/A	0.50
‡Bergamini and colleagues[39]	1995	Duplex vs. Angio	80	86	96	67	99	95	N/A
‡Karacagil and colleagues[19]	1994	Duplex vs. Angio	68	100	98	80	100	99	N/A
Superficial Femoral									
‡Löfberg and colleagues[11]	2001	Duplex vs. Angio	162	80	94	88	90	90	N/A
‡Allard and colleagues[40]	1994	Duplex vs. Angio	110	92	96	N/A	N/A	94	N/A
‡Karacagil and colleagues[19]	1994	Duplex vs. Angio	68	97	91	92	97	94	N/A
‡Moneta and colleagues[57]	1993	Duplex vs. IAPM	151	95	100	100	92	N/A	N/A
*Hatsukami and colleagues[18]	1992	Duplex vs. Angio	58	85	97	94	92	N/A	N/A
†Hatsukami and colleagues[18]	1992	Duplex vs. Angio	58	97	100	100	99	N/A	N/A
Deep Femoral									
‡Allard and colleagues[40]	1994	Duplex vs. Angio	110	92	44	N/A	N/A	97	N/A

Continued

TABLE 25-1. Summary of Duplex Ultrasound Performance—cont'd

Author	Year	Modality	n	Sensitivity	Specificity	PPV	NPV	Accuracy	Kappa
Popliteal									
‡Löfberg and colleagues[11]	2001	Duplex vs. Angio	162	49	97	83	85	85	N/A
‡Allard and colleagues[40]	1994	Duplex vs. Angio	110	37	92	N/A	N/A	88	N/A
‡Karacagil and colleagues[19]	1994	Duplex vs. Angio	66	89	77	38	98	79	N/A
‡Moneta and colleagues[57]	1993	Duplex vs. IAPM	151	78	99	98	86	N/A	N/A
*Hatsukami and colleagues[18]	1992	Duplex vs. Angio	58	100	92	80	100	N/A	N/A
†Hatsukami and colleagues[18]	1992	Duplex vs. Angio	58	100	93	70	100	N/A	N/A
Tibioperoneal									
‡Katsamouris and colleagues[14]	2001	Duplex vs. Angio	80	80	91	80	89	83	0.59
‡Löfberg and colleagues[11]	2001	Duplex vs. Angio	486	38	95	35	96	91	N/A
‡Karacagil and colleagues[20]	1996	Duplex vs. Angio	40	83	77	79	81	80	N/A
‡Bergamini and colleagues[39]	1995	Duplex vs. Angio	80	25	100	100	83	84	N/A
‡Karacagil and colleagues[19]	1994	Duplex vs. Angio	66	82	67	33	95	70	N/A
Anterior Tibial									
*Hatsukami and colleagues[17]	1992	Duplex vs. Angio	58	86	96	92	92	N/A	N/A
†Hatsukami and colleagues[17]	1992	Duplex vs. Angio	58	83	100	100	93	N/A	N/A
Posterior Tibial									
*Hatsukami and colleagues[17]	1992	Duplex vs. Angio	58	79	96	92	92	N/A	N/A
†Hatsukami and colleagues[17]	1992	Duplex vs. Angio	58	83	100	100	88	N/A	N/A

*Stenosis 50%; †Occlusion; ‡Stenosis 50% or Occlusion; ‖Suitability for PTA; n = number of limbs; PPV = positive predictive value; NPV = negative predictive value; IAPM = intra-arterial pressure measurement.

Duplex scanning provides accurate information for both the aortoiliac and femoropopliteal arterial segments and has been shown to diagnose effectively arterial disease in 80% to 100% of patients.[17-23] Some authors feel that duplex scanning is more accurate than angiography in predicting hemodynamically significant lesions.[23] Because the accuracy of color duplex scanning stems from its presentation of physiologic data in relation to anatomic structures, and contrast angiography provides only 2-dimensional information about vessel diameter in a single plane, numerous authors have suggested replacing percutaneous contrast angiography as a screening tool with duplex ultrasonography in selected patients.[13,15,22–29]

Benefits

Arterial mapping with color-duplex ultrasonography has numerous advantages. First, by using duplex scanning as a screening tool, diagnostic and therapeutic procedures may be combined, thus eliminating multiple angiograms. Second, revascularization strategies can be made in advance. With a roadmap of the diseased arterial segments, puncture site selection and catheterization route can be chosen in advance of intraoperative arteriography. Third, by targeting only diseased segments, both angiography time and contrast use can be reduced.[28]

Color-coded duplex scanning has established itself as a major clinical diagnostic tool because of its accuracy, low risk of complication, ease of repeatability, high patient acceptance, and cost-effectiveness. In contrast to angiography, duplex ultrasonography is risk-free. In one study the major complication rate of arteriography was calculated at 7% (with significant variations based on transaxillary or transfemoral approaches).[29] Most commonly, angiography results in problems such as hematoma, bleeding, adverse reactions to contrast, contrast extravasation, local neurovascular injury, pseudoaneurysm formation, thromboemboli, catheter and guidewire complications, and renal failure.[29–32]

Though avoidance of complications is desirable in all patients, candidates for endovascular procedures in particular may be considered in a separate category for risk aversion. First, those patients selected for percutaneous transluminal angioplasty (PTA) generally suffer from intermittent claudication rather than critical limb ischemia. Thus their lower risk of limb loss warrants a lower-risk diagnostic procedure. Second, the subset of high-risk PTA patients who cannot undergo open revascularization should be further shielded from any additional risks imposed by angiography.[33]

An approximately tenfold difference in cost may be found between angiography and duplex scanning. Excluding ancillary services and indirect costs, at the authors' institution an arterial duplex scan of the lower extremity is billed at $455; the charge for a lower extremity angiogram is $1800. Levy and colleagues analyzed the total hospital costs, with regard to arteriography versus duplex scanning and magnetic resonance arteriography (at another institution in 1998).[33] The savings of using noninvasive modalities was significant; the cost difference between duplex ultrasonography and preoperative angiography was calculated at $551 to $695 per case.[33] Accordingly, some authors suggest that duplex scanning replace angiography as a screening tool for lower extremity arterial disease (Table 25-2).[11,13,22,28,33–37]

TABLE 25-2. Benefits of Color Duplex Scanning

Avoids diagnostic angiography
Permits preoperative planning of catheterization
Reduces angiography time
Reduces contrast use
Provides accurate diagnosis
Noninvasive
Risk-free
Easily repeated
Performance unaffected by multisegment disease
Has high patient acceptance
Cost-effective

Limitations

Some of the limitations of color-flow scanning are linked to the intrinsic shortfalls of ultrasonography. Because the depth of sound-wave tissue penetration varies inversely with wave frequency, and because higher frequencies produce higher resolution images, image quality degrades when deeper structures are scanned. In addition, severe vessel calcification limits sound wave penetration such that images cannot be obtained from these arterial segments. Ramaswami and colleagues described a failure to visualize the iliac arteries in 20% of patients because of various reasons including obesity, bowel gas, abdominal tenderness, chronic obstructive airway disease, and the use of higher resolution transducers (4.5/3.5 MHz).[17] These variables, along with technician skill, have been cited as contributors to reduced diagnostic sensitivity and specificity.

Several authors have reported on the performance of duplex scanning in the presence of multisegment arterial disease, and the results have been varied. An early study by Jager and colleagues stated that the sensitivity, specificity, and accuracy of duplex scanning were unaffected by multiple lesions.[9] Furthermore, Sensier and colleagues analyzed the effect of multisegment disease by examining the concordance between arteriography and duplex scanning in arterial segments adjacent to an area of 50% or greater stenosis. Their results produced kappa values of 0.78 and 0.63 for segments adjacent and nonadjacent to severe stenoses, respectively. They concluded that duplex assessment was not adversely affected by adjacent disease.[38] However, other findings have revealed that low-flow velocities distal to lesions of greater than

50% stenosis (including total occlusions) reduce the performance of duplex scanning.[1,19,39] Allard and colleagues demonstrated that the sensitivity and specificity of duplex scanning in arterial segments without any adjacent lesions of 50% or greater lumen diameter were calculated at 80% and 98%, respectively; with the presence of a severe adjacent stenosis, sensitivity and specificity rates dropped to 66% and 94%, respectively.[40] Given the contrasting viewpoints regarding the effect of multiple lesions on the ability of duplex scanning to detect hemodynamically significant lesions, further investigation is warranted.

Several factors necessitate the continued use of perioperative angiography. In addition to those aforementioned issues (e.g., obesity, vessel calcification, and multiple stenoses), the location of the arterial segment in question has a significant impact on scanning performance. Numerous studies have indicated that duplex scanning alone is not sufficient for evaluation of the crural arteries (Table 25-3).[17,20,21,24,26,41] Moneta and colleagues demonstrated that 17% of the peroneal artery segments seen by angiography could not be seen with duplex scanning.[21] Larch and colleagues hypothesized that the deep location of the peroneal artery, as well as the multiple fascial layers that surround the vessels, may contribute to the imaging difficulties.[42] Several authors suggest that if patency of the tibial or peroneal arteries is questionable after duplex scanning, diagnostic angiography should be performed.[20,43,44] Alternatively, magnetic resonance imaging has been suggested as a preoperative modality to detect lesions below the popliteal artery trifurcation.[45,46]

What Information Does It Give You?

Once lower extremity arterial occlusive disease is suspected, the entire vascular tree from the iliac arteries to the tibioperoneal trunk can be assessed for plaque characterization, lumen diameter, and hemodynamic changes. Nonoccluding stenoses are demonstrated by a pathologic Doppler spectrum with high intrastenotic flow

TABLE 25-3. Limitations of Color Duplex Scanning

Poor visualization of deep structures
Unable to image calcified vessels
Image quality related to patient habitus, bowel preparation
Operator dependent
Reduced performance with multisegment disease
Reduced performance in infragenicular segments

velocities and spectral broadening; waveform analysis of flow patterns reveals prestenotic increased reverse-flow components and poststenotic dampened flow patterns.[47]

In addition to stenosis information, occlusion length can also be derived from duplex scanning.[48] Total occlusions are recognizable by an absence of color-flow signals within the vessel lumen, whereas distal runoff vessels would display a resumption of arterial filling. The segment without flow data thus may be used to approximate occlusion length. This ability proves to be another strength in an area of weakness for angiography. Several studies have found that arteriography inadequately estimates lesion length: both over- and underestimations have been found.[3,49,50] In addition, angiography often fails to visualize arterial segments both proximal and distal to total occlusions. These failures have been ascribed to poor timing, incorrect injection site, hemodynamic variables, and inadequate use of multiplane views.[3,17]

Screening for PTA using duplex scanning alone has been examined in several studies.[10,11,22,49,51,52] Various authors have found that the indication for PTA in patients with lower extremity arterial disease was correct in 84% to 94% of cases screened.[22,28,53] Böstrom-Ardin and colleagues further examined the role of duplex scanning in categorizing lesions as suitable or unsuitable for PTA, and revealed varying levels of accuracy based on the arterial segment. Superficial femoral lesions were correctly selected for PTA in 85% of cases, popliteal lesions in 66%, and crural lesions in 32%.[10] Thus duplex scanning can be used as a screening tool in the lower extremities; however, clinical judgment must still be applied to these findings.

How Does This Information Influence Your Treatment?

The duplex scan may be used to determine whether the patient is a candidate for endovascular intervention. The selection between PTA and surgical reconstruction is based on the location, severity, and length of the lesion in question. A special writing group of The American Heart Association has described morphologic characteristics of those lesions most amenable to angioplasty, and listed them as Category 1 (PTA alone is the procedure of choice); Category 2 (lesions well suited for PTA); Category 3 (lesions treatable with PTA, although a lower chance of initial technical success or long-term benefit is likely); or Category 4 (extensive vascular disease, for which PTA has a very limited role).[54] These categories are summarized in Table 25-4. By utilizing the morphologic, hemodynamic, and topographic information from color-flow duplex scanning to preoperatively determine occlusion length and stenosis, one may determine patient candidacy.

TABLE 25-4. **The American Heart Association Guidelines for Percutaneous Transluminal Angioplasty of the Abdominal Aorta and Lower Extremity Vessels**

Segment	Category 1*	Category 2†	Category 3‡	Category 4‖
Aorta (infrarenal)	Stenosis < 2 cm, with minimal atherosclerotic disease of the aorta otherwise	Stenosis from 2 to 4 cm, with mild atherosclerotic disease of the aorta otherwise	1. Stenosis > 4 cm 2. Stenosis with atheroembolic disease, or 3. Stenosis 2 to 4 cm of the infrarenal aorta with moderate to severe athero-sclerotic disease of the aorta otherwise	1. Occlusion, or 2. Stenosis associated with abdominal aortic aneurysm
Iliac	Stenosis < 3 cm, concentric, and noncalcified	Stenosis 1. 3 to 5 cm, or 2. < 3 cm, calcified or eccentric	1. Stenosis 5 to 10 cm, or 2. Occlusion < 5 cm after thrombolytic therapy	1. Stenosis >10 cm 2. Occlusion > 5 cm after thrombolytic therapy 3. Extensive bilateral aortoiliac atherosclerotic disease is present, or 4. Stenosis associated with abdominal aortic aneurysm
Femoro-popliteal	1. Stenosis 5 cm, and not at the superficial femoral origin or distal popliteal, or 2. Single occlusion 3 cm, not involving the superficial femoral origin or distal popliteal.	1. Stenosis 5–10 cm, not involving the distal popliteal 2. Occlusion 3–10 cm, not involving the distal popliteal 3. Heavily calcified stenosis 5 cm 4. Multiple lesions, either stenoses or occlusions, each < 3 cm, or 5. Single or multiple lesions without continuous tibial runoff	1. Single occlusion 3 to 10 cm 2. Multiple lesions, each 3 to 5 cm 3. Stenosis or occlusion > 10 cm	1. Common or superficial femoral artery occlusion 2. Popliteal and proximal trifurcation occlusion, or 3. Multiple lesions without intervening normal segments
Infrapopliteal	Stenosis 1cm of the tibial or peroneal vessels	1. Multiple focal stenoses, each 1 cm, of the tibial or peroneal vessels 2. One or two focal stenoses, 1 cm, of the tibial trifurcation, or 3. Tibial or peroneal stenosis dilated in combination with femoral popliteal bypass	1. Stenosis 1 to 4 cm or occlusion 1 to 2 cm of tibial or peroneal arteries, or 2. Stenosis of tibial trifurcation	1. Occlusion > 2 cm of tibial or peroneal arteries 2. Diffusely diseased tibial or peroneal arteries

*PTA alone is the procedure of choice; †Lesions well suited for PTA; ‡Lesions treatable with PTA, with a lower chance of initial technical success or long-term benefit; ‖Extensive vascular disease, for which PTA has a very limited role.

Once the lesions have been deemed suitable, duplex information may be used to plan sites for percutaneous transluminal angioplasty access. For example, with normal aortoiliac segments and infrainguinal disease, a direct antegrade femoral puncture should be used. Conversely, in the case of iliac artery disease, a contralateral retrograde puncture should be employed. Thus, as recommended by Elsman and colleagues, unilateral symptoms should be followed up with duplex scanning of both the affected limb and the contralateral aortoiliac segment for the purpose of ruling out asymptomatic disease that could potentially complicate any endovascular intervention.[28]

Conclusions

Duplex scanning is an accurate and noninvasive modality for the assessment of iliac, femoral, and popliteal arterial occlusive disease. In color-flow scanning, morphologic, topographic, and physiologic data are presented in a semiquantitative visual format, and more quantitative hemodynamic data may be interpreted by spectral wave analysis. Thus it is both an effective screening and planning tool for candidates of percutaneous transluminal angioplasty. However, despite this depth of information, intraoperative angiography is still necessary.

REFERENCES

1. Kohler TR, Nance DR, Cramer MM, et al: Duplex scanning for diagnosis of aortoiliac and femoropopliteal disease: A prospective study. Circulation 76:1074–1080, 1987.
2. Sensier Y, Hartshorne T, Thrush A, et al: A prospective comparison of lower limb colour-coded duplex scanning with arteriography. Eur J Vasc Endovasc Surg 11:170–175, 1996.
3. Cossman DV, Ellison JE, Wagner WH, et al: Comparison of contrast arteriography to arterial mapping with color-flow duplex imaging in the lower extremities. J Vasc Surg 10:522–528, 1989.
4. Leng GC, Whyman MR, Donnan PT, et al: Accuracy and reproducibility of duplex ultrasonography in grading femoropopliteal stenoses. J Vasc Surg 17:510–517, 1993.
5. Ranke C, Creutzig A, Alexander K: Duplex scanning of the peripheral arteries: Correlation of the peak velocity ratio with angiographic diameter reduction. Ultrasound Med Biol 18:433–440, 1992.
6. Legemate DA, Teeuwen C, Hoeneveld H, et al: Value of duplex scanning compared with angiography and pressure measurement in the assessment of aortoiliac arterial lesions. Br J Surg 78:1003–1008, 1991.
7. Hatsukami TS, Primozich J, Zierler RE, et al: Color Doppler characteristics in normal lower extremity arteries. Ultrasound Med Biol 18:167–171, 1992.
8. Zierler RE, Zierler BK: Duplex sonography of lower extremity arteries. Semin Ultrasound CT MR 18:39–56, 1997.
9. Jager KA, Phillips DJ, Martin RL, et al: Noninvasive mapping of lower limb arterial lesions. Ultrasound Med Biol 11:515–521, 1985.
10. Boström-Ardin A, Löfberg AM, Hellberg A, et al: Selection of patients with infrainguinal arterial occlusive disease for percutaneous transluminal angioplasty with duplex scanning. Acta Radiologica 43:391–395, 2002.
11. Löfberg AM, Karacagil S, Hellberg A, et al: The role of duplex scanning in the selection of patients with critical lower-limb ischemia for infrainguinal percutaneous transluminal angioplasty. Cardiovasc Intervent Radiol 24:229–232, 2001.
12. Mazzariol F, Ascher E, Hingorani A, et al: Lower-extremity revascularization without preoperative contrast arteriography in 185 cases: Lessons learned with duplex ultrasound arterial mapping. Eur J Vasc Endovasc Surg 19:509–515, 2000.
13. Aly S, Sommerville K, Adiseshiah M, et al: Comparison of duplex imaging and arteriography in the evaluation of lower limb arteries. Br J Surg 85:1099–1102, 1998.
14. Katsamouris AN, Giannoukas AD, Tsetis D, et al: Can ultrasound replace arteriography in the management of chronic arterial occlusive disease of the lower limb? Eur J Vasc Endovasc Surg 21:155–159, 2001.
15. Koelemay MJ, den Hartog D, Prins MH, et al: Diagnosis of arterial disease of the lower extremities with duplex ultrasonography. Br J Surg 83:404–409, 1996.
16. Kohler TR, Andros G, Porter JM, et al: Can duplex scanning replace arteriography for lower extremity arterial disease? Ann Vasc Surg 4:280–287, 1990.
17. Ramaswami G, Al-Kutoubi A, Nicolaides AN, et al: The role of duplex scanning in the diagnosis of lower limb arterial disease. Ann Vasc Surg 13:494–500, 1999.
18. Hatsukami TS, Primozich J, Zierler RE, et al: Color Doppler imaging of infrainguinal arterial occlusive disease. J Vasc Surg 16:527–533, 1992.
19. Karacagil S, Lofberg AM, Almgren B, et al: Duplex ultrasound scanning for diagnosis of aortoiliac and femoropopliteal arterial disease. Vasa 23:325–329, 1994.
20. Karacagil S, Lofberg AM, Granbo A, et al: Value of duplex scanning in evaluation of crural and foot arteries in limbs with severe lower limb ischaemia: A prospective comparison with angiography. Eur J Vasc Endovasc Surg 12:300–303, 1996.
21. Moneta GL, Yeager RA, Antonovic R, et al: Accuracy of lower extremity arterial duplex mapping. J Vasc Surg 15:275–284, 1992.
22. Edwards JM, Coldwell DM, Goldman ML, et al: The role of duplex scanning in the selection of patients for transluminal angioplasty. J Vasc Surg 13:69–74, 1991.
23. Pemberton M, London NJ: Colour-flow duplex imaging of occlusive arterial disease of the lower limb. Br J Surg 84(7):912–919, 1997.
24. Wain RA, Berdejo GL, Delvalle WN, et al: Can duplex scan arterial mapping replace contrast arteriography as the test of choice before infrainguinal revascularization? J Vasc Surg 29:100–109, 1999.
25. Legemate DA, Teeuwen C, Hoeneveld H, et al: The potential of duplex scanning to replace aorto-iliac and femoro-popliteal angiography. Eur J Vasc Surg 3:49–54, 1989.
26. Pemberton M, Nydahl S, Hartshorne T, et al: Colour-coded duplex imaging can safely replace diagnostic arteriography in patients with lower-limb arterial disease. Br J Surg 83:1725–1728, 1996.
27. Whelan JF, Barry MH, Moir JD: Color-flow Doppler ultrasonography: Comparison with peripheral arteriography for the investigation of peripheral vascular disease. J Clin Ultrasound 20:369–374, 1992.
28. Elsman BH, Legemate DA, van der Heyden FW, et al: The use of color-coded duplex scanning in the selection of patients with lower extremity arterial disease for percutaneous transluminal angioplasty: A prospective study. Cardiovasc Intervent Radiol 19:313–316, 1996.
29. AbuRahma AF, Robinson PA, Boland JP, et al: Complications of arteriography in a recent series of 707 cases: Factors affecting outcome. Ann Vasc Surg 7:122–129, 1993.
30. Nunn DB: Complications of peripheral arteriography. Am Surg 44:664–669, 1978.

31. Hessel SJ, Adams DF, Abrams HL: Complications of angiography. Radiology 138:273–281, 1981.

32. Sigstedt B, Lunderquist A: Complications of angiographic examinations. Am J Roentgenol 130:455–460, 1978.

33. Levy MM, Baum RA, Carpenter JP: Endovascular surgery based solely on noninvasive preprocedural imaging. J Vasc Surg 28:995–1005, 1998.

34. Ascher E, Hingorani A, Markevich N, et al: Lower extremity revascularization without preoperative contrast arteriography: Experience with duplex ultrasound arterial mapping in 485 cases. Ann of Vasc Surg 2002; online publication.

35. Bodily K, Buttorff J, Nordesgaard A, et al: Aorto-iliac reconstruction without arteriography. Am J Surg 171:505–507, 1996.

36. Schneider PA, Ogawa DY, Rush MP: Lower extremity revascularization without contrast arteriography: A prospective study of operation based upon duplex mapping. Cardiovasc Surg 7(7):699–703, 1999.

37. Boström A, Ljungman C, Hellberg A, et al: Duplex scanning as the sole preoperative imaging method for infrainguinal arterial surgery. Eur J Vasc Endovasc Surg 23:140–145, 2002.

38. Sensier Y, Hartshorne T, Thrush A, et al: The affect of adjacent segment disease on the accuracy of colour duplex scanning for the diagnosis of lower limb arterial disease. Eur J Vasc Endovasc Surg 12:238–242, 1996.

39. Bergamini TM, Tatum CM Jr., Marshall C, et al: Effect of multilevel sequential stenosis on lower extremity arterial duplex scanning. Am J Surg 169:564–566, 1995.

40. Allard L, Cloutier G, Durand LG, et al: Limitations of ultrasonic duplex scanning for diagnosing lower limb arterial stenoses in the presence of adjacent segment disease. J Vasc Surg 19:650–657, 1994.

41. Lingush JL Jr., Reavis SW, Preisser JS, et al: Duplex ultrasound scanning defines operative strategies for patients with limb-threatening ischemia. J Vasc Surg 28:482–491, 1998.

42. Larch E, Minar E, Ahmadi R, et al: Value of color duplex sonography for evaluation of tibioperoneal arteries in patients with femoropopliteal obstruction: A prospective comparison with anterograde intraarterial digital subtraction angiography. J Vasc Surg 25:629–636, 1997.

43. Sensier Y, Fishwick G, Owen R, et al: A comparison between colour duplex ultrasonography and arteriography for imaging infrapopliteal arterial lesions. Eur J Vasc Endovasc Surg 15:44–50, 1998.

44. Avenarius JK, Breek JC, Lampmann LE, et al: The additional value of angiography after colour-coded duplex on decision making in patients with critical limb ischaemia: A prospective study. Eur J Vasc Endovasc Surg 23:393–397, 2002.

45. Huber TS, Back MR, Ballinger RJ, et al: Utility of magnetic resonance arteriography for distal lower extremity revascularization. J Vasc Surg 26:415–423, 1997.

46. Carpenter JP, Baum RA, Holland GA, et al: Peripheral vascular surgery with magnetic resonance angiography as the sole preoperative imaging modality. J Vasc Surg 20:861–869, 1994.

47. Blackshear WM Jr., Philiips DJ, Thiele BL, et al: Detection of carotid occlusive disease by ultrasonic imaging and pulsed Doppler spectrum analysis. Surgery 86:698–706, 1979.

48. Karasch T, Rieser R, Grun B, et al: Determination of the length of the occlusion in extremity arteries: Color duplex ultrasound versus angiography. Ultraschall Med 14:247–254, 1993.

49. Collier P, Wilcox G, Brooks D, et al: Improved patient selection for angioplasty utilizing color Doppler imaging. Am J Surg 160:171–174, 1990.

50. Whyman MR, Gillespie I, Ruckley CV, et al: Screening patients with claudication from femoropopliteal disease before angioplasty using Doppler colour flow imaging. Br J Surg 79:907–909, 1992.

51. Elsman BH, Legemate DA, van der Heijden FH, et al: Impact of ultrasonographic duplex scanning on therapeutic decision making in lower-limb arterial disease. Br J Surg 82:630–633, 1995.

52. Lai DT, Huber D, Glasson R, et al: Colour-coded duplex ultrasonography in selection of patients for transluminal angioplasty. Australas Radiol 39:243–245, 1995.

53. van der Heijden FH, Legemate DA, van Leeuwen MS, et al: Value of duplex scanning in the selection of patients for percutaneous transluminal angioplasty. Eur J Vasc Surg 7:71–76, 1993.

54. Pentecost MJ, Criqui MH, Dorros G, et al: Guidelines for peripheral percutaneous transluminal angioplasty of the abdominal aorta and lower extremity vessels: A statement for health professionals from a special writing group of the Councils on Cardiovascular Radiology, Arteriosclerosis, Cardio-Thoracic and Vascular Surgery, Clinical Cardiology, and Epidemiology and Prevention, the American Heart Association. Circulation 89:511–532, 1994.

55. Lai DT, Huber D, Glasson R, et al: Colour duplex ultrasonography versus angiography in the diagnosis of lower-extremity arterial disease. Cardiovasc Surg 4:384–388, 1996.

56. Schneider PA, Ogawa DY: Is routine preoperative aortoiliac arteriography necessary in the treatment of lower extremity ischemia? J Vasc Surg 28:28–34, 1998.

57. Moneta GL, Yeager RA, Lee RW, et al: Noninvasive localization of arterial occlusive disease: A comparison of segmental Doppler pressures and arterial duplex mapping. J Vasc Surg 17:578–582, 1993.

Chapter 26

The Preoperative, Intraoperative, and Postoperative Noninvasive Evaluation of Infrainguinal Vein Bypass Grafts

SHEELA T. PATEL • JOSEPH L. MILLS SR.

Introduction

Thorough preoperative assessment, meticulous operative technique, intraoperative evaluation of the completed arterial reconstruction, and detailed long-term follow-up are essential components of vascular reconstructive surgery. Infrainguinal revascularization, however, is perhaps the most demanding of all vascular reconstructive procedures and requires utilization of multiple techniques to ensure that each of these essential components is accomplished. Invasive imaging modalities (e.g., preoperative contrast venography and intraoperative angioscopy to evaluate suitability of vein conduit) and intraoperative and postoperative contrast arteriography to detect graft-threatening lesions have all been of some clinical utility and are still of occasional benefit. However, there has been a significant trend toward completion of the necessary pre-, intra-, and postoperative evaluation of infrainguinal bypass grafts with noninvasive imaging techniques such as duplex ultrasound and impedance analysis. Although the various invasive and noninvasive studies generally provide useful anatomic data, noninvasive modalities offer the major advantages of allowing serial evaluations and providing important hemodynamic information of clinical and prognostic significance.

Preoperative Vein Graft Evaluation

Autogenous vein is the optimal infrainguinal bypass conduit. Vein availability and quality are of paramount importance when planning such a bypass and may become critical issues in patients undergoing reoperative lower extremity bypass or in those requiring lower extremity bypass who have had the greater saphenous vein stripped or harvested for coronary bypass. Ipsilateral greater saphenous vein is inadequate or absent in as many as 30% to 40% of patients needing lower extremity revascularization.[1-3] In relatively thin patients with minimal body fat, a reasonable estimation of available vein length and quality can often be made on physical examination. When performing a physical examination of a potential leg bypass candidate, special attention should be paid to the presence and location of previous extremity incisions and scars as well as signs of prior venipuncture over sites of potentially usable vein conduit. The course and continuity of the greater saphenous vein as well as the cephalic vein can sometimes be evaluated with the limb dependent or following the application of a light tourniquet. The transmission of a wave centrally along the course of the vein following percussion suggests continuity. Although all patients should undergo a thorough clinical inspection of potential vein conduits before infrainguinal bypass, the utility of clinical examination alone is often compromised by body habitus, limb edema, lack of visibility, and uncertainties regarding course and quality.

Physical examination is not usually sufficient to determine availability of venous conduit and is also often inadequate in the estimation of vein quality. Vein quality is a complex and incompletely defined entity but encompasses consideration of factors such as caliber, patency, wall thickness, compressibility or distensibility, and the presence or absence of intrinsic defects (e.g., calcification, valve leaflet or luminal sclerosis, postphlebitic occlusion with or without recanalization, and major varicosities). The patency and caliber of potential venous conduit are the two most salient matters, but the presence and extent of the other factors mentioned may mandate rejection of the entire conduit or, if the defect is focal, excision of the inadequate segment with vein splicing to create a conduit of sufficient length to perform the proposed reconstruction. In experienced hands, such conduit decisions can often be made at the time of operation; however, many vascular surgeons now routinely perform additional preoperative evaluation of potential vein conduit. Such anatomic information helps to formulate an operative plan with an algorithm of options should a longer bypass than planned be required or should initially harvested vein fall short of expectations.

Venography

Various techniques have been described to assess the availability and suitability of vein conduit for infrainguinal bypass. Sapala and Szilagyi[4] were among the first to propose the use of preoperative contrast venography to establish the availability and adequacy of vein conduit. However, venography is invasive, relatively expensive, associated with the potential of local and systemic contrast-induced toxicity, and may well yield an inaccurate estimation of conduit diameter. Veith and colleagues[5] observed that the saphenous vein at the time of operation dilated to a diameter 73% greater than that determined by venography. Shah and colleagues[6] reported that, in 80% of cases, preoperative venography underestimated saphenous vein diameter by an average of 1.1 mm compared with the final arterialized lumen measured at operation. It is clear that the preoperative venographic measurement of vein graft diameter is problematic. Venography allows estimation of luminal diameter but cannot be used to assess wall thickness. Several authors have also postulated that the injection of contrast material may adversely compromise the quality of the vein by damaging the endothelium and triggering a sclerotic reaction. For all these reasons, preoperative contrast venography is no longer widely utilized.

Duplex Scanning

Duplex scanning and cutaneous vein mapping before lower extremity revascularization provide useful information regarding aberrant venous anatomy (e.g., double or parallel venous systems or varicosities), caliber, and the presence of sclerotic or occluded segments. Such anatomic variations and anomalies can be found in up to 45% of patients.[5,6] This information, in conjunction with scanning data on vein depth and course, permits the surgeon to strategically place incisions and avoid extensive, subcutaneous, undermining dissection that might result in ischemic flaps with resultant wound complications. Preoperative vein mapping may also identify unsuitable vein unworthy of exploration. Panetta and colleagues[7] correlated preoperative duplex findings with operative evaluation of the saphenous vein in 21 patients and reported that duplex ultrasound had a sensitivity of 62% for identifying unsuspected intrinsic vein abnormalities and a prevalence rate of 12% for these conditions. One should generally avoid exploration of small-caliber, thick-walled, sclerotic, occluded, recanalized, calcified, or excessively varicose segments.

Among the various characteristics evaluated by duplex ultrasound, conduit diameter has been the most extensively studied. Numerous investigators have demonstrated that small-caliber grafts are at substantially increased risk for the development of graft stenosis or occlusion.[8-11] Wengerter and colleagues[8] demonstrated a pattern of progressively decreasing patency rates with vein graft diameters ranging from 4.0 mm down to 3.0 mm on duplex ultrasound. Particularly noteworthy was the observation that veins with a distended external diameter of less than 3 mm, when used for infrapopliteal bypasses, had a distinctly inferior 1-year patency rate (31%) compared with larger caliber veins (62%). Idu and colleagues[10] concluded that the only factor significantly affecting the development of vein graft stenoses was a minimum graft diameter less than 3.5 mm on duplex ultrasound. Darling and colleagues[12] reported higher revision rates at 25 months in vein grafts constructed with diameters less than 3.5 mm compared with grafts greater than 3.5 mm (12% vs. 8%). It has also been suggested that small-caliber grafts are more vulnerable to intraoperative damage during harvesting than are larger vein grafts, particularly during valve lysis required by the in situ technique. Injury may trigger a local myointimal hyperplastic response, resulting in subsequent stenosis.

Small-caliber veins may also be the result of previous episodes of phlebitis or other pre-existing pathology that can compromise overall conduit quality. These and other data suggest that search for and utilization of vein conduits of at least 3.5 to 4.0 mm is an important principle in the performance of infrainguinal bypass. Unfortunately, preoperative duplex measurements do not always precisely correlate with those obtained at operation following gentle distention or arterialization of the vein or with intraoperative angiography.[13,14] By necessity, evaluation of venous diameter at operation follows some dissection and tissue trauma. This results in medial smooth muscle contraction and subsequent decrease in intraluminal diameter. Furthermore, intraoperative assessment of vein by calipers or by comparison with catheters of known sizes determines the external diameter only. This may or may not correlate with luminal diameter, which is the real determinant of vein utilization. Therefore duplex ultrasound may well be more accurate than intraoperative evaluation in assessing vein diameter. In addition, it has been increasingly recognized that the vascular endothelium is a living organ in which the metabolism and synthetic activities of vasoactive factors regulating luminal diameter are altered in response to biochemical forces generated by bloodflow.[15-17] Fillinger and colleagues[17] demonstrated that conduit diameter following vein graft implantation is regulated by shear stress; in normally adapting vein conduit, small-caliber veins (high shear stress) will enlarge or dilate over time, and large-caliber veins (low shear stress) will constrict or thicken in order to normalize shear stress. This may explain the finding in one study that vein grafts less than 3 mm have excellent patency rates when used in situ.[18] Despite these caveats, bigger is better, and vein segments of at least 3.5 to 4.0 mm should be utilized whenever possible.

Although duplex ultrasound has become the preferred modality for preoperative vein mapping, the best technique for evaluating potential venous conduits has yet to be determined. The multiple vein scanning techniques previously reported in the literature lack prospective validation. The optimal position in which the patient should be examined and the utility of examination with a proximal tourniquet in place remain poorly defined and are not standardized. Clinical investigators have attempted to increase venous distention to maximize venous diameter by placing the patient in a progressively more upright position. Blebea and colleagues[19] reported a prospective, preoperative evaluation of the effects of patient position on the measurement of vein diameter. All subjects were examined in the supine position in bed; in the 20-degree, reversed Trendelenburg position; sitting on the edge of the bed; standing; and in the supine position with a high-thigh, low-pressure tourniquet. The authors concluded that the optimal position for venous mapping is with the patient supine, and further suggested repeat examination with tourniquet application when the vein diameter is below a minimal threshold of 2 mm. In the vascular unit at the University of Arizona, preoperative duplex vein mapping is routinely conducted with the patient supine. A 5- to 7-MHz linear probe is used to sequentially measure the internal diameter of the proposed vein conduit at multiple sites along its course. During examination of the greater saphenous vein, the technician specifically notes the vein diameter at six specific sites: just inferior to the saphenofemoral junction, midthigh, above the knee, below the knee, midcalf, and superior to the medial malleolus. Each measurement is taken with the patient supine, the hip externally rotated, and the knee slightly flexed. If this nondistended vein diameter falls beneath an acceptable minimal caliber (2 mm at the authors' institution), a narrow, high-thigh tourniquet is applied at a venous occlusion pressure of approximately 50 to 65 mmHg. If the venous diameter is still less than 2 to 2.5 mm, the authors would generally choose not to explore it and would search for alternate vein conduits such as the lesser saphenous, cephalic, or basilic vein. The authors routinely perform preoperative vein mapping in all patients before infrainguinal bypass; however, it is of greatest utility in the evaluation of reoperative patients and of those patients requiring the use of alternate vein conduits. In addition to marking the course of the main branch of the underlying vein on the skin surface and performing multiple diameter measurements, technicians at the authors' institution also evaluate compressibility, wall thickness, and note areas of sclerosis, calcification, and significant varicosity.

Intraoperative Vein Graft Evaluation

Early (les than 30 days) graft failure is most commonly attributed to technical and judgmental errors (e.g., inappropriate patient selection, failure to appreciate the significance of an inflow or outflow lesion, or inappropriate conduit selection). However, progression of an occult, pre-existing conduit abnormality; or subtle, anastomotic defect, unrecognized or unappreciated at the initial operation, may account for a significant number of intermediate bypass failures that occur from 1 to 18 months postoperatively. Depending on the intraoperative technique used to identify them, the incidence of residual anatomic defects after infrainguinal bypass ranges from 15% to 30%.[20,21] To ensure optimal graft function, intraoperative imaging to assess morphologic graft integrity is important; however, no diagnostic method has gained universal acceptance. Intraoperative completion arteriography, angioscopy, and duplex scanning have been the most commonly employed techniques to verify the absence of potential problems such as intimal flap, plaque dissection, anastomotic stricture, intrinsic graft defect, intraluminal thrombus, or platelet aggregation. Additionally, several reports have suggested that intraoperative determination of outflow resistance may have a high predictive value for graft failure but these reports are incompletely substantiated.[22-24]

Completion Arteriography

Arteriography, despite its imperfections, remains the gold standard for intraoperative infrainguinal bypass assessment. Mills and colleagues,[25] in a prospective study of the value of routine completion angiography, evaluated 214 consecutive infrainguinal bypass grafts and detected significant technical problems requiring immediate revision in 8%. The yield was significantly greater for femorotibial compared with femoropopliteal reconstructions. The 30-day primary patency rates were 99% for femoropopliteal grafts and 93% for femorodistal grafts.

Intraoperative angiography allows detection of gross anatomic and technical defects (e.g., anastomotic stenoses) and graft kinks and twists. It also offers the important advantage of permitting detailed evaluation of the arterial runoff. However, it does not always detect residual arteriovenous fistulae after in situ saphenous vein bypass grafting, and it may also be insufficiently sensitive to detect more subtle findings (e.g., valve leaflet-associated abnormalities in reversed grafts, incomplete valve lysis in in situ conduits, and sites of platelet aggregation). Another major shortfall of angiography, like angioscopy, is that neither method provides hemodynamic information.

Angioscopy

Although prospective controlled data are lacking to support the proposition that routine intraoperative angioscopy improves long-term graft patency, there is no question that it allows the identification of vein conduit defects of potential significance.[26-29] This is especially true when utilizing arm vein conduits.[27-29] Arm vein conduits may harbor stenoses; synechiae; webs; or other intrinsic, intraluminal abnormalities in 50% to 75% of patients. In contrast, such abnormalities have been identified in only 12% of saphenous veins.[7] These lesions are identifiable and sometimes correctable with angioscopy, allowing the surgeon to upgrade conduit quality.[27,30] Angioscopy may also be utilized as an adjunct to performing valve lysis during in situ bypass. However, angioscopy is somewhat cumbersome, may be difficult and potentially injurious with smaller diameter conduits, and is not especially useful in assessment of runoff.[31] It also provides no hemodynamic information. Excepting its use in centers performing a high volume of arm vein grafts, and by some surgeons who use it as an adjunct to valve lysis during in situ bypass, angioscopy is not widely employed.

Duplex Scanning

Intraoperative duplex scanning provides not only an anatomic assessment of the vein bypass and inflow and outflow vessels, it also provides hemodynamic information that may be useful in planning the rational application of adjunctive procedures to increase graft flow, postoperative anticoagulation, and graft surveillance. Disadvantages of intraoperative duplex scanning include the expense and availability of the scanner, increase in operative time, and the need for acquisition of the necessary skills and expertise to correctly perform and interpret the duplex study. Papanicolaou and colleagues[32] reported a series of 81 vein grafts in which they compared the use of color-flow duplex with peak systolic velocity (PSV) measurements to angiography for completion study of infrainguinal bypass. Among 49 intraoperative studies, duplex scan abnormalities were identified in 17 patients (34.7%), 9 (18.4%) of which were immediately revised. Specific criteria for revision included a focal PSV greater than 200 cm/sec or a low graft flow velocity less than 45 cm/sec. Unrepaired duplex-detected defects were followed to determine their contribution to the need for early or late graft revision. All of the grafts with unrepaired abnormalities required revision in the postoperative period. None of the grafts with normal intraoperative scans developed lesions requiring revision during a mean follow-up interval of 16.1 months. Bandyk and colleagues,[33] in a prospective study of 275 infrainguinal vein graft bypasses undergoing intraoperative color-duplex evaluation, identified abnormalities requiring immediate operative intervention in 16% of grafts. Criteria for intraoperative graft revision were a focal PSV greater than 180 cm/sec associated with a Vr greater than 2.5. Reversed vein grafts exhibited the lowest scan abnormality and revision requirement rates (7%), whereas translocated, in situ, and arm vein grafts harbored significant duplex-detectable flow abnormalities in 15% to 23% of patients. A normal intraoperative scan was associated with a 90-day thrombosis rate of

0.4%. In contrast, grafts with residual or unrepaired duplex abnormalities were associated with a thrombosis rate of 40%. These data suggest that a normal intraoperative duplex is predictive of early and intermediate graft patency; that intraoperative duplex scanning has a higher yield when applied to translocated, in situ, or arm vein conduits; and that significant unrepaired defects compromise subsequent graft patency.

Johnson and colleagues[34] proposed that vein grafts with low intraoperative PSV (less than 30 to 40 cm/sec) and high outflow resistance (absent diastolic flow) should undergo adjunctive procedures to augment flow (e.g., distal arteriovenous fistulae or sequential bypass grafting). If adjunctive procedures could not be performed, antithrombotic therapy was initiated. They used intraoperative color-duplex scanning to assess vein graft patency and hemodynamics in 626 infrainguinal vein bypass grafts. Criteria for intraoperative repair were PSV of more than 180 cm/sec with spectral broadening and velocity ratio greater than 3. Duplex scanning prompted revision of 104 lesions in 96 (15%) bypass grafts. A normal intraoperative scan on initial imaging or after revision was associated with a 30-day thrombosis rate of 0.2% and a revision rate of only 0.8%. In contrast, 29% of the grafts with residual or unrepaired stenoses or low flow required a subsequent corrective procedure for graft thrombosis or stenosis.

Intravascular ultrasound (IVUS) is another emerging method of possible utility in the intraoperative anatomic evaluation of lower extremity vein grafts.[35] IVUS may permit detection of luminal and anastomotic irregularities, vessel wall abnormalities, and inflow and outflow lesions; however, it is relatively expensive, is associated with a risk of catheter-induced injury, and provides no hemodynamic information.

Hydraulic Impedance

Bloodflow measurements have long been proposed as an effective means of confirming bypass patency and of documenting hemodynamic improvement at the completion of infrainguinal bypass procedures. Early studies focused on the measurement of bloodflow using electromagnetic flow monitoring; results suggested that grafts with adequate levels of bloodflow exhibited superior patency rates at 1 year.[36,37] More recent efforts have raised the concept of functional runoff assessment through determination of resistance.[22-24] The method for measuring outflow resistance was first described in the 1980s.[38,39] The vein graft is cannulated proximally with a 20-gauge intravenous catheter which is connected to an arteriographic injector. A 23-gauge needle is introduced into the hood of the distal anastomosis and is pressure transduced to a monitor. Pressure measurements are obtained from the hood of the distal anastomosis to confirm that no hemodynamically significant lesions exist in the graft or inflow source. Outflow resistance is

obtained by clamping the proximal graft, infusing normal saline solution at a rate of 60 mL/min through the proximal cannula, and measuring the resultant pressure generated at the distal anastomosis. The distal pressures typically reach an initial peak followed by a slightly lower plateau pressure. All measurements are done after the administration of 30 mg papaverine into the outflow bed via the vein graft to correct for differing amounts of vasospasm among patients. Applying Ohm's law, plateau pressure is used to calculate the outflow resistance:

$$\text{Outflow resistance} = \text{plateau pressure (mmHg)/infusion rate (mL/min)}$$

Peterkin and colleagues[40] have shown correlation between this outflow resistance and preoperative angiographic findings.

Although many investigators have found that intraoperative measurements of bloodflow, flow waveform contour, flow velocity, and resistance correlate with graft patency to some degree, the most physiologic parameter may be the impedance, which describes the total opposition to flow presented by a system. Schwartz and colleagues[41] reported that determination of longitudinal impedance is of greater prognostic significance than are calculations of bloodflow and resistance. Longitudinal impedance can be calculated using a complex Fourier transformation. In a series of 73 autologous infrainguinal bypass grafts, the study authors demonstrated that intraoperative longitudinal impedance in infrainguinal vein grafts was independent of outflow conditions and hence described the resistive properties of the conduit only. In addition, these preliminary data suggest that longitudinal impedance is predictive of short-term primary patency and may be a better predictor of graft patency than are other currently available methods. This technique, although of some interest, is unlikely to be widely adopted in the clinical setting.

Vein Biopsy

Preimplant vein morphology has been implicated as a risk factor for graft stenosis.[7,42-44] The aforementioned evidence that shear stress is the primary determinant of luminal diameter also implies that vein grafts fail when the vein does not adapt properly. Thus intrinsic vein disease may be even more important than vein diameter in determining ultimate graft patency. LoGerfo and colleagues[42] in 1977 reported that vein quality was associated with a significant reduction in graft patency, although no objective criteria were defined to categorize a vein as poor quality. Marin and colleagues[44] studied remnant vein specimens taken at the time of surgery and concluded that microscopic intimal thickening and increased cellularity were strongly associated with failed or failing vein grafts. They advocated random saphenous vein biopsy to detect vein at risk for subsequent graft failure. However, James and colleagues[45] found that preimplant vein intimal thickness, determined from a random vein biopsy at the time of primary leg bypass in a macroscopically normal preimplant vein, was not predictive of the subsequent development of vein graft stenosis. Further investigation is needed to resolve this issue.

Postoperative Vein Graft Evaluation

Serial vein graft attrition remains the most significant obstacle to long-term clinical success. Five years after implantation, in the absence of reintervention, only 50% to 70% of infrainguinal vein grafts will be patent, and only 40% to 50% will be primarily patent after the first decade.[46] The ultimate goal of infrainguinal vein graft surveillance is to prevent graft occlusion by accurate identification and timely repair of graft-threatening lesions. Vigilant surveillance and strategic surgical revision will avert the persistent threat of graft failure caused by anastomotic and conduit defects, myointimal hyperplasia, and progressive atherosclerosis and improves long-term graft patency and limb salvage rates. An improvement in 1-year patency rate of approximately 15% has been reported in patients who were prospectively followed by duplex scanning.[47,48] However, many concerns have been raised, including the efficacy of performing graft revision procedures on asymptomatic patients, the economic costs of surveillance, and the vascular laboratory manpower requirements. Nevertheless, graft occlusion is technically demanding for the vascular surgeon, potentially disastrous for the patient, and incurs significant healthcare costs. Most surgeons, therefore, feel that graft surveillance in some form is both necessary and justifiable.

Rationale for Surveillance

Failing infrainguinal autogenous venous conduits are often heralded by the development of intrinsic graft stenoses. Certain intrinsic lesions may progress to hemodynamic significance, reduce graft flow below the thrombotic threshold velocity, and culminate in graft thrombosis. In Szilagyi and colleagues[49] classic, serial angiographic study of 377 reversed lower extremity vein grafts, 33% of grafts developed stenosis within 5 years of implantation. More recent studies utilizing duplex surveillance have confirmed that 20% to 35% of grafts develop stenoses within the graft or in the native arterial inflow or outflow vessels within 2 years.[48,50-54] Numerous reports confirm that 60% to 80% of graft-threatening lesions are focal, identifiable, and potentially correctable. Donaldson and colleagues[55] reported a detailed analysis of the causes of graft failure in a consecutive series of 440 in situ vein grafts: Over 63% of failures were caused by intrinsic defects within the vein conduit itself or its anastomoses. Mills and colleagues[56] identified intrinsic graft lesions as the cause of failed or failing grafts in 60% of cases in a prospective duplex study of 227 consecutive reversed vein grafts. Intrinsic graft stenosis is thus the most common cause of both in situ and reversed vein graft failure following implantation.

The incidence of stenotic lesions in vein grafts differs between series depending on the diagnostic criteria for graft stenosis, the screening technique employed, and the duration of follow-up. In patients monitored by clinical means alone, with perhaps the addition of simple ankle-brachial index (ABI) measurement, the incidence ranges from 5% to 21%. Duplex scanning is much more sensitive and detects lesions in 20% to 37% of grafts.[48,56,57]

Clinical examination can only detect the presence or absence of a pulse in a graft or run-off vessel and gives no indication of the potential likelihood of thrombosis. Pulses may be enhanced by reflected waves from a very high-resistance peripheral bed, and pulses may be difficult to palpate in obese or edematous patients. Pulse palpation has serious limitations because the graft may be located in a deep anatomic compartment and may be inaccessible to direct palpation. Bandyk and colleagues[58] demonstrated that 68% of patients with preocclusive vein graft stenoses had no clinical symptoms. ABI is likewise a poor predictor of graft function. Recent studies have shown that up to 40% of grafts fail without a premonitory drop in ABI. Recurrence of symptoms and decreases in ABI are more likely the result of a failed graft unsuitable for surgical or endovascular intervention, rather than an indicator of a failing, potentially readily salvageable graft. Idu and colleagues[48] reported that clinical symptoms identified only 33% of stenotic grafts. A significant drop in ABI (greater than 0.15) was observed in only 38% of grafts with significant duplex-detected stenoses. The ABI can be a useful prognosticator, however, when used in conjunction with duplex graft surveillance data. Green and colleagues[59] found that grafts harboring duplex surveillance-detected stenoses associated with an ABI decrease of 10% or greater had a 66% incidence of thrombosis within 3 months; if the ABI was normal, but the duplex scan was abnormal, the corresponding risk of failure within 3 months was only 4%; no graft thrombosed if both scan and ABI were normal.

The function of autogenous vein grafts implanted into the arterial circulation is best monitored by serial duplex surveillance. Impedance analysis has been suggested as an alternative method to detect graft-related stenoses; however, its utility has yet to be proven.[60,61] Graft impedance can only be accurately measured during operation and is not widely performed.

Duplex graft surveillance is noninvasive, sensitive, accurate, reproducible, and economical. At least 80% of graft lesions develop within the first 2 postoperative years, with the highest risk incurred during the first 6 months. There are several studies indicating a high incidence of duplex-detected flow abnormalities in both in situ and reversed vein grafts studied within 30 days of implantation despite normal completion arteriograms. Such data suggest that maximizing the utility of graft surveillance would require increased surveillance intensity during this early period of particular graft vulnerability.

Vein graft stenoses developing during the first 3 to 6 postoperative months may behave in a particularly aggressive manner. Several investigators have suggested that these lesions are more prone to rapid progression and vein graft thrombosis than are later, more slow-to-develop lesions.[52,62–64] Early and late-appearing graft lesions may therefore exhibit different biologic behaviors. It has been hypothesized that early flow disturbances could be associated with platelet aggregation at sites of technical imperfection, areas of intimal injury, or at valve leaflet defects. During the period of adaptation to the arterial circulation, these early flow disturbances may be subjected to a different milieu of growth factors and cytokines compared with later lesions. Nielsen[64] reported that patients who developed stenoses within 3 months of surgery had a higher risk of graft thrombosis than did patients who developed stenoses at a later stage (12 month patency 40% vs. 83%, p = 0.01). They proposed that early stenoses exceeding specific velocity parameters (Vr > 2.5) should be revised even in the absence of ankle-brachial index reduction. Ihnat and colleagues[65] observed that grafts with early postoperative flow disturbances detected by means of duplex scanning were associated with a nearly threefold increase in subsequent development of graft-threatening stenosis and requirement for revision when compared with grafts with normal early scans.

Vein grafts with serial normal duplex studies exhibit an extremely low rate of graft occlusion during long-term follow-up. In contrast, the natural history of grafts harboring high-grade intrinsic stenoses, particularly those detected in the first 3 to 6 months after surgery, is sudden occlusion. Unrevised vein grafts with critical stenoses have a short-term rate of subsequent occlusion that is as high as 80%.[66] Prophylactic intervention for such high-grade lesions is justified because prophylactic revision of stenotic grafts is durable and the outcome of treatment for graft occlusion is poor. Robinson and colleagues[67] found that vein grafts requiring thrombectomy within 30 days of surgery had a twofold risk of developing stenosis as well as reduced secondary patency rates. Vein grafts that occlude in the intermediate and late postoperative periods also fare poorly. Numerous reports have confirmed dismal long-term patency rates (ranging from 19% to 28%) for grafts following thrombectomy and thrombolysis.[68–72] On the other hand, surgical correction of a failing vein graft before thrombosis occurs yields 5-year assisted patency rates (80% to 85%) comparable to those for nonstenotic grafts, effectively restoring the life-table curve to normal.[73,74]

Method of Graft Surveillance

The purpose of a graft surveillance program is to maximize the detection of graft-threatening lesions before the occurrence of graft thrombosis. The protocol design must take into account both the progression and natural history of vein graft stenosis. Nearly 80% of graft stenoses develop within 12 months of graft implantation; the majority of these are detectable within the first 6 postoperative months. Early graft lesions (less than 3 months) tend to progress more rapidly and are more threatening than are lesions developing at later intervals. Mills and colleagues[75] prospectively performed duplex surveillance, beginning in the intra- and early postoperative period, to determine the origin of vein graft lesions and delineate their propensity for progression. They found that significant stenoses appeared to develop at sites of preexisting or early-appearing conduit abnormalities or unrepaired technical defects; only 2% of stenoses developed de novo in graft segments that were entirely normal at the time of graft implantation. Of 42 grafts (32% of series) with abnormal scans within the first 3 months, 18 (43%) subsequently developed high-grade stenoses. In addition, 27 grafts (22% of series) demonstrated suspicious areas on the 1-week scan, and 8 of these (30%) subsequently developed hemodynamically significant stenoses requiring revision.

The authors recommend early postoperative scanning (one scan within 4 weeks of reconstruction, two scans within 3 months) because it allows the surgeon to stratify grafts into high, intermediate, and low-risk categories for thrombosis. The criteria we utilize consist of low-flow and high-velocity thresholds and are outlined in Table 26-1. Grafts with early flow disturbances require more intensive surveillance. Although the risk of developing a graft stenosis falls off significantly after 1 to 2 years, there persists an annual 2% to 4% incidence of late-appearing graft stenosis and a 5% to 10% lifetime risk of inflow/outflow disease progression requiring intervention.[65] Reifsnyder and colleagues[76] have demonstrated that venous conduits commonly develop significant lesions beyond 5 years. Landry and colleagues[74] reported that although most vein bypass revisions were required in the first year, 34% of revisions were performed between the first and fifth year, and 11% after 5 years. Long-term follow-up, albeit of diminished intensity, is therefore worthwhile.

We recommend a surveillance paradigm that incorporates available natural history and disease progression data (Fig. 26-1). The first postoperative scan is obtained before discharge from the hospital or at the time of the first postoperative clinic visit (within 4 weeks of graft implantation). A repeat study is performed 3 months after graft implantation. If these two studies are normal (about two thirds of grafts), the surveillance visits are extended to every 6 months until 2 years after surgery. After 2 years, annual studies are performed for the lifetime of the patient. If lesions are detected during inter-

TABLE 26-1. **Stratification of Risk of Graft Thrombosis Based on Surveillance Data**

Category	High Velocity Criteria		Low Velocity Criteria		Drop in ABI
I (Highest Risk)	PSV > 300 cm/s or Vr > 3.5	and	GSV < 45 cm/s	or	>0.15
II (High Risk)	PSV > 300 cm/s or Vr > 3.5	and	GSV > 45 cm/s	and	<0.15
III (Intermediate Risk)	180 < PSV > 300 cm/s or Vr > 2.0	and	GSV > 45 cm/s	and	<0.15
IV (Low Risk)	PSV < 180 cm/s and Vr < 2.0	and	GSV > 45 cm/s	and	<0.15

PSV = Duplex-derived peak systolic velocity at site of flow disturbance; GFV = graft flow velocity (global or distal); Vr = velocity ratio of stenosis to more proximal graft segment of same caliber; ABI = Doppler-derived ankle-brachial index.

mediate or late follow-up, scanning frequency is increased to identify grafts with progressive lesions. Low and intermediate-grade lesions are followed for progression. Duplex scanning is performed every 6 to 8 weeks until the lesion resolves or until it becomes high-grade. High-grade lesions mandate revision.

Graft surveillance consists of physical examination (pulse palpation); ABI determination; and complete color-duplex interrogation of the adjacent inflow and outflow arteries, both proximal and distal anastomoses, and the entire venous conduit. If there is a significant drop in ABI, or a low-flow graft is identified but duplex surveillance fails to detect a responsible lesion, further evaluation with conventional arteriography or MRA is indicated.

The most important component of graft surveillance is thorough duplex interrogation of the graft. Surveillance is simplified if the graft has been tunneled subcutaneously and when color-flow imaging is utilized. Doppler imaging with either a 5.0- or 7.5-MHz linear-array probe is initiated in the native artery proximal to the origin of the reconstruction. Velocity spectra measurements should be made at a Doppler angle less than or equal to 60 degrees. Arterial waveforms and velocities are recorded from the inflow artery, proximal anastomosis, the proximal graft, the midgraft, the distal graft, the distal anastomosis,

and the outflow artery. Findings suggestive of a possible inflow artery stenosis include a rounded upstroke on the waveform tracing and a clearly prolonged upstroke acceleration time.

If a focal, mosaic color-flow disturbance is identified, the peak systolic velocity (PSV) is measured and compared with a normal caliber, turbulence-free site in the graft proximal to the flow disturbance. The ratio of the stenosis PSV (V2) to normal proximal PSV (V1) is termed the velocity ratio (Vr). The advantage of employing a ratio is that changes in graft flow caused by alterations in peripheral resistance or cardiac output are annulled. The use of Vr allows accurate measurement and comparison of stenosis progression between visits. PSV and Vr determinations are the most useful duplex-derived surveillance measurements, but Vr is the single most accurate criterion for the determination of the presence and degree of graft stenosis.

The mean PSV in a normal infrainguinal vein graft is generally 60 to 80 cm/sec. A stenosis is defined as a PSV greaer than 180 cm/sec with a Vr greater than 1.5. A focal vein graft PSV greater than 300 cm/sec and a Vr greater than 3.5 indicate a high-grade stenosis. Measurements of end-diastolic velocity (EDV) can also be readily performed (Fig. 26-2). Although the EDV is less sensitive than PSV and Vr, an EDV exceeding 75 to 100 cm/sec

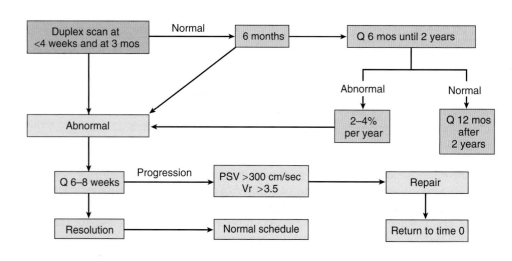

Figure 26-1. Surveillance algorithm detailing recommended timing of postoperative graft surveillance.

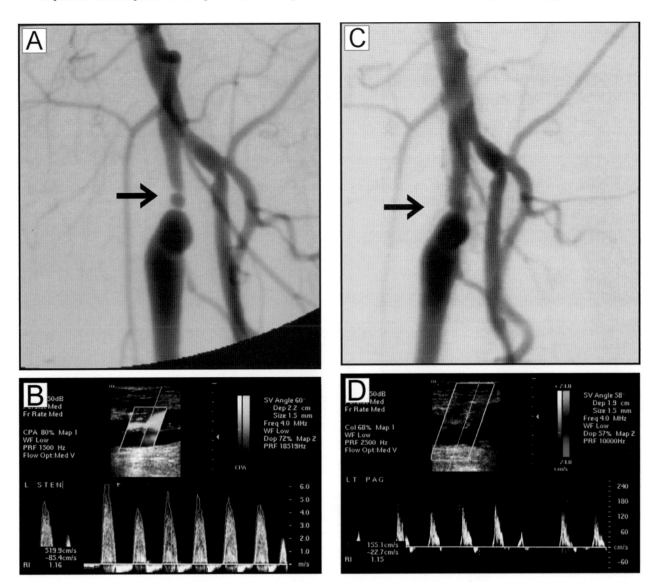

Figure 26-2. *A, Selective arteriogram demonstrates a severe proximal graft stenosis. B, Previous duplex examination revealed a focal stenosis associated with a peak systolic velocity of 520 cm/sec, Vr = 5, and reduced ABI = 0.75. C, Arteriogram after 6 mm PTA of vein graft stenosis. D, Duplex examination documents a reduction of peak systolic velocity to 155 cm/sec after PTA, restoration of triphasic waveform, and improved ABI = 0.93.*

at the site of flow disturbance is a very specific finding for a stenosis exceeding 75% diameter reduction.[77] As outlined in Table 26-1, the authors utilize both high- and low-flow/velocity criteria to guide intervention. High-velocity criteria include a PSV greater than 300 cm/sec at the site of stenosis and/or Vr greater than 3.5. Peak systolic graft flow velocity generally should exceed 45 cm/sec in a normal caliber infrainguinal vein graft. If the graft flow velocity falls below this critical threshold, the graft is more prone to thrombosis. The authors also perform ABI determinations at each surveillance visit. Low-velocity criteria include a global graft PSV less than 45 cm/sec as well as a decrease in ABI greater than 0.15.

Flow characteristics of a vein graft are influenced primarily by the outflow resistance and graft diameter. Belkin and colleagues[78,79] have suggested that vessel diameter be taken into account in the determination of abnormal PSV measurements. They noted a significant inverse correlation between PSV and diameter for tibial and popliteal grafts but not for inframalleolar level grafts. Fillinger and colleagues[17] suggest that it may be useful to calculate shear stress during graft surveillance because it is determined by both velocity and diameter. This may help eliminate the problem of detecting abnormalities caused by native vessel diameter rather than by focal stenosis (Fig. 26-4). Despite these limitations, it should be understood that no single threshold for PSV is accurate in identifying all grafts at risk for failure. Serial measurements should be used to detect deterioration in graft function.

Four categories of thrombotic risk are defined according to four hemodynamic parameters: PSV, Vr, GFV (distal or global flow velocity), and ABI (see Table 26-1). The

A Common femoral (inflow) artery waveform
7 years s/p femoropopliteal bypass

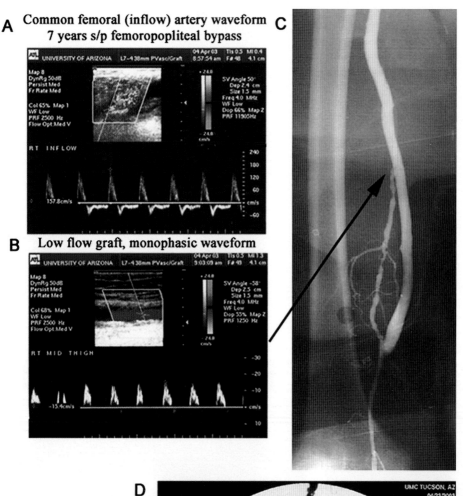

B Low flow graft, monophasic waveform

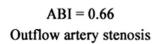

ABI = 0.66
Outflow artery stenosis

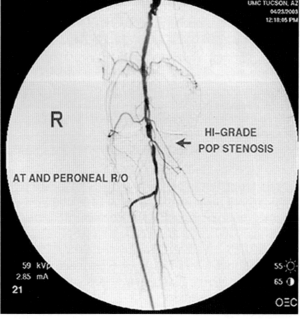

Figure 26-3. A, *Duplex examination of common femoral artery in a patient who underwent a femoral popliteal bypass with saphenous vein 7 years ago. There is a normal triphasic waveform.* **B,** *Duplex examination of midvein graft with low flow (peak systolic velocity = 15 cm/sec) and monophasic waveform.* **C,** *Selective arteriogram demonstrating the absence of significant vein graft lesions.* **D,** *Selective arteriogram demonstrating a high-grade outflow popliteal artery stenosis. This patient had an ABI = 0.66.*

highest risk category includes grafts with PSV greater than 300 cm/sec, Vr greater than 3.5, and a reduction in ABI. These graft lesions are unlikely to regress and mandate revision to prevent graft thrombosis. Lesions of intermediate hemodynamic significance (PSV greater than 180 cm/sec and Vr greater than 1.5) should be monitored by duplex every 4 to 6 weeks until resolution or progression to threshold for intervention occurs. Normal graft surveillance studies are associated with a very low risk of graft thrombosis. Sladen and colleagues[80]

A   Midgraft waveform post outflow popliteal artery angioplasty

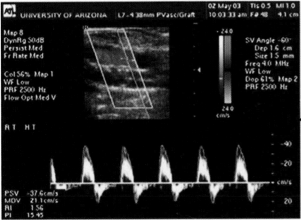

Triphasic graft waveform

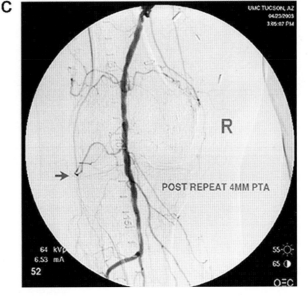

ABI = 0.96
Post popliteal PTA

Figure 26-4. The patient in Figure 26-3 underwent outflow popliteal artery PTA. **A,** Subsequent duplex examination indicates return of a triphasic waveform in the midgraft. **B,** Selective arteriogram demonstrating the absence of significant vein graft lesions. **C,** Selective arteriogram after popliteal PTA (magnified view) demonstrating successful resolution of the popliteal artery stenosis with an increase in ABI to 0.96.

described nearly identical criteria. There are minor variations in the literature concerning the definition of high-grade stenosis. In general, a PSV greater than 250 to 300 cm/sec or a Vr greater than 3 to 4 is felt by most clinicians to mandate either arteriography or intervention.

The surveillance program is most intense during the first 1 to 18 months, which is the period of greatest risk for graft stenosis and occlusion. Surveillance is continued for the lifetime of the patient to capture hemo-

dynamically significant atherosclerotic deteriorations in outflow and inflow arteries and late development of lesions within the graft conduit itself.

There have been minor inconsistencies in published reports with respect to the magnitude of stenosis mandating revision. Some understanding of the natural history of vein graft stenosis is critically important before recommending graft revision. Idu and colleagues[48] described the impact of a color-flow duplex surveillance program on infrainguinal vein graft patency. Two patient groups were followed for a median of 21 months: 160 bypass grafts were monitored with clinical assessment as well as duplex scanning, whereas 41 bypass grafts were followed by clinical assessment alone. Stenoses greater than 30% were identified in 29% of all vein grafts (32% in the surveillance group vs. 7% in clinical assessment only group, p = 0.005). None of the grafts with stenoses between 30% and 49% diameter-reduction failed during follow-up. Occlusion occurred in 57% of the nonrevised, vs. only 9% of the revised grafts (p = 0.047) harboring stenoses in the 50% to 69% category. Stenoses with greater than 70% diameter-reduction were associated with graft failure in 100% of nonrevised bypasses, vs. 10% of revised grafts (p = 0.004). Mills and colleagues[66] reported that 7 of 9 grafts with unrepaired critical stenoses (PSV greater than 300 cm/sec, or Vr greater than 4) thrombosed within 4 months.

Identification of subgroups of patients who may benefit from more intensive surveillance has been the subject of a number of clinical studies. However, clinical and technical variables appear to offer little prognostic value as to the risk of graft stenosis. The presence of severe comorbid illnesses (e.g., coronary artery disease, diabetes mellitus, and end-stage nephropathy) does not appear to significantly influence the development of graft stenosis. Operative technique, most specifically the controversy between reversed and in situ conduit configurations, has received considerable attention, but there has been no convincing evidence that either technique offers a significant patency advantage.[54,81,82] Tobacco smoking increases the risk of graft stenosis.[54] There are conflicting results as to whether female gender is a risk factor for graft stenosis.[83,84] Alternative venous grafts (e.g., arm, lesser saphenous, or spliced) are associated with an increased incidence of graft stenosis as well as poorer patencies, factors that mandate more aggressive surveillance.[65,85,86] Ihnat and colleagues[65] reported a 30-month assisted-primary patency rate of alternate vein conduits of 73%, compared with 93% for greater saphenous grafts. Interestingly, it also has been demonstrated that low graft flow is a predictor of graft stenosis after infrainguinal bypass.[87,88] Ihlberg and colleagues[87] suggested that it would be beneficial to devise flow criteria for risk group stratification for future surveillance programs.

Graft Revision

The rate of graft revision reported in the literature varies with the criteria used to determine the need for revision and the duration of follow-up. Natural history data support the efficacy of vein graft surveillance and prophylactic revision of grafts with high-grade stenosis. Mattos and colleagues[89] reported that when grafts with stenoses detected by duplex were left untreated, the patency rate at 1 year was 66% compared with 96% in revised grafts. Ihnat and colleagues[65] found that 34% of grafts followed for a mean period of 35 months required revision procedures; operative revision was durable.

Not all stenoses progress to occlusion, and the criteria for bypass revision remain in evaluation. Patients with early stenoses, most often caused by myointimal hyperplasia, appear to benefit from revision even in the absence of ABI reduction.[64,65] Stenoses reaching the threshold criteria in the early postoperative period represent rapidly progressing lesions, whereas stenoses identified later may represent more slowly developing lesions. Recent reports have questioned the necessity of correcting proximal inflow lesions in the absence of clinical symptoms. Some investigators have reported that these lesions do not have a negative impact on graft patency and thus surveillance of these areas may be unnecessary.[90] Moreover, regression may occur.[91]

Preoperative arteriography before graft revision has been a contentious issue. Landry and colleagues[50] observed that arteriography significantly contributed to operative planning in 42% of revision cases. Duplex surveillance criteria for arteriography suggested by these authors include a PSV greater than 200 cm/sec, Vr greater than 3.0, presence of a midgraft velocity less than 45 cm/sec, interval drop in ABI 0.2, and/or change in clinical status. Arteriography was critical for identifying significant lesions when the proximal anastomosis was to the profunda femoris artery or in the presence of tandem graft lesions. The authors repaired lesions with greater than 50% angiographically confirmed stenosis, which led to a 5-year–assisted primary patency rate of 91%. They concluded that preoperative arteriography was mandatory before revision of failing vein grafts. Idu and colleagues[92] recently published the results of a multicenter Dutch study assessing the role of angiography before graft revision. A standardized postoperative vein graft surveillance protocol was performed in 300 patients, of whom 84 (28%) subsequently underwent vein graft revision. These authors found a Vr greater than 3 to have a high correlation with greater than 70% angiographic stenosis. According to their proposed algorithm, patients with a Vr less than 2.5 underwent conservative treatment without angiography or revision, patients with a Vr greater than 4 underwent revision on the basis of duplex scan findings alone without angiography, and patients with a Vr between 2.5 and 4.0 underwent angiography before revision. This policy of selective arteriography resulted in a 5-year assisted-primary patency of 74%. Mills and colleagues[66] suggested that intermediate graft stenoses (PSV less than 300 cm/sec, Vr less than 4) could be safely followed with close serial duplex surveillance, and that high-grade lesions (Vr greater than 4, PSV greater than 300) could be repaired based on duplex-findings alone.

The type of graft revision procedure is dependent on the location of the stenosis. It is generally accepted that vein patch angioplasty is appropriate for focal graft body lesions, whereas interposition grafting is indicated for more diffuse disease. Jump grafts are favored for distal anastomotic stenoses. Successful revision normalizes graft hemodynamics.

The anatomic distribution of stenotic vein graft lesions has been reported by several authors. Interestingly, the location of the lesion may be dependent on the grafting technique. Mills and colleagues[56] prospectively studied 227 infrainguinal reversed vein grafts over a 5-year period and found 33 intrinsic graft stenoses in 29 grafts, of which the majority (53%) were juxta-anastomotic and only 29% of the lesions were in the middle of the graft. Similarly, Berkowitz and colleagues[93] reported anatomic data in a series of reversed saphenous vein graft stenoses in which the majority of lesions (40%) were just distal to the proximal anastomosis hood and 29% were juxta-anastomotic. In contradistinction, Donaldson and colleagues[94] detailed the causes of primary failure of 85 in situ bypass grafts and found that 63% of graft thromboses were caused by intrinsic graft lesions, with the majority being in the midgraft, whereas only 27% were juxta-anastomotic lesions. Some authors have suggested that proximal lesions are more common in reversed grafts and distal lesions more common in in situ grafts (Table 26-2), but the available data do not fully support this assertion.

A patent graft does not necessarily guarantee limb preservation. Most authors have suggested that graft surveillance improves both graft patency and limb salvage rates.[48,89,95,96] The only prospective randomized study in favor of an intensive surveillance program found an improvement of 25% in assisted-primary patency rate compared with routine clinical follow-up in patients with autogenous infrainguinal bypass grafts. The authors did not report limb salvage rates.[97] A meta-analysis of graft surveillance by Golledge and colleagues[96] concluded that although the patency of infrainguinal vein grafts was improved by surveillance, no improvement

could be demonstrated with respect to limb salvage rates. The lack of level I evidence and differing interpretations of available duplex surveillance data resulted in the initiation of a prospective, randomized trial in the United Kingdom to determine the efficacy of duplex ultrasound graft surveillance.[98] The study is under way, but the trial is incomplete and results are not yet available.

Economics of Graft Surveillance

Two studies, one in North America and one in western Europe, have carefully evaluated the economics of vein graft surveillance. Wixon and colleagues[99] analyzed 155 consecutive autogenous infrainguinal bypass grafts performed in 141 patients. Graft revision for duplex-detected stenosis, in comparison with revision after thrombosis, improved 1-year patency, resulted in fewer amputations, and generated fewer expenses at 12 months ($17,688 vs. $45,252). Visser and colleagues[100] also concluded that duplex surveillance was cost-effective in both claudicants and in those with critical limb ischemia, and that it reduced the risk of major limb amputation. Both studies suggest that the prevention of a small to moderate number of vein graft occlusions by judicious use of a duplex surveillance protocol makes clinical sense and yields substantial economic benefit.

Conclusions

The ultimate fate of an infrainguinal vein bypass depends in part on the philosophy and aggressiveness of the vascular surgeon. Adoption of a nihilistic approach to graft surveillance results in an unacceptable incidence of unexpected graft thrombosis. Every effort must be made to detect the failing vein graft before thrombosis

TABLE 26-2. Incidence and Location of Graft-Threatening Stenoses Detected by Duplex Surveillance

Author	Year	Graft Type	Number of Stenoses / Number of Grafts (%)	Inflow	Proximal Anastomosis	Midgraft	Distal Anastomosis	Outflow
Bandyk[58]	1991	In situ	83/372 (22%)	9	10	40	9	15
Buth[77]	1991	In situ	43/116 (37%)	-	17	23	3	-
Donaldson[94]	1992	In situ	85/455 (19%)	3	14	37	14	16
Mills[56]	1993	Reversed	38/227 (18%)	3	10	6	8	2
Mattos[89]	1993	Mixed	62/170 (36%)	2	10	40	7	3
Erickson[53]	1996	In situ	169/556 (30%)	13	6	61	9	11

occurs. The best available evidence supports a surveillance protocol utilizing duplex scanning for all patients undergoing infrainguinal bypass with autologous vein. There are no data suggesting that duplex surveillance of prosthetic grafts is worthwhile.[65,97,101,102]

REFERENCES

1. Taylor LM Jr, Edwards JM, Brant B, et al: Autogenous reversed vein bypass for lower extremity ischemia in patients with absent or inadequate greater saphenous vein. Am J Surg 153:505–510, 1987.
2. Gentile AT, Lee RW, Moneta GL, et al: Results of bypass to the popliteal and tibial arteries with alternative sources of autogenous vein. J Vasc Surg 23:272–280, 1996.
3. Halloran BG, Lilly MP, Cohn EJ, et al: Tibial bypass using complex autogenous conduit: Patency and limb salvage. Ann Vasc Surg 15:634–643, 2001.
4. Sapala JA, Szilagyi DE: A simple aid in greater saphenous phlebography. Surg Gynecol Obstet 140:265–267, 1975.
5. Veith FJ, Moss CM, Sprayregen S, et al: Preoperative venography in arterial reconstructive surgery of the lower extremity. Surgery 85:253–256, 1979.
6. Shah DM, Chang BB, Leopold PW, et al: The anatomy of the greater saphenous venous system. J Vasc Surg 3:273–283, 1986.
7. Panetta TF, Marin ML, Veith FJ, et al: Unsuspected preexisting saphenous vein disease: An unrecognized cause of vein bypass failure. J Vasc Surg 15:102–112, 1992.
8. Wengerter KR, Veith FJ, Gupta SK, et al: Influence of vein size (diameter) on infrapopliteal reversed vein graft patency. J Vasc Surg 11:525–531, 1990.
9. Meyerson SL, Moawad J, Loth F, et al: Effective hemodynamic diameter: An intrinsic property of vein grafts with predictive value for patency. J Vasc Surg 31:910–917, 2000.
10. Idu MM, Buth J, Hop WCJ, et al: Factors influencing the development of vein graft stenosis and their significance for clinical management. Eur J Vasc Endovasc Surg 17:15–27, 1999.
11. Davies AH, Magee TR, Sheffield E, et al: The aetiology of vein graft stenoses. Eur J Vasc Surg 8:389–394, 1994.
12. Darling RC III, Roddy SP, Chang BB, et al: Long-term results of revised infrainguinal arterial reconstructions. J Vasc Surg 35:773–778, 2002.
13. Ruoff BA, Cranley JJ, Hannan LW, et al: Real-time duplex ultrasound mapping of the greater saphenous vein before in situ infrainguinal revascularization. J Vasc Surg 6:107–113, 1987.
14. Leopold PW, Shandall AA, Corson JD, et al: Initial experience comparing B-mode imaging and venography of the saphenous vein before in situ bypass. Am J Surg 152:206–210, 1986.
15. Gimbrone MA Jr, Anderson KR, Topper JN, et al: The critical role of mechanical forces in blood vessel development, physiology, and pathology. J Vasc Surg 29:1104–1151, 1999.
16. Zarins CK, Zatina MA, Giddens DP, et al: Shear stress regulation of artery lumen diameter in experimental atherogenesis. J Vasc Surg 5:413–420, 1987.
17. Fillinger MF, Cronenwett JL, Besso S, et al: Vein adaptation to the hemodynamic environment of infrainguinal grafts. J Vasc Surg 19:970–979, 1994.
18. Towne JB, Schmitt DD, Seabrook GR, et al: The effect of vein diameter on patency of in situ grafts. J Cardiovasc Surg 32:192–196, 1991.
19. Blebea J, Schomaker WR, Hod G, et al: Preoperative duplex venous mapping: A comparison of positional techniques in patients with and without atherosclerosis. J Vasc Surg 20:226–234, 1994.
20. Miller A, Marcaccio EJ, Tannenbaum GA, et al: Comparison of angioscopy and angiography for monitoring infrainguinal vein grafts: Results of a prospective randomized trial. J Vasc Surg 17:382–388, 1993.
21. Bandyk DF, Jorgensen RA, Towne JB: Intraoperative assessment of in situ saphenous vein arterial grafts using pulsed Doppler spectral analysis. Arch Surg 121:292–299, 1986.
22. Ascer E, Veith FJ, White-Flores SA, et al: Intraoperative outflow resistance as a predictor of late patency of femoropopliteal and infrapopliteal arterial bypasses. J Vasc Surg 5:820–827, 1987.
23. Vos GA, Rauwerda JA, van der Broek TA, et al: The correlation of preoperative outflow resistance measurements with patency of 109 infrainguinal arterial reconstructions. Eur J Vasc Surg 3:539–542, 1989.
24. Schwartz LB, Belkin M, Donaldson MC, et al: Validation of a new and specific intraoperative measurement of vein graft resistance. J Vasc Surg 25:1033–1041, 1997.
25. Mills JL, Fujitani RM, Taylor SM: Contribution of routine intraoperative completion arteriography to early infrainguinal bypass patency. Am J Surg 164:506–511, 1992.
26. Clair DG, Golden MA, Mannick JA, et al: Randomized prospective study of angioscopically assisted in situ saphenous vein grafting. J Vasc Surg 19:992–1000, 1994.
27. Marcaccio EJ, Miller A, Tannenbaum GA, et al: Angioscopically directed interventions improve arm vein bypass grafts. J Vasc Surg 17:994–1004, 1993.
28. Faries PL, Arora S, Pomposelli FB Jr, et al: The use of arm vein in lower-extremity revascularization: Results of 520 procedures performed in 8 years. J Vasc Surg 31:50–59, 2000.
29. Miller A, Stonebridge PA, Tsoukas AI, et al: Angioscopically directed valvulotomy: A new valvulotome and technique. J Vasc Surg 13:813–821, 1991.
30. Holzenbein TJ, Pomposelli FB Jr, Miller A, et al: Results of a policy with arm veins used as the first alternative to an unavailable ipsilateral greater saphenous vein for infrainguinal bypass. J Vasc Surg 23:130–140, 1996.
31. Gilbertson JJ, Walsh DB, Zwolak RM, et al: A blinded comparison of angiography, angioscopy, and duplex scanning in the intraoperative evaluation of in situ saphenous vein bypass grafts. J Vasc Surg 15:121–129, 1992.
32. Papanicolaou G, Aziz I, Yellin AE, et al: Intraoperative color duplex scanning for infrainguinal vein grafts. Ann Vasc Surg 10:347–355, 1996.
33. Bandyk DF, Johnson BL, Gupta AK, et al: Nature and management of duplex abnormalities encountered during infrainguinal vein bypass grafting. J Vasc Surg 24:430–438, 1996.
34. Johnson BL, Bandyk DF, Back MR, et al: Intraoperative duplex monitoring of infrainguinal vein bypass procedures. J Vasc Surg 31:678–690, 2000.
35. van der Lugt A, Gussenhoven EJ, The SH, et al: Femorodistal venous bypass evaluated with intravascular ultrasound. Eur J Vasc Endovasc Surg 9:394–402, 1995.
36. Terry HJ, Allan JS, Taylor GW: The relationship between blood-flow and failure of femoropopliteal reconstructive arterial surgery. Br J Surg 59:549–551, 1972.
37. Albrechtsen D: Intraoperative hemodynamic findings and their prognostic significance in femoropopliteal reverse saphenous vein graft bypass operations. Scand J Thor Cardiovasc Surg 10:67–76, 1976.
38. Ascer E, Veith FJ, Morin L, et al: Quantitative assessment of outflow resistance in lower extremity arterial reconstructions. J Surg Res 37:8–15, 1984.
39. Menzoian JO, LaMorte WW, Cantelmo NL, et al: The preoperative angiogram as a predictor of peripheral vascular runoff. Am J Surg 150:346–352, 1985.
40. Peterkin GA, Manabe S, LaMorte WW, et al: Evaluation of a proposed standard reporting system for preoperative angiograms in infrainguinal bypass procedures: Angiographic correlates of measured runoff resistance. J Vasc Surg 7:379–385, 1988.

41. Schwartz LB, Purut CM, Craig DM, et al: Measurement of vascular input impedance in infrainguinal vein grafts. Ann Vasc Surg 11:35–43, 1997.

42. LoGerfo FW, Corson JD, Mannick JA: Improved results with femoropopliteal vein grafts for limb salvage. Arch Surg 112:567–570, 1977.

43. Davies AH: Vein factors that affect the outcome of femorodistal bypass. Ann R Coll Surg Engl 77:63–66, 1995.

44. Marin ML, Veith FJ, Panetta TF, et al: Saphenous vein biopsy: A predictor of vein graft failure. J Vasc Surg 18:407–415, 1993.

45. James DC, Durrani T, Wixon CL, et al: Preimplant vein intimal thickness is not a predictor of bypass graft stenosis. J Surg Res 96:1–5, 2001.

46. Veith FJ, Gupta SK, Ascer E, et al: Six-year prospective multicenter randomized comparison of autologous saphenous vein and expanded polytetrafluoroethylene grafts in infrainguinal arterial reconstructions. J Vasc Surg 3:104–114, 1986.

47. Moody P, Gould DA, Harris PL: Vein graft surveillance improves patency in femoro-popliteal bypass. Eur J Vasc Surg 4:117–121, 1990.

48. Idu MM, Blankstein JD, de Gier P, et al: Impact of a color-flow duplex surveillance program on infrainguinal vein graft patency: A 5-year experience. J Vasc Surg 17:42–53, 1993.

49. Szilagyi DE, Elliot JP, Hageman J, et al: Biologic fate of autogenous vein implants as arterial substitutes: Clinical, angiographic, and histopathologic observations in femoro-popliteal operations for atherosclerosis. Ann Surg 178:232–246, 1973.

50. Landry GJ, Moneta GL, Taylor LM Jr, et al: Duplex scanning alone is not sufficient imaging before secondary procedures after lower extremity reversed vein bypass graft. J Vasc Surg 29:270–281, 1999.

51. Nehler MR, Moneta GL, Yeager RA, et al: Surgical treatment of threatened reversed infrainguinal vein grafts. J Vasc Surg 20:558–565, 1994.

52. Caps MT, Cantwell-Gab K, Bergelin RO, et al: Vein graft lesions: Time of onset and rate of progression. J Vasc Surg 22:466–475, 1995.

53. Erickson CA, Towne JB, Seabrook GR, et al: Ongoing vascular laboratory surveillance is essential to maximize long-term in situ saphenous vein bypass patency. J Vasc Surg 23:18–27, 1996.

54. Gentile AT, Mills JL, Gooden MA, et al: Identification of predictors for lower extremity vein graft stenosis. Am J Surg 174:218–221, 1997.

55. Donaldson MC, Mannick JA, Whittemore AD: Femoral-distal bypass with in situ greater saphenous vein: Long-term results using the Mills valvulotome. Ann Surg 213:457–465, 1991.

56. Mills JL, Fujitani RM, Taylor SM: The characteristics and anatomic distribution of lesions that cause reversed vein graft failure: A 5-year prospective study. J Vasc Surg 17:195–206, 1993.

57. Laborde AL, Synn AY, Worsey MJ, et al: A prospective comparison of ankle/brachial indices and color duplex imaging in surveillance of the in situ saphenous vein bypass. J Cardiovasc Surg 33:420–425, 1992.

58. Bandyk DF, Bergamini TM, Towne JB, et al: Durability of vein graft revision: The outcome of secondary procedures. J Vasc Surg 13:200–210, 1991.

59. Green RM, McNamara J, Ouriel K, et al: Comparison of infrainguinal graft surveillance techniques. J Vasc Surg 11:207–215, 1990.

60. Zhang Q, Houghton AP, Derodua J, et al: Impedance analysis compared with quickscan in the detection of graft-related stenoses. Eur J Vasc Endovasc Surg 9:218–221, 1995.

61. Wyatt MG, Tennant WG, Scott DJA, et al: Impedance analysis to identify the "at risk" femorodistal graft. J Vasc Surg 13:284–293, 1991.

62. Ferris BL, Mills JL Sr, Hughes JD, et al: Is early postoperative duplex scan surveillance of leg bypass grafts clinically important? J Vasc Surg 37:495–500, 2003.

63. Wilson YG, Davies AH, Currie IC, et al: Vein graft stenosis: Incidence and intervention. Eur J Vasc Endovasc Surg 11:164–169, 1996.

64. Nielsen TG: Natural history of infrainguinal vein bypass stenoses: Early lesions increase the risk of thrombosis. Eur J Vasc Endovasc Surg 12:60–64, 1996.

65. Ihnat DM, Mills JL, Dawson DL, et al: The correlation of early flow disturbances with the development of infrainguinal graft stenosis: A 10-year study of 341 autogenous vein grafts. J Vasc Surg 30:8–15, 1999.

66. Mills JL Sr, Wixon CL, James DC, et al: The natural history of intermediate and critical vein graft stenosis: Recommendation for continued surveillance or repair. J Vasc Surg 33:273–280, 2001.

67. Robinson KD, Sato DT, Gregory RT, et al: Long-term outcome after early infrainguinal graft failure. J Vasc Surg 26:425–438, 1997.

68. Belkin M, Conte MS, Donaldson MI, et al: Preferred strategies for secondary infrainguinal bypass: Lessons learned from 300 consecutive reoperations. J Vasc Surg 21:282–295, 1995.

69. Belkin M, Donaldson MI, Whittemore AD, et al: Observations on the use of thrombolytic occlusion of infrainguinal vein grafts. J Vasc Surg 11:289–296, 1990.

70. Cohen JR, Mannick JA, Couch NP, et al: Recognition and management of impending vein-graft failure: Importance for long-term patency. Arch Surg 121:758–759, 1986.

71. Graor RA, Risius B, Young JR, et al: Thrombolysis of peripheral arterial bypass grafts: Surgical thrombectomy compared with thrombolysis: A preliminary report. J Vasc Surg 7:347–355, 1988.

72. Ouriel K, Shortell CK, DeWeese JA, et al: A comparison of thrombolytic therapy with operative revascularization in the initial treatment of acute peripheral arterial ischemia. J Vasc Surg 19:1021–1030, 1994.

73. Bandyk DF, Schmitt DD, Seabrook GR, et al: Monitoring functional patency of in situ saphenous vein bypasses: The impact of a surveillance protocol and elective revision. J Vasc Surg 9:286–296, 1989.

74. Landry GJ, Moneta GL, Taylor LM Jr, et al: Long-term outcome of revised lower-extremity bypass grafts. J Vasc Surg 35:56–63, 2002.

75. Mills JL, Bandyk DF, Gahtan V, et al: The origin of infrainguinal vein graft stenosis: A prospective study based on duplex surveillance. J Vasc Surg 21:16–25, 1995.

76. Reifsnyder T, Towne JB, Seabrook GR, et al: Biologic characteristics of long-term autogenous vein grafts: A dynamic evolution. J Vasc Surg 17:207–217, 1993.

77. Buth J, Disselhoff B, Sommeling C, et al: Color-flow duplex criteria for grading stenosis in infrainguinal vein grafts. J Vasc Surg 14:716–728, 1991.

78. Belkin M, Mackey WC, McLaughlin R, et al: The variation in vein graft flow velocity with luminal diameter and outflow level. J Vasc Surg 15:991–999, 1992.

79. Belkin M, Raftery KB, Mackey WC, et al: A prospective study of the determinants of vein graft flow velocity: Implications for graft surveillance. J Vasc Surg 19:259–267, 1994.

80. Sladen JG, Reid JD, Cooperberg PL, et al: Color-flow duplex screening of infrainguinal grafts combining low- and high-velocity criteria. Am J Surg 158:107–112, 1989.

81. Wengerter KR, Veith FJ, Gupta SK, et al: Prospective randomized multicenter comparison of in situ and reversed vein infrapopliteal bypasses. J Vasc Surg 13:189–199, 1991.

82. Moody AP, Edwards PR, Harris PL: In situ versus reversed femoropopliteal vein grafts: Long-term follow-up of a prospective, randomized trial. Br J Surg 79:750–752, 1992.

83. Harris EJ Jr, Taylor LM Jr, Moneta GL, et al: Outcome of infrainguinal arterial reconstruction in women. J Vasc Surg 18:627–636, 1993.

84. Magnant JG, Cronenwett JL, Walsh DB, et al: Surgical treatment of infrainguinal arterial occlusive disease in women. J Vasc Surg 17:67–78, 1993.

85. Chang BB, Darling RC III, Bock DEM, et al: The use of spliced vein bypasses for infrainguinal arterial reconstruction. J Vasc Surg 21:403–412, 1995.

86. Chew DKW, Conte MS, Donaldson MC, et al: Autogenous composite vein bypass graft for infrainguinal arterial reconstruction. J Vasc Surg 33:259–264, 2001.

87. Ihlberg LHM, Alback NA, Lassila R, et al: Intraoperative flow predicts the development of stenosis in infrainguinal vein grafts. J Vasc Surg 34:269–276, 2001.

88. Lundell A, Bergqvist D: Prediction of early graft occlusion in femoropopliteal and femorodistal reconstruction by measurement of volume flow with a transit time flowmeter and calculation of peripheral resistance. Eur J Vasc Surg 7:704–708, 1993.

89. Mattos MA, van Bemmelen PS, Hodgson KJ, et al: Does correction of stenoses identified with color duplex scanning improve infrainguinal graft patency? J Vasc Surg 17:54–66, 1993.

90. Treiman GS, Ashrafi A, Lawrence PF: Incidentally detected stenoses proximal to grafts originating below the common femoral artery: Do they affect graft patency or warrant repair in asymptomatic patients? J Vasc Surg 32:1180–1189, 2000.

91. Ryan SV, Dougherty MJ, Chang M, et al: Abnormal duplex findings at the proximal anastomosis of infrainguinal bypass grafts: Does revision enhance patency? Ann Vasc Surg 15:98–103, 2001.

92. Idu MM, Buth J, Hop WCJ, et al: Vein graft surveillance: Is graft revision without angiography justified and what criteria should be used? J Vasc Surg 27:399–413, 1998.

93. Berkowitz HD, Fox AD, Deaton DH: Reversed vein graft stenosis: Early diagnosis and management. J Vasc Surg 15:130–141, 1992.

94. Donaldson MC, Mannick JA, Whittemore AD: Causes of primary graft failure after in situ saphenous vein bypass grafting. J Vasc Surg 15:113–120, 1992.

95. Bergamini TM, George SM Sr, Massey HT, et al: Intensive surveillance of femoropopliteal-tibial autogenous vein bypasses improves long-term graft patency and limb salvage. Ann Surg 221:507–516, 1995.

96. Golledge J, Beattie DK, Greenhalgh RM, et al: Have the results of infrainguinal bypass improved with the widespread utilization of postoperative surveillance? Eur J Vasc Endovasc Surg 11:388–392, 1996.

97. Lundell A, Lindblad B, Bergqvist D, et al: Femoropopliteal-crural graft patency is improved by an intensive surveillance program. A prospective randomized study. J Vasc Surg 21:26–34, 1995.

98. Kirby PL, Brady AR, Thompson SG, et al: The Vein Graft Surveillance Trial: Rationale, design, and methods. VGST participants. Eur J Vasc Endovasc Surg 18:469–474, 1999.

99. Wixon CL, Mills JL, Westerband A, et al: An economic appraisal of lower extremity bypass graft maintenance. J Vasc Surg 32:1–12, 2000.

100. Visser K, Idu MM, Buth J, et al: Duplex scan surveillance during the first year after infrainguinal autologous vein bypass grafting surgery: Costs and clinical outcomes compared with other surveillance programs. J Vasc Surg 33:123–130, 2001.

101. Hoballah JJ, Nazzal MM, Ryan SM, et al: Is color duplex surveillance of infrainguinal polytetrafluoroethylene grafts worthwhile? Am J Surg 174:131–135, 1997.

102. Lalak NJ, Hanel KC, Hunt J, et al: Duplex scan surveillance of infrainguinal prosthetic bypass grafts. J Vasc Surg 20:637–641, 1994.

The Current Role of MRA in Planning Interventions for Lower Extremity Ischemia

MARK D. MORASCH • JEREMY COLLINS

Introduction

Lower extremity contrast-enhanced three-dimensional (3-D) magnetic resonance angiography (LE-CEMRA) is a valuable diagnostic tool in peripheral vascular occlusive disease,[1-4] although its acceptance as an alternative to digital subtraction angiography (DSA) clearly is not universal.[2-4] In fact, the use of DSA as a primary preoperative imaging modality continues to be the rule rather than the exception. In an attempt to supplant invasive imaging from this primary role, a number of different approaches have been applied to improve the quality and reproducibility of LE-CEMRA. Simultaneously, steps have been taken to decrease LE-CEMRA examination times in hopes of improving patient acceptance and increasing overall efficiency.

A number of different LE-CEMRA contrast-injection and acquisition schemes have been created in an attempt to eliminate the guesswork involved in imaging lower extremity vessels by measuring exact contrast arrival times to the pelvis, thighs, and calves.[5,6] Standardized protocols now consistently produce high-quality images and have allowed an almost complete elimination of DSA as the preoperative diagnostic test of choice at the authors' institution.

Hybrid MRA Technique

Between July and December 2001, 60 consecutive patients were imaged with a standard technique using 3-D FLASH gradient echo pulse sequences and a dedicated peripheral vascular coil. Two independent timing measurements were performed, one for the pelvis at the level of the aortic bifurcation and one at the calves at the level of the tibial trifurcation. Timing runs were performed with a flow-insensitive, T1-weighted gradient-echo sequence with an automated image-subtraction algorithm.[5]

After the precontrast mask acquisitions were obtained in the calves/feet, distal LE-CEMRA acquisitions were performed based on the calf timing run. All patients were asked to actively plantar flex the foot so that the pedal vessels were within the imaging volume. Using the measured contrast arrival time, a 20-mL contrast bolus administered at 2 mL per second was performed. Two consecutive 3-D acquisitions were then obtained.

Once calf imaging was complete, mask acquisitions for the pelvis and thigh stations were obtained. Pelvis and thigh stepping-table LE-CEMRA was performed with a second infusion of 30 to 35 mL of gadolinium contrast. The start of the pelvic acquisition was determined from the pelvic timing run in a manner similar to a single injection bolus chase technique. Imaging parameters at each station were optimized to permit rapid scanning while maximizing in-plane and through-plane resolution. Average total acquisition time was 33 seconds for the pelvis and thighs and 25 seconds for the calves. Total magnetic resonance (MR) examination time averaged 45 minutes (Fig. 27I-1).

Results

Compared to angiographic correlates as gold standards, the overall sensitivity, specificity, and accuracy of LE-CEMRA were 99%, 97%, and 98%, respectively. Sensitivity and specificity for the calf stations alone were 100% and 91% using this standardized technique. In addition, venous contamination was marginally reduced in the proximal stations and was virtually eliminated ($p < 0.01$) in the calf station.

The renal vessels were visualized in 44 (73%) of the 60 patients. In 96 of 118 patient limbs (81%), the ankle posterior tibial and the dorsalis pedis arteries were visualized or could be clearly diagnosed as occluded. In seven magnetic resonance arteriography (MRA) studies, the acquisition data identified patent target vessels in the foot that DSA labeled as occluded (Fig. 27I-2). Conversely, DSA identified patent vessels eight times when MRA missed them. MRA missed the patent foot vessels because of poor positioning, not because of contrast mistiming, in three of the eight. Metallic suspectibility artifacts from arterial stents, knee prostheses, or hip prostheses degraded images in 7 of the 60 examinations.

The authors successfully formulated a sound treatment plan, without further diagnostic imaging, based on the data set provided by MR imaging alone, in 58 patients (97%). A preoperative diagnostic angiogram was required to formulate a treatment plan in only 2 (3%) of the 60 study patients.

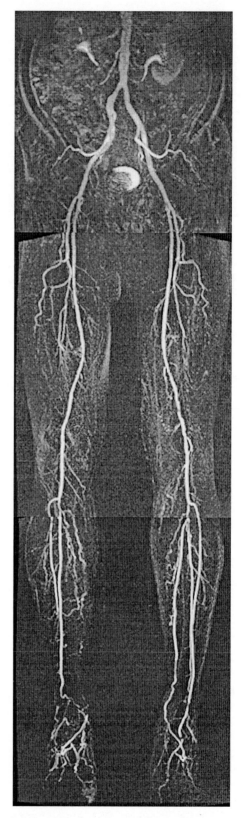

Figure 27I-1. Typical contrast-enhanced MRA using dual-timing dual-injection schemes on a standard automated stepping-table.

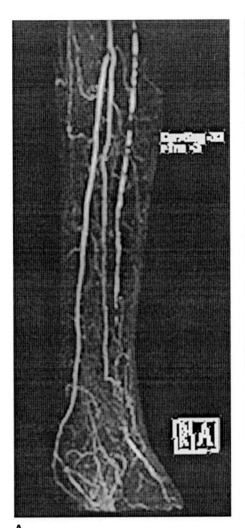

A

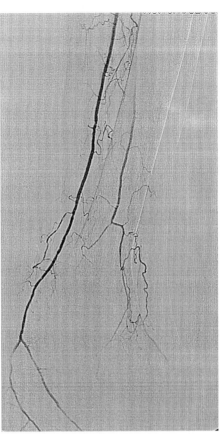

B

Figure 27I-2. Contrast-enhanced calf MRA clearly demonstrates patent tibial and pedal vessels prior to reconstruction. ***A****, Calf MRA;* ***B****, calf angiogram.*

Discussion

Early MR angiograms using contrast enhancement and signal reception from surface coils were completed by moving a phased array coil from station to station for separate acquisitions of the calves, thighs, and pelvis. These techniques, devised for stationary MR tables, required separate paramagnetic contrast injections for each of the three imaging stations, the calf being the last. Progressive accumulation of contrast in the soft tissues hampered optimal visualization of calf vessels.[6–9]

The development of an automated stepping-table[1,10–12] and newer dedicated peripheral array coils[13] has greatly improved the speed and image quality by capitalizing on bolus-chase contrast infusion. The implementation of simple single-injection bolus-chase techniques extended the quality of the images to all three regions (i.e., pelvis, thighs, and calves). Chasing the arterial bolus all the way to the calves and feet before venous contamination occurs remained challenging, however.[1] Although many techniques (e.g., cardiac gating,[14] fluoroscopic real-time bolus monitoring,[1] elliptical centric k-space acquisition,[15] projection reconstruction, and k-space undersampling) have improved LE-CEMRA, no single technique has been universally accepted.[16,17] Despite significant improvements, the quality of standard single-injection bolus-chase techniques remains inconsistent.[18,19] Alternative MRA techniques (e.g., 2-D time-of-flight acquisitions) that are based on thin axial slices and use no contrast are very sensitive to slow flow, and when performed properly can identify patent tibial and pedal runoff vessels more accurately than conventional DSA.[20,21] Unacceptably long acquisition times limit the clinical practicality of time-of-flight techniques, however.[22–25]

Digital subtraction angiography has its own limitations: it involves an arterial puncture, radiation exposure, and nephrotoxic iodinated contrast. Contrast angiography uses x-ray projection techniques, which are known to over- or underestimate nonconcentric stenoses unless multiple projections are used. Also, as seen with bolus-chase LE-CEMRA, timing differences exist between legs, and this can lead to poor imaging of distal segments with catheter angiography when mistiming occurs. In fact, when compared to certain MR techniques, DSA may provide inferior pedal vessel images unless a concerted effort is made to image with vasodilators. Similarly, CT angiography (CTA) is limited by the requirements for ionizing radiation and nephrotoxic iodinated contrast.

Hybrid dual-contrast injection and dual-acquisition LE-CEMRA schemes were developed to try to limit the variability involved in imaging the vessels of the lower extremities with MR. This newer technique eliminates venous contamination in the calf while enabling near-isotropic resolution where identification of distal bypass targets is critical. These techniques preserve both in-plane and through-plane spatial resolution in the pelvis and thighs to allow retrospective image reconstruction in an infinite number of projections. This is information that could be derived only from additional contrast-boluses and additional projections if DSA were used. When tibial contrast arrival times are discrepant, as seen in patients with asymmetric occlusive disease or in patients with a unilateral bypass graft, a separate timing run to the calves allows operators to tailor the MRA to allow optimal imaging of both extremities. Also, because of reduction in venous signal and tissue enhancement, pedal vessel visualization is better than with a single run bolus-chase technique. The authors have found that pedal vessel visualization can be improved significantly by stressing the importance of maintaining plantar flexion throughout the calf/foot acquisition.

This MRI protocol has allowed the successful replacement of invasive angiography in most cases. From clinical experience, the authors recommend that, when reviewing any LE-CEMRA examination that utilizes image-mask subtraction, the contrast-enhanced original partitions should always be viewed to avoid erroneous conclusions caused by misregistration artifacts that could be translated onto the subtracted data sets. Following this protocol, only 3% of the authors' study patients who went on to an intervention required any further diagnostic imaging. Such diagnostic confidence in MR echoes that described by prior authors.[2,4,19]

Although significantly safer than other accepted imaging modalities, there are a few well-recognized contraindications to MR imaging. Patients with pacemakers, ocular metallic foreign bodies, or ferromagnetic intracranial aneurysm clips should not be imaged. MR imaging may also suffer from artifacts around intravascular stents and near joint prostheses, limiting visualization in the vicinity of these ferromagnetic objects. Large doses of gadolinium have also been found to cause renal failure in patients with a prior history of chronic renal insufficiency, so caution must be exercised.

Conclusions

Hybrid LE-CEMRA is robust, accurate, and reproducible in clinical practice. This technique consistently provides high-quality images that satisfy the rigorous preoperative demands of vascular surgeons and interventional radiologists by providing data sufficient to formulate sound treatment plans, in most cases rendering conventional DSA unnecessary.

KEY POINTS

- Contrast-enhanced lower extremity magnetic resonance angiography is a valuable preoperative planning tool that will likely replace angiography.

- Techniques continue to be refined constantly, but it is important to standardize protocols so that institutional results are consistent.

- The authors' standardized protocol is presented as one option that has allowed imaging of inflow and target vessels with precision. As such, it has virtually eliminated invasive conventional angiography in the authors' practice.

REFERENCES

1. Wang Y, Lee H, Khilnani N, et al: Bolus-chase MR digital subtraction angiography in the lower extremity. Radiology 207(1):263–269, 1998.
2. Cambria R, Kaufman J, L'Italien G, et al: Magnetic resonance angiography in the management of lower extremity arterial occlusive disease: A prospective study. J Vasc Surg 25(2):380–389, 1997.
3. Nelemans P, Leiner T, de Vet H, et al: Peripheral arterial disease: Meta-analysis of the diagnostic performance of MR angiography. Radiology 217(1):105–114, 2000.
4. Huber T, Back M, Ballinger R, et al: Utility of magnetic resonance arteriography for distal lower extremity revascularization. J Vasc Surg 26(3):415–424, 1997.
5. Finn J, Francois C, Moore J, et al: Lower extremity MRA with full prior specification of bolus transit times. Paper presented at ISMRM, 10th Scientific Meeting and Exhibition, May 2002, Honolulu, HI.
6. Carr JC, Pereles FS, Collins JC, et al: Stepping-table lower extremity MR angiography with separate calf acquisition and dual-level bolus timing. ISMRM, 10th Scientific Meeting and Exhibition, May 2002, Honolulu, HI.
7. Aksit P, Frigo F, Polzin J, et al: Shoot and scoot: A segmented volume acquisition method of high-resolution multi-station imaging of peripheral vasculature. Paper presented at ISMRM 10th Annual Scientific Meeting and Exhibition, May 2002, Honolulu, HI.
8. Leiner T, Kessels A, Van Engelshoven J: Total runoff peripheral MRA in patients with critical ischemia and tissue loss can detect more patient arteries than IA-DSA. Paper presented at ISMRM 10th Annual Scientific Meeting and Exhibition, May 2002, Honolulu, HI.
9. Sabati M, Lauzon M, Frayne R: Interactive large field-of-view peripheral MRA. Paper presented at ISMRM 10th Annual Scientific Meeting and Exhibition, May 2002, Honolulu, HI.

10. Ho K, Leiner T, de Haan M, et al: Peripheral vascular tree stenoses: Evaluation with moving-bed infusion-tracing MR angiography. Radiology 206(3):683–692, 1998.

11. Leiner T, Ho K, Nelemans P, et al: Three-dimensional contrast-enhanced moving-bed infusion-tracking (MoBI-Track) Peripheral MR angiography with flexible choice of imaging parameters for each field of view. J Mag Res Imag 11:368–377, 2000.

12. Meaney J, Ridgway J, Chakraverty S, et al: Stepping-table gadolinium-enhanced digital subtraction MR angiography of the aorta and lower extremity arteries: Preliminary experience. Radiology 211(1):59–67, 1999.

13. Ruehm S, Hany T, Pfammatter T, et al: Pelvic and lower extremity arterial imaging: Diagnostic performance of three-dimensional contrast-enhanced MR angiography. Am J Roentgenol 174:1127–1135, 2000.

14. Glickerman D, Obregon R, Schmiedl U, et al: Cardiac-gated MR angiography of the entire lower extremity: A prospective comparison with conventional angiography. Am J Roentgenol 167:445–451, 1996.

15. Snidow J, MS J, Harris V, et al: Three-dimensional gadolinium-enhanced MR angiography for aortoiliac inflow assessment plus renal artery screening in a single breath hold. Radiol 198(3):725–732, 1996.

16. Du J, Block W, Carroll T, et al: Peripheral angiography with a time-resolved VIPR sequence. Paper presented at ISMRM 10th Annual Scientific Meeting and Exhibition, May 2002, Honolulu, HI.

17. Fain S, Du J, Browning F, et al: Floating table isotropic projection imaging (FLIPR): A technique for fast, extended FOV, contrast-enhanced MRA. Paper presented at ISMRM 10th Annual Scientific Meeting and Exhibition, May 2002, Honolulu, HI.

18. Kreitner K-F, Kalden P, Neufang A, et al: Diabetes and peripheral arterial occlusive disease. Am J Roentgenol 174:171–179, 2000.

19. Levy M, Baum R, Carpenter J: Endovascular surgery based solely on noninvasive preprocedural imaging. J Vasc Surg 28(6):995–1005, 1998.

20. Owen RS: Magnetic resonance imaging of angiographically occult runoff vessels in peripheral arterial occlusive disease. N Engl J Med 326:1577–1581, 1992.

21. Cortell ED, Kaufman JA, Geller SC, et al: MR angiography of tibial runoff vessels: Imaging with the head coil compared with conventional arteriography. Am J Roentgenol 167(1):147–151, 1996.

22. McCauley TR, Monib A, Dickey KW, et al: Peripheral vascular occlusive disease: Accuracy and reliability of time-of-flight MR angiography. Radiol 192(2):351–357, 1994.

23. Schmiedl UP, Yuan C, Nghiem HV, et al: MR angiography of the peripheral vasculature. Seminars in Ultrasound, CT & MR 17(4):404–411, 1996.

24. Snidow J, Harris V, Trerotola S, et al: Interpretations and treatment decisions based on MR angiography versus conventional arteriography in symptomatic lower extremity ischemia. J Vasc Intervent Radiol 6:595–603, 1995.

25. Yucel E, Silver M, Carter A: MR angiography of normal pelvic arteries: Comparison of signal intensity and contrast-to-noise ratio for three different inflow techniques. Am J Roentgenol 136:197–201, 1994.

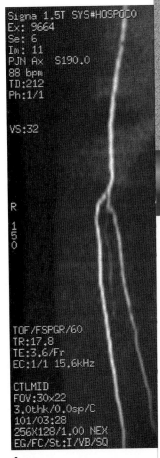

A

Figure 27II-1. **A**, *MRA in*
patient with left nonhealing
demonstrating areas of focal
the popliteal and proximal tib
The patient was at high card
open surgical revascularizati
treated with percutaneous a
B, *Arteriogram done at the*
confirms the focal lesions se

Chapter 27II

The Role of Magnetic Resonance Angiography in Peripheral Vascular Disease

SANDRA C. CARR • WILLIAM D. TURNIPSEED
• THOMAS M. GRIST

▦ Imaging Techniques

▦ Use of MRA for Lower Extremity Arterial
Occlusive Disease

▦ Use of MRA to Detect Restenosis Following
Lower Extremity Grafting

▦ Limitations of MRA

▦ Future of MRA

▦ Conclusions

I maging of the vascular system is an essential component in the preoperative and postoperative management of patients with peripheral vascular disease of the lower extremities. Traditionally, contrast angiography, especially digital subtraction angiography, has been the gold standard for imaging of the arterial system. Digital subtraction angiography (DSA) has many advantages and provides excellent visualization of the inflow and outflow vessels in most cases. Disadvantages of contrast angiography are that it is interventional, costly, and not completely safe.

Complications are rare but include contrast-related nephrotoxicity, arterial injury with hemorrhage, thrombosis, allergic reaction, and distal embolization. Because of this, there has been impetus for the development of noninvasive imaging techniques such as magnetic resonance arteriography (MRA). Magnetic resonance imaging (MRI) utilizes a magentic field to create differential atomic signals in soft tissues to obtain information about the morphology of the arterial system and functional assessment of its bloodflow.

Magnetic resonance arteriography has many advantages over traditional contrast arteriography. At the authors' institution, MRA costs nearly $800 less than a contrast arteriogram. More importantly, MRA is safer for many patients. This technique is noninvasive, thus avoiding arterial catheterization. Exposure to radiation is not required, and the use of high-volume ionic contrast agents is unnecessary. This is especially important for diabetic patients with peripheral vascular disease and pre-existing renal insufficiency, who are at especially high risk for contrast-induced nephrotoxicity. Various imaging techniques may be necessary to get the best anatomic and functional information for proper treatment. This chapter summarizes commonly used imaging techniques and clinical applications of MRI in the

diagnosis and managem
disease.

Imaging Techniq

The most common tecl
peripheral arterial system
three-dimensional (3-D)
CE-MRA). Two-dimensi(
gradient-recalled echo t
quency pulses to suppi
soft tissue.[1] Thin cross-s
thick) are repeatedly exp
this causes the soft tiss
appear dark, whereas t
blood, not exposed to re
appear bright (high sigr
this phenomenon, know
blood flowing rapidly t
the best (high signal,
Slow-flowing blood is p
through the slice, causin
advantages of 2-D TOF
effects for normal flov
time, and increased ser
flow states in the circul

3-D CE-MRA uses mi
(i.e., 3- to 8-mm thick) tł
than 1-mm thick) partiti(
tissue volume slabs, tht
The addition of paramag
3-D MRA imaging has
and clinical utility of M.
artifacts and flow void s(
Gadolinium, a heavy m
diethylenetriamine peni
contrast enhancement; i
tion and is not known t
a potent T_1-relaxing ag
lution by increasing tł
surrounding soft tissue
mined so that proper ti
calculated for the partic
Using gadolinium witł
significant imaging tim
of artifacts, eliminatioı
improved spatial resolu

In addition to TOF im
(PCA) is often perforn
stenotic lesions in are
PCA takes advantage o
change in the phase
through a magnetic fie
change is proportional
protons in the blood. B

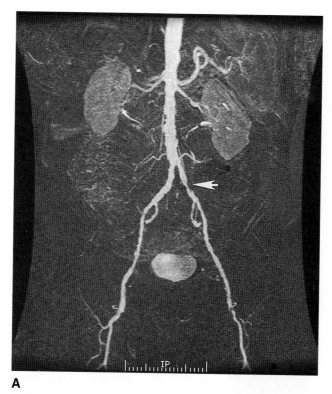

A

Figure 27II-2. **A**, MRA demonstrates a focal left iliac stenosis (arrow) treated intraoperatively with balloon angioplasty at the time of femoral popliteal bypass. **B**, Intraoperative arteriogram before (top) and after (bottom) angioplasty of this iliac lesion.

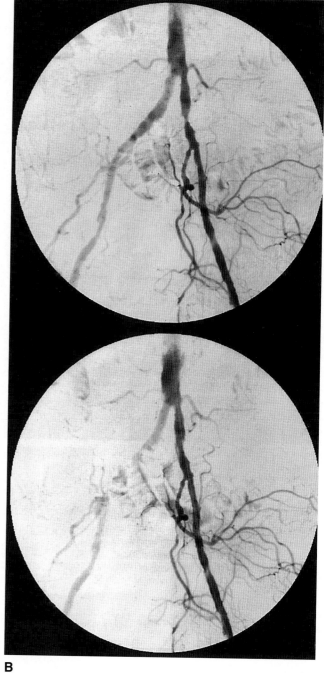

B

by MRA. Unlike contrast arteriography, MRA correctly identified all vessels found to be patent at surgery.[5] The use of MRA in these patients avoided the need for blind exploration of runoff vessels and led to limb salvage procedures that had not been previously regarded as possible, based on the preoperative contrast arteriogram. In a study by Hoch and colleagues, 50 ischemic lower limbs in 45 patients were examined with both conventional contrast DSA and 2-D TOF MRA. Interpretation of MRA and DSA studies correlated exactly in 315 (89.5%) of 352 arterial segments. The MRA and DSA interpreta-

tions disagreed in 28 (13.8%) of 203 infrageniculate arteries compared with only 8 (5.6%) disagreements in the suprageniculate arterial segments. MRA predicted the level of arterial reconstruction in all 23 limbs that required arterial bypass and in 18 of 19 (94.7%) limbs treated with percutaneous angioplasty. Importantly, they also noted a 31% ($756) cost savings with MRA compared with DSA angiography.[6] Because of problems with timing and low flow states in the distal infrageniculate arteries, DSA angiography may fail to identify a suitable distal target vessel, especially if the injection of contrast is

TABLE 27II-1. **MRA Compared With Contrast Angiography**

	Number of Patients (n)	Sensitivity	Specificity	Technique	Vascular Bed
Prince	43	74%	98%	3-D contrast	Aortoiliac
Snidow	32	100%	98%	3-D contrast	Aortoiliac
Hany	39	93% to 96%	96% to 100%	3-D contrast	Aortoiliac
Ho	38	93%	98%	3-D contrast	All
Winchester	22	90%	98%	2-D contrast	All
Meaney	20	95%	98%	3-D contrast	All
Bendib	23	91%	92%	3-D contrast	Bypass grafts
Turnipseed	20	95%	80%	2-D TOF	Bypass grafts
Baum	155	85%	81%	2-D TOF	Infrageniculate

From: Prince MR: Gadolinium-enhanced MR angiography. Radiology 191:155–164, 1994. Snidow J, Aison A, Harris V, et al: Iliac artery MR angiography comparison of 3-D gadolinium-enhanced and 2-D time of flight techniques. Radiology 196:371–378, 1995; Hany TF, Debatin JF, Leung DA, Pfammatter T: Evaluation of the aortoiliac and renal arteries: Comparison of breath-hold, contrast-enhanced, three-dimensional MR angiography with conventional catheter angiography. Radiology 204:357–362, 1997. Ho K, Leiner T, DeHaan M, et al: Peripheral vascular tree stenosis: Evaluation with moving-bed infusion-tracking MR angiography. Radiology 206:683–692, 1998; Winchester PA, Lee HM, Khilnan NM, et al: Comparison of 2-D MR digital subtraction angiography of the lower extremities with x-ray angiography. J Vasc Intervent Radiology 9:891–899, 1998; Meaney JF, Ridgway JP, Chakrquerty S: Stepping-table gadolinium-enhanced digital subtraction MR angiography of the aorta and lower extremity arteries: Preliminary experience. Radiology 211:59–67, 1999; Bendib K, Berthezene Y, Croisille P, et al: Assessment of complicated arterial bypass grafts: Value of contrast-enhanced subtraction magnetic resonance angiography. J Vasc Surg 26:1036–1042, 1997; Turnipseed WD, Sproat IA: A preliminary experience with use of magnetic resonance angiography in assessment of failing lower extremity bypass grafts. Surgery 112:664–669, 1992. Baum RA, Rutter CM, Sunshine JH, et al: Multicenter trial to evaluate vascular magnetic resonance angiography of the lower extremity. American College of Radiology Rapid Technology Assessment Group. JAMA 274:875–880, 1995.

made at the aortic level. Because of its ability to detect low flow states, MRA can be very useful in evaluating these difficult cases. In the authors' experience, distal runoff vessels not visualized by MRA are not suitable target vessels for surgical bypass (Fig. 27II-3).

Use of MRA to Detect Restenosis Following Lower Extremity Grafting

At the authors' institution, patients undergo routine pulse volume recording and duplex surveillance following lower extremity arterial bypass or percutaneous intervention. When noninvasive tests suggest impending graft failure, MRA is used to identify the location and severity of the occlusive lesions threatening graft function. Stenotic lesions caused by intimal hyperplasia at the anastomotic sites or within autogenous grafts can be identified and distinguished from disease progression in host vessels proximal or distal to the graft (Fig. 27II-4). Surgical revision is usually required for anastomotic or midautogenous graft stenoses, whereas focal stenoses secondary to progressive disease can often be treated with percutaneous angioplasty and/or stenting.

In 1990, Turnipseed and colleagues evaluated a series of failing bypass grafts identified by color-flow Doppler scanning using 2-D TOF MRA and digital subtraction angiography. MRA showed an exact correlation with DSA in 75% of patients. There were four false-positive MRA scans and one false-negative.[7] Interpretation errors in this study were most often caused by metallic clips and would likely be prevented by the use of 3-D TOF and the addition of gadolinium contrast. In a more recent report by Bendib and colleagues, gadolinium-enhanced MRA was found to be 91% sensitive and 97% specific for detecting graft stenosis.[8]

Limitations of MRA

Although the 2-D TOF techniques have been shown to be accurate for the assessment of infrainguinal disease, these methods have a few limitations.[1] Disadvantages include sensitivity to flow traveling in the same plane as the magnetic field, creating an imaging void[9] (Fig. 27II-5). Motion can severely degrade image quality and spatial resolution, resulting in overestimation of disease severity. Areas of turbulent arterial flow within a vessel can also result in signal loss, or a flow void, because of intervoxel dephasing. Most of these limitations have been overcome by the use of 3-D TOF and the addition of gadolinium contrast. Still, because of signal loss at or distal to a stenotic vascular lesion, there is a tendency to overestimate the degree of stenosis. In a report by Winterer and colleagues, no false-negative results were

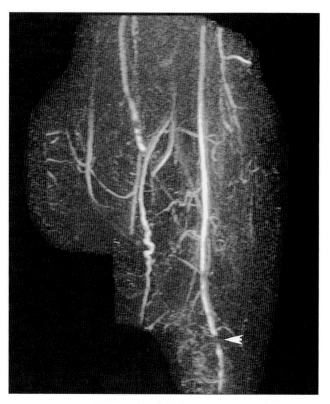

Figure 27II-4. *MRA demonstrates a stenosis at the distal anastamosis of a femoral popliteal graft.*

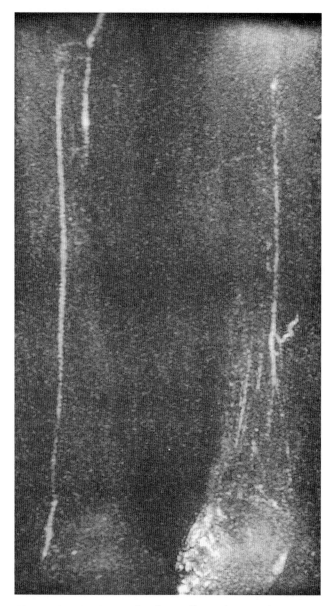

Figure 27II-3. *Patent distal runoff vessels were detected by MRA in this patient with limb threatening ischemia. Contrast arteriogram failed to detect an appropriate target for bypass.*

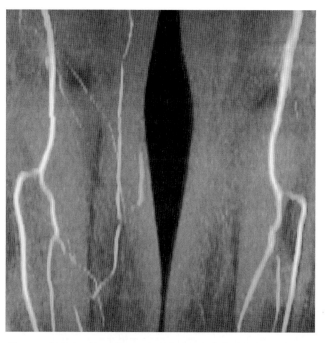

Figure 27II-5. *Two-dimensional time of flight MRA demonstrating a flow void at the origin of the anterior tibial artery. Blood moving in the same plane as the magnetic field may appear as an area of stenosis.*

found when comparing MRA to DSA in the iliac and femoropopliteal areas. MRA proved to be rather sensitive, however, with rates of 10% to 16% overgrading of the amount of stenosis.[10]

Unfortunately, not all patients are good candidates for MRA. Absolute contraindications to MRA include cardiac pacemakers, automatic cardiac defibrillator devices, cerebral aneurysm clips, and metal within the eyes (e.g., old shrapnel injuries). Although many patients have problems with claustrophobia, this is usually overcome with mild sedation.[1] With the equipment available at the authors' institution, patients larger than 380 pounds are unable to undergo MRA. Magnetic resonance imaging is adversely affected by movement during the radio frequency pulse sequences. Problems with swallowing, respiratory motion, and intestinal peristalsis decrease the image quality. When imaging the arterial system of the lower extremities, it is important to have a cooperative patient because physical movements greatly affect the image quality. Patients with severe respiratory disease may have problems lying flat for the examination. It is important to choose patients who are cooperative and able to follow instructions.[1]

Metallic stents such as the Palmaz stent, vena cava filters, ferromagnetic clips, and prosthetic joints cause significant artifacts and severely limit the ability to image the arterial system in that area. Artifacts are caused by the susceptibility effects of the metal, which causes signal dropout in the region of the metal. A metal artifact can be identified because of the signal void that has a characteristic build-up of signal on one side of the void.[8] A simple soft-tissue plain film can screen for metallic devices. Artifacts can be minimized but not completely eliminated using short TE sequences of 3-D contrast MRA.[11] Endovascular surgeons should use nitinol stents when possible, which are totally nonmagnetic.

Future of MRA

MRA currently provides a noninvasive, accurate, and sensitive method to image the vascular system. The spatial resolution of contrast-enhanced MRA has been improved but still does not equal that of contrast-enhanced DSA angiography. Current MRA techniques require a trade-off between spatial resolution and length of the examination. As the MR scanner hardware and software become more efficient, it will become possible to reconstruct high-resolution images relatively independent of the acquisition time. Unlike contrast-enhanced DSA, MRA often demonstrates signal loss at or distal to a stenosis because of complex flow in the area. This has led to problems with overestimation of the extent of disease. This is why noninvasive testing with duplex and pulse volume recording becomes important in MRA interpretation. Research in MRA techniques has been directed at shortening the short echo time (TE) to reduce this signal loss and improve image quality. Advances in postprocessing techniques may also further reduce the problems with overestimation of stenoses. Improvements in MRA software have allowed for the measurement of flow volumes and velocities, which will give vascular surgeons even more information about the functional significance of a particular vascular lesion.

The addition of gadolinium contrast has greatly improved the quality of MRA images. Research is also being done in the area of the development of improved contrast agents. Agents are being developed with higher relativity, which produces greater T1 shortening and results in improved signal-to-noise ratio. Other contrast agents are being produced that remain in the intravascular space for prolonged periods, thus allowing substantially higher resolution imaging.[12]

Currently, MRA is used for diagnostic road mapping and in the planning of therapy for lower extremity vascular occlusive disease. The relatively slow image reconstruction techniques for MRA have so far made it not suitable for real-time imaging. In the authors' practice, patients requiring an endovascular intervention must undergo contrast DSA at the time of the procedure. Research is currently being done to allow MR-guided interventions by combining MRA with fluoroscopic imaging to guide catheter manipulation. MRA-guided interventional procedures will eventually be possible when coupled with real-time reconstruction and display of MRA images.[12]

Conclusions

The addition of MRA imaging has greatly improved the vascular surgeon's ability to diagnose and properly treat lower extremity vascular disease. MRA has proven to be a noninvasive, safe, and accurate imaging modality when compared with traditional contrast DSA. Unlike DSA, MRA can provide not only anatomic information but physiologic information as well. Combinations of 2-D TOF and 3-D CE-MRA provide enough diagnostic information to plan for surgical or percutaneous intervention in the majority of patients. The limitations of MRA are gradually being overcome by improvements in coil design and software technology and by the addition of new contrast agents. Research in MRA-guided endovascular interventions will eventually make this modality even more useful.

REFERENCES

1. Turnipseed WD, Grist TM: Role of Magnetic Resonance Angiography in Peripheral Vascular Disease. In Whittemore AD, Bandyk D, Croenwett J, et al (eds): Advances in Vascular Surgery, vol 6. St. Louis: Mosby Year-Book, 1998.
2. Turnipseed WD: Magnetic Resonance Angiography Alone for Carotid Artery Surgery. In Yao JS, Pearce WH (eds): Current Techniques in Vascular Surgery. New York: McGraw-Hill, 2001.
3. Grist TM: MRA of the abdominal aorta and lower extremities. J Mag Res Imag 11:32–43, 2000.
4. Velazquez OC, Baum RA, Carpenter JP: Magnetic Resonance Angiography of Lower Extremity Arterial Disease. In Kerstein MD, White JV (eds): The Surgical Clinics of North America, vol 78. Philadelphia: WB Saunders, 1998.
5. Prince MR, Narasimham DL, Stanly JC, et al: Breath-hold gadolinium-enhanced MR angiography of the abdominal aorta and its major branches. Radiology 197:785–792, 1995.
6. Snidow J, Aison A, Harris V, et al: Iliac artery MR angiography comparison of 3-D gadolinium-enhanced and 2-D time of flight techniques. Radiology 196:371–378, 1995.

7. Winchester PA, Lee HM, Khilnan NM, et al: Comparison of 2-D MR digital subtraction angiography of the lower extremities with x-ray angiography. J Vasc Intervent Radiology 9:891–899, 1998.

8. Bendib K, Berthezene Y, Croisille P, et al: Assessment of complicated arterial bypass grafts: Value of contrast-enhanced subtraction magnetic resonance angiography. J Vasc Surg 26:1036–1042, 1997.

9. Grist TM: Peripheral MR angioplasty: Lower extremity. The Experts Guide 9–12, 2001.

10. Hang T, Debatin J, Leung D, et al: Evaluation of the aortoiliac and renal arteries: Comparison of breath-hold, contrast enhanced, 3-D MR angiography with conventional catheter angiography. Radiology 204:357–362, 1997.

11. Turnipseed WD, Sproat IA: A preliminary experience with use of magnetic resonance angiography in assessment of failing lower extremity bypass grafts. Surgery 112:664–669, 1992.

12. Baum RA, Rutter CM, Sunshine JH, et al: Multicenter trial to evaluate vascular magnetic resonance angiography of the lower extremity. American College of Radiology Rapid Technology Assessment Group. JAMA 274:875–880, 1995.

Chapter 28

Diagnosis of Congenital and Acquired AV Fistulas

ROBERT B. RUTHERFORD

Introduction

General Considerations

The vascular diagnostic laboratory (VDL) can provide much useful clinical decision-making information regarding peripheral arteriovenous fistulas, using much of the same instrumentation employed in diagnosing peripheral arterial occlusive disease (i.e., segmental limb pressures and plethysmography, velocity wave form analysis, and Duplex scanning).[1] A number of considerations govern how these diagnostic methods can or should be applied to greatest advantage. First, one needs to understand the hemodynamic characteristics of the arteriovenous fistula (AVF) in order to apply and interpret the various tests properly. Second, the diagnostic capabilities and limitations of the available tests differ and must be understood in applying them. Physiologic tests simply gauge the pressure, volume, or velocity changes associated with the arteriovenous fistula, and do not visualize the AVF as can ultrasonic and magnetic resonance imaging. Most of these tests are qualitative and not quantitative, and most can only be applied to peripheral or extremity AVFs, as will be evident in this chapter. Third, congenital and acquired AVFs differ from each other significantly in terms of their anatomic localizations. Congenital AVFs characteristically are much more diffuse, and as a result are often not as well localized by the so-called physiologic tests or are not completely visualized by Doppler ultrasonography. These differences deserve some preliminary comments. Fourth, the diagnostic goals may vary considerably in different clinical settings, and this significantly affects the application of the tests. The simplest diagnostic goal may be to determine the presence or absence of an AVF, but as often as not, the presence of an AVF is obvious and it is the relative magnitude of its peripheral hemodynamic effects that needs to be gauged (e.g., the presence of a distal steal and the severity of the associated ischemia).

The main focus of this chapter will be on diagnostic approaches that are available in most VDLs. The basic diagnostic methods and the instrumentation behind each of them is covered elsewhere in this book, and will not be described at length here; but the utility of these methods in this setting will be discussed, so that after each diagnostic method has been introduced (i.e., the instrumentation used and the interpretation or analysis of its output), its appropriate clinical applications as well as its limitations will be discussed.

Congenital AVFs

Congenital arteriovenous malformations (AVMs) are less common than congenital venous malformations. Nevertheless they make up over one third (vs. one half) of all congenital vascular defects and constitute the majority of those presenting clinically. Although much is made of the diagnostic triad of birthmark, varicose veins, and limb enlargement, a bare majority of patients presenting with congenital AVFs present with the complete triad, and those with purely venous malformations and no AVFs (e.g., the Klippel-Trenaunay syndrome) may present with the same triad. The vascular diagnostic techniques described in the following text can be valuable in ruling in or out the presence of AVFs in patients presenting with atypical (in location or age of onset) varicose veins and a birthmark, with or without limb enlargement.[2] Depending on their location and localization, the same simple physiologic tests used in diagnosing peripheral arterial occlusive disease can be employed in diagnosing congenital AVFs or AVMs. They also can do so quickly and inexpensively, avoiding the need for angiography, which is particularly important because many of the presenting patients are young children. Although qualitative in nature, the degree of abnormality associated with congenital AVFs on these tests gives the clinician a rough impression of their relative magnitude. Increasingly, the duplex scan, the current workhorse of the VDL, has found useful application in evaluating AVFs.

These noninvasive tests have been underutilized in the past in this clinical setting because many if not most physicians presented with these patients have persisted with a primary reliance on angiography. Unfortunately, this misguided "AGA" (always get an angiogram) approach is still prevalent today because many clinicians do not realize that angiography is only required if the need for therapeutic intervention for congenital arteriovenous fistulas has been determined and will be undertaken soon. They also don't realize that the presence or absence of congenital arteriovenous fistulas (and their relative severity) can be determined by noninvasive methods in most cases. This allows management decisions to be made on the basis of these tests alone, without angiography and its attendant discomfort and associated risks, which is a major consideration in infants and young children.

Although this "addiction" to contrast angiography deserves opposition, there are a number of noninvasive or minimally invasive imaging approaches that have emerged in recent years that deserve discussion in that they offer significant additional perspectives over that achieved by VDL diagnostic methods, particularly in the evaluation of congenital AVFs. These diagnostic modalities (e.g., radionuclide quantification of AV shunting, computed tomography, and magnetic resonance imaging) will also be discussed in detail in this chapter. A knowledge of their capabilities and clinical applications is important because these modalities provide additional diagnostic options that must be considered in this setting. On the other hand, these new imaging methods are considerably more expensive and time-consuming so that, if the dimension they add is not required for decision making, their use may be inappropriate in spite of the additional perspective they offer.

Acquired AVFs

The basic diagnostic methods described here also have application to acquired AVFs (whether caused by iatrogenic or other penetrating trauma) in detecting and localizing them and assessing their hemodynamic significance. As will become apparent, they also have specialized applications in the management of those acquired AVFs created by direct anastomosis or interposed shunts for hemodialysis access. Traditionally, most acquired arteriovenous fistulas have been traumatic in origin. Currently the most common traumatic form results as a complication of invasive catheter techniques, particularly those using a transfemoral artery approach. The standard Seldinger technique actually involves puncture of the posterior wall of the artery, and depending on the anatomic location (particularly in the groin), may enter the vein as well. It is not surprising then that AVFs can be inadvertently created iatrogenically, although pseudoaneurysms more commonly result. These arteriovenous fistulas can be readily visualize by duplex scanning, and duplex scanning can even aid in monitoring attempts at closure by compression and/or injection of thrombogenic material. There is little need for using noninvasive physiologic testing for acquired AVFs, with one major exception: monitoring hemodialysis AVFs and shunts. As will be seen, they have specialized applications in the management of those AVFs created by surgeons as direct anastomoses or interposed shunts for hemodialysis access. These have now become the most common acquired arteriovenous fistula, and this application will be separately discussed.

Hemodynamic Considerations

From a hemodynamic perspective, arteriovenous fistulas can be considered a "short-circuit" between the high-pressure arterial system and the low-pressure venous system. If the AVF (or, in the case of congenital disease, the AVFs) is significant enough hemodynamically, it will result in an arterial pressure drop; a significant diversion of flow into the venous system rather than through the microcirculation; and an increase in velocity, often with turbulence. These hemodynamic changes often increase with time. The mean arterial blood pressure distal to an arteriovenous fistula is always reduced to some degree: this is the result of blood being shunted away from the peripheral vascular bed into the low-resistance pathway offered by the arteriovenous communication.[3] The reduction in pressure is particularly severe when the fistula is large and the arterial collaterals are small. Even when collaterals are well developed, reversal of flow in the artery distal to the fistula(s) further decreases peripheral arterial pressure because much of the collateral flow is diverted back into the fistulous circuit and never reaches the periphery. On the other hand, when the fistula is small and the collaterals are large, there may be little or no perceptible effect on the peripheral pressure. Thus the magnitude of the pressure drop across a fistula, or the limb segment containing the fistula, can provide the surgeon with an objective assessment of its hemodynamic consequences. If the pressure drop is severe enough, there may be distal ischemia. If fistula flow is great enough, there will be associated venous hypertension. These two are responsible for the major peripheral manifestation and symptoms.

It should be pointed out that normal resting extremity circulation is characterized by low flow and high resistance, shifting to high flow and low resistance with exercise. The pattern of an arteriovenous fistula is similar to that of exercise and gives very different velocity patterns than those observed in the normal resting limb. Other conditions that can increase extremity flow include external heat, infection, certain vasodilating drugs, and sympathectomy. Fortunately, these conditions are rarely present in patients referred to a VDL, but the clinician must be aware of them as an occasional source of error.

The pressure, flow volume, and velocity changes associated with AVFs in an extremity can be readily detected, and their relative magnitude roughly assessed, by noninvasive physiologic tests, particularly when compared to the normal contralateral extremity. These noninvasive physiologic tests are the same as those used for close to four decades in the diagnosis of peripheral arterial occlusive disease and will be described in the following section.

Segmental Limb Pressures

Segmental limb pressure measurements are standard techniques described elsewhere in this book. Noninvasive methods of measuring systolic blood pressure are reasonably accurate and reproducible and are painless, rapid, and simple in application. A pneumatic cuff is placed around the limb segment at the required site and inflated to above systolic pressure. As the cuff is deflated, the point at which bloodflow returns distal to the cuff is noted on an aneroid or mercury manometer. Return of flow can be detected with a Doppler flow meter, a mercury-in-Silastic strain gauge, a photoplethysmograph, or a pulse volume recorder. In the upper extremity, pressure measurements can be made at the upper arm, forearm, wrist, or finger levels; in the lower extremity, pressure measurements can be made at the thigh, calf, ankle, foot, or toe. Cuffs should be applied bilaterally to allow comparison with the normal contralateral limb.

A hemodynamically significant AVF will reduce mean pressure in the limb or in the arterial tree close to the fistula. It must be remembered, however, that these cuffs measure systolic pressure, and even though mean pressure is reduced in the arterial tree as one approaches an arteriovenous fistula, the pressure swings between systolic and diastolic (i.e., the pulse pressure) may be increased, so that systolic pressure is likely to be elevated proximal to a fistula. The systolic pressure can be recognized as elevated by comparing it with that of the opposite limb at the same level.[4] Systolic pressure in that limb will also be found to be elevated if the pressure cuff has been placed directly over the site of the fistula or its afferent tributaries. In general, however, compared with the contralateral extremity, cuffs at or above a hemodynamically significant fistula or group of fistulas will usually a record a higher systolic pressure, whereas those below the fistula will record a normal or lower systolic pressure, depending on the magnitude of the fistula. Major fistulas are associated with a detectable degree of distal steal.

Limitations

Finding a normal peripheral arterial pressure does not rule out the presence of a congenital arteriovenous fistula or fistulas in the limb. Small fistulas (e.g., those transmitting less than 5% of total extremity flow) may not produce a detectable pressure effect. Furthermore, there is normally a pressure drop from cuff to cuff as one moves down the extremity; this has to be taken into account. A smaller fistula may simply produce less of a pressure drop than would normally be expected at the same anatomic level, but this subtlety may not be recognized.

Segmental Plethysmography

Segmental plethysmography is also a standard technology described elsewhere in this text; it employs cuffs of precise dimensions applied at various levels/locations along an extremity, much the same as when measuring segmental limb pressures. Air-filled cuffs are normally used. The resulting tracing contour is generally assessed in terms of magnitude in shape. When the pulse-sensing device is placed over the fistula or proximal to it, the pulse volume may actually be increased.[4,5] This is commonly seen in limbs with congenital AVMs, the increased pulsation being almost diagnostic in itself (Fig. 28-1). Although the pulse contour may be normal (or nearly so) in a limb distal to an arteriovenous fistula, its volume is often reduced, particularly in the presence of a steal (Fig. 28-2).[6] As in the case of segmental limb pressure measurements, the reduction in pulse volume depends on the size of the fistula and the adequacy of the collateral arteries. Therefore, very much as previously described for segmental limb pressures, plethysmography tracings are increased in magnitude above or at the level of an AV fistula or group of AV fistulas. Depending on the degree of distal steal, the tracings below the fistula

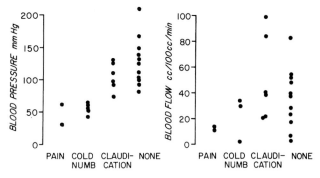

Figure 28-2. *Relationship between symptoms and hemodynamic measurements in the index fingers of patients with side-to-side radial artery-cephalic vein fistulas. Blood pressure was measured at the proximal phalanx, and bloodflow was measured in the distal phalanx. Note that pressure measurements correlate well with the patient's symptoms, whereas flow measurements do not. (From Rutherford RB [ed]: Vascular Surgery, 5th ed. Philadelphia: WB Saunders, 2000.)*

will be reduced or, at best, normal in magnitude. A study of the tracings compared with the contralateral extremity will often allow the general location or level of a significant arteriovenous fistula to be identified.

Velocity Waveform Analysis

Velocity tracings can be recorded over any extremity artery by a Doppler probe connected to the DC recorder and strip chart, or by the velocity readout of a Duplex scan. In evaluating for arteriovenous fistulas, the recording is taken over the major inflow artery (e.g., femoral or axillary). For many if not most clinical purposes, a qualitative estimate of flow velocity and the contour of the analog velocity tracings or "waveforms" obtained with a directional Doppler velocity detector provide sufficient information for clinical diagnosis. Finding a high-velocity flow pattern in an artery leading to a suspicious lesion is good evidence that the lesion is an arteriovenous fistula.[7,8]

The velocity tracings of a resting normal extremity are characterized by end-systolic reversal at the end of peak systolic flow; this is followed by low flow in early diastole and negligible flow in late diastole. Such a low-flow high-resistance pattern is most pronounced in the lower extremity. In the upper extremity there may be little end-systolic reversal. In contrast, high-flow low-resistance arterial velocity patterns are seen in many major organ artery beds (e.g., renal, carotid, and celiac arteries). In the extremities, high-flow patterns are seen after exercise and, importantly, in association with AVFs. In these settings, peak systolic velocity is not only high but there is continuous flow throughout diastole, and the drop between systole and diastole does not approach the 0 velocity baseline, let

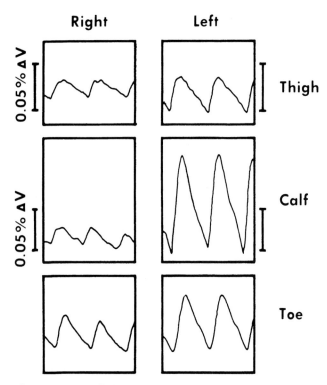

Figure 28-1. *Plethysmographic pulses obtained with a mercury-in-Silastic strain-gauge at thigh, calf, and toe levels in a 4-year-old girl with a congenital arteriovenous fistula of the left pelvic region. The pulses measured: right thigh, 0.02% DV; left thigh, 0.04% DV; right calf, 0.03% DV; and left calf, 0.11% DV. Increased pulses on the left side suggest the presence of further arteriovenous malformations at multiple levels in the leg. DV, difference in velocity.*

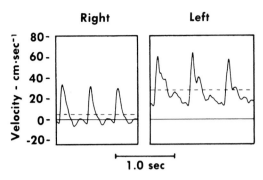

Figure 28-3. *Bloodflow in the common femoral arteries of a 4-year-old girl with a left iliofemoral arteriovenous fistula. The Doppler probe was held at a 45-degree angle to the underlying vessel. The right common femoral artery measured 0.45 cm in diameter and the left one measured 0.55 cm. Mean flow velocity (dashed line) was 5 cm/sec on the right and 28 cm/sec on the left. Total flow was estimated to be 48 mL/min on the right and 397 mL/min on the left. Contrast the reversal of flow on the right during diastole with the high velocty of the flow throughout diastole on the left. (From Rutherford RB [ed]: Vascular Surgery, 5th ed. Philadelphia: WB Saunders, 2000.)*

alone show an end-systolic reversal as it does in the normal resting extremity. The characteristic arterial pattern associated with AVFs, shown in Figure 28-3, thus consists of an elimination of end-systolic reversal and a marked increase in diastolic velocity that "elevates" the entire tracing above the 0 velocity baseline. The degree of elevation in end-diastolic velocity correlates directly with the flow increase caused by the AVF.[4,5] By using these characteristic Doppler velocity signals as a guide, the clinician can detect and localize congenital or traumatic arteriovenous communications that otherwise might escape detection.[9,10] Peripheral arteriovenous fistulas constituting 5% to 8% of extremity flow can be readily detected by this means.

Care must be taken to compare the signal from one limb with that from the other at the same anatomic location. Also, the clinician must appreciate the fact that hyperemic tissues can produce similar signals. Therefore, false positives can occur in other hyperemic settings (e.g., inflammation associated with superficial thrombophlebitis, lymphangitis, bacterial infection, and thermal or mechanical trauma). Inflammation of the limb is usually evident on clinical examination. Hyperdynamic flow associated with conditions such as beriberi or thyrotoxicosis is generalized and therefore should cause no confusion. Other causes of hyperemia isolated to an individual vessel or limb (e.g., exercise or reactive hyperemia following a period of ischemia) are transient, lasting only a few minutes. Externally applied heat, local infection (e.g., cellulitis or abscess), or sympathetic blockade can also increase flow. None of these creates any significant confusion in the usual patient referred to the VDL for evaluation of congenital or acquired AVFs.

Evaluation for Arteriovenous Fistulas Using These Three Physiologic Tests in Combination

Advantages

These three tests are inexpensive, quickly applied, and require little operator or interpretive skill. The instrumentation is simple and used on an everyday basis in most vascular diagnostic laboratories.

Limitations

These tests give qualitative rather than quantitative information and can be applied only to arteriovenous fistulas located in the extremity proper (at or below the highest cuff).

Primary Clinical Applications

1. Screening for congenital AVFs in patients presenting with suggestive signs (e.g., a birthmark, atypical varicose veins, and limb enlargement). Because this triad may be present not only in patients with congenital AVFs (e.g., Parks-Weber syndrome) but also in those with purely venous congenital malformations (e.g., Klippel-Trenaunay syndrome), simple noninvasive tests that can rule in or rule out AVFs have considerable clinical value.

2. Detecting, roughly localizing, and assessing the relative magnitude of congenital AVMs and traumatic AVFs. With anatomically localized lesions, these tests, with or without duplex scanning suffice for most clinical decision-making.

3. Evaluating patients with hemodialysis fistulas or shunts with hand complaints or digital lesions for arterial steal with distal ischemia. As will be seen later, this application is of practical value but is generally underutilized by the many specialists involved in hemodialysis access.

Duplex Scanning

The basic duplex scanner combines an ultrasound image with a focused directional Doppler probe. In modern instruments the velocity signal is color-coded so that red represents arterial flow and blue represents venous flow (going in opposite directions). The velocity signal is also displayed on the screen as needed for specific applications.

Because the duplex scanner provides velocity information, it can serve as a means of doing velocity waveform analysis. As previously described for a simple

Doppler probe connected to a DC recorder, the pattern serves as a simple yet sensitive means of diagnosing an AVF. Because of the additional information obtainable, the former has replaced the latter for this purpose in most VDLs. For example, the high peak mean velocity readings recorded over the main inflow artery of the involved extremity, compared with those at the same location of the contralateral normal extremity, will more accurately confirm the presence of an arteriovenous fistula in that limb. The software of some of today's duplex scanners also allows a rough estimation of volume flow, with diameter being used to estimate cross-sectional area and the velocity signals and the angle of incidence of the probe allowing the Doppler equation to be applied:

Flow = Velocity (frequency shift) × Cosine theta (angle of incidence of the ultrasound beam) × Cross-sectional area, divided by C (velocity of sound in tissue, a constant)

Turbulence is a major problem in using the duplex scan to interrogate AVFs directly to obtain velocity or flow measurements. On the other hand, a Doppler scan placed directly over an AVF will show flashes of yellow, representing turbulent fistula flow, and register high velocities. Traumatic arteriovenous fistulas, particularly the iatrogenic variety produced by the percutaneous introduction of catheters via the femoral vessels, are readily seen as multicolored, orange to white "flashes" between the red and blue artery and vein. The nearby tissues transmitting the thrill will appear to light up with each cardiac cycle because of a motion artifact. Congenital arteriovenous fistulas are more complex, but their high-flow patterns are readily recognized and the nature and extent of the more localized superficial lesions can be well characterized. This in itself can be diagnostic, and is particularly useful when applied to mass lesions, often presenting as a cluster of varicosities, the superficial evidence of an underlying congenital vascular malformation. The diagnostic dilemma, that these varicosities may either be part of a congenital venous malformation or be associated with an underlying arteriovenous malformation, can be resolved by this approach. The detection of high velocities or flashes of turbulence when viewed by a duplex scanner will often quickly identify the type of malformation with which one is dealing. Thus, the duplex scan can be valuable in detecting and localizing an acquired fistula or a localized AVM. Although it is not able to directly measure fistula flow, the duplex scan can do so indirectly by velocity readings over the major inflow artery, comparing the involved limb with the contralateral normal extremity at the same level.

Advantages

Duplex scanners are in everyday use in today's vascular diagnostic laboratories, so the instrumentation and the operator skills are there. It is rather versatile in evaluating AVFs and can be used to interrogate either a penetrating wound or groin hematoma following a catheterization procedure, or a mass lesion suspected of harboring congenital AVFs in a young patient. It may directly visualize and interrogate the AVF; provide velocity evidence of its existence (e.g., high flow in the artery leading to a suspected fistula area): or, as separately described in the section "Arteriovenous Fistulas for Hemodialysis: Diagnostic Considerations," be used in monitoring hemodialysis access fistulas or shunts.

Limitations

In the case of congenital arteriovenous malformations where the AV fistulas may be diffuse, the duplex scanner may not be able to directly visualize the fistulas, although it can supply direct information by interrogating the velocity characteristics of the inflow artery. Like the previously described physiologic tests, it can be applied to extremity lesions but not to central lesions in the trunk or pelvis. Much of its application is qualitative not quantitative, although flow estimates are possible.

Primary Clinical Applications

Detecting, localizing, and guiding thrombotic or embolic therapy in both traumatic and congenital AVFs, when superficially located, are the primary applications of the duplex scanner.

Radionuclide AV Shunt Quantification

Radionuclide-labeled albumen microspheres can be used to diagnose and quantitate arteriovenous shunting. The basic principle behind the study is simple: radionuclide-labeled albumen microspheres too large to pass through capillaries are injected into the inflow artery proximal to the suspected AVF. Those passing through arteriovenous communications are trapped in the next vascular bed in the lung, and may be quantified by counting over the lungs, or by a rectilinear scintillation scanner maintained in a fixed position over a limited pulmonary field.[5,11] The fraction of microspheres reaching the lungs is determined by comparing these counts with the lung counts following another injection of microspheres placed into any peripheral vein, 100% of which should lodge in the lungs. The agent usually used consists of a suspension of 35-μ human albumin microspheres labeled with technetium-99m (similar to that commonly used in lung scans). To ensure similar counting efficiencies, the suspension injected into the vein contains only one fourth to one third of the activity of that injected into the artery, approximately

1.0 mCi vs. 4 mCi. The relative radioactivity of the microsphere suspensions injected is measured by scintillation counting of the syringes before and after the microspheres have been administered.

The formula used to estimate the percentage of arteriovenous shunting is as follows:

$$Pa - Bg/Pv - Pa \times Ia_1 - Ia_2/Iv_1 - Iv_2 \times 100$$

where Bg is background pulmonary counts per unit time, Pa is pulmonary counts per unit time after arterial injection, Pv is pulmonary counts per unit time after venous injection, Iv_i is counts per unit time of venous syringe before injection, Iv_r is residual counts per unit time of venous syringe after injection, Ia_i is counts per unit time of arterial syringe before injection, and Ia_r is residual counts per unit time of arterial syringe after injection.[11] For example, if the pulmonary radioactivity following the arterial injection (Pa – Bg) was half that measured following the venous injection (Pv – Pa), and the ratio of the activity of the venous injectate (Iv_i – Iv_r) to that of the arterial injectate (Ia_i – Ia_r) was one fourth, the estimated shunt volume would be 12.5% of the total flow to the extremity, or

$$(1/2)(1/4)(100) = 12.5\%$$

Advantages

The study is minimally invasive, relatively simple to perform, causes little discomfort, and carries a negligible risk. It quantifies the degree of AV shunting, something none of the other tests do. Because shunt flow can be quantified, the results have prognostic value.[4,5] One can estimate the hemodynamic significance of an AVF or congenital AVM and thus be better able to predict the need for intervention.

Limitations

Although naturally occurring arteriovenous shunts are present in normal human extremities, less than 3% of the total bloodflow (and usually much less) is diverted through these communications.[11] However, measurements made during anesthesia are not accurate because anesthesia, both general and regional, increases shunting through naturally occurring arteriovenous communications. The examiner must be also aware that the percentage of blood shunted through arteriovenous communications can be as high as 40% in the limbs of patients with sympathetic denervation, cirrhosis, or hypertrophic pulmonary osteopathy.[12] Finally, this study shares the limitation of the physiologic studies previously described in that it does not ordinarily localize the lesion. However, several injections can be made at key locations at the time of arteriography and quantified against a later venous injection to give such information. For example, if one recorded 50% shunting following injection in the common iliac artery, 70% shunting following injection in the external iliac artery, 100% following injection in the profunda femoris, and 0% in the superficial femoral artery, the AVM is entirely localized to the distribution of the profunda femoris artery (actual case).

Clinical Applications

Radionuclide-labeled microspheres are most useful for studying patients with suspected congenital AVFs.[2,5] Arteriography occasionally may fail to demonstrate the fistula or fistulas, either because they are too small or because the flow is too rapid. Early venous filling may be the only clue to their existence. In such cases, injection of microspheres in conjunction with arteriography can be used to establish the diagnosis. The patient can be taken to the nuclear medicine lab later for pulmonary counting before and after a venous injection. In patients with diffuse or extensive congenital vascular malformations presenting with a birthmark, varicose veins, and/or limb overgrowth, it may be difficult to distinguish clinically between patients with multiple small AVFs, which cannot be visualized angiographically, and those with predominantly venous malformations (e.g., Klippel-Trenaunay syndrome). The labeled microsphere study solves this dilemma. Importantly, the success of surgical or endovascular interventions can be adequately gauged by pre- and postintervention studies. Finally, serial measurements will indicate whether the fistula is following a stable or progressive course, and whether previously dormant arteriovenous communications have begun to open up or grow.

Magnetic Resonance Imaging and Computed Tomography Scanning

Angiographic studies tend to underestimate the full anatomic extent of vascular malformations. Computed tomography (CT) will usually demonstrate the location and extent of the lesion and even the involvement of specific muscle groups and bone.[13,14] Deep intramuscular lesions give a mottled appearance, and with the bolus administration of contrast, there is enhancement that depends on the rate of arteriovenous shunting in, and the degree of cellularity of, the lesion. Offsetting these desirable features are the need for contrast, the lack of an optimum protocol for its administration, and the practical limitation of having to use multiple transverse images to reconstruct the anatomy of the lesion.

Magnetic resonance imaging (MRI) possesses a number of distinct advantages over CT in evaluating congenital vascular malformations (CVMs). There is no need for contrast, the anatomic extent is more clearly demon-

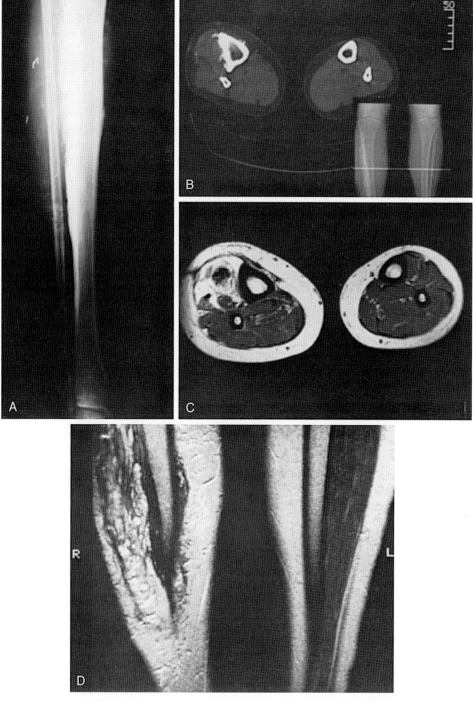

Figure 28-4. A, *Radiograph of the lower leg of a 29-year-old woman with a right anterior tibial mass present since birth shows speckled calcifications, metal clips from multiple previous operations, and tibial cortical irregularities. An arteriogram (not shown) revealed hypervascularity and one area of early venous filling.* **B**, *Computed tomographic scan also suggests bone involvement.* **C**, *Transverse magnetic resonance imaging (MRI) view shows lesion filling the anterior tibial compartment, but the margins of the tibia are clean.* **D**, *Longitudinal MRI view also demonstrates the lack of fast-flow voids. Total excision of the lesion was performed without difficulty or significant blood loss. Histologic study revealed a higly cellular and fibrotic cavernous (venous) malformation. (From Rutherford RB [ed]: Vascular Surgery, 5th ed. Philadelphia: WB Saunders, 2000.)*

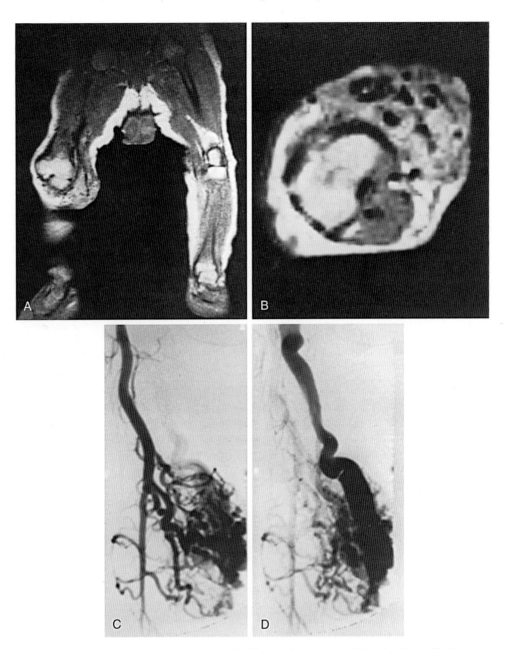

Figure 28-5. *A 4-day old infant who presented with a medial lower thigh mass with palpable thrill.* ***A,*** *Longitudinal magnetic resonance imaging (MRI) view shows the mass with a large, high-flow draining vein.* ***B,*** *Transverse MRI view shows multiple fast-flow voids with involvement of muscle and bone.* ***C,*** *After several months, this arteriogram was obtained because of the onset of high-output heart failure.* ***D,*** *Later-phase view shows the same large draining vein seen on MRI. Therapeutic embolization was carried out, resulting in transient disseminated intravascular coagulation but with a diminution of the mass and control of heart failure. (From Rutherford RB [ed]: Vascular Surgery, 5th ed. Philadelphia: WB Saunders, 2000.)*

strated, longitudinal as well as transverse sections may be obtained, and the flow patterns in the CVM can be characterized. As a result, MRI has become the pivotal diagnostic study in the evaluation of most CVMs. The MRI signal intensity depends on the proton density, the magnetic relaxation times (T1 and T2), and the bulk proton flux (the last-named reflecting bloodflow). If an image is obtained after the pulsed protons (in rapidly moving blood) have left the field, a (black) flow void appears on T2-weighted scans, identifying high-flow vascular spaces and their feeding arteries and draining veins. In contrast, a predominantly venous malformation with its slow flow would appear white. Cellularity can be appreciated because stromal tissues "relax" at different rates. Thus cellularity produces a higher-intensity signal than that from blood-filled spaces.[15] Clinical examples of the value of MRI in the setting of CVMs are illustrated in Figures 28-4 to 28-6.

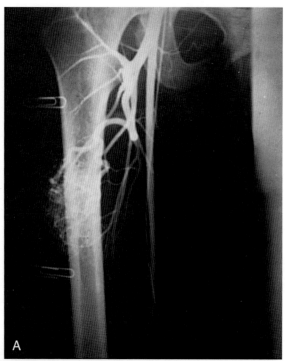

Figure 28-6. *This 24-year-old man had been aware of a painless soft mass on his upper anterolateral thigh for many years.* **A,** *An arteriogram was obtained and showed a localized arteriovenous malformation fed by the profunda femoris artery. The patient was referred for operation.* **B,** *Sagittal magnetic resonance imaging (MRI) view shows high-flow voids and large draining veins.* **C,** *Transverse MRI view shows not only the high-flow voids but also diffuse involvement of the anterior thigh muscles. Operation was withheld in this asymptomatic man because excision would have produced immediate neuromuscular disability. There was no distal steal or cardiac embarrassment. (From Rutherford RB [ed]: Vascular Surgery, 5th ed. Philadelphia, WB Saunders, 2000.)*

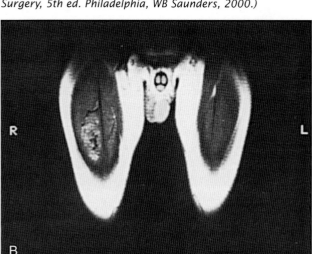

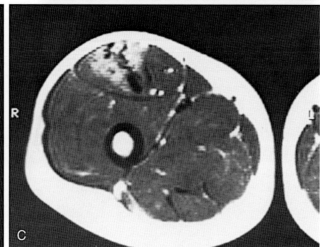

Arteriovenous Fistulas for Hemodialysis: Diagnostic Considerations

Noninvasive diagnostic studies can be useful in evaluating patients before AV fistulas or shunts are constructed, in diagnosing the cause of dysfunction, and in evaluating patients with established hemodialysis fistulas and shunts.[16]

Preoperative Studies

For primary access procedures, or the initial procedure in a new limb, normal arteries and adequate veins may be presumed by palpating bounding peripheral pulses,

obtaining a normal Allen's test, and seeing adequate veins distended by tourniquet application. If this clinical assessment is not obviously normal, the arterial tree can be objectively evaluated, noninvasively, by segmental pressure measurements and plethysmography.[4,5] Normal digital pressures and plethysmography not only indicate open major arteries but rule out digital artery disease, common in patients with end-stage renal disease (ESRD). Patients with debilitating diseases require frequent admissions, during which intravenous infusions may have produced obliterative phlebitis of the superficial arm veins. The adequacy of superficial veins can be determined by duplex scanning.[17] In addition, those with previous dialysis through proximal sites in the neck may have occult stenotic lesions or even thrombosis in the subclavian vein, which may greatly complicate attempts to create an arteriovenous fistula distally in the same extremity. These can and should be detected by duplex scanning before the creation of a shunt or fistula.[18]

Postoperative Studies

Palpation of a prominent thrill over the outflow vein after creation of an arteriovenous fistula or a shunt may suffice when present, but Doppler interrogation offers more objective evidence of adequate fistula flow in the perioperative period. Actual flow rates may be estimated by the previously described approach using the Doppler equation; however, reproducible measurements require special software and exacting technique. Thus at the present time, serial study to detect a failing fistula cannot be justified as a routine, even though it can be predictive.[19] More commonly, dialysis flow rates, venous and arterial pressures on either side of the dialysis machine at increasing flow rates, and percent urea recirculation are observed during dialysis in an attempt to predict access failure.[20] However, by following up with duplex scanning any abnormal observations made during dialysis that are suggestive of access failure, flow-reducing occlusive lesions can be detected with reasonable accuracy.[21]

In patients presenting with hand symptoms such as pain, numbness, or swelling, digital pressures and plethysmography (and their response to collateral compression maneuvers) can be extremely helpful. Late complications of radial artery-cephalic vein fistulas are relatively rare; however, some patients will develop ischemic symptoms in the hand or fingers secondary to distal steal, whereas others may complain of pain and swelling as a result of elevated peripheral venous pressure or secondary carpal tunnel syndrome.[22–24] These symptoms can be readily investigated.[25]

First, digital pressures and plethysmography are monitored. It must be remembered that these will always be reduced to some degree distal to a significant fistula or shunt. Although some degree of distal steal is commonplace, ischemic hand symptoms are uncommon and should not be presumed from these tests unless the digital pressures are below 40 mmHg and the pulse volume recordings (PVRs) are flat. If not abnormal to this degree, other causes of the hand symptoms must be sought. If digital pressures and plethysmography are this low, they should be repeated while carrying out collateral compression maneuvers. Compressing a wrist or radiocephalic fistula, or the radial artery distal to it, should improve digital perfusion and be reflected in increasing digital pressures and PVRs. Conversely, compressing the contralateral (e.g., ulnar) artery will further reduce digital perfusion because this artery is the main collateral inflow into the hand in the presence of a mature radiocephalic fistula. These additional findings are of clinical value because they would lead logically to ligation of the radial artery distal to the fistula, where flow can be shown to be reversed, to relieve the digital ischemia. Digital pressures and plethysmography, plus similar compressive maneuvers, applied to fistulas and shunts at other locations may also confirm the diagnosis of digital ischemia secondary to distal steal and guide appropriate therapy (e.g., a distal revascularization-inflow ligation [DRIL] procedure). If pressure is low in the digital arteries, but unevenly so, there may be occlusion of digital arteries in some fingers and not others because of peripheral arteriosclerosis.[26] This can be confirmed by individual interrogation of these arteries with the Doppler probe. Their perfusion may be improved sufficiently by inflow ligation to relieve symptoms, and monitoring the effect of compressing the inflow artery distally can attest to this.

Although no longer common in wrist fistulas, fistulas or shunts that are anastomosed into the side of a major vein may produce hand symptoms from distal venous hypertension if the proximal outflow vein becomes obstructed.[24] Digital pressures and plethysmography may be reduced (though not to the point of ischemia), and may be improved by compression of the major outflow vein. If this occurs with compression of the distal rather than the proximal vein, then distal venous hypertension as the cause of the hand symptoms is likely and, because edema often results in compression of the median nerve in the carpal tunnel, carpal tunnel release may be required. Through thoughtful application of these simple noninvasive tests, the cause of bothersome hand symptoms associated with hemodialysis AV fistulas can be diagnosed and appropriate treatment initiated.

REFERENCES

1. Rutherford RB, Sumner DS: Diagnostic Evaluation of Arteriovenous Fistulae. In Rutherford RB (ed): Vascular Surgery, 5th ed. Philadelphia: WB Saunders, 2000.
2. Rutherford RB: Congenital Vascular Malformations of the Extremities. In Moore WS (ed): Vascular Surgery: A Comprehensive Review, 5th ed. Philadelphia: WB Saunders, 2000.
3. Strandness DE Jr, Sumner DS (eds): Arteriovenous fistula. In Hemodynamics for Surgeons. New York: Grune & Stratton, 1975.
4. Rutherford RB, Fleming PW, Mcleod FD: Vascular diagnostic methods for evaluating patients with arteriovenous fistulas. In Diethrich EB (ed): Noninvasive Cardiovascular Diagnosis: Current Concepts. Baltimore: University Park Press, 1978.
5. Rutherford RB: Noninvasive testing in the diagnosis and assessment of arteriovenous fistula. In Bernstein EF (ed): Noninvasive Diagnostic Techniques in Vascular Disease. St. Louis: CV Mosby, 1982.
6. Brener BJ, Brief DK, Alpert J, et al: The effect of vascular access procedures on digital hemodynamics. In Diethrich EB (ed): Noninvasive Cardiovascular Diagnosis: Current Concepts. Baltimore: University Park Press, 1978.
7. Barnes RW: Noninvasive assessment of arteriovenous fistula. Angiology 29:691, 1978.
8. Stella A, Pedrini LD, Curti T: Use of ultrasound technique in diagnosis and therapy of congenital arteriovenous fistulas. Vasc Surg 15:77, 1981.
9. Bingham HG, Lichti EL: Doppler as an aid in predicting the behavior of congenital cutaneous hemangioma. Plast Reconstr Surg 47:580, 1971.

10. Pisko-Dubienski ZA, Baird RJ, Bayliss CE, et al: Identification and successful treatment of congenital microfistulas with the aid of directional Doppler. Surgery 78:564, 1975.

11. Rhodes BA, Rutherford RB. Lopez-Majano V, et al: Arteriovenous shunt measurement in extremities. J Nucl Med 13:357, 1972.

12. Rutherford RB: Clinical applications of a method of quantitating arteriovenous shunting in extremities. In Vascular Surgery, 1st ed. Philadelphia: WB Saunders, 1977.

13. Rauch RF, Silverman PM, Korobkin M, et al: Computed tomography of benign angiomatous lesions of the extremities. J Comput Assist Tomogr 8:1143, 1984.

14. Pearce WH, Rutherford RB, Whitehill TA, et al: Nuclear magnetic resonance imaging: Its diagnostic value in patients with congenital vascular malformations of the limbs. J Vasc Surg 8:64, 1988.

15. Mills CM, Brant-Zawadzki M, Crooks LE: Nuclear magnetic resonance: Principles of blood flow imaging. Am J Roentgenol 142:165, 1984.

16. Rutherford RB: The value of noninvasive testing before and after hemodialysis access in the prevention and management of complications. Semin Vasc Surg 10:157–161, 1997.

17. Salles-Cunha SX, Andros G, Harris RW, et al: Preoperative noninvasive assessment of arm veins to be used as bypass grafts in the lower extremities. J Vasc Surg 3:813, 1986.

18. Passman MA, Criado E, Farber MA, et al: Efficacy of color-flow duplex imaging for proximal upper extremity venous outflow obstruction in hemodialysis patients. J Vasc Surg 28:869–875, 1998.

19. Bosman PJ, Boereboom FT, Eikelboom BC, et al: Craft flow as a predictor of thrombosis in hemodialysis grafts. Kidney Int 54:1726–1730, 1998.

20. May RE, Himmelfarb J, Yenicesu M, et al: Predicting measures of vascular access thrombosis: A prospective study. Kidney Int 52:1656–1662, 2001.

21. Bay WH, Henry ML, Lazarus JM, et al: Predicting hemodialysis access failure with color-flow Doppler ultrasound. Am J Nephrol 18:296–394, 1998.

22. Bussell JA, Abbott JA, Lim RC: A radial steal syndrome with arteriovenous fistula for hemodialysis. Ann Intern Med 75:387, 1971.

23. Kinnaert P, Struyven J, Mathieu J, et al: Intermittent claudication of the hand after creation of an arteriovenous fistula in the forearm. Am J Surg 139:838, 1980.

24. Delpin EAS: Swelling of the hand after arteriovenous fistula for hemodialysis. Am J Surg 132:373, 1976.

25. Strandness DE Jr, Gibbons GE, Bell JW: Mercury strain gauge plethysmography: Evaluation of patients with acquired arteriovenous fistula. Arch Surg 85:215, 1962.

26. Yeager RA, Moneta GL, Edwards JM, et al: Relationship of hemodialysis access to finger gangrene in patients with end-stage renal disease. J Vasc Surg 36:245–249, 2002.

Chapter 29

Pseudoaneurysm: Diagnosis and Treatment

STEVEN S. KANG

- Diagnosis
- Ultrasound-Guided Thrombin Injection
- Technique
- Results
- Conclusions

Diagnosis

A femoral pseudoaneurysm is suspected when there is a hematoma, especially an enlarging one, at a puncture site hours or days after the procedure. There is often significant ecchymosis of the overlying skin. There may be a bruit, but a continuous bruit is usually associated with an arteriovenous fistula. There may be pain or neuralgia, and the site is often tender. A pulsatile mass is usually palpable, but a simple hematoma overlying the artery may give the same impression. Only a minority of pseudoaneurysms are unequivocally diagnosed by physical examination.

The diagnosis of a femoral pseudoaneurysm has become very easy with duplex ultrasound, especially with color-flow. Before refinements in ultrasound technology, pseudoaneurysms were evaluated using a variety of techniques including intra-arterial angiography, intravenous digital subtraction angiography, CT scanning, and labeled red cell nuclear scans.

On B-mode ultrasound examination, an echolucent cavity is seen overlying the artery. It can be difficult to differentiate a hematoma from a pseudoaneurysm with B-mode only. A pseudoaneurysm may exhibit pulsatile expansion and contraction of the suspected echolucent area. Spontaneously occurring thrombus might be detectable within the cavity, most commonly on the outer margins of the cavity. On Doppler examination, bidirectional flow is detectable at the neck of the pseudoaneurysm because some blood flows in and out of the aneurysm cavity with each systole and diastole. This flow pattern is pathognomonic for pseudoaneurysms. The cavity itself may show a swirling flow pattern on color mode.

Ultrasound-Guided Thrombin Injection

In 1996 the author developed a method for treating postcatheterization femoral pseudoaneurysms using ultrasound-guided thrombin injection. This was spurred by the shortcomings of ultrasound-guided compression repair (UGCR). Universally, UGCR was painful and time-consuming. The author found UGCR usually effective in patients with normal coagulation parameters; however, no success was seen in patients who were anticoagulated at the time of compression.[1] This was understandable because UGCR requires spontaneous thrombosis of blood within the pseudoaneurysm cavity while flow is temporarily arrested by compressing the neck. It was thought that compression would have a higher success rate and require less time if the clinician could locally alter the coagulability of the blood within the pseudoaneurysm. The initial protocol proposed performing compression after ultrasound-guided injection of thrombin into the pseudoaneurysm cavity. After the first injection caused immediate thrombosis of the pseudoaneurysm, it was realized that compression would not be necessary. The author's first paper reported successful treatment of 20 out of 21 femoral pseudoaneurysms.[2] A follow-up report confirmed the efficacy of the procedure, with overall success in 80 out of 83 patients, which included 29 patients who were anticoagulated and 9 nonfemoral pseudoaneurysms.[3] Since then, others using the same technique have reported good results with few complications.[4–12] The procedure has gained widespread acceptance and has become the primary treatment option. Reflecting this development, in 2002 the American Medical Association assigned a new current procedural terminology (CPT) code for percutaneous thrombin injection of pseudoaneurysms.

Technique

The author has found that most pseudoaneurysms are amenable to thrombin injection, which is not true for UGCR. Patients with evidence of local infection, overlying skin or distal limb ischemia, or a history of allergic responses to thrombin or bovine products are excluded. Before thrombin injection, distal pulses and ankle-brachial indices should be measured for comparison after thrombin injection; this should allow detection of most cases of intra-arterial thrombus formation or embolization.

The transducer is placed directly over the pseudoaneurysm (Fig. 29-1). The orientation of the transducer is not important; it is placed so that there is a convenient location next to the transducer for needle insertion. A 21- or 22-gauge spinal needle is attached to a small syringe containing thrombin at 1000 U/mL. The skin along the short edge of the transducer is cleaned with alcohol. With color-flow off, the needle is placed percutaneously into the center of the pseudoaneurysm along the same plane as the ultrasound image (Fig. 29-2). This can be done free-hand or with a biopsy guide. Although the shaft of the needle is not always visible, the echogenic thrombus that forms on the bevel of the needle can be identified once it is within the pseudoaneurysm cavity (Fig. 29-3). When the location of the tip is certain, color-flow is turned on and thrombin is slowly injected.

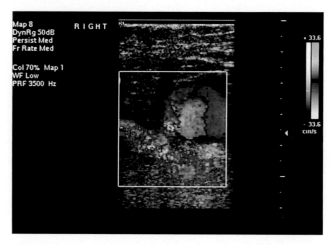

Figure 29-1. Duplex ultrasound of the pseudoaneurysm before needle insertion. The femoral artery is visible below the pseudoaneurysm.

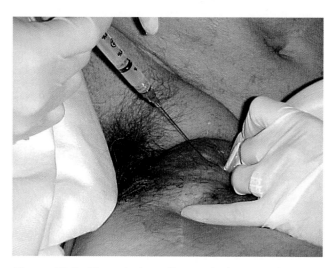

Figure 29-2. The spinal needle attached to a syringe containing thrombin solution is percutaneously inserted into the pseudoaneurysm.

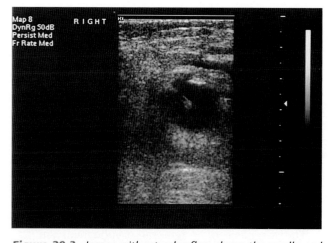

Figure 29-3. Image without color-flow shows the needle and the thrombus that forms on the tip of the needle within the pseudoaneurysm. Once the tip is localized in the center of the pseudoaneurysm, color-flow is turned back on before thrombin injection.

This results in rapid thrombosis of the aneurysm cavity as seen by the disappearance of the color-flow (Fig. 29-4). Usually, less than 0.5 mL of thrombin solution is sufficient. If only partial thrombosis is seen, the needle is redirected into the remaining flow cavity and additional thrombin is injected.

A similar procedure had been described in five patients by Liau.[13] After application of local anesthesia, an intravenous catheter was introduced into the pseudoaneurysm. Because this catheter was not visible on ultrasound, saline containing micro-air bubbles was injected through the catheter to detect the location of the catheter tip and to guide positioning. This was followed by injection of thrombin. The author's technique of using a spinal needle with thrombin already in the needle seems simpler.

Patients do not require any sedation or analgesia. Because no compression is used, there is only minor discomfort from the needle. After successful thrombin injection, patients are allowed to ambulate immediately. As with UGCR, the author recommends repeating the duplex examination within a few days to detect any recurrences. Unlike UGCR, there appears to be no need to discontinue anticoagulation to improve results.

Results

From February 1996 to December 2002, 149 pseudoaneurysms were treated with ultrasound-guided thrombin injection. There were 136 femoral, 6 brachial, 2 radial, 2 subclavian, 1 posterior tibial, 1 distal SFA pseudoaneurysms, and 1 arm arteriovenous fistula. Thrombin injection was initially successful in 145 of 149 patients. The other four, all of whom had femoral pseudoaneurysms, had partial thrombosis. One of them had complete thrombosis 3 days later when brought back for repeat injection; three had surgical repair. There were early recurrences in 11 that had initially successful thrombin injections. Seven were successfully reinjected at the time the recurrence was diagnosed. One had spontaneous thrombosis several days after recurrence was identified. Two failed repeat injections and had surgical repair. One underwent surgical repair without an attempt at repeat injection. Overall only 6 of 149 required surgical repair. Of 45 patients who were anticoagulated with heparin or coumadin at the time of thrombin injection, 42 had successful treatment.

Three patients experienced complications. (1) A brachial artery pseudoaneurysm had injection of thrombin directly into the neck, which caused thrombosis of the brachial artery.[14] The thrombosis resolved in a few minutes after intravenous heparin. (2) A femoral pseudoaneurysm was successfully injected with thrombin. The ankle-brachial index was noted to be decreased after thrombin injection. Arterial duplex revealed thrombus in the posterior tibial artery. Intravenous heparin was administered immediately. The thrombus was gone when the artery was scanned later in the day. (3) A femoral pseudoaneurysm with a neck that was about 10 mm in width (Fig. 29-5) had partial thrombosis of the aneurysm after initial injection. Further injection was not able to thrombose the remaining cavity but instead caused a tail of thrombus to form in the superficial femoral artery. The patient underwent surgical thrombectomy and repair of the aneurysm.

Results from other institutions have confirmed that thrombin injection is safe and effective. Some of the early larger series that have been published are shown in Table 29-1. The cumulative success rate of these series and the author's was 453 out of 475 (95%). There were only eight complications (1.7%), which were all thromboses of the feeding artery or distal embolism. A

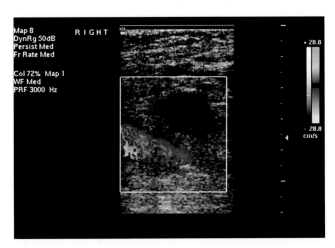

Figure 29-4. Color-flow image after thrombin injection shows complete thrombosis of the pseudoaneurysm.

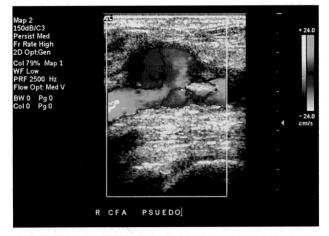

Figure 29-5. Femoral pseudoaneurysm with a wide neck, which may be more likely to develop arterial thrombosis with thrombin injection.

TABLE 29-1. Results of Ultrasound-Guided Thrombin Injection

Study	Cases	Successes (%)	Anticoagulated (%)	Complications (%)
Taylor, et al[4]	29	27 (93)	3	0
Paulson, et al[5]	26	25 (96)	9	0
Lennox, et al[6]	30	30 (100)	18	0
Pezzullo, et al[7]	23	22 (96)	12	1
Sackett, et al[8]	30	27 (90)	11	1
Morrison, et al[9]	39	38 (97)	7	3
La Perna, et al[10]	70	66 (94)	21	0
Owen, et al[11]	25	25 (100)	7	0
Sheiman, et al[12]	54	50 (93)	25	0
Current	149	143 (96)	45	3
Totals	475	453 (95)	158 (33)	8 (1.7)

few other case reports have described similar thromboembolic complications.[15-17] They are most likely caused by inadvertent injection of the thrombin solution into the artery, either by incorrect needle placement or by injecting too much thrombin, especially in the presence of a wide neck, as in the author's series. There are also single case reports of allergic reactions to thrombin causing anaphylactic shock[18] and prolonged pruritus.[19]

As has been shown, nonfemoral pseudoaneurysms can also be treated by this method. Besides the subclavian, brachial, radial, tibial, and distal SFA pseudoaneurysms that the author reported,[3] the literature now also includes treatment of axillary,[20] vein graft,[21] pancreatic,[22] and splanchnic artery pseudoaneurysms,[23] among others. As suggested in the author's paper,[3] thrombin has also been injected under CT guidance into the aneurysm sac of an abdominal aortic aneurysm previously treated by an endograft to obliterate an endoleak.[24]

Conclusions

Ultrasound-guided thrombin injection has become the preferred treatment for most iatrogenic pseudoaneurysms. It appears to have significant advantages over compression therapy or surgery.

REFERENCES

1. Hodgett DA, Kang SS, Baker WH: Ultrasound-guided compression repair of catheter-related femoral artery pseudoaneurysms is impaired by anticoagulation. Vasc Surg 31:639–644, 1997.
2. Kang SS, Labropoulos N, Mansour MA, et al: Percutaneous ultrasound-guided thrombin injection: A new method for treating postcatheterization femoral pseudoaneurysms. J Vasc Surg 27:1032–1038, 1998.
3. Kang SS, Labropoulos N, Mansour MA, et al: Expanded indications for ultrasound-guided thrombin injection of pseudoaneurysms. J Vasc Surg 31:289–298, 2000.
4. Taylor BS, Rhee RY, Muluk S, et al: Thrombin injection versus compression of femoral artery pseudoaneurysms. J Vasc Surg 30:1052–1059, 1999.
5. Paulson EK, Sheafor DH, Kliewer MA, et al: Treatment of iatrogenic femoral arterial pseudoaneurysms: Comparison of US-guided thrombin injection with compression repair. Radiology 215:403–408, 2000.
6. Lennox AF, Delis KT, Szendro G, et al: Duplex-guided thrombin injection for iatrogenic femoral artery pseudoaneurysm is effective even in anticoagulated patients. Br J Surg 87:796–801, 2000.
7. Pezzullo JA, Dupuy DE, Cronan JJ: Percutaneous injection of thrombin for the treatment of pseudoaneurysms after catheterization: An alternative to sonographically guided compression. Am J Roentgenol 175:1035–1040, 2000.
8. Sackett WR, Taylor SM, Coffey CB, et al: Ultrasound-guided thrombin injection of iatrogenic femoral pseudoaneurysms: A prospective analysis. Am Surg 66:937–942, 2000.
9. Morrison SL, Obrand DA, Steinmetz OK, et al: Treatment of femoral artery pseudoaneurysms with percutaneous thrombin injection. Ann Vasc Surg 14:634–639, 2000.
10. La Perna L, Olin JW, Goines D, et al: Ultrasound-guided thrombin injection for the treatment of postcatheterization pseudoaneurysms. Circulation 102:2391–2395, 2000.
11. Owen RJ, Haslam PJ, Elliott ST, et al: Percutaneous ablation of peripheral pseudoaneurysms using thrombin: A simple and effective solution. Cardiovasc Intervent Radiol 23:441–446, 2000.
12. Sheiman RG, Brophy DP: Treatment of iatrogenic femoral pseudoaneurysms with percutaneous thrombin injection: Experience in 54 patients. Radiology 219:123–127, 2001.
13. Liau CS, Ho FM, Chen MF, et al: Treatment of iatrogenic femoral artery pseudoaneurysm with percutaneous thrombin injection. J Vasc Surg 26:18–23, 1997.

14. Kang SS: Reply regarding: Percutaneous ultrasound guided thrombin injection: A new method for treating postcatheterization femoral pseudoaneurysms. J Vasc Surg 28:1121, 1998.

15. Forbes TL, Millward SF: Femoral artery thrombosis after percutaneous thrombin injection of an external iliac artery pseudoaneurysm. J Vasc Surg 33:1093–1096, 2001.

16. Lennox A, Griffin M, Nicolaides A, et al: Letter regarding: Percutaneous ultrasound guided thrombin injection: A new method for treating postcatheterization femoral pseudoaneurysms. J Vasc Surg 28:1120–1121, 1998.

17. Sadiq S, Ibrahim W: Thromboembolism complicating thrombin injection of femoral artery pseudoaneurysm: Management with intra-arterial thrombolysis. J Vasc Interv Radiol 12:633–636, 2001.

18. Pope M, Johnston KW: Anaphylaxis after thrombin injection of a femoral pseudoaneurysm: Recommendations for prevention. J Vasc Surg 32:190–191, 2000.

19. Sheldon PJ, Oglevie SB, Kaplan LA: Prolonged generalized urticarial reaction after percutaneous thrombin injection for treatment of a femoral artery pseudoaneurysm. J Vasc Interv Radiol 11:759–761, 2000.

20. Elford J, Burrell C, Roobottom C: Ultrasound-guided percutaneous thrombin injection for the treatment of iatrogenic pseudoaneurysms. Heart 82:526–527, 1999.

21. Farrell MA, Douglas BR, Bower TC: Sonographically guided percutaneous thrombin injection for treatment of a vein graft pseudoaneurysm. Am J Roentgenol 176:1032–1034, 2001.

22. Luchs SG, Antonacci VP, Reid SK, et al: Vascular and interventional case of the day. Pancreatic head pseudoaneurysm treated with percutaneous thrombin injection. Am J Roentgenol 173:830, 833–834, 1999.

23. Kemmeter P, Bonnell B, VanderKolk W, et al: Percutaneous thrombin injection of splanchnic artery aneurysms: Two case reports. J Vasc Interv Radiol 11:469–472, 2000.

24. van den Berg JC, Nolthenius RP, Casparie JW, et al: CT-Guided thrombin injection into aneurysm sac in a patient with endoleak after endovascular abdominal aortic aneurysm repair. Am J Roentgenol 175:1649–1651, 2000.

Upper Extremity Ischemia: Diagnostic Techniques and Clinical Applications

JOHN K. KARWOWSKI • BONNIE JOHNSON • RONALD L. DALMAN

Introduction

Upper extremity ischemia is a common and debilitating condition, often occurring in young, relatively healthy, and productive individuals. Thorough diagnostic evaluation expedites effective treatment and often reveals significant medical comorbidities. The etiology of upper extremity ischemia may be divided into intrinsic occlusive disease secondary to atherosclerosis; or collagen vascular or autoimmune diseases, embolic disease, and steal syndromes associated with ipsilateral hemodialysis access procedures. A range of indirect and direct noninvasive imaging and catheter-based imaging studies are used to quantify disease severity and to localize obstructing or embolizing lesions.

Office Examination

Evaluation of the ischemic upper extremity begins with a thorough and focused history and physical examination. Episodic digital discoloration and pain evoked by exposure to cold environments or stress suggests the presence of Raynaud's disease. This disorder occurs either as a consequence of increased sensitivity to cold stimuli in normal digital arteries (primary Raynaud's syndrome), or normal response to cold stimuli in the setting of underlying digital occlusive disease (secondary Raynaud's syndrome). In the setting of cold-induced digital vasospasm the medical history should focus on the possibility of coexisting collagen vascular disorders (e.g., scleroderma); autoimmune conditions (e.g., systemic lupus erythematosus [SLE], dermatomyositis, polymyositis, or rheumatoid arthritis); primary pulmonary hypertension; blood dyscrasias; hepatitis; occupational use of vibratory tools; frostbite; or treatment with ergot preparations, beta blockers, or cytotoxic chemotherapeutic agents. Even after the diagnosis of primary Raynaud's syndrome is established in the absence of coexisting conditions, patients may need future re-evaluation because a significant minority of young women with this condition go on to develop underlying collagen vascular or autoimmune conditions months or years after the onset of symptoms.[1] Digital ulceration is clearly a marker of comorbidity because it occurs almost exclusively in patients with serious underlying medical conditions such as scleroderma or SLE. Consideration of the full range of diagnostic and therapeutic modalities available for patients with Raynaud's disease is beyond the scope of this chapter[2]: These concepts are outlined only to emphasize the importance of a complete medical history as part of the diagnostic assessment of upper extremity occlusive disease.[3]

Physical examination should highlight the location and laterality of symptoms and signs of ischemia. As a general rule, bilateral symptoms increase the likelihood of intrinsic arterial disorders and underlying medical conditions (e.g., scleroderma). Unilateral symptoms or signs occur more commonly with proximal embolizing lesions such as subclavian aneurysms. Aortic or mitral valve lesions, patent foramen ovale, or myocardial rhythm disturbances can throw emboli to one or both upper extremities. Toward this end, the precordium should be auscultated for rhythm disorders or murmurs. Similarly, the presence of upper extremity arteriovenous fistulas, shunts, or central venous catheters should be noted and correlated with symptom laterality. Characteristic cutaneous conditions such as rashes, jaundice, or petechial lesions suggest the possibility of underlying comorbid medical conditions and should prompt more extensive systemic assessment.

Establishing symptomatic unilaterality facilitates diagnostic precision. Auscultation and palpation of the juxtaclavicular region may identify relevant murmurs or prominent or aneurysmal pulsations. Similarly, the brachial, ulnar, and radial pulse status should be noted. Arm-arm brachial and forearm pressures are obtained and indexed to the highest value with segmental pressures recorded on the affected limb. In patients with possible thoracic outlet disease, pressure and pulse examinations are repeated during evocative maneuvers such as the Adson test, military brace, or the elevated arm stress test (EAST).[4]

Application-Specific Diagnostic Modalities

Beyond laterality and localization techniques, specific diagnostic tests are best considered in the context of their most common applications.

Cold Intolerance/Finger Discoloration and Occlusive Disease

When historical information or physical examination suggests the presence of cold intolerance or discoloration,

bilateral upper extremity pressure testing and digital plethysmography are performed. These tests are useful in differentiating normal from obstructive or vasospastic arterial waveforms. Photoplethysmography (PPG) uses a photocell to acquire an analog recording of the pulse contour as the flow of blood passes through the capillary bed from the arterial side to the venous return. Mercury plethymography employs miniaturized strain gauges around the digit to record volume changes. Digital pressure is modified via 2.5-cm pressure cuffs placed simultaneously at the base of each digit. Normal digital pressures are within 20 to 30 mmHg of brachial pressures, or a digital/brachial index of greater than 0.80. Finger pulse/volume recordings are obtained at rest and are categorized by waveform phasicity. The finding of multiple bilateral monophasic and obstructive digital signals at room temperature supports the diagnosis of secondary Raynaud's syndrome.

The presence of normal pulse volume recordings and coloration at room temperature in patients with symptoms suggestive of cold intolerance may be investigated further via cold challenge. As described by Nielsen and Lassen,[5] this can be accomplished by either immersion in an ice bath or by perfusion of cold water through the digital pressure cuffs. More recently, Carter and associates have emphasized the importance of whole body cooling to improve test sensitivity.[6] These tests are elaborate and, in the case of cold immersion, potentially painful. The simplest test involves immersing the affected hand in ice water for 30 seconds. After the hand is dried, a temperature probe measures digital temperature every 5 minutes for 45 minutes, or until it reaches preimmersion levels (30 °C minimum). Despite obvious limitations associated with these methods, more sophisticated testing modalities have not gained widespread acceptance. As a general rule, pulse contours tend to be less sensitive than reduced finger blood pressures for confirmation of disease.

When obtaining baseline measurements in patients with obvious digital ischemia, it is important to ensure that the finger temperature is at 28 to 30 °C. Lower temperatures may induce vasospasm and skew results. Healthy individuals will demonstrate normal waveforms with an upstroke of less than 0.2 seconds both at room temperature and following rapid cooling. A slower upstroke denotes an obstructive pattern, although not necessarily specific to the level of the palmar and digital arteries. Cold-induced vasospasm presents with a different abnormal waveform altogether, known as a peaked pulse, where a vessel does not demonstrate normal elasticity (Fig. 30-1). Similar methods can be used to follow efficacy of therapy. Plain soft-tissue hand films (x-ray) may reveal calcinosis, supporting the diagnosis of secondary etiologies such as CREST syndrome and diabetic or azotemic arteriopathy. Current guidelines regarding the necessary elements of a cold-sensitivity

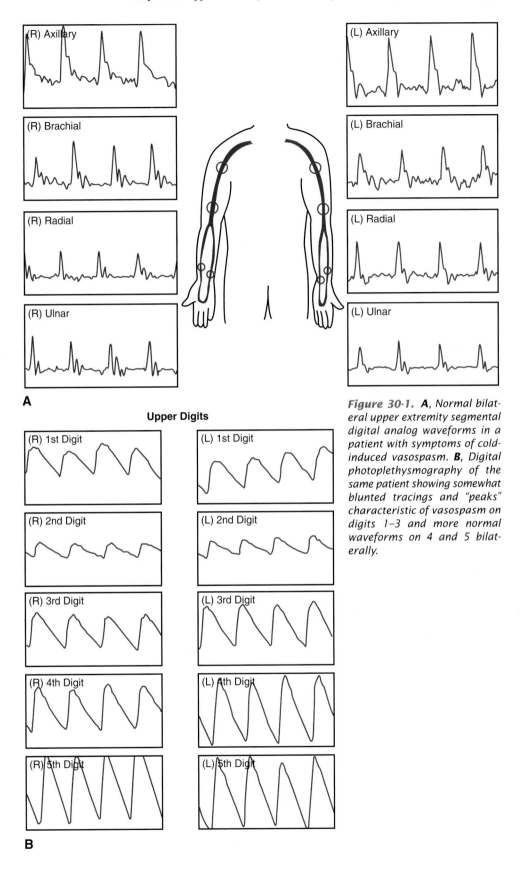

Upper Digits

A

B

Figure 30-1. **A**, *Normal bilateral upper extremity segmental digital analog waveforms in a patient with symptoms of cold-induced vasospasm.* **B**, *Digital photoplethysmography of the same patient showing somewhat blunted tracings and "peaks" characteristic of vasospasm on digits 1–3 and more normal waveforms on 4 and 5 bilaterally.*

examination in the vascular laboratory can be found on the Society of Vascular Ultrasound Web site at www. svunet.org/about/positions/index.htm.

Evidence of obstructive waveforms warrants further investigation of more proximal vessels from the wrist to the level of the aortic and mitral valves. Chronic embolic disease may mimic digital vasospasm or obstructive conditions, even in otherwise healthy young women or high-performance athletes.[7] Duplex scanning is not useful in diagnosis of primary Raynaud's disease, per se, but is helpful at performing the necessary investigation of any proximal lesions that may present with episodic digital ischemia.

Any discernable large vessel pathology that lends itself to operative repair will ultimately be evaluated by contrast angiography, either via magnetic resonance or selective intra-arterial injection. Angiography is also indicated in the setting of digital gangrene, in which advanced distal atherosclerosis[8] or secondary Raynaud's syndrome is likely. Although of limited value today in diagnostic assessment, angiography remains essential for planning revascularization strategies. Angiographic examinations must opacify all regions of interest from the ascending aorta to the proper digital arteries. Bilateral examinations are crucial in determining the role of anatomic variability vs. underlying disease. The palmar arch, for example, is complete in less than half of patients undergoing upper extremity arteriography.

Focal Upper Extremity Aneurysmal Degeneration and Distal Embolization

Upper extremity arterial aneurysms occur in predictable and reproducible locations, including the subclavian artery or its branches at the thoracic outlet (Fig. 30-2); the axillary artery; the brachial artery at or above the antecubital fossa (Fig. 30-3); and the ulnar artery where it crosses the hook of the hamate bone.

Arterial and venous injuries occur at the thoracic outlet secondary primarily because of bony trauma (e.g., cervical rib and interactions between the first rib and clavicle or the head of the humerus).[9,10] The most common clinical manifestation of these injuries is distal embolization, followed by secondary axillosubclavian thrombosis. Diagnosis is established by bilateral proximal arterial color duplex imaging using 4- to 7-MHz transducers.

More subtle but equally debilitating injuries can occur to branches of the axillary artery just distal to the humeral head. These injuries may present as obvious distal emboli or ipsilateral cold sensitivity, or may be indirectly recognized by reduced strength, sensation, or neuromuscular control in the involved arm. Thrombosed aneurysms of the common, anterior, or posterior circumflex arteries may not opacify or may not be recognized during upper extremity arteriography, high-

lighting the importance of careful duplex ultrasonic interrogation as an integral component of the diagnostic evaluation.[11]

Brachial and radial artery aneurysms occur either as a sequela of trauma (e.g., posterior elbow dislocations) or as complications of brachial catheterizations or other iatrogenic injuries. The superficial location of the brachial artery usually ensures prompt recognition and evaluation. Distal ulnar artery aneurysms, however, are also subtle and often unrecognized sources of digital embolization. These aneurysms represent another manifestation of repetitive motion injuries, occurring most commonly in the modern era in vocational or avocational athletes.[8,12] The short segment of the superficial branch of the ulnar artery that forms the origin of the superficial palmar arch is prone to injury from acute and chronic blunt trauma to the hypothenar eminence, where it lies relatively unprotected between skin and bone. These aneurysms may occlude or chronically embolize. Angiographic abnormalities are subtle and easily overlooked, often demonstrating corkscrew luminal deformities or subtle contour irregularities in the absence of obvious aneurysmal degeneration. Preprocedural duplex insonation at higher frequencies (10 MHz and above) easily identifies aneurysms with and without luminal thrombus in younger, active patients with symptoms of ipsilateral digital ischemia. In a fashion similar to ischemic conditions caused by more proximal embolizing lesions, ulnar aneurysms and their digital sequelae are definitively treated by autogenous vein reconstruction preceded in selected cases by preoperative intra-arterial catheter-directed thrombolysis.[13]

Hand Ischemia/Digital Gangrene in End-Stage Renal Disease

Hand and finger ischemia occurs commonly in end-stage renal disease patients undergoing hemodialysis as renal replacement therapy. The presence of hand pain and numbness ipsilateral to surgically created fistulas and shunts suggests the possibility of arterial steal syndromes. The most common remedies for steal syndromes include the DRIL (distal revascularization and interval ligation)[14] procedure or similar surgical solutions. When gangrene is present, however, it almost invariably identifies the presence of severe distal atherosclerotic disease not amenable to revascularization.[15] The diagnostic assessment and categorization of steal or distal pain syndromes is most commonly performed by evaluation of distal arterial perfusion with or without temporary occlusion of the access conduit during distal digital PPG tracings, in addition to digital pressure and waveform assessment. Current guidelines regarding the necessary components for noninvasive assessment of hemodialysis-related upper extremity ischemia are posted and updated on the Society of Vascular Ultrasound Web site www.svunet.org/about/positions/index.htm.

Upper Digits

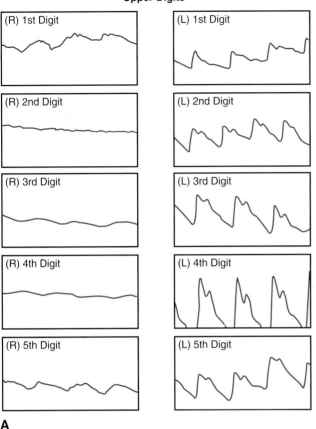

A

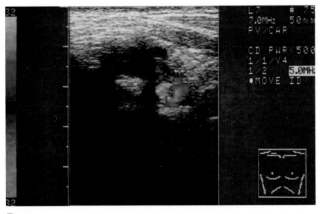

B

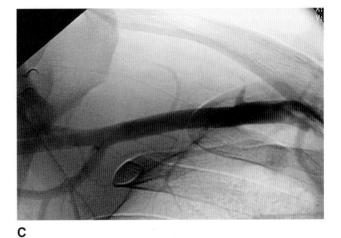

C

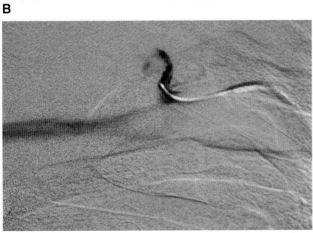

D

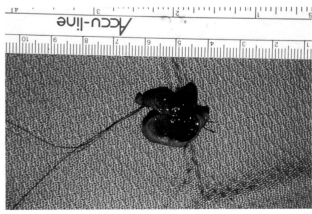

E

Figure 30-2. **A**, *Unilateral blunted PPG tracings in right-hand dominant professional athlete with discolored, cold-intolerant hand and intact ipsilateral radial, ulnar, and brachial pulses.* **B**, *Duplex scan showing aneurysmal right subscapular artery with intraluminal thrombus.* **C**, *Subclavian injection-contrast arteriography showing subtle filling defects of the subscapular artery.* **D**, *Selective subscapular injection showing thrombus-filled aneurysm.* **E**, *Surgical specimen open showing luminal thrombus. (All images courtesy of Cornelius Olcott IV, MD.)*

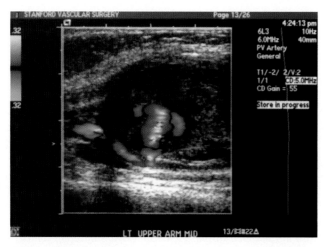

Figure 30-3. *Midforearm brachial pseudoaneurysm. These lesions are often successfully treated at the time of diagnosis by thrombin injection under ultrasound guidance. Although reported to be more often accompanied by distal embolization than femoral artery pseudoaneurysms, the authors have treated several similar brachial lesions successfully without embolic sequelae.*

Conclusions

The etiology of upper extremity ischemia varies widely from autoimmune conditions to overuse and repetitive motion injuries. Familiarity with the full range of diagnostic tests available in the vascular laboratory helps physicians and vascular surgeons promptly address and resolve what are often long-standing and debilitating conditions. Somewhat contrary to current trends in vascular diagnosis, a combination of imaging and indirect testing modalities is still required to optimize outcome in many patients suffering from finger and hand discoloration, pain, and digital gangrene.

REFERENCES

1. Landry GJ, Edwards JM, McLafferty RB, et al: Long-term outcome of Raynaud's syndrome in a prospectively analyzed patient cohort. J Vasc Surg 23:76–85, 1996.
2. Bowling JC, Dowd PM: Raynaud's disease. Lancet 361:2078–2080, 2003.
3. Landry GJ, Edwards JM, Porter JM: Current management of Raynaud's syndrome. Adv Surg 30:333–347, 1996;
4. Schneider DB, Stoney RJ: Diagnosis of Thoracic Outlet Syndrome. In Ernst CB, Stanley JC (eds): Current Therapy in Vascular Surgery, 4th ed. St. Louis, Mosby, 2001.
5. Nielsen SL, Lassen NA: Measurements of digital blood pressure after local cooling. J Appl Physiol 43:907–910, 1977.
6. Carter SA, Dean E, Kroeger EA: Apparent finger systolic pressures during cooling in patients with Raynaud's syndrome. Circulation 77:988–996, 1988.
7. Arko FR, Harris EJ, Zarins CK, et al: Vascular complications in high performance athletes. J Vasc Surg 33:935–942, 2001.
8. Nehler MR, Dalman RL, Harris EJ Jr, et al: Upper extremity arterial bypass distal to the wrist. J Vasc Surg 16:633–642, 1992.
9. Cormier JM, Amrane M, Ward A, et al: Arterial complications of the thoracic outlet syndrome: 55 operative cases. J Vasc Surg 9:778–787, 1989.
10. Durham JR, Yao JS, Pearce WH, et al: Arterial injuries in the thoracic outlet syndrome. J Vasc Surg 21:57–69, 1995.
11. Dalman RL, Olcott C IV: Upper extremity revascularization proximal to the wrist. Ann Vasc Surg 11:643–650, 1997.
12. Dalman RL: Hypothenar Hammer Syndrome. In Ernst CB, Stanley JC (eds): Current Therapy in Vascular Surgery, 4th ed. St. Louis, Mosby, 2001.
13. Dalman RL: Upper extremity arterial bypass distal to the wrist. Ann Vasc Surg 11:550–557, 1997.
14. Knox RC, Berman SS, Hughes JD, et al: Distal revascularization—interval ligation: A durable and effective for ischemic steal syndrome after hemodialysis access. J Vasc Surg 36:250–256, 2002.
15. Yeager RA, Moneta GL, Edwards JM, et al: Relationship of hemodialysis access to finger gangrene in patients with end stage renal disease. J Vasc Surg 36:245–249, 2002.

INTRA-ABDOMINAL OCCLUSIVE DISEASE

Chapter 31

Vascular Diagnosis of Renovascular Disease

R. EUGENE ZIERLER

- Introduction
- Screening for Renovascular Disease
- Interpretation and Results of Renal Duplex Ultrasound
- Prediction of Clinical Outcome
- Clinical and Research Applications
- Conclusions

Introduction

Although the broad topic of renovascular disease can be considered to include the thoracoabdominal aorta, renal arteries, parenchymal vessels, and renal veins, the most common and clinically significant renovascular disorders involve the renal arteries. Occlusive disease of the renal arteries may result in hypertension or ischemic nephropathy. Hypertension affects about 50 million individuals in the United States, and the proportion with a renovascular etiology is in the range of 1% to 6%.[1,2] However, the prevalence of renovascular hypertension in patients with severe hypertension (i.e., diastolic blood pressure greater than 105 mmHg) may be as high as 30% to 40%.[3] Ischemic nephropathy can be defined as a progressive decline in renal function secondary to global renal ischemia. It has been estimated that 60,000 to 120,000 patients in the United States have azotemia on this basis, and ischemic nephropathy may account for 5% to 15% of the patients who develop end-stage renal disease (ESRD) each year and require renal replacement therapy.[4,5]

The principal lesions associated with renal artery stenosis are atherosclerosis and fibromuscular dysplasia. Atherosclerosis is by far the most common cause of renovascular disease. These lesions are typically located at the origins or in the proximal segments of the renal arteries and are found in patients over 50 years of age with significant aortoiliac or lower extremity arterial occlusive disease (Fig. 31-1). The lesions of fibromuscular dysplasia are usually found in patients under the age of 40 years and affect the middle or distal segments of the renal arteries with a characteristic "string of beads" appearance (Fig. 31-2).

Renal artery stenosis is relatively common, particularly in patients with atherosclerosis in other arterial segments. In a study of 395 patients undergoing routine arteriography for peripheral arterial disease, a renal artery stenosis of more than 50% diameter reduction was found in 38% with abdominal aortic aneurysms, in 33% with aortoiliac occlusive disease, and in 39% with lower extremity occlusive disease.[6] Because many patients are found to have unilateral or bilateral renal artery stenosis without severe hypertension or renal insufficiency, it is clear that not all renal artery lesions

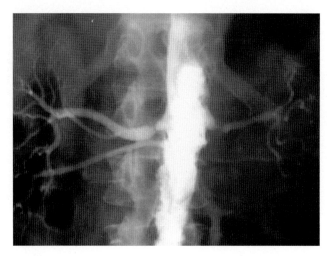

Figure 31-1. Arteriogram of atherosclerotic renal artery stenosis. The lesions are located in the proximal renal artery segments and are associated with significant aortic involvement. There is poststenotic dilatation on the right side.

are physiologically significant. Therefore, in order to be most useful, diagnostic tests must address both the anatomy and physiology of renovascular disease.

Screening for Renovascular Disease

The rationale for screening in patients with suspected renal artery stenosis is to identify those individuals who are most likely to benefit from renal artery interventions for management of hypertension or renal insufficiency. Severe hypertension occurring in children or young adults is particularly likely to be renovascular. Some other general features that suggest the presence of renovascular hypertension rather than essential hypertension are sudden or recent onset of hypertension, an abdominal bruit, resistance to standard antihypertensive therapy with multiple medications, and acute azotemia during treatment with angiotensin-converting enzyme inhibitors. Although these features can be used to increase the positive yield of screening tests, they do not have sufficient discriminative value to exclude patients from further diagnostic evaluation. Therefore, the principal criterion for screening remains the severity of hypertension, particularly the diastolic component.

Screening for renovascular hypertension or ischemic nephropathy is particularly complicated because these conditions involve physiologic as well as anatomic abnormalities. Historically, a variety of screening tests have been used for this purpose. Peripheral plasma renin assays, rapid-sequence intravenous pyelography, and isotope renography have all been tried, but they lack sufficient sensitivity to serve as reliable screening tests.[7]

Captopril renal scintigraphy is based on the pathophysiology of renovascular hypertension, and it has been advocated as a valid screening test.[8] Contrast arteriography remains the "gold standard" for the anatomic diagnosis of renal artery disease, but it is unsuitable for use as a screening test because of its high cost and invasive nature. The potential nephrotoxicity of radiographic contrast is another factor that has limited the use of arteriography in patients with renal artery disease and renal insufficiency. Spiral computed tomography (CT) and magnetic resonance angiography (MRA) are also being used as screening tests for renal artery disease. Although sensitivities and specificities of greater than 90% have been reported for detection of main renal artery stenoses by spiral CT, this approach may not be suitable for many patients because it requires relatively large volumes (up to 150 mL) of iodinated contrast.[9,10] Calcification in atherosclerotic plaques interferes with arterial imaging by spiral CT, and accessory renal arteries may not be reliably identified.[11] MRA does not require injection of iodinated contrast and can produce images that appear similar to standard arteriograms. Gadolinium is a non-nephrotoxic contrast agent that may enhance the ability of MRA to identify accessory renal arteries. Excellent sensitivities and specificities have been reported for imaging main renal artery stenoses by MRA.[12,13] The main disadvantage of MRA is that it may overestimate the severity of stenosis and produce false-positive results. As with all magnetic resonance studies, the test cannot be performed on patients with pacemakers, stents, or other metal devices.

When a hemodynamically significant renal artery stenosis is found, functional studies may be indicated

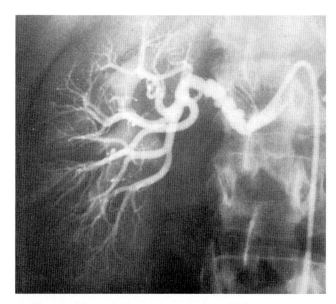

Figure 31-2. Arteriogram of renal artery fibromuscular dysplasia. The "string of beads" lesion involves the middle and distal segments of the renal artery, as well as the segmental branches.

to determine whether the lesion is truly responsible for the clinical findings. This can be accomplished by either renal vein renin determinations or split renal function studies; however, both of these methods are complex and invasive. The most commonly used approach is to measure the renin concentration in blood sampled from each renal vein to detect unilateral renin hypersecretion. The test is considered positive if there is a ratio of at least 1.5 to 1.0 when the stenotic and nonstenotic sides are compared. Split renal function studies are rarely used and require cystoscopy with ureteral catheterization to measure urine flow and urinary concentration from each kidney. Unfortunately, these functional studies have numerous sources for error and the results are not uniformly reliable, particularly in the presence of bilateral renal artery disease or renal artery stenosis involving a solitary kidney.[4]

Duplex ultrasound scanning was developed in the 1970s as a direct noninvasive method for evaluating the extracranial carotid artery. Subsequent advances in ultrasound technology, particularly the availability of improved B-mode systems, color-flow imaging, and lower frequency ultrasound transducers, have extended the applications of duplex scanning to the more complex and deeply located vessels of the abdomen. Duplex scanning is currently the only method available in the noninvasive vascular laboratory for evaluating the renal arteries.

Interpretation and Results of Renal Duplex Ultrasound

The general principles of renal duplex scanning are identical to those for other arterial sites. After the renal artery is visualized by B-mode and color-flow imaging, the pulsed Doppler sample volume is placed within the vessel and spectral waveform analysis is used to characterize the flow pattern and to classify the severity of disease. A localized flow disturbance with a high velocity jet indicates the presence of a high-grade stenosis. The main challenge in renal artery duplex scanning is to locate the vessels and obtain satisfactory pulsed Doppler signals. Renal arteries are especially difficult to examine because of their small size, deep location, and variable anatomy. The effects of respiratory motion and overlying bowel gas can also limit the success of renal duplex scanning.

The classification of renal artery disease by duplex scanning is based on spectral waveforms from the renal artery and adjacent abdominal aorta. The triphasic flow pattern seen in the aortoiliac and lower extremity arteries is a result of the relatively high vascular resistance of the normal peripheral circulation. In contrast, the normal kidney offers a low vascular resistance, and the renal artery velocity waveform is monophasic with forward flow throughout the cardiac cycle (Fig. 31-3). Renal artery

narrowing results in a focally increased renal artery peak systolic velocity (PSV). Normal renal arteries typically show PSV values of less than 180 cm/sec.[14] Because the PSV associated with a hemodynamically significant renal artery stenosis increases relative to aortic PSV, the ratio of peak systolic velocities in the renal artery and aorta can be used as an index of renal artery stenosis severity (Fig. 31-4). This is referred to as the renal/aortic ratio or RAR. Renal artery occlusion is present when the artery is visualized but no flow signal can be detected in the proximal segment. A set of criteria for classification of renal artery disease by duplex scanning is given in Table 31-1.

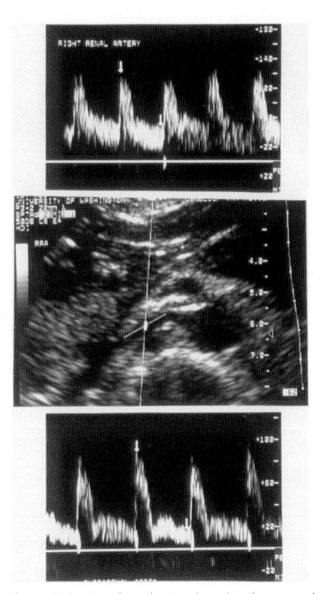

Figure 31-3. Normal renal artery (upper) and suprarenal aortic (lower) spectral waveforms. The renal artery waveform indicates low vascular resistance, with relatively high velocities in diastole. The pulsed Doppler sample volume is located in the right renal artery on the B-mode image.

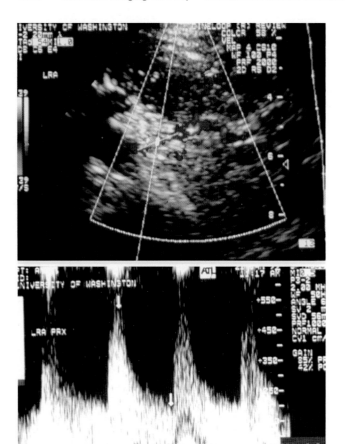

Figure 31-4. B-mode image of a stenotic left renal artery (top) and the corresponding spectral waveform from the proximal renal artery (bottom). Calcification is seen on the B-mode image at the site of stenosis. The renal artery PSV is 530 cm/sec. Based on an aortic peak systolic velocity of 75 cm/sec, the renal/aortic ratio (RAR) is 7.1, indicating a 60% or greater stenosis.

TABLE 31-1. Criteria for Classification of Renal Artery Disease by Duplex Scanning

Renal Artery Diameter Reduction	Renal Artery PSV	RAR
Normal	< 180 cm/sec	< 3.5
< 60%	180 cm/sec	< 3.5
60%	180 cm/sec	3.5
Occlusion (100%)	No signal	No signal

PSV, peak systolic velocity; RAR, renal/aortic ratio (ratio of the PSV in the renal artery to the PSV in the adjacent abdominal aorta).

These criteria were validated by Hoffman and colleagues in a series of 41 patients with 74 renal arteries that were evaluated by both duplex scanning and arteriography.[14] A renal artery PSV of 180 cm/sec or greater discriminated between normal and diseased renal arteries with a sensitivity of 95% and specificity of 90%. Based on 60% diameter reduction as the threshold for a hemodynamically significant stenosis, a RAR of 3.5 or greater identified high-grade renal artery stenoses with a sensitivity of 92% and a specificity of 62%. This relatively low specificity was caused by a large number of borderline lesions which had RAR values greater than 3.5 but were interpreted as being in the range of 50% to 60% diameter reduction by arteriography. It is noteworthy that several of these borderline renal artery lesions were treated by angioplasty or surgery with a successful clinical outcome, suggesting that the stenoses were hemodynamically significant, as predicted by the duplex scan. Occluded renal arteries were correctly identified by duplex scanning in 10 of 11 cases; however, accessory or branch renal artery stenoses were not reliably detected.

Other researchers have used similar methods and interpretation criteria to validate renal duplex scanning, with reported sensitivities and specificities in the range of 93% to 98%.[15,16] Hansen and colleagues found that a focal renal artery PSV of 200 cm/sec or greater in combination with a "turbulent" distal velocity waveform correlated highly with an arteriographic renal artery stenosis of 60% or greater diameter reduction.[15] Among 122 kidneys with single renal arteries in 74 patients, duplex scanning correctly identified 67 of 68 arteries that were normal or had less than 60% stenosis and 35 of 39 arteries with 60% to 99% stenosis. All 15 renal artery occlusions were correctly identified. This resulted in a sensitivity of 93%, a specificity of 98%, a positive predictive value of 98%, a negative predictive value of 94%, and an overall accuracy of 96%. However, among the 14 patients who had 20 kidneys with multiple renal arteries, the sensitivity of duplex scanning decreased to 67%, with a corresponding negative predictive value of 79%.

The rationale for renal hilar duplex scanning is that velocity waveforms obtained distal to a hemodynamically significant renal artery stenosis should become damped and have a more gradual systolic upstroke. Because pulsed Doppler signals are relatively quick and easy to obtain from the renal hilum using a flank approach, it has been suggested that a hilar duplex scan could serve as a rapid screening test for renal artery stenosis. The renal hilar waveform parameters that have been described include the acceleration time (AT), acceleration index (AI), early systolic peak (ESP), and tardus/parvus pattern (TPP). Although the reported specificity of the hilar parameters is typically greater than 90%, the sensitivity is more variable, with a range of 32% to 93%.[17-19] Consequently, the renal hilar scan appears to be reliable when it is positive; however, false-negative results are relatively common, and the low sensitivity makes it unsuitable for use as a primary screening test.

Prediction of Clinical Outcome

Although the applications and techniques of renal duplex scanning have emphasized the main renal arteries, important clinical information can also be obtained by ultrasound evaluation of the renal parenchyma. Measurements of kidney length and evaluation of parenchymal flow patterns have been used to assess the status of the kidney and to predict the clinical response to renal artery interventions. Velocity waveforms taken from within the kidney reflect renovascular resistance. Parameters that have been used to quantify renovascular resistance include the end-diastolic ratio or EDR (parenchymal end-diastolic velocity/parenchymal peak systolic velocity); and the renal resistive index or RRI, which is the inverse of the EDR ([parenchymal peak systolic velocity – parenchymal end-diastolic velocity]/parenchymal peak systolic velocity). Elevated renal parenchymal resistance, which is associated with low EDR or high RRI values, occurs in kidneys with severe parenchymal disease; this may be a factor in failures of renal artery interventions.[20–22] An example of normal and abnormal renal parenchymal waveforms is shown in Figure 31-5.

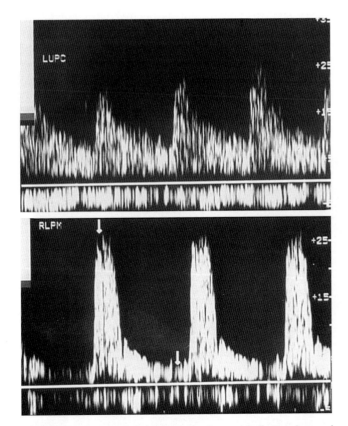

Figure 31-5. Normal (top) and abnormal (bottom) renal parenchymal velocity waveforms. The normal waveform has low resistance flow with high velocities in diastole and an EDR of 0.40 (RRI 0.60), whereas the abnormal waveform indicates a high vascular resistance with low end-diastolic velocities and an EDR of 0.13 (RRI 0.87). Arrows on the abnormal waveform indicate peak systolic and end-diastolic velocities.

In a review of 23 patients undergoing 31 renal revascularizations, Cohn and colleagues found that the mean preintervention EDR was significantly higher in those patients who had a favorable blood pressure response or an improvement in renal function.[21] A preintervention EDR of less than 0.30 correlated with a poor clinical outcome. Radermacher and colleagues reported similar results using the RRI in a cohort of 138 hypertensive patients with unilateral or bilateral renal artery stenosis who had 131 technically successful interventions.[20] Among the 35 patients with a RRI of .80 or greater, 34 showed no significant decrease in blood pressure, and renal function deteriorated in 28. However, 90 of 96 patients with a RRI of less than .80 showed a decrease in blood pressure of 10% or more. These authors concluded that a RRI value of .80 or greater identifies a group of patients unlikely to respond to renal revascularization.

Clinical and Research Applications

Current applications of renal duplex scanning include screening of patients with hypertension or renal failure, intraoperative assessment, follow-up after renal artery interventions, evaluation of renal transplants, and natural history studies. The value of duplex ultrasound is that it provides both anatomic information and an assessment of the hemodynamic significance of any renal artery lesions, as well as information on kidney size and the status of the renal parenchyma.

Screening

The general approach to screening for renovascular disease has already been discussed. Ideally, a screening test for renal artery stenosis should be able to detect and classify lesions in all segments of the main renal arteries and in accessory renal arteries. As previously mentioned, renal duplex scanning is generally reliable for assessing the main renal arteries, but it does not consistently identify accessory renal arteries or lesions in the segmental branches. When renovascular hypertension is suspected, the status of the main renal arteries and any accessory or polar arteries must be evaluated because hypertension can result from isolated accessory renal artery stenosis. In this situation, failure to detect a hemodynamically significant stenosis in an accessory renal artery could result in a false-negative screening test. Therefore additional imaging studies should be considered when a duplex scan shows nonstenotic renal arteries and there is a strong clinical suspicion for renovascular hypertension. Ischemic nephropathy results from "total" renal ischemia, so there must be hemodynamically significant stenoses in both main renal arteries (or in a single main renal artery in patients with a solitary kidney) for this condition to be present.

Consequently, if one or both main renal arteries are shown to be widely patent, ischemic nephropathy can be ruled out.

Follow-Up

Duplex ultrasound provides a practical noninvasive method for assessing the results of renal artery interventions. In 1989 Taylor and colleagues reported on 16 renal artery stenoses of 60% or greater diameter reduction that were followed after interventions.[23] Six arteries in five patients were treated by percutaneous transluminal angioplasty (PTA), and surgical bypass was performed on 10 arteries in 7 patients. The PTA group was followed for a mean of 6.5 months. Duplex scanning documented relief of renal artery stenosis in two patients whose hypertension improved after PTA, and persistent stenosis in three patients whose hypertension did not improve. Follow-up of the surgical bypass group for a mean of 9 months showed 8 patent and 2 occluded grafts. In another follow-up study of 51 renal artery interventions in 36 patients, including 8 PTAs, the diagnostic accuracy of duplex scanning was 86%, with a sensitivity of 80% and a specificity of 87%.[24] A larger study of 61 renal artery interventions (44 surgical repairs, 17 PTAs) indicated that duplex scanning had an overall accuracy of 92%, a sensitivity of 69%, and a specificity of 98%.[25] The duplex scan results were adversely affected by the presence of branch renal artery disease, and a separate analysis of the 50 interventions for main renal artery lesions yielded an accuracy of 96%, a sensitivity of 89%, and a specificity of 98%.

In a prospective but nonrandomized study, Baumgartner and colleagues compared primary PTA to primary stenting for ostial, proximal, and isolated truncal atherosclerotic renal artery stenosis.[26] Duplex scanning was used to follow 163 patients with 200 treated renal artery lesions for a median of 12 months. Primary patency rates at 12 months for PTA alone were 34% for ostial stenoses, 65% for proximal stenoses, and 83% for truncal stenoses. The corresponding primary patency rates for the stented renal arteries were 80%, 72%, and 66%. A significant reduction in the rate of restenosis for the stented renal arteries was observed only for the ostial stenoses.

Experience with duplex scanning for follow-up after renal artery interventions indicates that the velocity criteria developed for classification of native renal artery disease can also be applied after PTA or surgical revascularization. The presence of a stent does not limit ultrasound interrogation of the vessel (Fig. 31-6).

Natural History Studies

The value of renal revascularization in patients with severe renal artery disease and established renovascular hypertension or ischemic renal failure is generally accepted. However, the role of intervention for renal artery stenosis that is not associated with uncontrollable hypertension or decreased renal function remains uncertain. The ultimate goal of natural history studies of renal artery disease is to provide a rationale for managing patients with asymptomatic or minimally symptomatic renal artery stenosis. A prospective study on the natural history of atherosclerotic renal artery stenosis was ini-

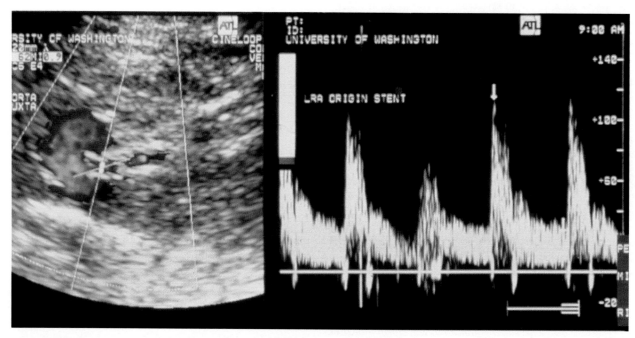

Figure 31-6. Duplex ultrasound evaluation of a left renal artery after PTA and stenting. The stent is well visualized on the B-mode image protruding slightly into the aortic lumen. The pulsed Doppler sample volume is positioned at the origin of the renal artery, and the spectral waveform indicates normal renal artery flow.

Prediction of Clinical Outcome

Although the applications and techniques of renal duplex scanning have emphasized the main renal arteries, important clinical information can also be obtained by ultrasound evaluation of the renal parenchyma. Measurements of kidney length and evaluation of parenchymal flow patterns have been used to assess the status of the kidney and to predict the clinical response to renal artery interventions. Velocity waveforms taken from within the kidney reflect renovascular resistance. Parameters that have been used to quantify renovascular resistance include the end-diastolic ratio or EDR (parenchymal end-diastolic velocity/parenchymal peak systolic velocity); and the renal resistive index or RRI, which is the inverse of the EDR ([parenchymal peak systolic velocity − parenchymal end-diastolic velocity]/parenchymal peak systolic velocity). Elevated renal parenchymal resistance, which is associated with low EDR or high RRI values, occurs in kidneys with severe parenchymal disease; this may be a factor in failures of renal artery interventions.[20–22] An example of normal and abnormal renal parenchymal waveforms is shown in Figure 31-5.

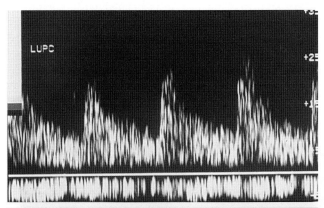

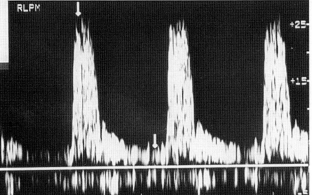

Figure 31-5. Normal (top) and abnormal (bottom) renal parenchymal velocity waveforms. The normal waveform has low resistance flow with high velocities in diastole and an EDR of 0.40 (RRI 0.60), whereas the abnormal waveform indicates a high vascular resistance with low end-diastolic velocities and an EDR of 0.13 (RRI 0.87). Arrows on the abnormal waveform indicate peak systolic and end-diastolic velocities.

In a review of 23 patients undergoing 31 renal revascularizations, Cohn and colleagues found that the mean preintervention EDR was significantly higher in those patients who had a favorable blood pressure response or an improvement in renal function.[21] A preintervention EDR of less than 0.30 correlated with a poor clinical outcome. Radermacher and colleagues reported similar results using the RRI in a cohort of 138 hypertensive patients with unilateral or bilateral renal artery stenosis who had 131 technically successful interventions.[20] Among the 35 patients with a RRI of .80 or greater, 34 showed no significant decrease in blood pressure, and renal function deteriorated in 28. However, 90 of 96 patients with a RRI of less than .80 showed a decrease in blood pressure of 10% or more. These authors concluded that a RRI value of .80 or greater identifies a group of patients unlikely to respond to renal revascularization.

Clinical and Research Applications

Current applications of renal duplex scanning include screening of patients with hypertension or renal failure, intraoperative assessment, follow-up after renal artery interventions, evaluation of renal transplants, and natural history studies. The value of duplex ultrasound is that it provides both anatomic information and an assessment of the hemodynamic significance of any renal artery lesions, as well as information on kidney size and the status of the renal parenchyma.

Screening

The general approach to screening for renovascular disease has already been discussed. Ideally, a screening test for renal artery stenosis should be able to detect and classify lesions in all segments of the main renal arteries and in accessory renal arteries. As previously mentioned, renal duplex scanning is generally reliable for assessing the main renal arteries, but it does not consistently identify accessory renal arteries or lesions in the segmental branches. When renovascular hypertension is suspected, the status of the main renal arteries and any accessory or polar arteries must be evaluated because hypertension can result from isolated accessory renal artery stenosis. In this situation, failure to detect a hemodynamically significant stenosis in an accessory renal artery could result in a false-negative screening test. Therefore additional imaging studies should be considered when a duplex scan shows nonstenotic renal arteries and there is a strong clinical suspicion for renovascular hypertension. Ischemic nephropathy results from "total" renal ischemia, so there must be hemodynamically significant stenoses in both main renal arteries (or in a single main renal artery in patients with a solitary kidney) for this condition to be present.

Consequently, if one or both main renal arteries are shown to be widely patent, ischemic nephropathy can be ruled out.

Follow-Up

Duplex ultrasound provides a practical noninvasive method for assessing the results of renal artery interventions. In 1989 Taylor and colleagues reported on 16 renal artery stenoses of 60% or greater diameter reduction that were followed after interventions.[23] Six arteries in five patients were treated by percutaneous transluminal angioplasty (PTA), and surgical bypass was performed on 10 arteries in 7 patients. The PTA group was followed for a mean of 6.5 months. Duplex scanning documented relief of renal artery stenosis in two patients whose hypertension improved after PTA, and persistent stenosis in three patients whose hypertension did not improve. Follow-up of the surgical bypass group for a mean of 9 months showed 8 patent and 2 occluded grafts. In another follow-up study of 51 renal artery interventions in 36 patients, including 8 PTAs, the diagnostic accuracy of duplex scanning was 86%, with a sensitivity of 80% and a specificity of 87%.[24] A larger study of 61 renal artery interventions (44 surgical repairs, 17 PTAs) indicated that duplex scanning had an overall accuracy of 92%, a sensitivity of 69%, and a specificity of 98%.[25] The duplex scan results were adversely affected by the presence of branch renal artery disease, and a separate analysis of the 50 interventions for main renal artery lesions yielded an accuracy of 96%, a sensitivity of 89%, and a specificity of 98%.

In a prospective but nonrandomized study, Baumgartner and colleagues compared primary PTA to primary stenting for ostial, proximal, and isolated truncal atherosclerotic renal artery stenosis.[26] Duplex scanning was used to follow 163 patients with 200 treated renal artery lesions for a median of 12 months. Primary patency rates at 12 months for PTA alone were 34% for ostial stenoses, 65% for proximal stenoses, and 83% for truncal stenoses. The corresponding primary patency rates for the stented renal arteries were 80%, 72%, and 66%. A significant reduction in the rate of restenosis for the stented renal arteries was observed only for the ostial stenoses.

Experience with duplex scanning for follow-up after renal artery interventions indicates that the velocity criteria developed for classification of native renal artery disease can also be applied after PTA or surgical revascularization. The presence of a stent does not limit ultrasound interrogation of the vessel (Fig. 31-6).

Natural History Studies

The value of renal revascularization in patients with severe renal artery disease and established renovascular hypertension or ischemic renal failure is generally accepted. However, the role of intervention for renal artery stenosis that is not associated with uncontrollable hypertension or decreased renal function remains uncertain. The ultimate goal of natural history studies of renal artery disease is to provide a rationale for managing patients with asymptomatic or minimally symptomatic renal artery stenosis. A prospective study on the natural history of atherosclerotic renal artery stenosis was ini-

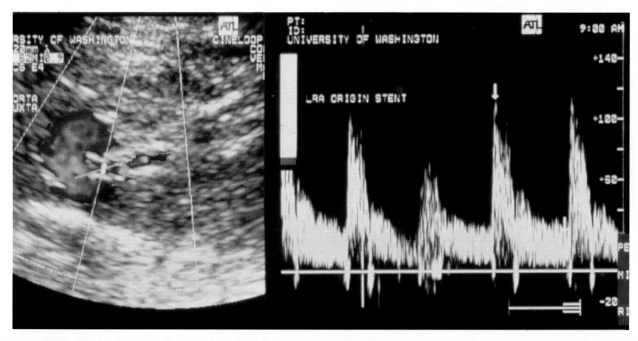

Figure 31-6. *Duplex ultrasound evaluation of a left renal artery after PTA and stenting. The stent is well visualized on the B-mode image protruding slightly into the aortic lumen. The pulsed Doppler sample volume is positioned at the origin of the renal artery, and the spectral waveform indicates normal renal artery flow.*

tiated in the vascular research laboratory at the University of Washington in 1990. The study population included patients with renal artery disease who did not require immediate intervention. All renal arteries were classified by duplex scanning as normal, less than 60% stenosis, 60% stenosis or greater, or occluded. Eligible patients had at least one abnormal renal artery with a PSV of 180 cm/sec or more; or a RAR of 3.5 or more. Disease progression in a renal artery was defined as either (1) an increase in renal artery PSV of 100 cm/sec or more relative to prior examinations (hemodynamic); (2) an increase in renal artery stenosis severity to 60% or more diameter reduction (anatomic); or (3) occlusion of a previously patent renal artery.

Caps and colleagues reported on 170 patients (85 males, 85 females, with a mean age of 68 years) who were followed for a mean of 33 months (range, 3 months to 7.2 years).[27] The baseline status of the 295 eligible renal arteries was normal in 56, less than 60% stenosis in 96, and 60% or greater stenosis in 143. Hemodynamic disease progression was detected in 91 of the 295 renal arteries (31%), and the 3-year cumulative incidence was 18%, 28%, and 49% for renal arteries initially classified as normal, less than 60% stenosis, and 60% or greater stenosis, respectively. Based on the duplex criteria, the 3-year cumulative incidence of anatomic renal artery disease progression was 13% from normal to 60% or greater stenosis and 56% from less than 60% to 60% or greater stenosis. Only 9 of the 295 renal arteries progressed to occlusion during the follow-up period, and all of these either had 60% or greater stenosis at the baseline examination or progressed to 60% or greater stenosis before occlusion.

Analysis of baseline risk factors indicated that the following four were independently associated with hemodynamic renal artery disease progression: increased systolic blood pressure, diabetes mellitus, presence of a high-grade ipsilateral renal artery stenosis, and a high-grade contralateral renal artery stenosis (Table 31-2). Systolic hypertension showed the strongest association, with a 2.1-fold increase in risk of progression for a value of 160 or greater mmHg. Renal arteries exposed to all four of the baseline risk factors listed in Table 31-2 would have a predicted 2-year cumulative incidence of disease progression of 65%; however, if none of these factors were present, the cumulative incidence would be only 7%.

Changes in renal size were also documented in 122 patients with a total of 204 eligible kidneys over a mean follow-up interval of 33 months.[28] Renal atrophy was defined as a decrease in kidney length of more than 1 cm during follow-up compared with the baseline length measurement. The 1 cm threshold was based on an analysis showing that a measured change in length of 1 cm would be unlikely to occur in a kidney that was not truly changing in size. A decrease in kidney length of more than 1 cm was observed in 33 (16%) of the 204

kidneys. The cumulative incidence of renal atrophy at 2 years was 6% for kidneys with normal renal arteries, 12% for kidneys having less than 60% stenosis, and 21% for kidneys having 60% or greater stenosis at baseline. Three baseline factors were strongly associated with renal atrophy: systolic hypertension, severity of renal artery stenosis, and diminished renal cortical bloodflow velocity. Each 20 mmHg increase in baseline systolic blood pressure was associated with a 2.1-fold increase in risk for renal atrophy. Decreases in both renal cortical peak and end-diastolic blood flow velocities were associated with an increased risk for renal atrophy, but the cortical end-diastolic velocity was more predictive, with a 2.1-fold increase in risk for each 2 cm/sec decrease in velocity. There was a statistically significant association between the number of kidneys per patient that showed atrophy and the observed change in the serum creatinine concentration. The mean change in serum creatinine was + .08 mg/dL per year among patients with atrophy detected in one kidney and + .33 mg/dL per year among those with atrophy detected in both kidneys.

Although no definitive clinical recommendations can be made on the basis of the current natural history data, it is clear that this patient population has a high incidence of renal artery disease progression and renal atrophy. These results suggest that early renal revascularization could be beneficial for selected patients with severe renal artery stenoses in terms of improved blood pressure control and preservation of renal function. However, the effect of such intervention on further disease progression and overall clinical outcome remains to be shown.

Conclusions

Renovascular disease presents a complex diagnostic and therapeutic challenge to the clinician. Duplex ultrasound is a reliable anatomic screening method that provides

TABLE 31-2. Stepwise Cox Proportional Hazards Analysis of Baseline Risk Factors for Renal Artery Disease Progression

Risk Factor	RR	95% CI	p value
Systolic blood pressure 160 mmHg	2.1	(1.2, 3.5)	0.006
Diabetes mellitus	2.0	(1.2, 3.3)	0.009
60% ipsilateral renal artery stenosis	1.9	(1.2, 3.0)	0.004
60% contralateral renal artery stenosis	1.7	(1.0, 2.8)	0.04

RR, relative risk, 95%; CI, 95% confidence interval.

distinct advantages in terms of cost and risk compared with alternative imaging techniques. Ultrasound also permits an evaluation of the renal parenchyma and may be valuable in predicting the functional response to renal artery interventions. However, renal duplex scanning is arguably the most difficult examination performed in the vascular laboratory, and not all laboratories have been able to achieve a high level of accuracy. Further experience and training, as well as continued advances in ultrasound technology, should increase the general availability of this approach.

When properly applied, duplex scanning can be used to screen patients for renovascular hypertension and ischemic nephropathy. It is also ideally suited for follow-up after renal artery interventions. Natural history studies of atherosclerotic renal artery stenosis have defined the clinical risk factors for disease progression and renal atrophy. Randomized clinical trials will be necessary to establish the role of early renal revascularization in the management of patients with renal artery disease.

REFERENCES

1. Chobanian AV, Bakris GL, Black HR, et al: The seventh report of the Joint National Committee on Prevention, Detection, Evaluation, and Treatment, of High Blood Pressure (The JNC 7 Report). JAMA 289:2560–2572, 2003.
2. Simon N, Franklin SS, Bleifer KH, et al: Clinical characteristics of renovascular hypertension. JAMA 220:1209–1218, 1972.
3. Dean RH: Screening and diagnosis of renal vascular hypertension. In Novick A (ed): Renovascular Disease. Philadelphia: WB Saunders, 1998.
4. Jacobson HR: Ischemic renal disease: An overlooked clinical entity. Kidney Int 34:729–743, 1988.
5. Rimmer JM, Gennari J: Atherosclerotic renovascular disease and progressive renal failure. Ann Intern Med 118:712–719, 1993.
6. Olin JW, Melia M, Young JR, et al: Prevalence of atherosclerotic renal artery stenosis in patients with atherosclerosis elsewhere. Am J Med 88:46N–51N, 1990.
7. Grim CE, Luft FC, Weinberger MH: Sensitivity and specificity of screening tests for renal vascular hypertension. Ann Intern Med 91:617–622, 1979.
8. Meier GH, Sumpio B, Black HR, et al: Captopril renal scintigraphy: An advance in the detection and treatment of renovascular hypertension. J Vasc Surg 11:770–777, 1990.
9. Olbricht CJ, Prokop M, Chavin A, et al: Minimally invasive diagnosis of renal artery stenosis by spiral computed tomography angiography. Kidney Int 48:1332–1337, 1995.
10. Beregi JP, Elkohen M, Deklunder G, et al: Helical CT angiography compared with arteriography in the detection of renal artery stenosis. Am J Roentgenol 167:495–501, 1996.
11. Elkohen M, Beregi JP, Deklunder G, et al: A prospective study of helical computed tomography angiography versus angiography for the detection of renal artery stenoses in hypertensive patients. J Hypertens 14:525–528, 1996.
12. Kent KC, Edelman RR, Kim D, et al: Magnetic resonance imaging: A reliable test for the evaluation of proximal atherosclerotic renal artery stenosis. J Vasc Surg 13:311–317, 1991.
13. Gedroyc WMW, Neerhut P, Negus R, et al: Magnetic resonance angiography of renal artery stenosis. Clin Radiol 50:436–439, 1995.
14. Hoffman U, Edwards JM, Carter S, et al: Role of duplex scanning for the detection of atherosclerotic renal artery disease. Kid Int 39:1232–1239, 1991.
15. Hansen KJ, Tribble RW, Reavis S, et al: Renal duplex sonography: Evaluation of clinical utility. J Vasc Surg 12:227–236, 1990.
16. Olin JW, Piedmonte MR, Young JR, et al: The utility of duplex ultrasound scanning of the renal arteries for diagnosing significant renal artery stenosis. Ann Intern Med 122:833–838, 1995.
17. Motew SJ, Cherr GS, Craven TE, et al: Renal duplex sonography: Main renal artery versus hilar analyisis. J Vasc Surg 32:462–471, 2000.
18. Stavros TA, Parker SH, Yakes WF, et al: Segmental stenosis of the renal artery: Pattern recognition of tardus and parvus abnormalities with duplex sonography. Radiology 184:487–492, 1992.
19. Kliewer, MA, Tupler RH, Carroll BA, et al: Renal artery stenosis: Analysis of Doppler waveform parameters and tardus-parvus pattern. Radiology 189:779–787, 1993.
20. Radermacher J, Chiavan A, Bleck B, et al: Use of Doppler ultrasonography to predict the outcome of therapy for renal artery stenosis. N Engl J Med 344:410–417, 2001.
21. Cohn EJ, Benjamin ME, Sandager GP, et al: Can intrarenal duplex waveform analysis predict successful renal artery revascularization? J Vasc Surg 28:471–480, 1998.
22. Frauchiger B, Zierler RE, Bergelin RO, et al: Prognostic significance of intrarenal resistance indices in patients with renal artery interventions: A preliminary study with duplex ultrasound. Cardiovasc Surg 4:324–330, 1996.
23. Taylor DC, Moneta GL, Strandness DE Jr: Follow-up of renal artery stenosis by duplex ultrasound. J Vasc Surg 9:410–415, 1989.
24. Eidt JF, Fry RE, Clagett P, et al: Postoperative follow-up of renal artery reconstruction with duplex ultrasound. J Vasc Surg 8:667–673, 1988.
25. Hudspeth DA, Hansen KJ, Reavis SW, et al: Renal duplex sonography after treatment of renovascular disease. J Vasc Surg 18:381–390, 1993.
26. Baumgartner I, von Aesch K, Do D, et al: Stent placement in ostial and nonostial atherosclerotic renal artery stenoses: A prospective follow-up study. Radiology 216:498–505, 2000.
27. Caps MT, Perissinotto C, Zierler RE, et al: A prospective study of atherosclerotic disease progression in the renal artery. Circulation 98:2866–2872, 1998.
28. Caps MT, Zierler RE, Polissar NL, et al: The risk of atrophy in kidneys with atherosclerotic renal artery stenosis. Kidney Int 53:735–742, 1998.

Chapter 32

Renal Artery Color-Flow Scanning: Technique and Applications

MARC CAIROLS

■ Introduction

■ Renal Artery Scanning Technique

■ Applications

Introduction

Detecting lesions in the renal arteries is important because in many patients they may cause secondary renovascular hypertension. As is well known, the advent of endovascular techniques has expanded the population that can be amenable to therapy.

Color-flow duplex scanning (CFDS) was developed in the '70s for carotid artery disease; however, later advances in ultrasound technology allowed a wider application to other fields. One of those newer fields was the renal arteries. Screening for renal artery diseases is often complicated because morphologic and hemodynamic abnormalities are usually involved. Also, the deep anatomic location of the renal arteries increases the difficulties.

In the past, a variety of screening tests have been advocated as useful tools for diagnosing renal diseases (e.g., renin plasma assays, intravenous pyolographies, and

isotope renograms); unfortunately, none of these has become the definitive test because of reliability.

Main pathologies are of atherosclerotic origin and stenosis secondary to fibromuscular dysplasia (FMD); other pathologies (e.g., aneurysms and arteritis) are a rarity.

There are diagnostic problems of paramount importance that must be solved before an adequate therapy can be established.

1. Establishing the renovascular origin of the hypertension or renal insufficiency. The fact that so many tests have been developed indicates the difficulties in settling this question. In too many occasions the diagnosis is made ex juvantibus once the therapy has been applied.

2. If there is a strong suspicion of renovascular hypertension, a proper mapping must be obtained in order to plan a correct interventional approach. Because there are so many variations in the type of lesion, the presence of polar renal arteries, and other morphologic abnormalities, the mapping information becomes of utmost importance.

3. Is duplex as reliable after percutaneous transluminal renal angioplasty (PTRA) as it is in a non-operated renal artery? It is well known that the

rate of restenosis after PTRA is high, but with aggressive reintervention protocols it is possible to obtain high secondary patency rates if restenosis is appropriately diagnosed.

4. Renal insufficiency tends to worsen along different timelines. Is duplex ultrasound reliable enough to establish prognostic criteria for detecting those kidneys at risk? By detecting renal artery stenosis (RAS) progression, although hypertension may not be of renovascular origin, the end-point is usually a kidney loss.

5. It is not uncommon that a renal stenosis is seen when performing an arteriogram for diagnosing a limb ischemia or because of an aortic aneurysm. The question then becomes whether or not it is of functional relevance. Captopril renal scintigraphy, which is based on this pathophysiology, has been advocated as the valid test.

Despite all these advances, arteriography remains the gold standard for anatomic diagnosis of RAS, but it is unsuitable for screening because it is invasive, costly, and potentially dangerous. Although not suitable for screening, wide application of PTRA has given arteriography a prominent place in the diagnostic/therapeutic algorithm.

Renal Artery Scanning Technique

Description

Duplex/color Doppler sonography of renal arteries is a demanding technique and should be approached only by those willing to understand the procedure and to do a complete examination. It is one of the most difficult examinations carried out in a vascular lab, and the usefulness and reliability of its results depend more than any other on the capacity and expertise of the technologist.

Provided these preliminary aspects are fulfilled, this technique offers an excellent means of evaluating renal artery disease.

To perform a renal duplex, the author uses a low frequency transducer (2.5 to 3 MHz). To scan main renal arteries, settings are adjusted to display high velocity signals; for parenchyma studies, a low flow set-up is used. Renal arteries lie deep in the abdomen, and motion imposed by respiration or by the interposition of intra-abdominal gas may contribute to problems doing the examination. For this reason, patients should be scheduled for renal duplex early in the morning after 12 hours fasting. Special bowel preparation has been proposed, but in the author's experience this adds very little to the feasibility of the study and represents a serious disturbance for the patient. In difficult cases, it is usually better to either repeat the examination after a brief walk, which will probably redistribute bowel gas and yield remarkably

improved results; or reschedule the patient and try again after a few days. Recently, the use of a sonographic contrast agent seems promising in diminishing the rate of technically inadequate examinations.

Normal Anatomy and Scanning Technique

The procedure begins by positioning the patient in the supine position, with the head of the bed elevated about 30 degrees. From the anterior midline approach, a longitudinal image of the aorta is obtained and a representative aortic velocity waveform is recorded at the level of the renal arteries, just below the origin of superior mesenteric artery (SMA). Peak systolic velocity (PSV) of the aorta will be used as a reference for comparison with those recorded in the renal arteries.

Right Renal Artery (RRA)

To localize the renal arteries the scanhead is rotated 90 degrees and the left renal vein (LRV) is easily identified crossing over the aorta below the SMA (Fig. 32-1). This vein is an important landmark to start searching for the origin of both renal arteries. The origin of the RRA is located in the anterolateral aspect of the aorta very close to the point where the LRV drains to the inferior vena cava (IVC). Insonation at this point is difficult because the artery lies perpendicular to Doppler beam and flow signal from the LRV interferes with the recording.

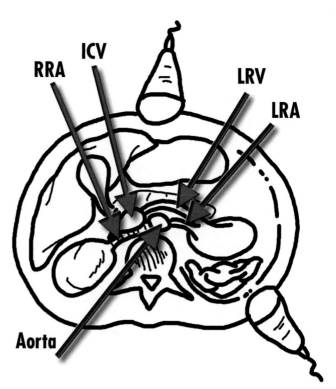

Figure 32-1. *Schema of insonation sites. RRA, Right renal artery; ICV, inferior vena cava; LRV, left renal vein; LRA, left renal artery.*

Immediately after its origin, the artery turns posteriorly to course beneath the IVC. It is important to obtain signals from the whole length of the vessel to avoid missing any lesion, but this is not always possible from a midline approach. Some authors[1] have proposed a modified flank approach in which scanning is done through the anterolateral abdomen, somewhat lower than when the liver is used as a window to image the kidney.

By placing the patient in left lateral decubitus position, the RRA we can be insonated through the kidney itself for almost its whole length.

Left Renal Artery (LRA)

The LRA tends to originate from the aorta somewhat lower than the RRA and from the posterolateral surface. It usually lies behind the LRV, which is larger and easier to identify in the midline transabdominal approach. After its origin it runs posteriorly over the psoas muscle (Fig. 32-2). It is important to realize that it is often difficult to know the precise angle of insonation, and that this may result in mistaken velocity measures. It is also important to be aware of the possibility of multiple renal arteries that might be located by scanning along the aorta above and below the main artery. Another way to image the LRA is through a flank approach, placing the patient in a right lateral decubitus position. This way, it is possible to scan the LRA, through the kidney, from the hilus back to the aorta. This position is very helpful in obese patients in whom, from the midline approach, the artery lies too deep to be adequately insonated. It is also helpful in cases of massive interposition of bowel gas.

Intrarenal Vessels

For estimation of renal size, and to assess the flow patterns from the renal medulla and the cortex of the kidney,

the patient is rolled onto the side and the kidney is approached from the flank.

The main renal artery and vein can be visualized by entering the kidney in the area of the hilus. The artery divides into anterior and posterior branches, and then into segmental arteries. The segmental arteries further bifurcate into lobar and then interlobar arteries that travel directly toward the transducer in the columns of Bertin between the medullary pyramids. The interlobar arteries give rise to arcuate arteries that traverse the corticomedullary junction and give rise to the interlobular arteries (Fig. 32-3).

Normal spectral waveforms of renal parenchyma show a low resistance pattern. For a quantitative evaluation of peripheral resistance, two similar ratios have been used. Strandness[2] has proposed the use of the ratio between end-diastolic velocity (EDV) and PSV, referred to as the end-diastolic ratio. This is usually measured in the interlobar and interlobular arteries of the superior and inferior poles of the kidney. Other authors[3] have proposed the use of the resistive index (RI), which is the PSV minus EDV divided by PSV (1 − EDV/PSV) (Table 32-1). The end-diastolic ratio increases as resistance decreases, whereas the RI is high when parenchymal resistance is increased. The usefulness of these two measures will be discussed later in this chapter.

Diagnostic Criteria of Renal Artery Stenosis

Main Renal Artery Duplex Scanning

The effects of narrowing the lumen of the renal artery are similar to those in other areas of the circulation: there is an increase in the velocity within the narrowed segment that reflects the degree of stenosis. Therefore the major goals of the study will be to identify the velocity changes that are consistent with a RAS.

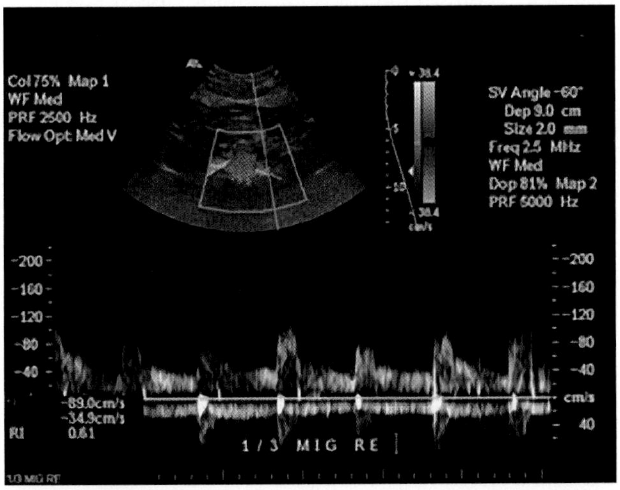

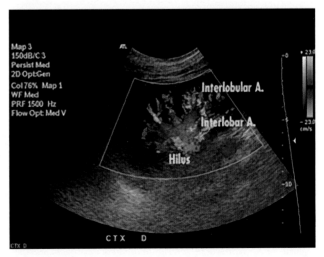

Figure 32-2. Transverse view of the aorta at the origin of renal arteries.

Figure 32-3. Parenchyma study. Flank approach to visualize the kidney and its vessels.

TABLE 32-1. **Description of Commonly Used Ratios**

Ratio		Description
RAR		PSV (renal artery)
		PSV (aorta)
EDR		EDV
		PSV
RI	$1-$	EDV
		PSV

RAR, renal aortic ratio; EDR, end-diastolic ratio; RI, resistive index; PSV, peak systolic velocity; EDV, end-diastolic velocity.

Duplex criteria for RAS have been set to identify stenoses that are hemodynamically significant; this appears to happen when the diameter reduction exceeds 60%. To achieve good diagnostic results, Doppler samples must be obtained directly at the point of maximum stenosis (Fig. 32-4). Two different parameters have been used. The first one is the absolute value of PSV at the stenosis (Fig. 32-5). Threshold values for PSV consistent with a 60% or greater diameter reduction of the renal artery obtained in most studies are 180 to 190 cm/sec. In some cases, when Doppler angle is difficult or impossible to adjust, or when flow velocity in the aorta is decreased because of age or atherosclerotic disease, it is useful to use the ratio between the velocity of the renal artery and the aorta (renal aortic ratio, RAR). Threshold values of this ratio diagnostic of a 60% or greater RAS vary in different studies from 3 to 3.5. In order to evaluate the predictive value and optimal cut-off points of Doppler parameters for detecting RAS in the author's center, 47 hypertensive patients were prospectively studied with renal duplex and intraarterial contrast angiography.[4] The

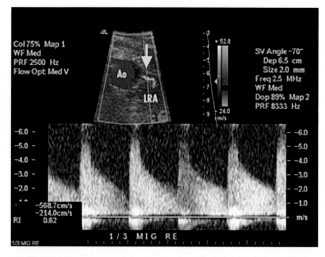

Figure 32-5. *Transverse anterior abdominal approach. Stenosis at the origin of left renal artery (arrow). Ao, Aorta; LRA, left renal artery. Increased PSV at the stenosis (568 cm/sec).*

results are summarized in Table 32-2. Duplex examination was not possible in three patients (6%) because of bowel gas or extreme obesity. By means of receiving operator characteristic curves (Fig. 32-6) it was established that the best threshold value for PSV at the stenosis was 180 cm/sec with a sensibility of 90.4%, negative predictive value of 96%, and kappa value of 0.76. RAR also showed very good correlation with RAS, and the best threshold value was 3 (sensibility 90.4, negative predictive value 96.6, and correlation kappa 0.73). In this study, five renal artery occlusions were correctly diagnosed with duplex.

The main criteria used to identify renal artery occlusion were: no signal at the location of the renal artery orifice and kidney size of less than 9 cm. Accessory renal arteries were present in three patients, and none was detected with duplex. These results are similar to those reported previously[5] and also to those of other authors,[6,7] confirming that renal duplex is an ideal test for screening provided that the population studied has a high prevalence of renovascular disease (40% in the author's study). This point is extremely important and might have influenced the poor results obtained by some authors.[8,9] It is well established that prevalence affects the predictive value of any test, and that if we apply it to a population with a very low probability of disease, the likelihood for an individual with a positive result to have the disease decreases or, in other words, the chance to have a false-positive increases. This subject was clearly established by Berqvist and colleagues[10] and is shown in Table 32-3. In a population of patients with hypertension, the prevalence of renovascular hypertension may vary greatly depending on selection criteria. Consequently, comparing different studies may be a waste of time because the patient may have been selected either on a RAS basis or on a clinical set-up.

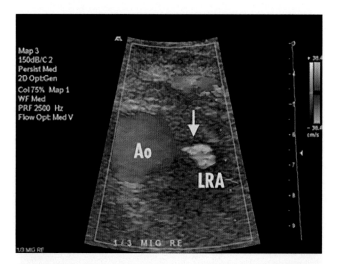

Figure 32-4. *Transverse anterior abdominal approach. Stenosis at the origin of left renal artery (arrow). Ao, Aorta; LRA, left renal artery.*

TABLE 32-2. **Results for Diagnostic Criteria of Renal Artery Stenosis as Compared With Angiography**

	Sensibility	Specificity	PPV	NPV	Accuracy
PSV > 180 cm/sec	90.4	90.7	76	96.7	90.6
RAR > 3	90.4	89.2	73	96.6	89.5

PSV, peak systolic velocity; RAR, renal aortic ratio; PPV, positive predictive value; NPV, negative predictive value.

Hiliar Duplex Scanning

Renal artery duplex scanning has not gained wide acceptance as a screening test for detection of RAS because it is time consuming and requires expertise for a proper examination. Renal hilar duplex scanning from a flank or translumbar approach has been suggested as a simplified alternative for screening, especially in those patients in whom conventional renal duplex examination is difficult to perform. Because of the difficulties in performing the standard renal artery duplex study, some authors have proposed to identify RAS indirectly by using intrarenal waveform analysis. Handa and colleagues[11] observed that systolic upstroke was abnormal distal to a hemodinamically significant stenosis. This observation has been called the "tardus-parvus" effect to describe that systolic upstroke is delayed (tardus) and dampened (parvus) distal to the stenosis. These criteria are based on measurements of acceleration time and acceleration index (Fig. 32-7), although some proponents of this technique think that simply looking at the waveform is enough. The criteria proposed by Handa for a significant RAS are an acceleration time of 100 ms or greater (normal, less than 70 ms) and an acceleration index of 291 cm/sec² or less (normal, greater than 300 cm/sec²). If any one of these is found to be positive, then a complete duplex scan should be carried out.

The main problem with this method is its lack of sensitivity,[12,13] but spectral abnormalities also may be subtle and differentiation between normal and abnormal waveforms is not always easy. Strandness[2] compared this method with the standard direct duplex study and demonstrated a sensitivity of 62% and an overall accuracy of 85%. This means that by using only the tardus-parvus pattern, more than one third of stenoses would have been missed; therefore, the waveform pattern criteria are commonly considered inappropriate for screening RAS.

Renal Parenchyma Studies

As previously explained, the study of Doppler waveforms in the renal parenchyma allows an evaluation of the resistance to flow within the kidney. This increased resistance itself may be the cause of hypertension and preclude the success of renal artery revascularization.[14] On the other hand, it has been established that patients with an increased RI are more prone to progression to renal failure even without RAS. Radermacher and colleagues[15] followed 162 patients with renal disease during 3 +/− 1.4 years and showed that those presenting a baseline RI of 80 or greater had a poorer evolution, with progression to renal failure and dialysis in 64% vs. 5%. Finally, the study of RI or EDR may be used to follow renal transplants, as will be discussed later.

Renal Artery Occlusion

Absence of flow in a visualized renal artery or within the kidney are the main criteria for diagnosing renal artery occlusion. Parenchymal Doppler velocity less than 10 cm/sec with dampened configuration and a kidney length less than 9 cm have been suggested as additional criteria for diagnosing occlusion. Although some studies have demonstrated very satisfactory results regarding the diagnosis of renal artery occlusion, false-negative studies

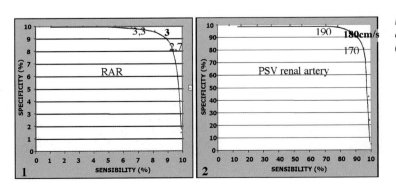

Figure 32-6. *Receiver-operating characteristic (ROC) curves obtained for (1) renal aortic ratio (RAR) and (2) peak systolic velocity (PSV) at the stenosis.*

TABLE 32-3. The Influence of Prevalence on Positive Predictive Values

Prevalence	Sensitivity and Specificity (%)			
	99	*95*	*90*	*80*
20.0	96.1	82.1	69.2	50.0
10.0	91.7	67.9	50.0	30.8
5.0	83.9	67.9	32.1	3.9
1.0	50.0	16.1	8.3	3.9
0.1	9.0	8.7	4.3	2.0

are mainly caused by misinterpretation of collateral arteries because patent renal arteries seem to cast doubt on the role of duplex imaging for exclusion of renal artery occlusion.

Technical Pitfalls

The main criticisms of renal duplex are related to the fact that its quality is so dependent on the examiner. This is one of the fields in which validation studies are imperative if we want to use the test in clinical practice. Apart from this, the examiner should be able to determine the reliability of each examination and give an estimation of it in the final report.

Feasibility of studies varies from one center to another, ranging from 78% to 94%.[4-16] The major causes for incomplete studies are the presence of bowel gas and obesity. Reproducibility of the studies, considering both intraobserver and interobserver variability, is acceptably high, with correlation coefficients of 0.64 to 0.82 for intraobserver PSV measurements and 0.79 to 0.80 for interobserver evaluations.[17]

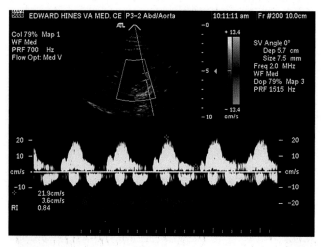

Figure 32-7. Example of tardus-parvus.

Apart from feasibility, the principal limitation of renal duplex scanning is failure to identify accessory renal arteries. The finding of one or more widely patent main renal arteries makes ischaemic nephropathy unlikely because this condition results from "total" renal ischemia. However, renovascular hypertension can be present with normal main renal arteries when there are isolated stenoses involving accessory renal arteries, so further testing by duplex scanning may be indicated in selected hypertensive patients with normal main renal arteries.

Functional Tests (Captopril Test)

Suppression of the renin-angiotensin system with captopril in patients with renovascular hypertension causes a hypersecretion of renin in response to the drug and decreases the glomerular filtration rate in the kidney ipsilateral to the RAS, particularly in the setting of unilateral RAS. This decrease correlates with a marked reduction of PSV in intrarenal vessels and can be used as a mean to increase the accuracy of CFDS to diagnose renal artery stenosis.

The test is performed in a manner similar to captopril-enhanced scintigraphy. The patient is scanned to obtain basal values of Doppler waveform at the renal cortex and medulla in both kidneys. Then a single oral dose of 50 mg of captopril is administered and the examination is repeated after 60 minutes. The observation of a decrease in PSV in the renal parenchyma is considered a positive response and is highly suggestive of RAS.

To assess the usefulness of captopril-enhanced sonography, the author performed a study that compared basal and postcaptopril CFDS with captopril-enhanced renal scintigraphy with Technetium-99m (DTPA), plasma renin levels (basal and postcaptopril), and renal angiography.[18] This study showed that the ratio between PSV in both renal parenchyma correlates well with the ratio between individual DPTA uptake in the isotope renogram. This ratio, based on Doppler data, may be an alternate noninvasive method of evaluating relative renal perfusion.

In the author's study, only 5 of 23 hypertensive patients with a RAS greater than 60% had both captopril enhanced test positive. These findings confirm the need to prove a renovascular origin for the hypertension, because simultaneous occurring RAS and hypertension does not always mean that it is of renovascular origin. Therefore, it seems appropriate to recommend the captopril test to reduce the number of patients submitted to arteriography for treating RAS for hypertension. Nevertheless, caution must be used in patients with bilateral lesions or impaired renal function because these are a major cause of a false-negative captopril tests and worsening of renal function, to the point that some authors contraindicate this test in bilateral RAS and high serum creatinine level.

Applications

Renal Transplant Evaluation

Renal transplant is the treatment of choice for patients with end-stage renal disease. Vascular complications posttransplantation may be related to organ harvest, donor vessel, surgical technique of transplantation, immunosuppression, or the recipient's disease. The interpretation of complications requires proper knowledge of the surgical technique used as well as an experienced technician.

Although the role of CFDS in detecting rejection has been questioned, it may be possible to monitor the change in resistance to flow found in the parenchyma. The basis for such a study is the observation that causes other than rejection will not result in an increased resistance to bloodflow. Also, it is important to notice that duplex findings can be modified or changed by the therapy being given.

Ultrasonic studies include the whole arterial renal tree from the main renal vessel to the corticomedullar level. The study also should include an estimate of the renal parenchyma RI or its equivalent, the end-diastolic resistance (EDR). Either will reflect the changes that have occurred in the kidney and its subsections. The major problem with renal transplant is documenting the role of either RI or EDR. In the study by Fleischer,[19] 16 out of 21 patients had acute rejection. It was important to be able to differentiate acute rejection from control patients as well as acute from chronic rejection. It appears that, as rejection occurs, the value of RI tended to approach 1, which would be the point at which the end-diastolic velocity would go to 0. Unfortunately, other authors using the same method have not been able to give such a promising results. As a consequence, more work is needed to assess the role of measurements using RI and EDR in evaluating the renal transplant function.

If rejection is in question, other complications may be detected by using CFDS.[20] Vascular complications after renal transplant have been observed in less than 10% of patients. Identifying these complications is important because of their high morbidity and mortality in comparison with other causes of renal transplant dysfunction. Once detected, they usually can be repaired and the graft function restored. Among the relevant vascular complications, stenosis of the renal transplant artery is an important cause of severe hypertension and late dysfunction of the transplanted kidney.

The stenosis can also be preanastomotic as a consequence of the recipient's arteriosclerotic disease progression. Anastomotic stenoses are most often related to graft changes, technical difficulties, and suture reaction. Postanastomotic stenoses are also the most common; they are related to iatrogenic arterial trauma and allograft rejection. In a retrospective study, Grenier and colleagues[21] used measurements of non–angle-corrected PSV with a cut-off point of 190 cm/sec, obtaining a 100% sensitivity and 90% specificity for stenosis above 50%. By analyzing the intrarenal waveforms instead of direct imaging of arterial stenosis, the difficulties in imaging the native and also transplanted arteries are avoided. A pressure drop across the stenosis is reflected distally by diminished systolic velocity and prolonged systolic acceleration time. Using a threshold of AT of 100 milliseconds or the subjective assessment of dampening of the waveforms, Gottlieb and colleagues[22] obtained a 95% accuracy in detecting a significant proximal RAS of the transplant.

Other significant complications, although uncommon, are transplant artery thrombosis and transplant vein obstruction or stenosis. Thrombosis of transplant artery is an early complication that can easily be diagnosed with CDFS because it reveals no arterial or venous flow. Transplant vein obstruction and stenosis is suspected when the renal arterial Doppler spectrum exhibits markedly high resistance with diastolic plateau-like flow reversal, while no renal flow can be demonstrated by any imaging modalities. A flow reversal in an allograft is a sign of poor prognosis. It is important to verify the absence of venous flow because it is the combination of arterial flow with high resistance and absent venous flow that is pathognomonic of renal vein thrombosis.

Finally, renal transplant biopsies may cause intrarenal arteriovenous fistulas or pseudoaneurysms, both of which are clearly underdiagnosed but tend to resolve spontaneously. On CFDS, arteriovenous fistulas and pseudoaneurysms appear as a disorganized coloring beyond the normal renal vessels configuration shown by high resolution equipment (Fig. 32-8).

Follow-Up Studies

Renal ischemia may produce two main consequences: systemic arterial hypertension difficult to control, which in turns give way to main cardiovascular events; and renal atrophy progressing toward end-stage renal disease needing dialysis or renal transplant. CFDS is considered an adequate method to assess arteriosclerotic renal progression and establish an appropriate management. The fact of being noninvasive and having a high accuracy makes renal duplex scanning the ideal test to follow up patients with or without revascularization of renal artery. Nevertheless, potential limitations of CFDS must be emphasized. As said previously, the imaging of renal arteries has inherent technical difficulties and, therefore, variable accuracy and reproducibility. In some labs it can be performed with a high rate of reliability, but in any case CFDS has so many advantages over arteriography that it is the best available tool for studying the natural history of RAS.

Zierler and colleagues[23] showed that this disease progresses at an average rate of 7% per year for all studied categories. However, if we consider only those having a moderate stenosis at baseline study, the cumulative incidence of progression to a 60% or greater RAS was

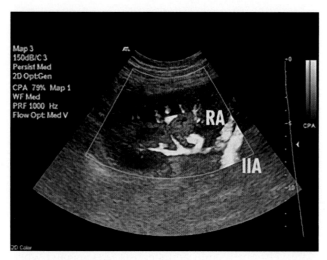

Figure 32-8. *Color-flow image of a transplanted kidney. RA, renal artery; IIA, iliac artery.*

as high as 75% in 5 years. Patients found to have 60% or greater RAS, diabetes, or systolic hypertension, and also those having decreased ankle-brachial indices in baseline study, were more prone to progression than were normal ones. Furthermore, renal artery occlusion, although rare, was also more common in patients with 60% or greater RAS.

Another interesting aspect indicated by follow-up studies is the fact that RAS is not only a possible cause of hypertension but also a cause of renal ischemia that may subsequently progress to renal atrophy and end-stage renal insufficiency. This was confirmed by Caps and colleagues,[24] who showed a clear relationship between RAS and a loss of renal mass as determined by ultrasound measurements of renal diameter. This study followed 122 patients for 3 years with renal duplex and reported a reduction of renal length of more than 1 cm in 20.8% of patients with RAS of 60% or greater, compared with only 5.5% in patients with normal baseline examinations. The study also showed that renal atrophy had a strong association with patients who had systolic hypertension and diminished cortical bloodflow velocities in baseline studies.

PTRA has been widely used for treating RAS; however, the short- and long-term anatomic results of PTRA have been poorly documented because of the lack of follow-up arteriography; this is mainly because radiologists are performing those procedures. Unfortunately, not all patients in whom a PTRA has been performed are properly evaluated in the postprocedure period by an accredited vascular laboratory. The parameters for assessing the degree of restenosis are similar to those of primary lesions. A prospective study carried out by Tullis and colleagues[25] with a mean follow-up of 34 months found that the cumulative incidence of restenosis from normal to above 60% was 13% at 1 year and 19% at 2 years. The cumulative incidence of restenosis from less than 60% to greater

than 60% was 44% at 1 year and 55% at years. The cumulative incidence of progression from more than 60% to occlusion was 10% at 2 years.

These figures should alert our colleagues as to the need for a strict follow-up as well as a more selective criteria for indicating PTRA because conventional open renal artery revascularization can be more effective despite the inherent rate of complication of this surgical therapy.

In summary, although CFDS has some pitfalls and limitations, as well as some areas of controversy, it represents a tremendous advantage in the diagnostic field for the majority of patients with renovascular hypertension, chronic renal insufficiency, and renal transplant, and should be included in all diagnostic algorithms.

REFERENCES

1. Lee HY, Grant EG: Sonography in renovascular hypertension. J Ultrasound Med 21:431–441, 2002.
2. Strandness DE Jr: Duplex scanning in vascular disorders. New York: Raven Press, 1993.
3. Schwerck WB, Restrepo IK, Stellwaag M, et al: Renal artery stenosis: Grading with image-directed Doppler US evaluation of resistive index. Radiology 190(3):785–790, 1994.
4. Hernandez E, Martinez Amenos A, Vila Coll R, et al: Diagnostico de la hipertensión arterial renovascular mediante eco-Doppler. Hipertensión 17(5):35–47, 2000.
5. Miralles M, Cairols MA, Cotillas J, et al: Value of Doppler parameters in the diagnosis of renovascular disease. J Vasc Surg 23:428–435, 1996.
6. Taylor DC, Kerrler MD, Moneta GL, et al: Duplex ultrasound scanning in the diagnosis of renal artery stenosis: A prospective evaluation. J Vasc Surg 7:363–369, 1988.
7. Olin JW, Piedmonte MR, Young JR, et al: The utility of duplex ultrasound scanning of the renal arteries for diagnosing significant renal artery stenosis. Ann Intern Med 122(11):833–838, 1995.
8. Desberg AL, Paushter DM, Lammert GK, et al: Renal artery stenosis: Evaluation with color Doppler-flow imaging. Radiology 177:749–753, 1990.
9. Berland LL, Koslin DB, Routh WD, et al: Renal artery stenosis: Prospective evaluation of diagnosis with color duplex US compared with angiography. Radiology 174:421–423, 1990.
10. Berqvist D, Karacagil S, Lörelius LE: Imaging for Renovascular Hypertensión: The Value of Duplex Against Angiography. In Greenhalgh R (ed): Vascular Imaging for Surgeons. London: WB Saunders, 1995.
11. Handa N, Fukunaga R, Etani H, et al: Efficacy of echo-Doppler examination for the evaluation of renovascular hypertension. Ultrasound Med Biol 14:1–5, 1988;
12. Motew SJ, Cherr GS, Craven TE, et al: Renal Duplex sonography: Main renal artery versus hiliar analysis. J Vasc Surg 32(3):462–469, 2000;
13. Hua Hong T, Hood Douglas B, Jensen Chris C, et al: The use of color-flow Duplex to detect significant renal artery stenosis. Ann Vasc Surg 14:118–124, 2000.
14. Radermacher J, Chavan J, Bleck J, et al: Use of Doppler ultrasonography to predict the outcome of therapy for renal artery stenosis. N Engl J Med 344:410–417, 2001.
15. Radermacher J, Ellis S, Haller H: Renal resistance index and progression of renal disease. Hypertension 39:699–703, 2002.
16. Mollo M, Pelet V, Mouawad J, et al: Evaluation of colour duplex ultrasound scanning in diagnosis of renal artery stenosis, compared to angiography: A prospective study. Eur J Vasc Endovasc Surg 14:305–309, 1997.

17. Baumgartner I, Behrendt P, Rohner O, et al: A validation study on the interobserver and interobserver reproducibility of renal artery duplex ultrasound. Ultrasound Med Biol 25(2):225–231, 1999.

18. Miralles M, Santiso A, Gimenez A, et al: Renal duplex scanning: Correlation with angiography and isotopic renography. Eur J Vasc Surg 7:188–194, 1993.

19. Fleischer AC, Hinton AA, Glick AD, et al: Duplex sonography or renal transplants: Correlation with histopathology. J Ultrasound Med 8:89–94, 1989.

20. Miralles M, Bestard J, Gasco J, et al: Vascular complications in the transplanted kidney: Detection with Doppler ultrasonography. Arch Esp Urol 48:1001–1008, 1995.

21. Grenier N, Douws C, Morel D, et al: Detection of vascular complications in renal allografts with colour-flow doppler imaging. Radiology 178:217–223, 1991.

22. Gottlieb RH, Lieberman JL, Pabico RC, et al: Diagnosis of renal artery stenosis in transplanted kidneys: Value of Doppler waveform analysis of the intrarenal arteries. Am J Roentgenol 165(6):1441–1446, 1995.

23. Zierler RE, Bergelin RO, Davidson RC, et al: A prospective study of disease progression in patients with atherosclerotic renal artery stenosis. Am J Hypertens 9(11):1055–1061, 1996.

24. Caps MT, Zierler RE, Polissar NL, et al: Risk of atrophy in kidneys with atherosclerotic renal artery stenosis. Kidney Int 53:735–742, 1998.

25. Tullis MJ, Zierler RE, Glickerman DJ, et al: Results of percutaneous transluminal angioplasty for atherosclerotic renal artery stenosis: A follow-up study with duplex ultrasonography. J Vasc Surg 25:46–54, 1997.

Chapter 33

Color-Flow Scanning of the Mesenteric Arteries: Techniques and Applications

EVERETT Y. LAM • GREGORY L. MONETA

Introduction

Duplex ultrasonography of intra-abdominal vessels is among the most technically challenging of all duplex studies in clinical use. When performed accurately, it serves as a valuable noninvasive screening test for splanchnic artery stenosis and for follow-up in patients with mesenteric artery reconstructions. Despite the accuracy of duplex detection of mesenteric artery stenoses, angiographic confirmation of high-grade stenoses or occlusion of the splanchnic vessels and appropriate history and physical examination are still required for the diagnosis of chronic mesenteric ischemia.

Technique

Respiratory motion, excessive bowel gas, previous abdominal surgery, obesity, and anatomic variation of the splanchnic vessels contribute to the technical difficulty of obtaining clinically relevant studies. Ideally, the patient is placed on a clear liquid diet the day before the examination. The patient must take nothing by mouth 8 hours before the study. The study is then performed early in the morning when intra-abdominal gas is minimal. Administration of 40 milligrams of simethicone orally and/or a mild cathartic before the study can also decrease the amount of bowel gas.[1]

The examination is performed with the patient supine and the head of the bed elevated to 30 degrees. Low-frequency scan heads (2.5 to 3.5 MHz) are used for duplex interrogation of the splanchnic vessels. In rare instances, a 5.0-MHz linear probe may be used in extremely thin individuals. An anterior midline approach, just below the xyphoid process, is used. Using the aorta as a landmark, the celiac artery (CA) and the superior mesenteric artery (SMA) are visualized by varying the angulation and position of the scan head (Fig. 33-1). Transverse imaging of the aorta may aid in the visualization of the celiac axis. The common hepatic and splenic arteries can be interrogated as they branch from the CA. The inferior mesenteric artery (IMA) is not easily visualized in most splanchnic artery examinations. Easy detection and ultrasonographic dominance of the IMA (Fig. 33-2) may suggest occlusion or high-grade stenosis of the SMA and the development of a functional arc of Riolan.

The B-mode image is important in placing the Doppler sample volume within the vessel to be examined. Atherosclerotic changes may appear as focal areas of increased echogenicity and irregular wall thickening. Color-flow imaging helps to locate the splanchnic vessels (see Fig. 33-2). A speckled color pattern indicating turbulent flow may suggest an area of stenosis; however, B-mode and color-flow imaging can only aid in locating vessels and cannot reliably grade stenoses. The only validated duplex criteria for identifying mesenteric artery stenoses are based on interpretation of Doppler-derived waveforms from the SMA and CA. Doppler waveforms must be insonated at a constant angle, generally accepted as 60 degrees. Increasing the Doppler angle 20 degrees can produce a peak systolic velocity increase of 120% on the SMA and 56% on the CA.[2] Because atherosclerotic lesions of the CA and SMA occur most commonly at the origins of these vessels, velocity waveforms from the CA and SMA should include recordings as close as possible to their origins from the aorta. For any suspected stenosis, velocity waveform recordings should be obtained from within the stenosis as well as proximally and distally.

Fasting and Postprandial Velocity Waveforms

In healthy individuals, fasting bloodflow velocity waveforms differ in the SMA vs. the CA. Arterial waveforms reflect end-organ vascular resistance. The liver and spleen have relatively high constant metabolic requirements and are therefore low-resistance organs. As a result, CA waveforms are generally biphasic, with a peak systolic component, no reversal of diastolic flow, and a relatively high end-diastolic velocity (Fig. 33-3). The normal fasting SMA velocity waveform is triphasic, reflecting the high vascular resistance of the intestinal tract at rest. There is a peak systolic component, often an end-systolic reverse flow component, and a minimal diastolic flow component (Fig. 33-4).

Changes in Doppler-derived arterial waveforms in response to feeding are also different in the CA and SMA. Because the liver and spleen have basically fixed metabolic demands, there is no significant change in CA velocity waveform after eating. Bloodflow in the SMA, however, increases markedly after a meal, reflecting a marked decrease in intestinal arterial resistance. The waveform changes in the SMA seen postprandially include a near doubling of systolic velocity, tripling of the end-diastolic velocity, and loss of reversal of bloodflow (Fig. 33-5). In addition, there is a detectable increase in the diameter of the SMA postprandially. The diameter of the SMA has been shown to be 0.60 ± 0.09 cm in the fasting state and 0.67 ± 0.09 cm after a meal (p < 0.0001). These changes are maximal at 45 minutes after ingestion of a test meal.[3]

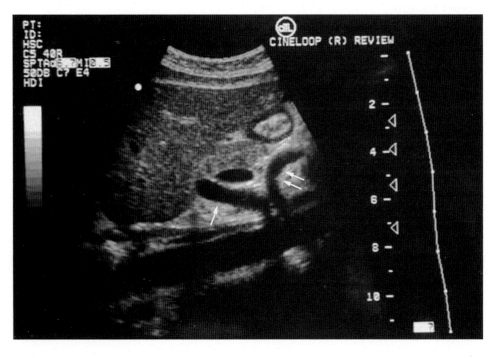

Figure 33-1. B-mode longitudinal image of the aorta with the origins of the celiac axis (single arrow) and SMA (double arrows) visualized.

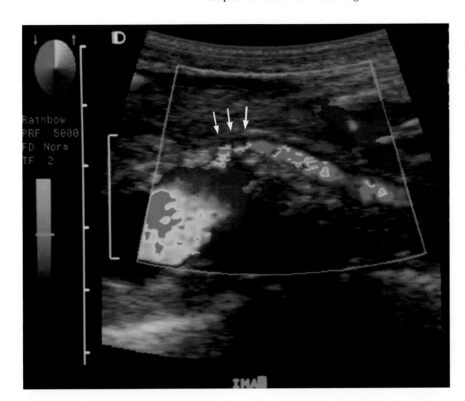

Figure 33-2. Color flow Doppler image of a dominant inferior mesenteric artery (arrows) in a patient with high-grade superior mesenteric artery stenosis.

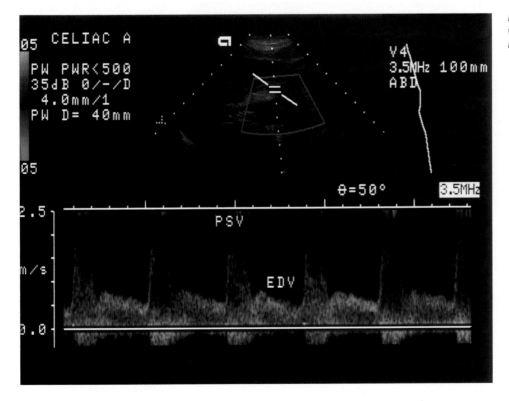

Figure 33-3. Duplex velocity waveform of the celiac artery. Note the relatively high EDV.

The magnitude of the postprandial hyperemic response in the SMA is dependent on the composition of the meal ingested. Intestinal absorption is required to elicit a hyperemic intestinal response. In a study evaluating SMA bloodflow after ingestion of either glucose or lactulose, SMA bloodflow increased 53% after a glucose load and no change in SMA bloodflow was noted with a lactulose load.[4] Mixed composition meals produce the greatest flow increase in the SMA when compared with equal caloric meals composed solely of fat, glucose, or protein.[5]

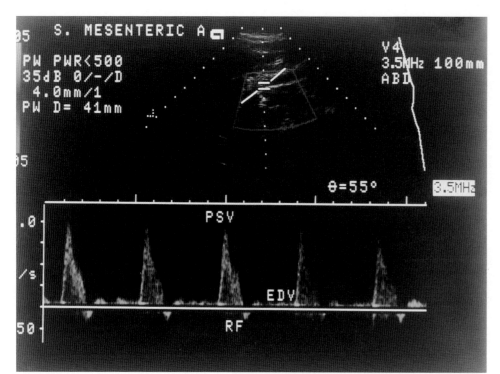

Figure 33-4. Duplex velocity waveform of the superior mesenteric artery. Note the systolic reverse flow component and the relatively low EDV.

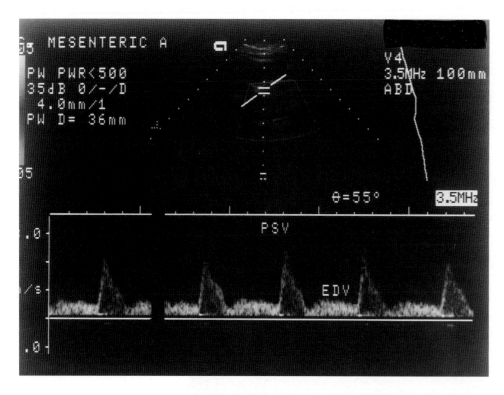

Figure 33-5. Duplex velocity waveform of the superior mesenteric artery in the postprandial state. Note the lack of reverse flow and the relatively high EDV.

Detection of Splanchnic Arterial Stenosis

After identification of duplex characteristics for SMA and CA in normal fasting and postprandial patients, duplex criteria were developed for detecting hemody-namically significant stenoses in splanchnic vessels. In 1986, investigators at the University of Washington found that flow velocities in stenotic SMA and CA were significantly increased when compared with normal controls.[6] To develop quantitative criteria for splanchnic artery stenosis, the authors' laboratory compared SMA and CA mesenteric duplex studies and lateral abdominal aortography of 34 patients who underwent both studies within 2 weeks.[7] Data from this study suggested that peak systolic velocity (PSV) could be an accurate predictor of a 70% or greater angiographic stenosis in both the SMA and CA. An SMA PSV of 275 cm/sec or greater, or no bloodflow, yielded a sensitivity of 89%, a specificity of 92%, a negative predictive value of 96%, and a positive predictive value of 80% for detection of a 70% or greater SMA stenosis. For the CA, a PSV of 200 cm/sec or greater correlated with a 70% or greater CA angiographic stenosis with a sensitivity of 75%, a specificity of 89%, a negative predictive value of 80%, and a positive predictive value of 85%. End-diastolic velocities and velocity ratios offered no improvement in accuracy in the detection of 70% or greater stenosis in either the CA or SMA.

The above criteria were then validated in a prospective study of 100 patients who underwent mesenteric artery duplex scanning and lateral aortography.[8] In this study, 100% of the CAs and 99% of the SMAs were able to be adequately examined with aortography, whereas 93% of the SMAs and 83% of the CAs were studied successfully with duplex scanning. A PSV in the SMA of 275 cm/sec or more detected a 70% or greater SMA stenosis with a sensitivity of 92%, a specificity of 96%, a positive predictive value of 80%, a negative predictive value of 99%, and an accuracy of 96% (Fig. 33-6A and B). For the CA, a PSV of 200 cm/sec or greater identified a 70% or greater angiographic stenosis with a sensitivity of 87%, a specificity of 80%, a positive predictive value of 63%, a negative predictive value of 94%, and an accuracy of 82%.

Other investigators have also developed duplex criteria for mesenteric artery stenoses. In one study,[9] an SMA end-diastolic velocity (EDV) greater than 45 cm/sec correlated with a 50% or greater SMA stenosis with a specificity of 92% and a sensitivity of 100%. An SMA PSV greater than 300 cm/sec predicted a 50% or greater stenosis with a sensitivity of 63% and specificity of 100%. A CA EDV of 55 cm/sec or greater predicted a 50% or greater CA stenosis with a sensitivity of 93%, a specificity of 100%, and an accuracy of 95%. These results were subsequently validated in a follow-up study from the same institution.[10]

Food Challenges in the Diagnosis of Mesenteric Arterial Stenosis

The value of postprandial mesenteric duplex scanning as an adjunct for the diagnosis of mesenteric ischemia has been evaluated at the authors' institution.[11] Fasting and postprandial duplex scans were performed on 25 healthy controls and 80 patients with vascular disease who underwent aortography. Patients without arterial disease did not undergo aortography. Patients with arterial disease were grouped according to their degree of angiographic stenosis. A fasting SMA PSV of 275 cm/sec or greater was considered indicative of a 70% or greater SMA stenosis. In this study, preprandial SMA PSVs in controls and patients with less than 70% SMA stenosis did not differ, and postprandial SMA PSVs in controls and patients with less than 70% SMA stenosis did not differ. Fasting SMA PSVs were, however, significantly higher in patients with 70% or greater SMA stenosis. The absolute increase in SMA PSV was lower in patients with 70% or greater SMA stenosis than in controls. A positive postprandial duplex study was defined as a failure of the postprandial SMA PSV to increase more than 20% over baseline.

In this study, fasting mesenteric duplex scanning predicted 70% to 99% SMA stenosis with 89% sensitivity and 97% specificity. Corresponding values for postprandial scanning were 67% and 94%, and for the combination of fasting and postprandial scanning, 67% and 100%. This information indicated that both fasting SMA PSVs and postprandial SMA PSVs can detect 70% or greater stenosis. The combination of fasting SMA PSVs and postprandial PSVs, however, only marginally improves upon fasting duplex scan specificity. Therefore postprandial duplex scanning offered no definite improvement over fasting mesenteric duplex scanning and is not routinely utilized in the authors' vascular laboratory. Postprandial examinations are, however, occasionally useful in difficult examinations, in that if there is a postprandial response, the insonated vessel can be confirmed as being the SMA.

Additional Uses of Splanchnic Artery Duplex Scanning

Although duplex scanning can detect mesenteric artery stenosis, it is important to differentiate high-grade mesenteric artery stenosis from the clinical entity of chronic mesenteric ischemia. Not all patients with mesenteric artery obstruction have mesenteric insufficiency. Asymptomatic patients with angiographically documented occlusions of the CA and SMA are well-recognized. Duplex ultrasonography offers a valuable initial screening study to evaluate for visceral artery stenosis in patients with chronic abdominal pain consistent with chronic mesenteric ischemia. The accuracy of duplex ultrasonography as a noninvasive test for mesenteric artery stenosis makes the evaluation of patients with possible mesenteric ischemia time- and cost-efficient.

Duplex scanning has been used in the evaluation of CA compression (median arcuate ligament syndrome).[12] However, the significance of this syndrome causing clinical visceral ischemia is controversial. CA PSVs have been shown to be increased during expiration and decreased during inspiration in patients who have reversible compression of the CA by the median arcuate ligament.

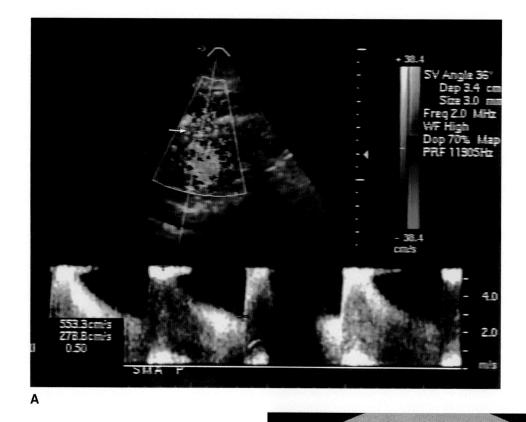

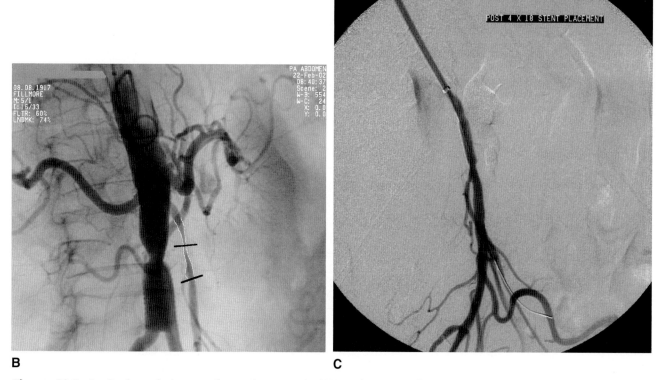

Figure 33-6. A, Duplex velocity waveform of a stenotic SMA with a PSV of 553 cm/sec (arrow indicates origin of the SMA). **B,** Confirmation with angiography of a highly stenotic SMA. **C,** Angiography of the SMA after angioplasty and stent placement.

Another application of splanchnic artery duplex scanning is postoperative surveillance of mesenteric revascularizations. There are currently no validated criteria for assessing flow in mesenteric artery bypass grafts. At the authors' institution, serial follow-up studies are obtained. Changes in PSV or EDV in serial examinations may suggest a stenosis in a graft and prompt angiographic evaluation of the bypass graft (Fig. 33-7).

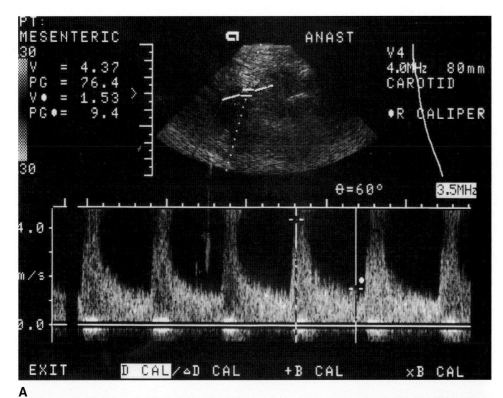

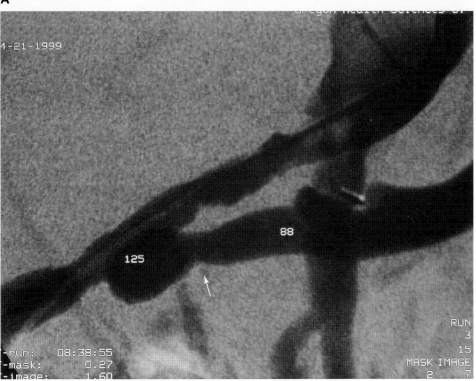

Figure 33-7. A, Duplex surveillance examination of an SMA bypass graft showing a PSV of 437 cm/sec near the anastomosis. **B,** Confirmation angiogram showing a 37-mmHg pressure gradient across the stenosis.

Conclusions

Duplex ultrasonography has proven to be an accurate noninvasive examination to study the mesenteric vasculature. With adequate patient preparation, the CA and SMA can be identified and the bloodflow velocity within these vessels measured. CA PSVs of 200 cm/sec and greater and SMA PSVs of 275 cm/sec or greater are suggestive of high-grade stenoses within these vessels. Postprandial studies may help identify the SMA in technically difficult examinations but are no more sensitive than fasting studies in the identification of SMA stenoses. In addition, duplex studies are important in the surveillance of mesenteric artery bypass grafts. Changes in velocity from the baseline postoperative examination may indicate a stenosis within the graft. Arteriography is indicated to confirm positive findings on duplex in patients with appropriate signs and symptoms. Prompt intervention in patients with chronic mesenteric ischemia and failing bypass grafts is necessary to avoid the morbidity and mortality associated with splanchnic artery obstruction.

REFERENCES

1. Moneta GL, Taylor DC, Yeager RA, et al: Duplex ultrasound: Application to intra-abdominal vessels. Perspectives in Vascular Surgery 2:133–148, 1989.
2. Rizzo RJ, Sandager G, Astleford P, et al: Mesenteric flow velocity variations as a function of angle of insonation. J Vasc Surg 11(5):688–694, 1990.
3. Jager K, Bollinger A, Valli C, et al: Measurement of mesenteric bloodflow by duplex scanning. J Vasc Surg 3(3):462–469, 1986.
4. Qamar MI, Read AE, Skidmore R, et al: Transcutaneous Doppler ultrasound measurement of superior mesenteric artery bloodflow in man. Gut 27(1):100–105, 1986.
5. Moneta GL, Taylor DC, Helton WS, et al: Duplex ultrasound measurement of postprandial intestinal bloodflow: Effect of meal composition. Gastroenterology 95(5):1294–1301, 1988.
6. Nicholls SC, Kohler TR, Martin RL, et al: Use of hemodynamic parameters in the diagnosis of mesenteric insufficiency. J Vasc Surg 3(3):507–510, 1986.
7. Moneta GL, Yeager RA, Dalman R, et al: Duplex ultrasound criteria for diagnosis of splanchnic artery stenosis or occlusion (see comments). J Vasc Surg 14(4):511–518; discussion 518–520, 1991.
8. Moneta GL, Lee RW, Yeager RA, et al: Mesenteric duplex scanning: A blinded prospective study. J Vasc Surg 17(1):79–84; discussion 85–86, 1993.
9. Bowersox JC, Zwolak RM, Walsh DB, et al: Duplex ultrasonography in the diagnosis of celiac and mesenteric artery occlusive disease. J Vasc Surg 14(6):780–786; discussion 786–788, 1991.
10. Zwolak RM, Fillinger MF, Walsh DB, et al: Mesenteric and celiac duplex scanning: A validation study. J Vasc Surg 27(6):1078–1087; discussion 1088, 1998.
11. Gentile AT, Moneta GL, Lee RW, et al: Usefulness of fasting and postprandial duplex ultrasound examinations for predicting high-grade superior mesenteric artery stenosis. Am J Surg 169(5):476–479, 1995.
12. Taylor DC, Moneta GL, Cramer MM, et al: Extrinsic compression of the celiac artery by the median arcuate ligament of the diaphragm: Diagnosis by duplex ultrasound. J Vasc Tech 11:236–238, 1987.

Chapter 34

Intraoperative and Postoperative Imaging of Renal and Mesenteric Revascularizations

GUSTAVO S. ODERICH • THANILA A. MACEDO •
JEAN M. PANNETON • PETER GLOVICZKI

Introduction

Open surgical techniques to reconstruct the renal and the mesenteric arteries for occlusive or aneurysmal disease have undergone significant evolution in recent years. The success of endovascular management of renal artery occlusive disease with angioplasty and stents has decreased the number of surgical candidates (Fig. 34-1). Indications for renal artery reconstructions include renal artery occlusive disease caused by fibromuscular dysplasia (FMD) or atherosclerosis, with clinical manifestations of renovascular hypertension (refractory to medical management), ischemic nephropathy or "flush," or recurrent pulmonary edema. Less commonly, renal artery aneurysm or trauma to the renal artery requires surgical treatment.[1] Those who undergo renal artery surgery have either failed percutaneous therapy or are not candidates because of renal artery occlusion, extensive stenoses, renal artery aneurysmal disease, multiple small renal arteries, lack of suitable access for angioplasty, or high risk of atheroembolization because of a shaggy abdominal aorta. Surgical candidates are commonly older, have bilateral renal and associated aortic disease, and have more medical comorbidities. Patients who undergo open renal artery surgery today in the authors' practice often undergo simultaneous aortic reconstruction (Fig. 34-2). Intraoperative imaging with duplex scanning has made open renal artery reconstructions safer, transforming the effectiveness of renal artery endarterectomy. It is because of the routine use of intraoperative duplex scanning that transaortic endarterectomy of the renal arteries has become an excellent and safe reconstruction.

Open revascularization remains the gold standard in the contemporary management of mesenteric disease, although the number of open mesenteric reconstructions has also diminished recently (Fig. 34-3) and stenting is

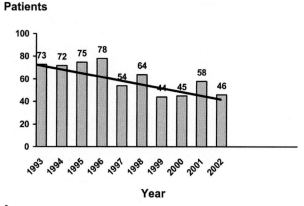

A

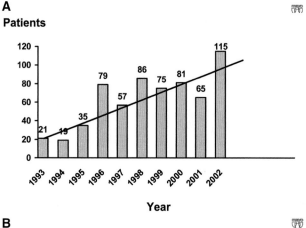

B

Figure 34-1. A, *Open surgical reconstruction of the renal arteries in 611 patients at the Mayo Clinic between 1993 and 2002.* **B,** *Percutaneous renal artery angioplasty and stenting in 633 patients at the Mayo Clinic between 1993 and 2002. (Courtesy of Michael McKusick, MD.)*

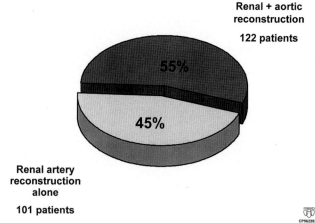

Figure 34-2. *Open renal artery reconstruction with and without concomitant aortic reconstruction in 233 patients. Data from one surgical service (PG, from 1987 to 2002).*

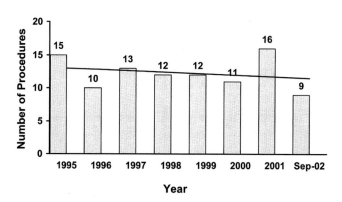

Figure 34-3. *Open surgical revascularization in 96 patients from chronic mesenteric ischemia between January 1, 1995 and September 30, 2002.*

performed more commonly than at any time before. Aortomesenteric bypass grafting, either antegrade or retrograde, is the most common type of revascularization performed today for chronic mesenteric ischemia.[2] Endovascular treatment, mostly angioplasty, has been reported for treatment of symptomatic mesenteric stenoses with 86% technical and 90% clinical success rate.[3] There are reports on stenting in the mesenteric circulation, but long-term data are not yet available.[4]

To optimize clinical outcome following renal and mesenteric revascularizations, intraoperative and postoperative imaging modalities have been added to the vascular surgeon's armamentarium. The aim of these studies is to identify technical problems that can be corrected at the time of operation, and to detect recurrent lesions that can lead to failure of revascularization. This chapter reviews the authors' experience with intraoperative ultrasound used during renal and mesenteric arterial revascularizations. It also discusses the available imaging modalities for postoperative surveillance of these patients.

Intraoperative Imaging

Absence of technical problems is a prerequisite to durable success of any arterial revascularization. Intraoperative assessment of the reconstruction should be safe, easy to use, versatile, accurate, and should provide high anatomic resolution and reliable physiologic data. Direct visual inspection, pulse palpation, continuous-wave Doppler signal analysis, arterial pressure measurements, and electromagnetic flow measurements are rapid, safe, and easy to perform, but lack sensitivity and cannot localize intraluminal defects. Although angiography can accurately detect small arterial abnormalities, it carries the disadvantages of being more invasive; time-consuming; adding radiation exposure; and carrying the risk of arterial injury, embolization, contrast-induced toxicity, and allergic reactions. Intraoperative duplex scanning has rapidly emerged as the method of choice to evaluate the adequacy of renal and mesenteric reconstructions.[5,6]

Intraoperative Duplex Scanning

Ultrasound has distinct advantages over other methods of intraoperative monitoring, including angiography and electromagnetic flow measurements. It is safe, noninvasive, expeditious, and provides both anatomic (gray scale) and hemodynamic (bidirectional Doppler) information with very high sensitivity, specificity, and negative predictive rates. Intraoperative duplex ultrasound has been shown to accurately identify technical problems, and to improve early and late outcome following carotid, renal, mesenteric, and infrainguinal arterial reconstructions.[7-12]

Scanning Technique

The examination is performed intraoperatively following completion of the revascularization. At the authors' institution, a staff radiologist performs the test assisted by an ultrasound technician. An Acuson XP 128 or Sequoia 512 (Acuson Inc., Mountain View, CA) with 6-15MHz linear array probes is used. The total scan time usually varies from 5 to 15 minutes. The probe is placed in a sterile plastic sheath previously filled with acoustic gel. Normal saline solution is poured into the abdominal cavity for acoustic coupling between the probe and the vessel. Occasionally, sterile acoustic gel is used. The probe is submerged in saline solution and positioned 1 to 2 centimeters from the vessel for optimal imaging and resolution. Initially, transverse and longitudinal gray scale images of the entire graft/endarterectomy segment and proximal and distal anastomoses are obtained. Next, color Doppler images are obtained in the longitudinal plane, and spectral waveforms are sampled in the vessel proximal to the revascularization, at the proximal anastomosis, in the revascularized segment, at the distal anastomosis, and in the vessel distal to the anastomosis. Peak systolic velocities (PSV), end-diastolic velocities (EDV), and velocity ratio ($Vr = PSV_{at\ lesion} / PSV_{proximal}$) are generated. For renal reconstructions, the velocities are measured to enable the calculation of the renal/aortic velocity ratio and renal resistive index ($RRI = PSV - [EDV / PSV]$).

Interpretation of the Ultrasound Findings

There is no uniform classification of intraoperative ultrasound results in the vascular literature. At the Mayo Clinic, ultrasound examinations are classified into normal or abnormal based on gray scale and Doppler analysis. A normal examination is defined as no evidence of technical defects on gray scale images and normal or nonfocal PSV elevations. The authors use a PSV of less than 2.75 m/sec for the superior mesenteric artery, 2.0 m/sec for the celiac axis, and 2.0 for the renal arteries as the upper limits of normal. More important than isolated velocity measurements, a Vr of greater than 2 is suggestive of a hemodynamically significant lesion. Nonfocal

PSV elevation without evidence of technical defect can have different causes (e.g., hyperdynamic state or graft-vessel mismatch) and is considered a normal finding. Abnormal ultrasounds are further classified into minor or major arterial defects. A minor defect consists of technical problems with normal PSV or Vr and usually includes mild residual plaque or small intimal flaps and kinks. Conversely, a major defect consists of hemodynamically significant defects (i.e., elevated PSV or Vr) including significant residual stenosis, thrombus, intimal flap, dissection, kink, or abnormal flow (decreased or reverse flow).

Clinical Results

Dougherty and colleagues and Okuhn and colleagues have reported excellent sensitivity and specificity rates with use of renal intraoperative duplex ultrasound.[8-9] The authors' initial experience was recently updated with intraoperative ultrasound of 164 renal artery reconstructions performed in 98 patients.[5] Abnormal duplex scanning was found in 22 reconstructions (13.4%), 11 (6.7%) had major defects, and 11 (6.7%) had minor defects (Figs. 34-4 and 34-5). Immediate operative revision was performed in all 11 cases with major defects. Operative revision included transection of the renal artery distal to the endarterectomy in one patient, removal of the intimal flap or residual plaque and end-to-end reanastomosis in three patients, vein patch angioplasty in 4, nephrectomy because of extensive distal disease in one, and excision of intimal flap in two. Repeat duplex ultrasound confirmed improvement in flow pattern and disappearance of turbulence or normalization of flow velocities in 10 patients. The 11 minor defects included small intimal flaps (7) and mild residual stenoses (4). Only one defect was immediately revised and there were no graft failures in this group of patients. Similarly, all cases of repaired major defects had patent grafts on follow-up studies.

Some 89% of the patients were followed with postoperative imaging studies to assess graft patency. The sensitivity of intraoperative ultrasound to identify a technical defect was 85%. The duplex study was falsely negative in 2 patients who developed postoperative bypass graft thrombosis as confirmed by postoperative angiography. In these patients it was assumed that duplex scanning failed to identify the technical defect responsible for this early graft thrombosis, although it is possible that this thrombosis might have been caused by hypercoagulability or more distal occlusive disease causing high resistance. The specificity of color-flow duplex scanning was 99%, with a negative predictive value of 98%, a positive predictive value of 92%, and an overall accuracy of 98%.

The authors have recently reviewed the impact of the renal resistive index (RRI) on clinical outcome after renal artery revascularization.[10] Intraoperative RRI was lower

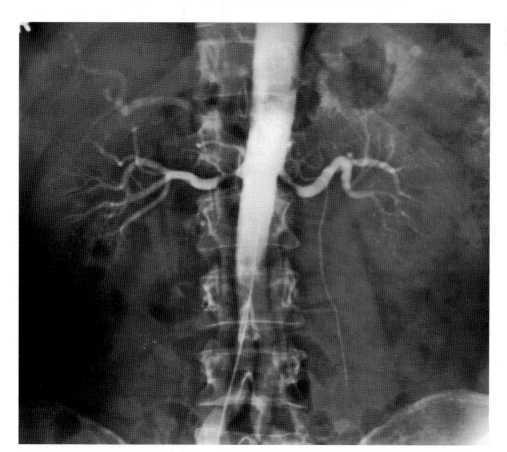

Figure 34-4. Contrast aortography demonstrates bilateral high-grade renal artery stenosis.

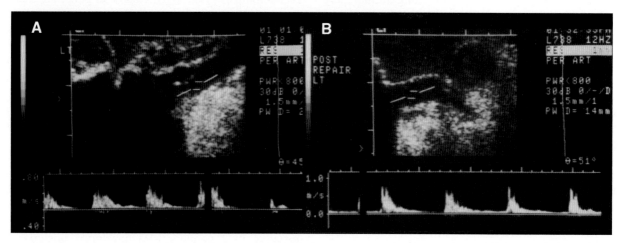

Figure 34-5. **A,** Intraoperative duplex scanning following transaortic endarterectomy reveals intimal flap at the origin of the left renal artery with dampened waveform distal to the flap (arrow). **B,** After surgical revision and removal of the intimal flap, Doppler interrogation was normal.

in patients with a low postoperative creatinine than in those with high postoperative creatinine (0.75 vs. 0.83, p < 0.01). Patients with a low RRI had better outcome than those with high RRI (i.e., lower long-term increase in creatinine and less need for chronic dialysis)

Similar benefit of intraoperative duplex scanning was noted in patients who underwent mesenteric revascularization (Figs. 34-6 and 34-7), and these results were

recently reported by Oderich and colleagues.[11] A total of 120 revascularized arteries were examined in 68 patients. Mesenteric reconstruction was performed using bypass grafting (84%), endarterectomy (10%), and medial arcuate ligament release with patch angioplasty (6%). Some 102 arteries (85%) had normal ultrasound examinations. Of these, 13 (10.8%) had nonfocal PSV elevation because of graft-vessel mismatch. Another 8

(6.6%) arteries had minor defects, including 4 mild graft/vessel kinks, 3 mild residual stenoses, and 1 small intimal flap. Another 10 arteries (8.4%) had major defects, which consisted of severe residual stenosis (4), thrombus (2), kink (2), bidirectional flow (1), and intimal flap (1). Minor defects were left untreated, and all 10 major defects prompted immediate operative revision. Immediate repair was performed using anastomotic revi-

sion (4), thrombectomy (3), patch angioplasty (3), removal of residual plaque (1), tacking sutures (1), resection of residual intimal flap (1), and resection of redundant artery (1). Postrevision ultrasound revealed six normal revascularizations, two mild residual stenoses, one bidirectional flow, and one dissection. With the exception of the dissection, all the other defects were left unrepaired. Patients with persistent abnormal ultrasounds

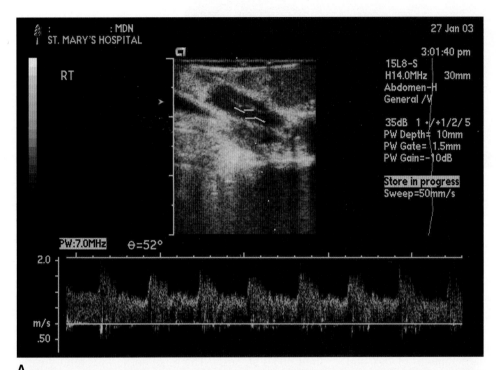

A

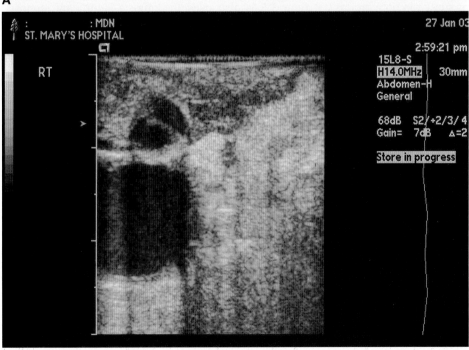

B

Figure 34-6. A, *Intraoperative duplex scanning following aorto-superior mesenteric artery bypass reveals intimal flap (arrow) and turbulent flow consistent with dissection.* **B,** *Transverse view at the level of the dissection reveals the intimal flap.*

Continued

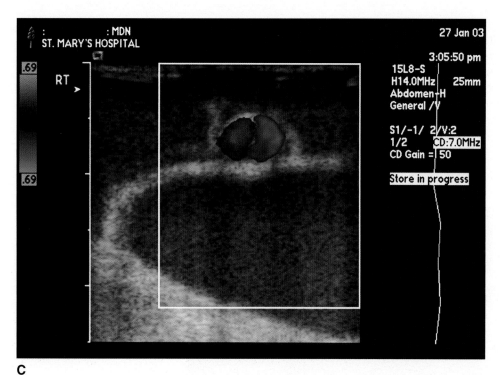

C

Figure 34-6, cont'd. C, Color Doppler reveals reversed flow in the false lumen.

had increased risk of graft-related complications (45.5% vs. 10.5%; p = 0.01), early graft thrombosis (11.7% vs. 0.97%, respectively; p = 0.04), graft-related death (27.3% vs. 3.5%, respectively; p = 0.02), and reintervention (17.6% vs. 3.9%; p = 0.04) as compared with patients with normal ultrasounds. The incidence of late restenoses (4% for normal and 13.3% for abnormal; p = 0.14)) and recurrent ischemic symptoms (5.45% and 10%, respectively; p = 0.38) was similar in both groups.

Postoperative Imaging

Recurrent renal and mesenteric arterial disease is often asymptomatic. Following renal revascularization, clinical evidence of deterioration in blood pressure control, loss of renal parenchyma, or reduction of renal function should prompt further evaluation with imaging studies to rule out recurrent disease. Conversely, clinical symptoms have limited sensitivity (as low as 33%) to assess patency following mesenteric revascularization, so that graft occlusions are likely to be missed and patency overestimated based on symptoms alone.[13] There are several imaging modalities but no standardized protocol to follow up patients with renal and mesenteric revascularizations.

Duplex Ultrasound

Duplex ultrasound provides both anatomic and functional assessment of renal and mesenteric arteries; however, the examination can be technically difficult because of the patient's body habitus, overlying bowel gas, abdominal scars, or the inability of the patient to cooperate with breathing instructions. The normal renal artery PSV is typically less than 1.8 m/sec. A PSV of 1.8 to 2.0 m/sec is considered borderline, but a PSV greater than 2.0 m/sec is suggestive of a hemodynamically significant (greater than 60%) stenosis. The renal-aortic PSV ratio greater than 3.5 is also used to define a significant stenosis. Using velocity criteria, the sensitivity of renal duplex ultrasound ranges from 91% to 95%, and specificity ranges from 90% to 97%.[14]

Similar to renal arterial disease, duplex ultrasound diagnosis of mesenteric artery stenosis is based on velocity criteria. The authors use a PSV of 2.75 m/sec for the superior mesenteric artery and 2.0 m/sec for the celiac axis as the upper limits of normal. The Oregon group prospectively validated this velocity criteria and found a sensitivity of 89%, a specificity of 92%, a positive predictive value of 80%, and a negative predictive value of 96% for a 70% or greater angiographic stenosis.[15] Although these velocity criteria were established for native renal and mesenteric arterial disease, the same values are applied to diagnose recurrent "graft" stenoses. The authors recommend a duplex ultrasound before dismissal or at the first visit at 1 to 3 months so that a baseline PSV is available for follow-up purposes. When recurrent disease is identified based on duplex scanning, further decisions are made regarding the need for angiographic and/or endovascular intervention.

Magnetic Resonance Angiography

Magnetic resonance angiography (MRA) has gained acceptance as one of the preferred imaging modalities to evaluate renal artery disease. The sensitivity ranges from 90% to 100% and specificity ranges from 71% to 100%.[16] The main advantages are noninvasiveness, nonionizing radiation, and avoidance of iodinated contrast. The gadolinium-based contrast has a very low risk of allergic reactions (1:20,000) and virtually no nephrotoxicity. In addition, renal MRA provides information about kidney length, parenchymal thickness, and concomitant intra-abdominal pathology. Contraindications

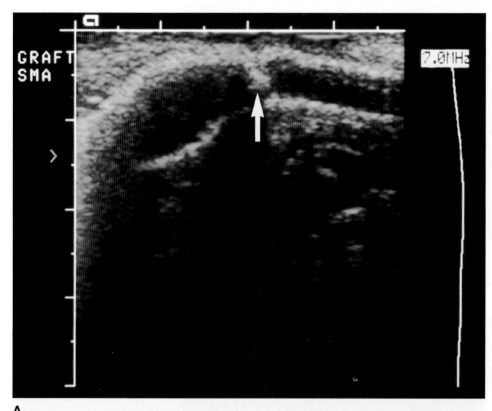

A

Figure 34-7. **A,** *Intraoperative duplex scanning reveals an intraluminal filling defect at the proximal anastomosis of a graft to the superior mesenteric artery.* **B,** *Doppler interrogation in the region of the intraluminal defect reveals elevated peak systolic velocity.*

Continued

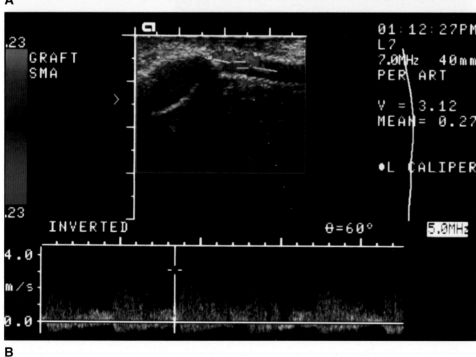

B

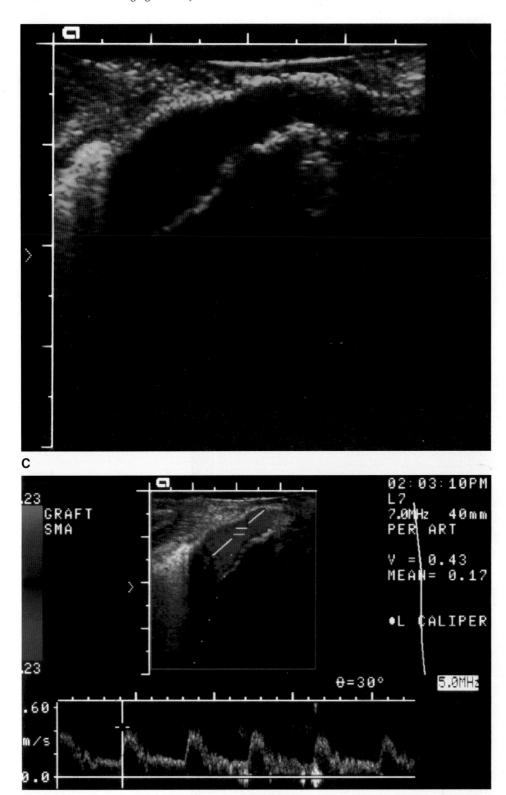

Figure 34-7, cont'd. C, Postrevision ultrasound scanning reveals that the filling defect is no longer present. **D,** Doppler interrogation after revision reveals normalization of peak systolic velocity.

for MRA include presence of MR-incompatible devices such as a pacemaker and orbital and cochlear metal implants. Although pregnancy is not an absolute contraindication for MRA, gadolinium-based contrast should be avoided. Patients with claustrophobia or anxiety disorders often require use of benzodiazepines. Although recent sequences have shortened the time for image acquisition, patient cooperation and ability to stay still remain a limiting factor of examination. Images can also be compromised by artifact from surgical clips.

Computed Tomography Angiography

Computed tomography angiography (CTA) has emerged as an important modality to evaluate the vascular system (Fig. 34-8). New helical CT scanners with multiple detectors have made feasible rapid image acquisition and evaluation of the arterial system. This modality has potential imaging capability comparable to that of MRA; however, the patient's collaboration with the examination is less of an issue because the examination can be as fast as 13 seconds and claustrophobia is almost never a problem. Three-dimensional reconstructions can be performed and angiography-like images can be generated. The disadvantages are related to the need of iodinated contrast and ionizing radiation.

Contrast Angiography

Angiography is considered the gold standard for evaluation of renal and mesenteric arterial disease. The authors generally reserve angiography for reoperation planning in certain cases, or when endovascular treatment is contemplated. Most often, a noninvasive study (e.g., ultrasound, MRA, or CTA) precedes this modality. The main disadvantages of angiography are its invasive nature, cost, ionizing radiation, and use of iodinated contrast. For renal angiography, a small volume of iso-osmolar nonionic contrast agent and digital subtraction are used, especially in patients at high risk for acute renal failure. On certain occasions, digital subtraction angiography (DSA) using gadolinium can be performed to avoid the complications associated with iodinated contrast. The examination usually begins with an aortogram to determine the number and location of renal arteries, followed by selective views of the renal arteries. For mesenteric angiography, lateral and frontal aortograms are performed. The most common type of reconstruction in the authors' practice is an antegrade aorto-celiac-superior mesenteric artery bypass, which can be well visualized using this technique. The contrast agent is usually injected just above the celiac axis or the proximal graft anastomosis, and the origins of the celiac axis, superior mesenteric artery, renal arteries, and inferior mesenteric artery are documented. Collateral flow is demonstrated, and selective mesenteric angiography is also obtained.

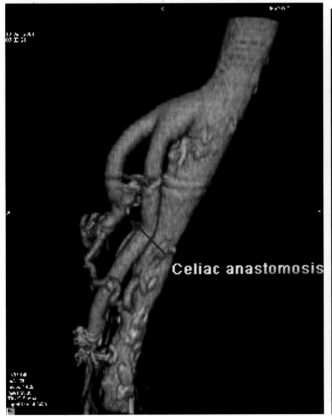 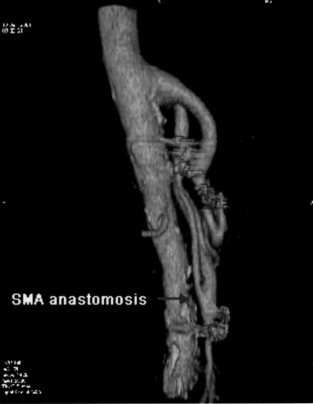

Celiac anastomosis

SMA anastomosis

A   **B**

Figure 34-8. *Volume rendered 3-D–computed tomography angiography images of the abdominal aorta reveals a widely patent bifurcated aorto-celiac-superior mesenteric artery bypass graft.* **A,** *Normal celiac trunk anastomosis and* **B,** *SMA anastomosis are well demonstrated.*

Conclusions

The authors advocate routine intraoperative duplex ultrasound monitoring during open surgical renal and mesenteric revascularizations. A normal ultrasound correlates with excellent early and late clinical outcome. Surgical judgment is still very important to determine the need for re-exploration if an abnormal finding is observed with duplex scanning. Based on current experience, the authors proceed with revision if there is both an abnormal gray scale image and an abnormal Doppler examination, suggesting a hemodynamically significant lesion. Minor defects, which do not decrease flow significantly, are not repaired; however, the fate of these defects is still unknown, and their impact on long-term patency will need further evaluation. Postoperatively, a duplex ultrasound is obtained before dismissal or at the first visit and yearly thereafter. CTA and or MRA are obtained if ultrasound is not technically feasible. When recurrent disease is identified on noninvasive studies, the risk-benefit ratio of angiography and possible reintervention must be weighed against the risks of not intervening.

REFERENCES

1. Safian RD, Textor SC: Renal-artery stenosis. N Engl J Med 344(6):431–444, 2001.
2. Park WM, Cherry KJ Jr., Chua HK, et al: Current results of open revascularization for chronic mesenteric ischemia: A standard for comparison. J Vasc Surg 35(5):853–859, 2002.
3. Matsumoto AH, Angle JF, Spinosa DJ, et al: Percutaneous transluminal angioplasty and stenting in the treatment of chronic mesenteric ischemia: Results and long-term follow-up. J Am Coll Surg 194(1 Suppl):S22–31, 2002.
4. Steinmetz E, Tatou E, Favier-Blavoux C, et al: Endovascular treatment as first choice in chronic intestinal ischemia. Ann Vasc Surg 16(6):693–699, 2002.
5. Oderich GS, Panneton JM: Mayo Clinic experience with intraoperative ultrasound during carotid endarterectomy and renal and splanchnic arterial reconstructions. Angiologie 53(4):15–21, 2001.
6. Gloviczki P, Panneton JM: Intraoperative Assessment of Renal and Splanchnic Arterial Reconstruction With Color-Flow Duplex Ultrasonography. In Branchereau A, Magman P-E (eds): Methods de Controle per-Operatoire des Restaurations Vasculaires. Marseille: Editions Chirurgie Vasculaire Nouvelle, 1994.
7. Bandyk DF, Mills JL, Gahtan V, et al: Intraoperative duplex scanning of arterial reconstructions: Fate of repaired and unrepaired defects. J Vasc Surg 20:426–433, 1994.
8. Dougherty MJ, Hallett JW Jr., Naessens JM, et al: Optimizing technical success of renal revascularization: The impact of intraoperative color-flow duplex ultrasonography. J Vasc Surg 17:849–857, 1993.
9. Okuhn SP, Reilly LM, Bennett JB III, et al: Intraoperative assessment of renal and visceral artery reconstruction: The role of duplex scanning and spectral analysis. J Vasc Surg 5:137–147, 1987.
10. Hallett JW, Loftus JP, Harmsen WS, et al: The value of intraoperative renal duplex ultrasound in predicting renal preservation. Twenty-second annual meeting of the Midwestern Vascular Surgical Society, Dearborn, Michigan, 1998 (Abstract book).
11. Oderich GS, Panneton JM, Macedo TA, et al: Intraoperative duplex ultrasound of visceral revascularizations: Optimizing technical success and outcome. J Vasc Surg 34:684–691, 2003.
12. Bandyk DF, Johnson BL, Gupta AK, et al: Nature and management of duplex abnormalities encountered during infrainguinal vein bypass grafting. J Vasc Surg 24:430–438, 1996.
13. McMillan WD, McCarthy WJ, Bresticker MR, et al: Mesenteric artery bypass: Objective patency determination. J Vasc Surg 21(5):729–740, 1995.
14. Riehl J, Schmitt H, Bongartz D, et al: Renal artery stenosis: Evaluation with colour duplex ultrasonography. Nephrol Dial Transplant 12(8):1608–1614, 1997.
15. Moneta GL, Lee RW, Yeager RA, et al: Mesenteric duplex scanning: A blinded prospective study. J Vasc Surg 17:79–86, 1993.
16. Tan KT, van Beek EJ, Brown PW, et al: Magnetic resonance angiography for the diagnosis of renal artery stenosis: A meta-analysis. Clin Radiol 57(7):617–624, 2002.

ANEURYSMS

Chapter 35

Vascular Diagnosis of Abdominal and Peripheral Aneurysms

M. ASHRAF MANSOUR

An aneurysm is described as a local dilatation of a blood vessel exceeding 150% of the diameter of the normal vessel proximal or distal to it.[1] Aneurysms may be saccular or fusiform in morphology and can occur in any artery of the body. There are a few case reports in the literature describing venous aneurysms. False aneurysms, or pseudoaneurysms, are a separate entity with a different etiology. False aneurysms usually develop as a result of trauma, infection, or anastomotic disruption at the junction of a graft and native vessel.[2] The precise cellular mechanism of aneurysmal formation is still being investigated.[3] Once an aneurysm reaches a certain size, complications can occur, usually as a consequence of wall rupture leading to hemorrhage; or by thrombus formation in the lumen, causing vessel occlusion or more distal embolization and impaired bloodflow.

This chapter is an overview of diagnostic methods used for the evaluation of intra-abdominal aneurysms involving the aorta, iliacs, and visceral arteries, and also peripheral aneurysms found in the neck and extremities.

Aneurysms of the Abdominal Aorta and Its Branches

Abdominal Aortic Aneurysms

Abdominal aortic aneurysms (AAAs) are the most common aneurysms encountered in vascular practice. There is a heightened awareness among physicians and the lay public about aneurysms because of their potential lethality, especially after sudden rupture (Fig. 35-1). The incidence of AAA ranges between 6% and 9% in men over 65 years of age in the United States.[3]

The majority of AAAs are asymptomatic. A common scenario is the discovery of an AAA on routine abdominal sonography or computed tomographic (CT) scan obtained to investigate a different presenting problem. Occasionally, a pulsatile abdominal mass is discovered on routine physical examination. Patients who have a ruptured AAA often present with the triad of abdominal, back, or flank pain; hypotension; and a pulsatile mass on abdominal examination.

There are several diagnostic modalities that may be used for the diagnosis of AAA, depending on the clinical situation. In an elective intact AAA, the choice of diagnostic testing will depend on what type of procedure is being entertained. For example, if the patient is being evaluated for endovascular repair, after the initial abdominal sonogram confirming the presence and size of the AAA, a spiral CT scan is obtained to determine eligibility for endovascular repair[4] (see Chapters 37 and 38). Angiography is usually obtained on a selective basis.

With open repair, preoperative CT scan is usually sufficient. A few investigators have advocated proceeding with open repair based on abdominal ultrasound only

(Fig. 35-2, *A*). Angiography is required before open repair to investigate renovascular hypertension, suspected mesenteric ischemia, or in cases of thoracoabdominal aneurysms.

Iliac Aneurysms

Iliac aneurysms develop most often in the common and internal arteries, and rarely in the external iliacs[5] (see Fig. 35-2, *B*). Iliac aneurysms are usually seen in conjunction with AAAs. It is estimated that isolated iliac aneurysms represent only 1% of abdominal aneurysms. As with AAA, iliac aneurysms may increase in size and rupture. The precise diameter at which they rupture has not been determined, and there have been reports of rupture of iliac arteries as small as 3.5 cm in diameter.

Although iliac aneurysms can be detected by ultrasonography, additional tests are often required for complete evaluation. CT scans are very helpful for the detection

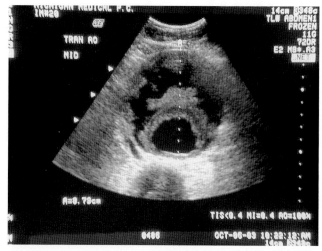

A

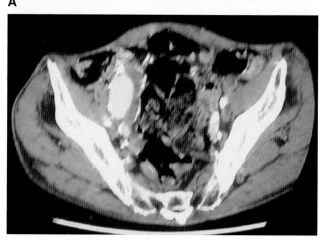

B

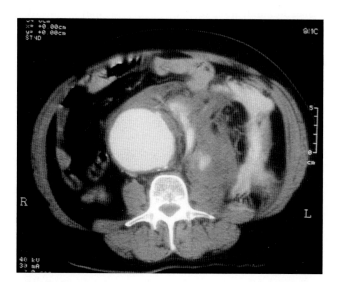

Figure 35-1. *CT scan showing a ruptured abdominal aortic aneurysm with a large retroperitoneal hematoma of the left side.*

Figure 35-2. *A, B-mode ultrasound of a large abdominal aortic aneurysm. B, CT scan of large right iliac aneurysm.*

of iliac aneurysms and also to follow patients after successful repair.[6,7] When iliac aneurysms are found with AAA, they are usually repaired in the same sitting, whether this is done with a conventional open procedure or an endovascular approach.[8,9] Unilateral internal iliac artery aneurysms can be ligated. Although coil embolization has been used to thrombose internal iliac aneurysms, continued growth and potential rupture may occur if some of the collateral flow is left open.

Abdominal Ultrasonography

Abdominal ultrasonography is used to evaluate patients with AAA in all phases. This means that a simple ultrasound is obtained for screening (diagnosis and sizing) and for preoperative and postoperative evaluation. Intraoperative duplex scan may be used to image visceral arterial reconstruction performed in conjunction with AAA repair.

The goal of abdominal ultrasonography is to confirm and to size the AAA. Ultrasonography is the ideal method for screening patients for AAA or for following individuals with smaller, not yet operable AAAs. In most cases, a simple B-mode ultrasound is all that is needed to image and measure the diameter of the AAA. There are rare cases when color-flow duplex scanning is helpful in identifying complicated AAA (e.g., with aorta-caval fistula).[10] When the left renal vein is located posterior to the aorta, or in the rare case of aorta left renal vein fistula, duplex can be diagnostic.[11,12] This type of patient presents with unusual clinical findings such as hematuria, congestive heart failure, or loud abdominal bruit.

Technique of Abdominal Ultrasonography

As with most abdominal sonograms, it is important to examine patients in a fasting state to diminish shadowing from bowel gas. Ideally, the aorta, from the renal arteries to the external iliacs, should be imaged in multiple longitudinal and transverse planes. The information to be acquired includes maximum diameter of the AAA, length and diameter of the proximal neck, diameter of the common iliacs, and also the diameter of the hypogastrics if they are aneurysmal. Of course, if the study is being obtained in a critically ill AAA patient, the presence of a retroperitoneal hematoma is diagnostic of rupture. Color-flow scans can be also quite helpful to determine if mesenteric or renovascular disease is present. In some cases, unsuspected findings (e.g., congenital renal anomalies, accessory renal arteries, or aortovenous fistulas) may be noted and lead to additional diagnostic studies.[11,12]

Color-flow scans also play an important role in postoperative studies, especially after endovascular repair. Endoleaks can be detected, and in type II or III endoleaks,

it is often possible to identify the precise location of the defect[13] (Fig. 35-3). Many investigators rely on color-flow scanning as the main test to follow patients after endovascular AAA repair.

Computed Tomography

Despite the widespread use of ultrasonography in emergency rooms and physicians' offices, the quality of the test will largely depend on the experience of the operator. Therefore, in a setting where a qualified sonographer is not available, or in cases where the ultrasonography is technically challenging, CT scans become the method of choice for evaluating iliac and AAA.[4] The complete evaluation of iliac and AAA requires an abdominal and pelvic CT scan.[5] If the patient has uncompromised renal function, it is desirable to use intravenous contrast for the CT scan, but oral contrast is usually not necessary.

As with the abdominal ultrasound, important information about the diameter of the AAA, the proximal and distal extent, the relationship to the renal vasculature, and the size and quality of the iliac vessels is to be gained from the study. Most of these anatomic relationships can be gleaned from 5-mm slices. When patients are being considered for endovascular repair, and when 3-D reconstruction is anticipated, thinner (3-mm or less) slices are needed (Fig. 35-4). New software can assign colors with 3-D reconstructions to highlight areas of interest (e.g., endoleaks). Occasionally, physicians will be faced with surprises that may alter their management of a particular patient, such as the discovery of metastatic nodules in the liver or congenital renal anomalies.

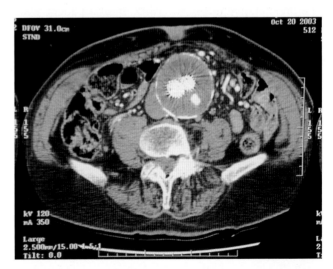

Figure 35-3. Postoperative CT scan, after endovascular AAA repair. Note contrast within the endograft and evidence of contrast outside the graft in the aneurysm sac. This is a type II endoleak from a patent lumbar artery.

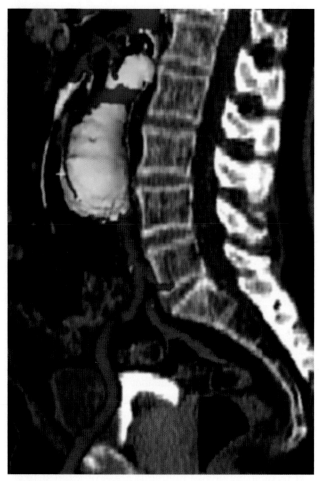

Figure 35-4. *3-D reconstruction of CT scan of AAA with specialized software (MMS).*

Angiography

The preoperative diagnostic work-up of a patient with AAA depends on the clinical presentation and the proposed method of treatment. In the majority of patients undergoing open AAA repair, a preoperative CT scan is sufficient. Angiography is obtained selectively to investigate specific problems such as renovascular hypertension, chronic mesenteric ischemia, or significant iliofemoral occlusive disease. About 20% of patients being evaluated for AAA repair will have clinically important evidence of visceral or renal pathology that requires careful imaging. Angiography helps in the planning of the operation. Angiography may also be needed in patients with renal anomalies such as horseshoe or pancake kidney. In the latter cases, multiple renal arteries may be present, and it is important to identify their precise locations before repair. Now that endovascular AAA repair is considered in an increasing proportion of patients, angiography is performed preoperatively to evaluate tortuous proximal aneurysm necks and iliac arteries, or to do selective coil embolization of a hypogatsric artery in preparation

for EVAR[14] (Fig. 35-5). Isolated iliac aneurysms or pseudoaneurysms can be repaired using covered stents or grafts (Fig. 35-6).

Visceral Aneurysms

Aneurysms occur in visceral arteries. In a contemporary vascular surgery practice, only a handful of these aneurysms are encountered yearly. Anatomically, visceral aneurysms have been identified in the celiac trunk and its branches, the superior mesenteric artery (SMA) and its branches, and the renal arteries.

Aneurysms of the Celiac Trunk, SMA, and Branches

In order of frequency, visceral aneurysms are detected in the splenic, hepatic, superior mesenteric (SMA), celiac trunk, and renal arteries.[15,16] The majority of visceral aneurysms are atherosclerotic (Fig. 35-7); however, mycotic aneurysms tend to occur in the SMA, and pseudoaneurysms may develop after surgical reconstruction of visceral arteries, other abdominal operations, or trauma.

As with AAA, visceral aneurysms may rupture and lead to fatal intra-abdominal hemorrhage. Splenic and renal aneurysms may occur in women of childbearing age, and these aneurysms have a propensity to rupture.

The incidence and natural history of visceral aneurysms is outlined in Table 35-1.

Renal Aneurysms

Renal aneurysms are detected in 0.1% to 0.75% of the population. Ruptured renal aneurysms in pregnant women can cause up to 80% fetal mortality and 50% maternal mortality[16] (Fig. 35-8).

The diagnosis of visceral artery aneurysms can be suspected on a plain film of the abdomen. When calcifications are present in the aneurysm wall, a "signet ring" appearance is observed, most often in splenic and renal aneurysms. Small visceral aneurysms are usually silent and most often are discovered accidentally. As the aneurysms enlarge, pressure on adjacent structures can cause symptoms, such as hematuria with a hilar renal aneurysm or vague abdominal pain with other aneurysms.

Duplex Scan

Confirmation of the presence of a visceral aneurysm and its location is usually done by duplex scan. Documen-

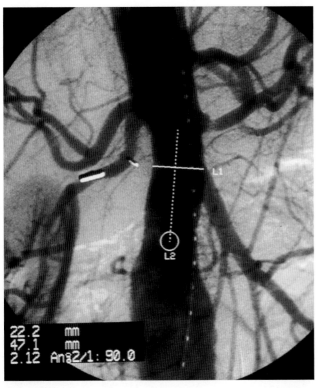

A

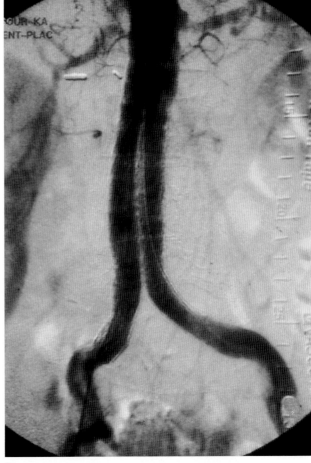

B

Figure 35-5. **A**, *Preoperative angiogram of AAA, with measurement of aneurysm neck length and diameter, in preparation for EVAR.* **B**, *Intraoperative completion angiogram after EVAR showing satisfactory graft placement with no endoleak.*

tation of the precise size and relationship with adjacent structures is important. If the aneurysm is asymptomatic or less than 1.5 cm in diameter, clinical observation is recommended. A follow-up duplex scan on a semi-annual or annual basis is useful to check for growth.

As with any abdominal ultrasound examination, it is best to examine the patient in a fasting state: this diminishes the possibility of bowel gas shadowing. Technical details of scanning are covered in Chapters 22, 32, and 33.

CT Scan and Angiography

Many patients are discovered to have a visceral aneurysm on a diagnostic CT scan obtained to investigate other clinical problems. CT and CT angiography with 3-D reconstruction are extremely useful to obtain precise measurements of the aneurysm as well as its relationship to branch vessels and adjacent structures.

Angiography is usually reserved for planning therapy in patients who are symptomatic or who present with

an enlarging visceral aneurysm. Poor surgical risk patients can be evaluated for coil embolization of the aneurysm at the same sitting. This is performed most commonly for splenic, renal, and distal hepatic aneurysms. If focal infarction occurs from small branch occlusion, it can be tolerated in the spleen and kidney. For other visceral aneurysms, especially in the SMA, infarction is a more serious complication. Coil embolization is also an important adjunct in symptomatic patients who are stable hemodynamically despite a contained rupture.

Surgical Management

Because visceral aneurysms are less common than AAAs, it is important to understand the available management options. A working knowledge of the natural history of these aneurysms and the goals of treatment will help the clinician obtain the appropriate diagnostic tests.[15,16] Surgical repair or ligation of visceral aneurysms is the only treatment if the patient presents in hemorrhagic shock. The death rate from a ruptured splenic aneurysm

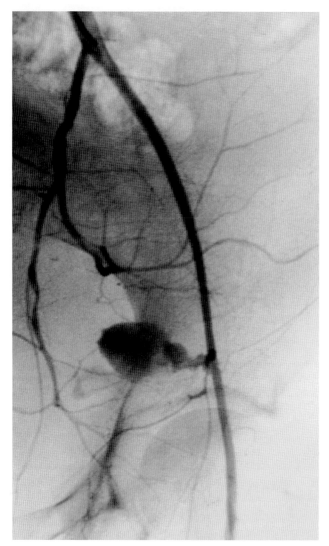

A

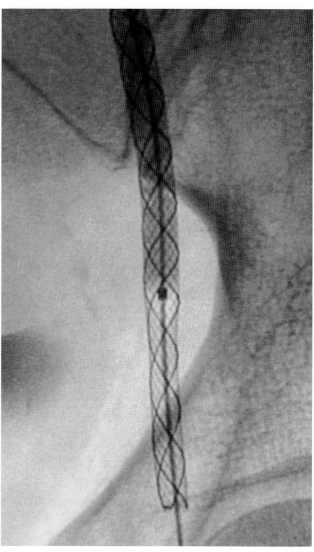

B

Figure 35-6. **A**, *Angiogram of left external iliac pseudoaneurysm, a complication of renal angiography. The patient had hypotension and a large retroperitoneal hematoma.* **B**, *Completion angiogram showing a Wallstent graft placed to repair left external iliac pseudoaneurysm with satisfactory exclusion of the pseudoaneurysm.*

can be as high as 25%. The mortality rate associated with the rupture of other aneurysms is also significant (see Table 35-1). The reason for increased mortality is commonly caused by the delay in diagnosis and treatment. The goal of surgical management is to stop the hemorrhage. In most cases, this will consist of a splenectomy for splenic aneurysms and a nephrectomy for renal aneurysms. Other aneurysms can be ligated. In the case of an SMA aneurysm rupture, urgent reconstruction may be needed to prevent bowel infarction. Autogenous material (e.g., saphenous vein) is preferred in cases where contamination is present or mycotic aneurysms are suspected.

Elective repair of visceral aneurysms can be complicated and require advanced skills. For renal aneurysms located in the hilum and involving branch vessels, ex-vivo reconstruction is necessary.

Aneurysms in the Neck

Carotid aneurysms are uncommon. In a contemporary clinical practice, it is more likely to encounter a carotid pseudoaneurysm or mycotic aneurysm, especially in patients who have undergone a previous carotid endarterectomy with synthetic patch closure.

Carotid aneurysms and pseudoaneurysms may be asymptomatic. Some patients present with neck pain or a pulsatile tender mass in the neck (Fig. 35-9). Rarely, particularly with an infected pseudoaneurysm or mycotic aneurysm, local swelling, redness, and a sinus tract may be present. The diagnosis can be confirmed by duplex scan. Angiography is obtained to plan repair. Surgical treatment is aimed at excision of the aneurysm and bypass with autogenous material. In selected cases, especially

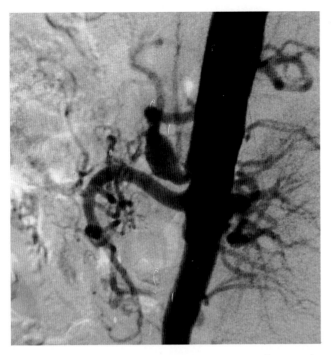

Figure 35-7. Angiogram, lateral projection, confirming the presence of common hepatic aneurysm.

if infection can be ruled out, a covered stent can be placed using endovascular techniques.

Aneurysms of the Upper Extremity

Subclavian and Axillary Aneurysms

Atherosclerotic aneurysms develop in the subclavian and axillary arteries. Subclavian and axillary aneurysms are rare. In a large series reporting on aneurysms, less than 1% of true aneurysms were in the subclavian arteries.[17]

Subclavian artery aneurysms are more common on the right side. The majority of subclavian aneurysms are found in conjunction with thoracic outlet syndrome. Some patients with subclavian aneurysms present with hand or digital ischemia caused by embolization. True brachial aneurysms are rare. Pseudoaneurysms are much more common, especially in patients who have arteriovenous fistulas or grafts for dialysis.

Traumatic pseudoaneurysms can also develop anywhere in the upper extremity as a consequence of penetrating or blunt injury.

Noninvasive diagnostic evaluation of subclavian and axillary aneurysms is often hampered by the bony structures surrounding those vessels. Most surgeons obtain angiograms for complete definition of the aneurysm and to plan repair, whether that is by an endovascular approach or open surgical correction. Endovascular repair usually consists of placement of a covered stent. Open repair of a right subclavian aneurysm is usually approached through a median sternotomy for proximal control, whereas a left subclavian aneurysm is most commonly approached through a left posterolateral thoracotomy. Most isolated axillary aneurysms can be treated with a combined supra and infraclavicular approach.

Brachial, Radial, and Ulnar Aneurysms

Aneurysms in the brachial, radial, and ulnar arteries are most commonly false aneurysms. Postcatherization pseudoaneurysms can develop after diagnostic cardiac catherization performed through the brachial or radial approach. Radial pseudoaneurysms can occur after a puncture for arterial pressure measurement or for arterial blood gas sampling. Ulnar aneurysm can occur as an occupational disease in patients with the "hypothenar hammer syndrome." These patients use their hand for repeated pounding on objects, resulting in trauma to this artery near the hook of the hamate. By far, the most common etiology of brachial and radial pseudoaneurysms is pre-

TABLE 35-1. Visceral Aneurysms

Location	Incidence	Male:Female Ratio	Mortality With Rupture
Splenic	60%	1:4	30%
Hepatic	20%	2:1	35%
SMA	5.5%	1:1	60%
Celiac	4%	1:1	40%
Gastric and gastroepiploic	4%	3:1	70%
Intestinal	3%	1:1	20%
Pancreatoduodenal	2%	4:1	50%
Gastroduodenal	1.5%	4:1	50%

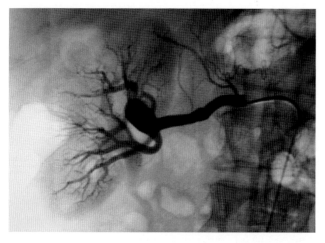

Figure 35-8. Preoperative angiogram of symptomatic right renal aneurysm.

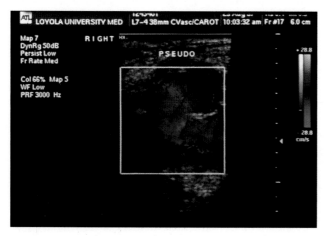

Figure 35-9. Color-flow ultrasound of a right carotid pseudo-aneurysm. The patient had an infected Dacron patch 6 months after carotid endarterectomy.

vious surgical procedures for arteriovenous access for dialysis.

As with aneurysms and pseudoaneurysms of the lower extremity, upper extremity aneurysms cause extremity ischemia from acute occlusion or distal embolization to the digits. Asymptomatic patients present with a pulsatile mass at the site of previous surgery or puncture.

Although a history and physical examination can lead to the correct diagnosis in most patients, color-flow scanning is most helpful in patients who do not provide a clear mechanism. Color-flow scanning can also identify the presence of a traumatic arteriovenous fistula with the false aneurysm. For upper extremity postcatheterization pseudoaneurysms, thrombin injection can be used, providing a narrow suitable neck is identified. In most other cases, open surgical repair is required; thus preoperative angiography is necessary to outline the precise anatomy as well as the status of the distal runoff.

Aneurysms of the Lower Extremity

Femoral and Popliteal Aneurysms

After AAA, the most common peripheral aneurysms encountered in practice are in the femoral and popliteal arteries.[18–20] In patients presenting with a true femoral or popliteal aneurysm, there is an increased likelihood that an aneurysm is present on the opposite side or in the aorta. It is thus good clinical practice to check the size of the popliteal and femoral arteries bilaterally, as well as the size of the aorta.

In contradistinction to AAAs, which tend to rupture with expansion, femoral and popliteal aneurysms tend to thrombose and rarely rupture. The most serious complication of a thrombosed femoral or popliteal aneurysm is acute limb ischemia. For this reason femoropopliteal aneurysms should be treated if they are symptomatic or if they expand to more than 2.5 to 3.0 cm in diameter (Fig. 35-10).

Color-Flow Duplex Scanning

In the average-sized patient, a femoral aneurysm can be palpated. Popliteal aneurysms are more difficult to detect by physical examination. Therefore, all pulsatile masses in the groin or the popliteal fossa should be examined by duplex. The study should include longitudinal and transverse views to obtain accurate diameter measurements and to document the presence of lining thrombus (see Fig. 35-10). It is also useful to determine the exact location of the aneurysm in relation to the knee joint. Commonly, additional information can be gathered from a popliteal duplex (e.g., Baker's cyst or venous problems). With duplex arterial mapping, the status of the runoff vessels can also be checked. Duplex is also very useful to follow the growth of smaller aneurysms in these locations on serial examinations.

CT and Angiography

Femoral aneurysms can be detected by CT scans if the cuts include the pelvis and groin (Fig. 35-11). CT scans are usually obtained to complete the evaluation of AAA. Because endovascular repair is now offered to an increasing number of patients, the iliofemoral segments should be fully evaluated. Many endovascular grafts require a minimum diameter of 7 mm (21 French) for introduction through the femoral approach.

Angiography is used to plan repair. The extent of the femoral aneurysm and involvement of the profunda

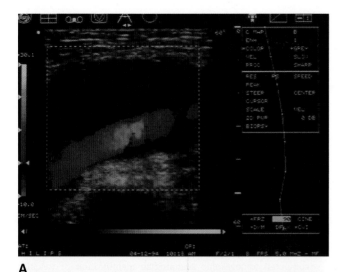

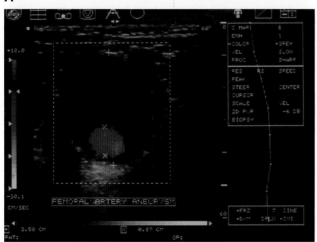

Figure 35-10. **A**, *Color-flow duplex of true right femoral aneurysm (longitudinal view).* **B**, *Color-flow duplex of the same true right femoral aneurysm (transverse view).*

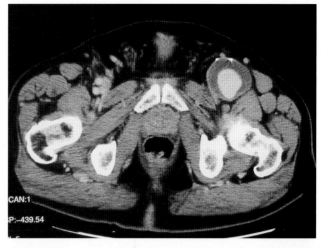

Figure 35-11. *CT scan of pelvis showing left femoral pseudoaneurysm developing several years after aortobifemoral bypass.*

femoris should be determined preoperatively. Similarly, the complete evaluation of popliteal aneurysms will include angiography. This is especially helpful to plan operative repair.

Aneurysms located above the knee can be repaired with prosthetic material with an above-knee incision. Aneurysms located at the knee joint can be approached posteriorly, with the patient in the prone position on the operating room table. Many aneurysms, however, involve both the above- and below-knee segments of the artery; thus they are approached through the familiar medial thigh and proximal leg incision. In rare cases, when angiography is contraindicated because of contrast allergy or poor renal function, MRA or duplex arterial mapping may be sufficient. In the future, MRAs may replace conventional digital subtraction angiography for the evaluation of lower extremity aneurysmal and occlusive disease (see Chapter 27I).

Femoral Pseudoaneurysms

With the increasing number of percutaneous procedures for both coronary and peripheral arteries, the number of postcatheterization pseudoaneurysms is on the rise. Many of these patients are placed on anticoagulants and antiplatelet therapy, thus increasing the chances of pseudoaneurysm formation. Pseudoaneurysms also may form after aortofemoral or femoropopliteal bypass. Although clinical examination can detect a pulsatile groin mass, often it is obscured by surrounding hematoma. Duplex is the first test obtained to confirm the presence of the pseudoaneurysm.

Most postcatheterization pseudoaneurysms can be treated by thrombin injection (see Chapter 29). Post-bypass pseudoaneurysms are treated surgically with graft replacement. Angiography is obtained to plan repair (Fig. 35-12). CT scans are helpful if graft infection is suspected.

Dorsalis Pedis Aneurysms

Although quite rare, aneurysms can develop in the pedal vessels. Because the vessels are close to the skin surface, it is usually possible to palpate and image the arteries. Color-flow scanning is used to confirm the diagnosis and also for postoperative follow-up.[21] In patients who have an intact posterior tibial artery and pedal arch, simple ligation of a dorsalis pedis aneurysm can be performed; however, repair of the aneurysm is mandatory in some cases to avoid forefoot ischemia.

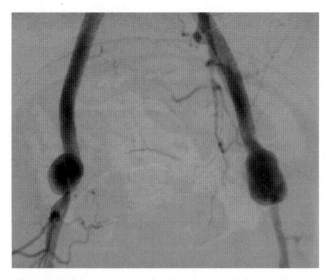

Figure 35-12. *Angiogram demonstrating bilateral femoral pseudoaneurysms.*

Conclusions

Aneurysms can develop at many locations in the arterial tree. This chapter focuses on aneurysms of the abdominal aorta and its branches; and on aneurysms developing in the neck and upper and lower extremities. Various diagnostic methods are employed to find the precise location and size of aneurysms and to help plan for repair. Noninvasive methods are typically selected as a first line. More invasive tests are selected as a second line, and often can be therapeutic. Management options are discussed in general terms.

KEY POINTS

▪ Aneurysms can occur in any location of the arterial tree.

▪ Pseudoaneurysms can develop after iatrogenic or noniatrogenic trauma to blood vessels.

▪ Noninvasive methods are very helpful in screening patients for the presence of aneurysms and for following the growth of aneurysms.

▪ CT scan and angiography are usually obtained before planning treatment.

▪ Aneurysms can be treated with open surgical repair or with newer endovascular techniques.

REFERENCES

1. Johnston KW, Rutherford RB, Tilson MD, et al: Suggested standards for reporting on arterial aneurysms. J Vasc Surg 13:452–458, 1991.
2. Seabrook GR, Schmidt DD, Bandyk DF, et al: Anastomotic femoral pseudoaneurysm: An investigation of occult infection as an etiologic factor. J Vasc Surg 11:629–634, 1990.
3. Thompson RW, Geraghty PJ, Lee JK: Abdominal aortic aneurysms: Basic mechanisms and clinical implications. Curr Probl Surg 39(2):110–230, 2002.
4. Bayle O, Branchereau A, Rosset E, et al: Morphologic assessment of abdominal aortic aneurysms by spiral computed tomographic scanning. J Vasc Surg 26:238–246, 1997.
5. Krupski WC, Selzman CH, Floridia R, et al: Contemporary management of isolated iliac aneurysms. J Vasc Surg 28:1–13, 1998.
6. Treiman GS, Weaver FA, Cossman DV, et al: Anastomotic false aneurysms of the abdominal aorta and iliac arteries. J Vasc Surg 8:268–273, 1988.
7. Kalman PG, Rappaport DC, Merchant N, et al: The value of late computed tomographic scanning in identification of vascular abnormalities after abdominal aortic aneurysms repair. J Vasc Surg 29:442–450, 1999.
8. Sanchez LA, Patel AV, Ohki T, et al: Midterm experience with the endovascular treatment of isolated iliac aneurysms. J Vasc Surg 30:907–914, 1999.
9. Morrissey NJ, Yano OJ, Soundararajan K, et al: Endovascular repair of para-anastomotic aneurysms of the aorta and iliac arteries: Preferred treatment for a complex problem. J Vasc Surg 34:503–512, 2001.
10. Baker WH, Mansour MA: Arteriovenous Fistulae of the Aorta and its Major Branches. In Rutherford RB (ed): Vascular Surgery. Philadelphia: WB Saunders, 1999.
11. Mansour MA, Russ PD, Subber SW, et al: Aorto-left renal vein fistula: Diagnosis by duplex sonography. Am J Roentgenol 152:1107–1108, 1989.
12. Mansour MA, Rutherford RB, Metcalf RK, et al: Spontaneous aorto-left renal vein fistula: The abdominal pain, hematuria, silent left kidney syndrome. Surgery 109:101–106, 1991.
13. Bendick PJ, Bove PG, Long GW, et al: Efficacy of ultrasound scan contrast agents in the noninvasive follow-up of aortic stent grafts. J Vasc Surg 37:381–385, 2003.
14. Ouriel K, Greenberg RK, Clair DG: Endovascular treatment of aortic aneurysms. Curr Probl Surg 39:233–348, 2002.
15. Stanley JC: Aneurysms of the Celiac and Mesenteric Circulations. In Yao JST, Pearce WH (eds): Aneurysms: New Findings and Treatments. Norwalk, CT: Appleton & Lange, 1994.
16. Dean RH: Renal artery aneurysms. In Yao JST, Pearce WH (eds): Aneurysms: New Findings and Treatments. Norwalk, CT: Appleton & Lange, 1994.
17. Clagett GP: Upper Extremity Aneurysms. In Rutherford RB (ed): Vascular Surgery. Philadelphia: WB Saunders, 1999.
18. Shortell CK, DeWeese JA, Ouriel K, et al: Popliteal artery aneurysms: A 25-year surgical experience. J Vasc Surg 14:771–779, 1991.
19. Carpenter JP, Barker CF, Roberts B, et al: Popliteal artery aneurysms: Current management and outcome. J Vasc Surg 19:65–73, 1994.
20. Diwan A, Sarkar R, Stanley JC, et al: Incidence of femoral and popliteal aneurysms in patients with abdominal aortic aneurysms. J Vasc Surg 31:863–869, 2000.
21. Taylor DT, Mansour MA, Bergin JT, et al: Aneurysm of the dorsalis pedis artery. Vasc Endovasc Surg 36:241–245, 2002.

Chapter 36

Screening for Abdominal Aortic Aneurysms

FRED N. LITTOOY

- ▨ Screening Methods
- ▨ Screening
- ▨ Follow-Up
- ▨ Cost-Effectiveness and Mortality Reduction
- ▨ Treatment of Coexisting Vascular Disease

Because aortic aneurysm ranks as the tenth leading cause of death in the older male population,[1] detection and treatment before rupture (the primary cause of death from infrarenal abdominal aortic aneurysm) is of paramount importance. According to the National Center for Health Statistics, about 15,000 patients presented to hospitals in the United States in 1999 with the diagnosis of ruptured abdominal aortic aneurysm (AAA).[1] This is definitely an under-representation of the actual number, because many such patients may die before reaching the hospital. The United States has an aging population, and because the prevalence of abdominal aortic aneurysms increases with age, we will be identifying more patients in the future. Endovascular repair of abdominal aortic aneurysm, which has lesser morbidity, has been available since 1990. As this technology continues to advance, it will become feasible for more and more patients. Also, higher-risk patients previously deemed inoperable now have the potential for definitive treatment of their abdominal aortic aneurysms.

Screening programs for the detection of abdominal aortic aneurysm have a great potential to be lifesaving because the primary serious outcome of abdominal aortic aneurysm is rupture and death. Nevertheless, mass screening is not likely to be cost-effective; therefore, pinpointing target populations for screening has considerable importance. Then the appropriate, cost-effective follow-up for patients found to have an aortic abdominal aneurysm is essential; it requires an understanding of the natural history of small abdominal aortic aneurysms. Consideration of and treatment of the other medical problems in these patients may also further affect the long-term outcome of these patients.

This chapter addresses screening methods, means of improving yields from a screening program, and cost-effective programs for follow-up. Identification and management of coexisting vascular disease will be touched on as well.

Screening Methods

Determining the population to screen requires an understanding of the expected prevalence of AAA in that population. Time and cost expended in the screening process need to be allocated so that it is cost-effective and beneficial to the patients affected with abdominal aortic aneurysm. Studies that have examined the risk factors associated with AAA will be discussed in detail. Reviewing these studies helps determine target populations and helps determine methods to screen those target populations. Invitations to participate in a large screening process are usually generalized, and positive responses range from 30%[2] to as high as 76%.[3] These response rates are highly dependent on the particular population queried and the particular health care system and cost. Other approaches to screening take a more targeted approach and utilize a quick screen of the infrarenal abdominal aorta as an add-on to other noninvasive laboratory examinations in patients with arterial occlusive disease in the coronaries, carotids, or lower extremity. Another approach invites first-degree relatives of patients with a family history of AAA. These approaches will provide a higher yield of patients with abdominal aortic aneurysm.

The tool of choice for screening is B-mode ultrasound examination of the infrarenal aorta (Figs. 36-1, 36-2, and 36-3). It is reasonably cheap, noninvasive, and does not expose the patient to radiation. Dedicated ultrasound machines may be used for large-scale population screenings. In the noninvasive vascular laboratory, the duplex ultrasound is the machine of choice and will often be utilized as a quick scan after the primary testing is complete. However, successful imaging of the entire infrarenal aorta requires an overnight fast and experienced technologists. Adequate visualization of the entire infrarenal aorta is reported to be 89% to 100%.[4,5]

Accuracy of ultrasound readings is important and becomes critical in the follow-up and decision making for patients detected to have infrarenal abdominal aortic aneurysms. Variability in the measurement of abdominal aortic aneurysms is reported in two studies. The Veterans Administration Aneurysm Detection and Management Trial (ADAM)[6] carefully studied 258 ultrasound-measured and centrally read CT pairs. Researchers reported that ultrasound measurements were smaller than CT measurements by an average of 0.27 cm. The difference was 0.2 cm or less in 44% but at least 0.5 cm in 37%. They recommended that these differences could be minimized by limiting the number of radiologists reading the ultrasound (intraobserver differences were less than interobserver differences) and by the use of calipers for measurements. Intraobserver and interobserver variability in the reading of ultrasounds was closely monitored in the Multicenter Aneurysm Screening Study (MASS)[7] as well. Researchers noted an intraobserver variability of 2.60 mm and an interobserver variability of 3.27 mm in the transverse plane.

Screening

Multiple screening studies, large and small, utilizing abdominal ultrasound have helped identify groups of patients in whom we can expect to find an increased prevalence of AAA. Populations with a higher prevalence include males, especially those who smoke; those over

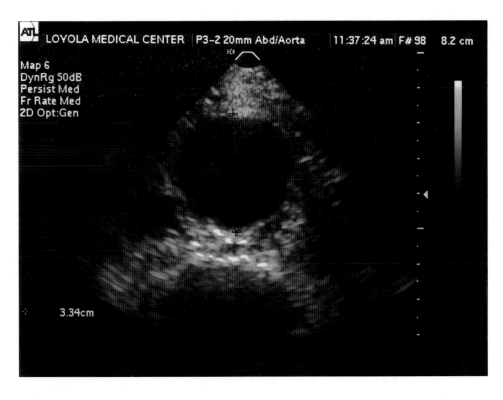

Figure 36-1. Duplex ultrasound of a 3-cm abdominal aortic aneurysm utilizing ATL HDI 3000 with a 3-MHz probe.

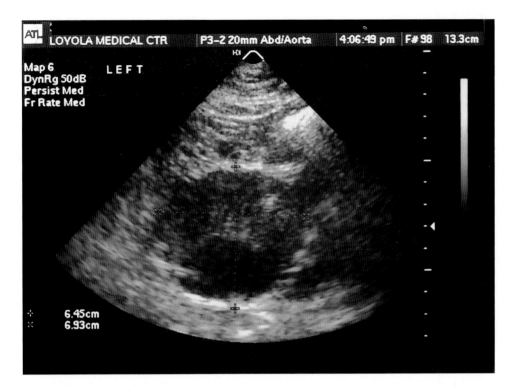

Figure 36-2. Duplex ultrasound, cross-sectional view, of a 5.6-cm abdominal aortic aneurysm.

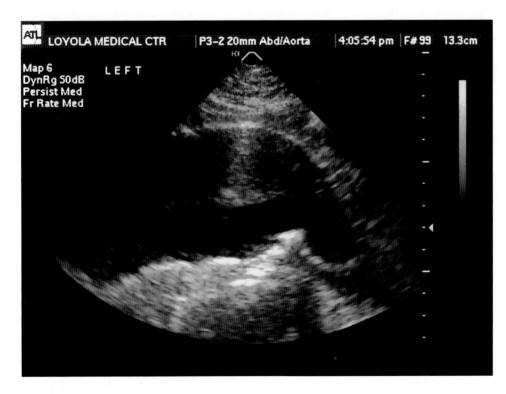

Figure 36-3. Duplex ultrasound, longitudinal view of a 5.6-cm abdominal aortic aneurysm (same patient as Figure 36-2).

65 years of age; patients with a family history of AAA; and patients with other vascular disease (e.g., coronary artery disease, lower extremity occlusive disease, and carotid stenosis). Some studies have reported an increased association with other risk factors such as hypertension, hypercholesterolemia, and chronic obstructive pulmonary disease, although to a lesser extent. Interestingly, female sex, African American race, and diabetes have often been shown to have a negative association with the presence of abdominal aortic aneurysms.

Lederle and colleagues[8] reported on the largest reported screening program in ADAM. AAA was defined as 3.0 cm or more in greatest diameter of the infrarenal aorta. In this study, 126,196 veteran patients aged 50 to 79 years underwent abdominal ultrasound screening for AAA. Prevalence of abdominal aortic aneurysm by diameter is illustrated in Table 36-1. As shown, the overall prevalence was 4.26%, but only 0.45% were 5.0 cm or greater. Smoking, age, family history of AAA, and atherosclerotic diseases were the principal positive associations with abdominal aortic aneurysms. Smoking accounted for 75% of all abdominal aortic aneurysms 4.0 cm or more in diameter with an odds ratio of 5.07 (4.13 to 6.21).

The MASS study[7] carried out in England and Wales screened 27,147 men aged 65 to 74 years for abdominal aortic aneurysm and produced similar findings in AAA prevalence (see Table 36-1). Total aneurysms detected were 4.9% (0.8% were between 4.5 and 5.4 cm and 0.58% were greater than 5.5 cm).

Three other large-scale screening studies from Norway, Denmark, and the United Kingdom[3,9,10] bring forth helpful data to better focus screening of patients. The Norwegian Study[9] of 6386 men and women aged 25 to 84 years noted a prevalence of 8.9% in men and 2.2% in women. No patient less than 48 years old had an abdominal aortic aneurysm. Smoking for 40 years vs. never smoked increased the odds ratio to 8.0 (5.0 to 12.0) for detection of AAA. Other risk factors for atherosclerosis were associated with an increased risk for AAA.

In the Denmark study[3] of 65- to 73-year-old men, 4.8% had an abdominal aortic aneurysm but only 0.6% were above 4.9 cm. Of note, 76% of invited patients responded to the invitation for screening and the scans were complete (entire infrarenal aorta visualized) in 97.6%.

The United Kingdom study[10] includes 11,666 men and women aged 65 to 80 years. With age, the prevalence increased from 5.4% to 10.4% in men and 0.67% to 2.17% in women. Data from district registrars gave information on probable deaths from ruptured abdominal aortic aneurysm. Only 4.4% of the deaths from rupture occurred before age 65, but 85% of the deaths occurred over age 70. The researchers, therefore, advocate a single screening at the age of 65 as well as 70.

Family history is a well-recognized univariable risk factor for AAA. In the ADAM trial, 5.1% reported a family member with an abdominal aortic aneurysm.[2]

However, testing of family members of patients with abdominal aortic aneurysms; and review of population registers, death certificates, and hospital records leads to a higher prevalence, as demonstrated by a study in Finland. The prevalence of families with at least two affected persons was 16%.[11]

Other screening strategies have targeted patients with other atherosclerotic disease involving the coronaries, carotids, and lower extremities. Wolf and colleagues[4] studied 501 patients who came for evaluation of lower extremity arterial disease with B-mode ultrasound of the infrarenal aorta as well. Scans were successful in 89% of patients. Of the successful scans, 6.7% had an abdominal aortic aneurysm (3 cm or greater). Aneurysms larger than 4.0 cm were found in 3.2%. A smoking history in males increased the overall incidence of abdominal aortic aneurysm to 15.2% (8.8% of which were larger than 4.0 cm). Limited scanning increased the length of the vascular lab examination by only 5 minutes on the average.

In a smaller study of 192 patients scheduled for elective coronary artery bypass graft (CABG),[12] the prevalence

TABLE 36-1. Prevalence of Abdominal Aortic Aneurysm by Diameter

ADAM Trial (8)		MASS Trial (7)	
Diameter (cm)	Combined Group n = 126, 196 n (%)	Diameter (cm)	Study Group n = 27, 147 n (%)
3.0	5283 (4.2)	3.0	1333 (4.9)
4.0	1644 (1.3)	3.0–4.4	944 (3.5)
5.0	571 (0.45)	4.5–5.4	223 (0.83)
5.5	342 (0.27)	5.5	166 (0.58)
6.0	212 (0.17)		
7.0	76 (0.06)		
8.0	32 (0.03)		

of new abdominal aortic aneurysm (3 cm or larger) was 13.0% (5.2% were larger than 5 cm). Risk factors identified were age 65 years or more and a history of smoking.

Kang and colleagues[13] screened 374 patients for AAA during evaluation for carotid disease where a 50% stenosis of the carotid artery was detected. An AAA 3.0 cm or larger was found in 18.2% and an AAA 4.0 cm or larger was found in 8.3% Absence of diabetes increased these prevalences to 21.97% and 9.2%, respectively. In this study, patients with a greater than 50% carotid artery stenosis and absence of diabetes had a relative risk of AAA that was two to three times greater than patients undergoing routine screening.

In summary, based on the aforementioned studies, it is possible to select populations with an increased prevalence and, therefore, increase the cost-effectiveness and benefit to the patient. Male smokers older than 65 years constitute a group of patients in whom a quick abdominal aortic ultrasound scan during other noninvasive vascular testing will also yield a significant number of patients with a family history of AAA. First-degree family members of patients with a family history of AAA often have a high prevalence. Patients younger than 50 years should not be screened. Benefits of screening patients older than 83 years are questionable, as noted in the Markov model of Lee and colleagues.[5] This will be discussed later. A single screening of all males 65 years old is advocated by some.[14]

Follow-Up

Screening programs, either general or targeted, will detect a larger number of abdominal aortic aneurysms between 3.0 and 3.9 cm. By no criteria should these patients be offered an operation at that time. Will they become operable candidates? The ADAM[15] and United Kingdom[16] trials enrolling patients with AAA between 4.0 and 5.4 cm in diameter demonstrated the safety of surveillance with operation withheld until the AAA reaches 5.5 cm. Rupture rate in these initially observed groups of AAA between 4.0 and 5.4 were 0.7% and 1% per year in the respective studies.[15,16] Operative mortalities do not approach these rates. On the other hand, approximately two thirds of the patients in the initially observed groups in both studies had an AAA eventually reach a diameter greater than 5.4 cm and underwent surgical repair. Follow-up (i.e., compliance) is extremely important. Patient compliance as part of a study approaches 90%, but compliance in the everyday practice may lag, and measures to keep track of the patient are necessary.

But what about all these detected small aneurysms (less than 4.0 cm)? Santilli and colleagues[17] reported on the largest number of such patients (790 men) followed with ultrasound. The patients were divided into two subgroups, I (3.0 to 3.4 cm) and II (3.5 to 3.9 cm) at initial detection. Average follow-up was 3.89 ± 1.93 years with a median expansion rate of 0.11 cm/year. Groups I and II expanded at 0.09 cm/year and 0.15 cm/year, respectively. Interestingly, 25% of the patients exhibited no expansion during the study. Only 2.6% of the patients came to operative repair. This differs from other studies but likely reflects the authors' bias to delay repair until a diameter of 5.5 cm is reached. No deaths caused by ruptured abdominal aortic aneurysms were detected among 140 deaths. Hypertension was the only risk factor associated with moderate expansion. Lifetable analysis survival was 84% at 7 years; therefore, some program for follow-up is required. This study determined that 3.0 to 3.9 cm abdominal aortic aneurysms expand slowly, do not rupture, infrequently grow to 5.0 cm or more within 4 years of follow-up, and rarely require operative repair. The authors recommend a follow-up ultrasound in 3 years, although they reasoned that elderly males without hypertension in group I needed no further follow-up ultrasound.

Follow-up ultrasound in the 4.0 to 5.4 cm group should be every 6 months, although nonhypertensive patients in the 4.0 to 4.4 cm range could be followed safely in 1 year. Endovascular surgical techniques will likely continue to improve and push the envelope for repair to something less than 5.5 cm, but even then interventional repair must have a mortality rate less than 1%.

Cost-Effectiveness and Mortality Reduction

How does screening affect mortality, and is screening cost-effective? Several studies address these issues and are important to the patient population and the health care system at large. The MASS study in the United Kingdom addressed both cost-effectiveness and affect on mortality in men with AAA.[7,18] In the cost-effectiveness aspect of the study, 67,800 men aged 65 to 74 years were studied over a 4-year period.[18] One half of the patients were invited for an ultrasound screening of the abdominal aorta (27,147 responded), and one half were not invited for ultrasound screening. They calculated patient-specific costs related to AAA including screening and follow-up ultrasounds, and surgical costs including evaluation and operative repair of elective or ruptured AAA. Details are in the paper.[18] Effectiveness was determined as survival free from mortality related to AAA for an individual up to 4 years. Cost-effectiveness was expressed as the incremental cost per additional life-year gained. Probability for cost-effectiveness is represented by cost-effectiveness acceptability curves. The authors placed those probabilities at a value of £30,000. At 4 years, the estimated cost-effectiveness ratio was £28,400 per life-year gained. The projected effectiveness at 10 years would be about £8000 per life-year saved. Although the

4-year incremental cost effectiveness is at the margin of the National Health Service acceptability, it projects to be much lower at 10 years.

Lee and colleagues[5] evaluated utilization of a "quick screen" as a cost-effective tool for detecting AAA. Because cost-effectiveness is directly linked to the detection rate of the screening program for AAA, they developed a strict set of criteria for screening patients. The criteria included a family history of AAA or three or more of the following risk factors: male gender, age over 60 years, current or former smoker, hypertension, hyperlipidemia, coronary disease, history of lower extremity bypass, claudication, ischemic rest pain, or carotid artery disease. Their "quick scan" took an upper limit of 5 minutes and was 100% accurate. They used a Markov model to determine cost-effective ratio (CER) or cost/QALY (quality adjusted life-year). They evaluated the cost of the ultrasound and then developed the model for various prevalences of AAA, probability of incidentally detected AAA in a nonscreened group, and age at initial screening. With their model they determined a CER of $11,215, which is well below the accepted CER of $60,000 society is willing to pay for interventions. Patients over 83 years of age increased the CER threshold to over $60,000.

A positive effect of screening in the United Kingdom was seen on mortality reduction from AAA.[7] In the MASS trial, patients screened vs. patients not screened demonstrated a 42% mortality reduction from aneurysm-related causes. Mortality reduction increased to 53% for the patients who actually attended the screening examination.

From a smaller randomized study of 6058 men aged 64 to 81 in Chichester, United Kingdom,[14] similar mortality reductions in AAA-related deaths were noted. Reduction was 68% at 5 years in those screened compared to those in the control group. The conclusion of this study included a recommendation that all men should receive screening at age 65 years because that one screening will identify the majority of abdominal aortic aneurysms that are of clinical significance.

Treatment of Coexisting Vascular Disease

Screening programs that invite the general population set new concerns into motion. As we know, AAA is a marker for coronary artery disease and significant numbers of these patients will have hypertension, diabetes mellitus, and hyperlipidemia. Many patients may be candidates for antiplatelet medication, statins, and/or beta blockers.

Treatment aimed at these medical problems has the potential of a long-term medical benefit for these patients as well.

Potential for medical treatment utilizing doxycycline to stop the growth of small abdominal aortic aneurysms has been suggested in pilot studies.[19] Doxycycline has the effect of decreasing MMP-9 and other metalloproteinases that are found in aneurysm walls and may weaken the wall; therefore treatment with doxycycline may prevent aneurysm growth. If this holds up in a clinical trial, the possibility of further decreasing health care costs and mortality exists.

REFERENCES

1. National Center for Health Statistics: Deaths, percent of total deaths, and death rates for 15 leading causes of death: United States and each state, 1999. CDC/NCHS, National Vital Statistics System, 2001.
2. Lederle FA, Johnson GR, Wilson SE, et al for the Aneurysm Detection and Management (ADAM) Veterans Affairs Cooperative Study Group: Prevalence and associations of abdominal aortic aneurysm detected through screening. Ann Intern Med 126:441–449, 1997.
3. Lindholt JS, Henneber EW, Fasting H, et al: Hospital-based screening of 65- to 73-year-old men for abdominal aortic aneurysms in the county of Viborg, Denmark. J Med Screen 3(1):43–46, 1996.
4. Wolf YG, Otis SM, Schwend RB, et al: Screening for abdominal aortic aneurysms during lower extremity arterial evaluation in the vascular laboratory. J Vasc Surg 22:417–423, 1995.
5. Lee TY, Korn P, Heller JA, et al: The cost-effectiveness of a "quick screen" program for aortic abdominal aneurysms. Surg 132:399–407, 2002.
6. Lederle FA, Wilson SE, Johnson GR, et al for the Abdominal Aortic Aneurysm Detection and Management (ADAM) Veterans Administration Cooperative Study Group: Variability in measurement of abdominal aortic aneurysms. J Vasc Surg 21:945–952, 1995.
7. The Multicenter Aneurysm Screening Study Group: The multicenter aneurysm screening study (MASS) into the effect of abdominal aortic aneurysm screening on mortality in men: A randomized controlled trial. Lancet 360:1531–1539, 2002.
8. Lederle FA, Johnson GR, Wilson SE, et al and the Aneurysm Detection and Management Veterans Affairs Cooperative Study Investigators: The aneurysm detection and management screening program: Validation cohort and final results. Arch Intern Med 160:1425–1430, 2000.
9. Singh K, Bonoa KH, Jacobsen BK, et al: Prevalence of and risk factors for abdominal aortic aneurysms in a population-based study: The Tromso Study. Am J Epidemiol 154(3):236–244, 2001.
10. Khoo DE, Ashton H, Scott RA: Is screening once at age 65 an effective method for detection of abdominal aortic aneurysms? J Med Screen 1(4):223–225, 1994.
11. Jaakkola P, Kuivaniemi H, Partanen K, et al: Familial abdominal aortic aneurysms: Screening of 71 families. Eur J Surg 162(8):611–617, 1996.
12. Bergersen L, Kiernan MS, McFarlane G, et al: Prevalence of abdominal aortic aneurysms in patients undergoing coronary artery bypass. Ann Vasc Surgy 12(2):101–105, 1998.
13. Kang SS, Littooy FN, Gupta SR, et al: Higher prevalence of abdominal aortic aneurysms in patients with carotid stenosis but without diabetes. Surg 126:687–692, 1999.
14. Scott RA, Vardulaki KA, Walker NM, et al: The long-term benefits of a single scan for abdominal aortic aneurysm (AAA) at age 65. Eur J Vasc Endovasc Surg 21(6):535–540, 2001.
15. Lederle FA, Wilson SE, Johnson GR, et al for the Aneurysm Detection and Management (ADAM) Veterans Affair Cooperative Study Investigators: Immediate repair compared with surveillance

of small abdominal aortic aneurysms. N Engl J Med 346:1437–1444, 2002.

16. The United Kingdom Small Aneurysm Trial Participants: Mortality results for randomized controlled trial of early elective surgery or ultrasonographic surveillance for small abdominal aortic aneurysms. Lancet 352:1649–1655, 1998.

17. Santilli SM, Littooy FN, Cambria RA, et al: Expansion rates and outcomes of the 3.0-cm to 3.9-cm infrarenal abdominal aortic aneurysm. J Vasc Surg 35:666–676, 2002.

18. Multicenter Aneurysm Screening Study Group: Multicenter aneurysm screening study (MASS): Cost-effectiveness analysis of screening for abdominal aortic aneurysms based on 4-year results from randomized controlled trial. BMJ 325:1135–1141, 2002.

19. Baxter BT, Pearce WH, Thompson R, et al: Prolonged administration of doxycycline in patients with small asymptomatic abdominal aortic aneurysms: Report of a prospective (Phase II) multicenter study. J Vasc Surg 36(1):1–12, 2002.

Chapter 37

Preoperative Imaging for Open Repair of Abdominal Aortic Aneurysm

BRIAN G. PETERSON • WILLIAM H. PEARCE

Introduction

The first open repair of an abdominal aortic aneurysm (AAA) was performed on March 29, 1951, when Dubost performed successful resection of an aortic aneurysm and homograft replacement.[1] Since then, advances in the field of vascular surgery have minimized the operative mortality rate for the elective repair of AAA to an acceptable level of 2% to 5%.[2-4] In addition to the significant advancements in anesthesia and surgical management of AAA in the past 50 years, preoperative imaging techniques have dramatically changed, enhancing our ability to care for AAA patients. Before the surgical repair of an AAA, several factors, including the anatomic features of the aneurysm, the contiguous vasculature, and the appearance of other intra-abdominal structures must be taken into consideration. The proximal and distal extent of the aneurysm (particularly, the involvement of the renal mesenteric) must be known preoperatively. In addition, the identification of the presence of other intra-abdominal anomalies (e.g., horseshoe kidneys or masses) plays an important role in planning the open repair of an AAA. Furthermore, the timing of the repair itself is determined by aneurysm size, progression, or the presence of rupture based on these imaging studies. The approach, whether thoracoabdominal, retroperitoneal, or transabdominal, is also determined by preoperative findings. Various imaging modalities can be used in the preoperative workup of AAA; however, the choice of a given study depends on the available technology and on certain patient characteristics (e.g., renal function).

Ultrasound

Ultrasound (US) is a useful and inexpensive method to screen and follow AAA. Ultrasonography can effectively be used to document the presence of an AAA with a sensitivity of 100% (Fig. 37-1).[5-9] Ultrasound has also been shown to accurately determine aneurysm size to within 0.3 to 0.6 cm in comparison with intraoperative findings.[10,11] The main advantages of US in comparison with other modalities are: (1) a lack of need for intravenous contrast or ionizing radiation; and (2) a relatively low cost. Despite these advantages, the use of US as the sole imaging modality for preoperative planning for the open repair of AAA is inadequate for several reasons. First, US provides only limited information regarding the anatomy of an AAA. US is unable to demonstrate the proximal extent of the AAA with respect to the renal arteries and cannot reliably demonstrate the presence or absence of associated internal iliac artery aneurysms.[12,13] Second, there is an inherent operator-dependent discrepancy with ultrasonographic imaging of AAA. Images of aneurysm size and morphology may vary according to the experience of the ultrasonographer. Finally, ultrasound quality is limited by patient body habitus and overlying bowel gas. In certain patient populations (i.e., in thin individuals and those with preimaging bowel preparation) ultrasonography with surface reconstruction, using a combination of 2-D ultrasound and Doppler flow studies of the renal, superior mesenteric, and iliac arteries, may be adequate in supplying the preoperative information necessary for the open repair.[14-16]

Computed Tomographic Scanning

Computed tomographic (CT) imaging is currently the imaging technique of choice for AAA. This noninvasive radiographic imaging modality determines aneurysm size more accurately than does US, and it also has the ability to differentiate thrombus seen within the aneurysm from its outer diameter. Angiography may grossly underestimate the size of an AAA because of its failure to demonstrate the presence of an intraluminal thrombus. In addition to demonstrating the AAA, CT also accurately detects both the extension of aneurysmal dilatation into the iliac vessels and any associated femoral aneurysms.[17] With concomitant occlusive disease of the lower extremities, symptoms of mesenteric ischemia, or uncontrolled hypertension, angiography may be indicated. The presence of concomitant vascular disease can safely and effectively be addressed at the time of aneurysm repair only if information regarding these vessels is known preoperatively.

CT is also helpful in determining the proximal extent of the AAA in relationship to the renal arteries, and it can be used to anticipate the need for suprarenal clamping during open operative repair (Fig. 37-2). A recent study demonstrated that when a distance of 26 mm between the proximal extent of the aneurysmal aorta and the orifices of the renal arteries was used as a cutoff for determining the site of proximal aortic cross clamping, CT successfully predicted the ability to repair the aneurysm using infrarenal clamping in 62% of cases.[18] Conversely, distances shorter than 26 mm will likely require suprarenal aortic cross clamping. Retroaortic renal veins are easily detected by CT (Fig. 37-3). Prior knowledge of a retro aortic left renal vein will decrease the chance for intraoperative injury. Other findings that CT is able to reliably demonstrate preoperatively include renal abnormalities (e.g., horseshoe and pelvic kidneys) (Figs. 37-4 and 37-5); intraabdominal masses; inflammatory aneurysms; gallstones; and diverticulitis.

Despite these advantages of CT scanning in planning open repair of AAA, there are several features of CT that may make this imaging modality less attractive in certain patient populations. CT requires the use of intravenous contrast material and subjects the patients to potentially harmful ionizing radiation. In addition, in patients with spinal instrumentation, the presence of metallic artifact interferes with AAA imaging (Fig. 37-6).

Angiography

The use of angiography has historically been regarded as the "gold standard" for imaging AAAs before open repair.[19,20] The ability of angiography to demonstrate stenotic lesions of the renal arteries and occlusive disease of the iliofemoral vessels makes this imaging modality extremely useful before surgical intervention in patients suspected to have concomitant vascular disease. Studies have shown that the presence of peripheral occlusive disease in patients with known AAA is high, and the suspicion of extra-aortic disease necessitates further workup with angiography.[19,21] In patients with uncontrolled hypertension or unexplained renal dysfunction, renal artery stenosis should be suspected. Although CT

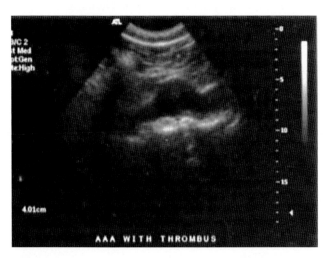

Figure 37-1. Ultrasound depicting 4.2-cm abdominal aortic aneurysm.

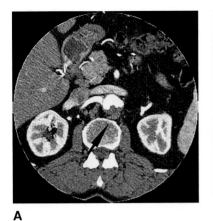

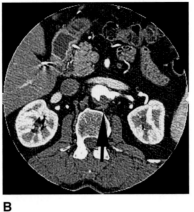

Figure 37-2. *CT of aorta with intravenous contrast demonstrating extensive thrombus within the aorta seen posteriorly at level of (**A**) left renal and (**B**) right renal arteries.*

A   **B**

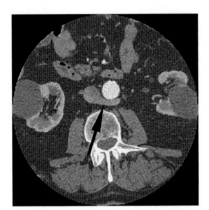

Figure 37-3. *CT of aorta with intravenous contrast demonstrating the presence of a retroaortic left renal vein.*

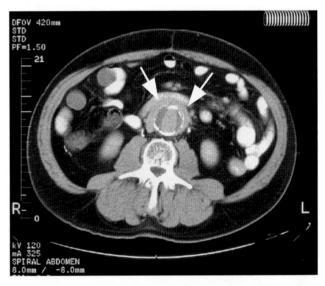

Figure 37-5. *CT of aorta with intravenous contrast demonstrating an inflammatory aneurysm (arrows). Note enhancing rim.*

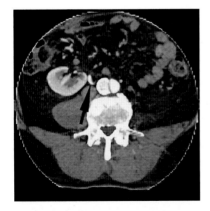

Figure 37-4. *CT of abdomen and pelvis demonstrating AAA and presence of pelvic kidney with a renal artery rising from the aortic bifurcation.*

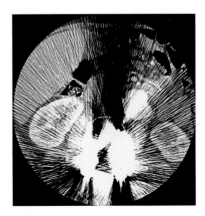

Figure 37-6. *CT of aorta with intravenous contrast suboptimally demonstrating AAA obscured by metallic artifact created by patient's spinal hardware.*

has been shown to accurately demonstrate the location of the renal arteries, their origins off the aorta (where stenotic lesions are likely to occur) are less easily demonstrable.[22] Additionally, patients with AAAs with symptoms of intestinal angina should undergo preoperative angiography to assess the status of the mesenteric circulation. Mesenteric revascularization should be undertaken at the time of AAA repair. Preoperative angiography is needed before AAA repair in patients with symptoms of peripheral artery occlusive disease, peripheral artery aneurysms, symptoms of intestinal ischemia, uncontrolled hypertension, unexplained renal dysfunction, chronic aortic dissection, and horseshoe kidney (Fig. 37-7).[21,23,24] Using these criteria, studies have shown that angiography will demonstrate associated pathology in 28% of cases, as opposed to only about 5% of the time when these criteria are not used.[25,26] Angiography does not come without complications, however, and the need for this invasive study must be addressed critically. Like CT, patients are exposed to intravenous contrast material (perhaps worsening renal dysfunction) as well as ionizing radiation. As previously discussed, angiography may grossly underestimate aneurysm size by only demon-

strating the inner diameter of the aneurysm, neglecting the outer diameter because of the presence of thrombus within the AAA. Arterial puncture used for angiography, although relatively safe, is associated with a complication rate of 1% to 2%.[25,27,28]

CT Angiography

CT angiography (CTA), made possible by advancements in helical CT technology, has developed out of this desire for less invasive testing. Several studies have compared spiral CTA with conventional angiography in demonstrating those characteristics of AAA that help surgeons in preoperative planning. One such study demonstrated that spiral CTA is equally efficacious as conventional angiography in demonstrating the presence of severe (70% to 99%) stenosis or occlusion of the renal arteries.[29] This same study, however, also revealed that spiral CTA poorly demonstrated occlusive disease involving the iliac arteries. Therefore the authors have advocated the use of spiral CTA in the preoperative workup of nonclaudicants who are candidates for AAA repair. In comparison with conventional angiography, size determination of AAA by spiral CT angiography has been shown to be more accurate, making CTA more valuable in determining the timing for operative intervention.[30,31] Additionally, CTA is comparable to conventional angiography in its ability to accurately demonstrate both proximal and distal extent of AAA.

Although the amount of intravenous contrast material and radiation exposure is slightly higher with CTA as compared with conventional angiography,[29] the noninvasive nature of CTA, the relative safety in performing this test, and the comparable information it provides in the preoperative assessment of patients with AAA make this radiographic imaging modality the ideal complement to routine CT scanning. CT angiography and 3-D reconstruction have all but voided the need for catheter-based angiography.

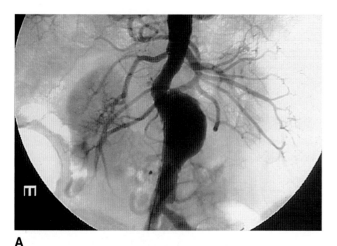

A

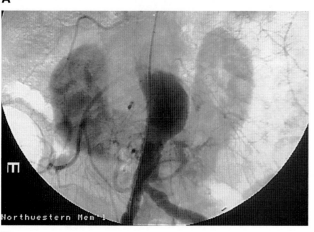

B

*Figure 37-7. **A** and **B**, Arteriogram depicting the presence of an AAA and horseshoe kidney.*

Magnetic Resonance Imaging

Magnetic resonance imaging (MRI) and magnetic resonance angiography (MRA) have been used as noninvasive modalities for imaging AAAs before open repair. With improvements in gating technology (both electrocardiographic and respiratory gating, to reduce the amount of artifact produced by cardiac and respiratory motion) and fast scanning (which allows for image acquisition with a single breath-hold), MRI and MRA have become more commonly utilized tools in planning open repair of AAA (Fig. 37-8). Unlike CT angiography and conventional angiography, MRA is not dependent on the use

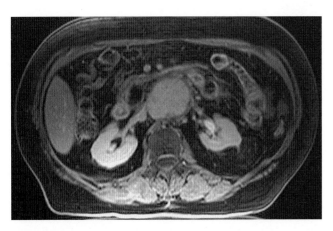

Figure 37-8. *MRI demonstrating AAA at level of renal arteries (transverse image).*

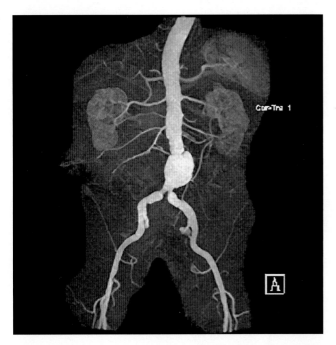

Figure 37-9. *MR angiogram demonstrating 5.5-cm fusiform infrarenal AAA with concomitant mild to moderate ostial stenosis of right renal artery and diminutive left renal artery.*

of iodinated contrast material, and therefore is indicated to evaluate AAA in patients with known contrast allergy or renal insufficiency. In patients in whom catheter angiography is deemed dangerous or in whom vascular access is difficult, MRA may be a suitable alternative to conventional angiography (Fig. 37-9). MRI and CT (the two main cross-sectional modalities used to image AAAs) share the advantages over other techniques of being able to demonstrate the presence of intraluminal thrombus and to detect perianeurysmal inflammation and hemorrhage.

Various reports have confirmed the abilities of MRI and MRA to accurately define the proximal neck of AAAs, to determine the number of renal arteries present, to demonstrate the presence of stenoses greater than 50% at the origin of the renal arteries, and to assess the patency

of the superior mesenteric artery.[32–36] In comparison with conventional angiography, however, MRA is less accurate in determining the patency of the inferior mesenteric artery and concomitant iliofemoral disease. One group has demonstrated that the use of MRA in combination with Doppler arterial flow studies, in patients without evidence of mesenteric, renal, or iliac artery occlusive disease, may be an effective alternative to conventional angiography and CT in preoperative planning for AAA repair.[37]

Despite the inherent advantages of MRI and MRA, the use of magnetic resonance (MR) has been limited for a variety of reasons. The uniform use of MR for imaging AAAs before operative repair (among all institutions performing such procedures) has been limited by the cost of MR hardware and the implementation of software specifically used for angiography and 3-D reconstruction. However, the use of outpatient facilities with the capability of MRI and MRA appears to be increasing. Despite technical advances made in the field of MR, some traditional constraints still apply. For instance, the presence of certain types of intracranial aneurysm clips and indwelling pacemakers limits the use of MR. Additionally, patient claustrophobia and long acquisition times further prohibit the universal use of MRI and MRA for preoperative AAA imaging. Further advancements in the field of MR will likely make this imaging modality more attractive to the vascular surgeon planning open repair of AAA in the future.

Conclusions

As technological advancements continue to be made in imaging AAA, surgeons are becoming more informed about the characteristics that influence their approach to the open repair of AAA. These advancements make surgical management of AAA and the postoperative care of patients with AAA more predictable and efficient. The use of ultrasonography, computed tomography, angiography, CTA, and MR in the preoperative work-up of AAA is ultimately dictated by the patient's presenting signs and symptoms and by local technology. Further developments in these areas will continue to make open repair of AAA a safe and effective management option in dealing with this potentially lethal disease.

The quality of imaging techniques will continually improve. Today the goal of imaging is to define anatomy; in the future, arterial physiology and hemodynamics will be determined by this same technology, and new information will be available on aneurysm rupture. Work by Fillinger[38,39] and Vorp[40,41] using finite element analysis and standard CT scans is leading to the ability to determine areas of high shear stress and high wall tension (Fig. 37-10). Such factors may be predictive in aneurysm rupture.

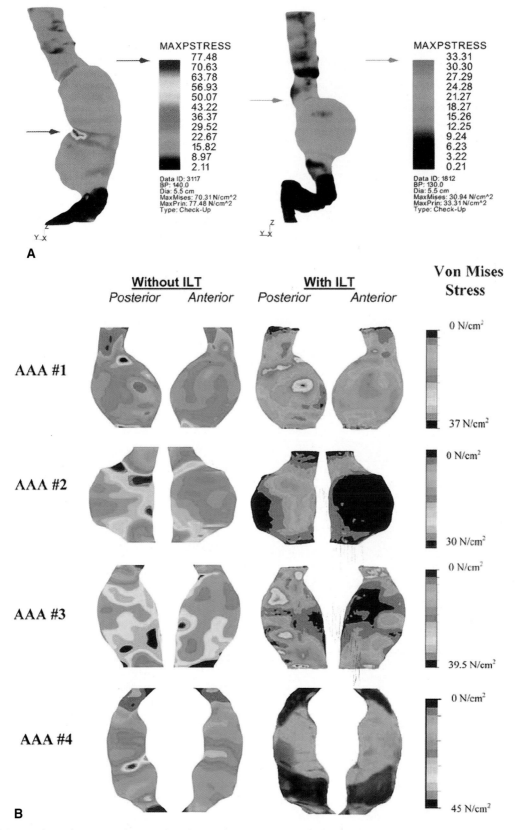

Figure 37-10. A, *Three-dimensional stress distribution for maximum wall stress at peak systolic blood pressure for two 5.5-cm aneurysms. Stress is mapped to corresponding color, with highest stress shown in red and lowest stress shown in blue. Stress map for patient on the right has been color-coded to correspond with stress map for patient on the left, for ease of comparison.* **B**, *Finite element (computational stress) analysis may be useful in determining the degree and distribution of mechanical forces or stresses acting on the wall of individual AAA. Shown here are the distributions of wall stresses on the posterior and anterior abdominal aortic walls of six different 3-D reconstructed AAA and one nonaneurysmal control aorta. Gray regions are those with artificially high stress concentrations because of edge effects. The common color scale provides stress magnitude. In all cases, blue represents the lowest stress magnitude and red the highest. Note the comparatively lower range of stress in the control aorta. Reprinted with permission from Mosby.[39,40]*

REFERENCES

1. Dubost C, Allary M, Oeconomos N: Resection of an aneurysm of the abdominal aorta: Reestablishment of the continuity by a preserved human arterial graft, with results after 5 months. Arch Surg 64:405–408, 1952.
2. Hertzer NR, Avellone JC, Farrell CJ, et al: The risk of vascular surgery in a metropolitan community, with observations on surgeon's experience and hospital size. J Vasc Surg 1:13, 1984.
3. Johnston KW, Scobie TK: Multicenter prospective study of non-ruptured abdominal aortic aneurysms: Population and operative management. J Vasc Surg 7:69, 1988.
4. Pilcher DB, Davis JH, Ashikaga T, et al: Treatment of abdominal aortic aneurysm in an entire state over 7.5 years. Am J Surg 139:487, 1980.
5. Laroy LL, Cormier PJ, Matalon TAS, et al: Imaging of abdominal aortic aneurysms. Am J Radiol 152:785–792, 1989.
6. Ernst CB: Abdominal aortic aneurysm. N Engl J Med 328:1167–1172, 1993.
7. Rose WM, Ernst CB: Abdominal aortic aneurysm. Compr Ther 21:339–433, 1995.
8. Lamah M, Drake S: Value of routine computed tomography in the preoperative assessment of abdominal aortic aneurysm replacement. World J Surg 23:1076–1081, 1999.
9. Vowden P, Wilkinson D, Ausobsky JR, et al: A comparison of three imagining techniques in the assessment of an abdominal aortic aneurysm. J Cardiovasc Surg 30:891–896, 1989.
10. Sternbergh WC, Gonze MD, Garrerd CL, et al: Abdominal and thoracoabdominal aortic aneurysm. Surg Clin North Am 78:827–843, 1998.
11. Myers K, Devine T: Abdominal aortic aneurysms. The old and the new. Aust Fam Physician 26:418–425, 1997.
12. Amparo EG, Hoddick WK, Hricak H, et al: Comparison of magnetic imaging and ultrasonography in the evaluation of abdominal aortic aneurysms. Radiol 154:451, 1985.
13. Wheeler WE, Beachley MC, Ranninger K: Angiography and ultrasonography: A comparative study of abdominal aortic aneurysms. Am J Radiol 126:95, 1976.
14. Leotta DF, Paun M, Beach KW, et al: Measurement of abdominal aortic aneurysms with three-dimensional ultrasound imaging: preliminary report. J Vasc Surg 33:700–707, 2001.
15. Johnson BL, Harris EJ Jr, Fogarty TJ, et al: Color duplex evaluation of endoluminal aortic stent grafts. J Vascular Tech 22:97–104, 1998.
16. Berdejo GL, Lyon RT, Ohki T, et al: Color duplex ultrasound evaluation of transluminally placed endovascular grafts for aneurysm repair. J Vascular Tech 22:201–207, 1998.
17. Gomes MN, Choyke PL: Preoperative evaluation of abdominal aortic aneurysms: Ultrasound or computed tomography? J Cardiovasc Surg 28:159, 1987.
18. Posacioglu H, Islamoglu F, Apaydin AZ, et al: Predictive value of conventional computed tomography in determining proximal extent of abdominal aortic aneurysms and possibility of infrarenal clamping. Tex Heart Inst J 29:172–175, 2002.
19. Kwaan JH, Conolly JE, Molen RV, et al: The value of aortography before abdominal aneurysmectomy. Am J Surg 121:542, 1977.
20. Robicsek F, Daugherty HK, Mullen DC, et al: The value of angiography in the diagnosis of unruptured aneurysms of the abdominal aorta. Ann Thorac Surg 11:538, 1971.
21. Brewster DC, Retana A, Waltman AC, et al: Angiography in the management of aneurysms of the abdominal aorta: Its value and safety. N Engl J Med 292:822–825, 1975.

22. Papanicolaou N, Wittenberg J, Ferrucci JT, et al: Preoperative evaluation of abdominal aortic aneurysms by computed tomography. Am J Roentgenol 146:711–715, 1986.
23. Bell DD, Gaspar MR: Routine aortography before abdominal aortic aneurysmectomy. Am J Surg 144:191, 1982.
24. Thompson JE, Hollier LH, Patman RD, et al: Surgical management of abdominal aortic aneurysms: Factors influencing mortality and morbidity: A 20-year experience. Ann Surg 181:654, 1975.
25. Couch NP, O'Mahoney J, McIrvine A, et al: The place of abdominal aortography in abdominal aortic aneurysm resection. Arch Surg 118:1029–1034, 1983.
26. Bandyk DF: Preoperative imaging of aortic aneurysms: Conventional and digital angiography, computed tomography scanning, and magnetic resonance imaging. Surg Clin North Am 69:721–735, 1989.
27. Lang EK: Prevention and treatment of complications following arteriography. Radiology 88:950, 1968.
28. Szilagyi DE, Smith RF, Mackgood AJ, et al: Abdominal aortography: Values and hazards. Arch Surg 85:41, 1962.
29. Errington ML, Ferguson JM, Gillespie IN, et al: Complete preoperative imaging assessment of abdominal aortic aneurysm with spiral CT angiography. Clin Radiol 52:369–377, 1997.
30. Gomes MN, Schellinger D, Hufnagel CA: Abdominal aortic aneurysms: Diagnostic review and new technique. Ann Thorac Surg 27:479–488, 1979.
31. Brewster DC, Darling RC, Raines JK, et al: Assessment of abdominal aortic aneurysm size. Circulation 56(Supp 2):164–167, 1977.
32. Tennant WG, Hartnell GG, Baird RN, et al: Radiological investigation of abdominal aortic aneurysm disease: Comparison of three modalities in staging and the detection of inflammatory change. J Vasc Surg 17:703–709, 1993.
33. Arlart IP, Guhl L, Edelman RE: Magnetic resonance angiography of the abdominal aorta. Cardiovasc Intervent Radiol 15:43–50, 1992.
34. Kim D, Edelman RR, Kent KC, et al: Abdominal aorta and renal artery stenosis: Evaluation with MR angiography. Radiology 174:727–731, 1990.
35. Gedrovc WMW, Neerhut P, Negus R, et al: Magnetic resonance angiography of renal artery stenosis. Clin Radiol 50:436–439, 1995.
36. Debatin JF, Spritzer CE, Grist TM, et al: Imaging of the renal arteries: Value of MR angiography. Am J Roentgenol 157:981–990, 1991.
37. Durham JR, Hackworth CA, Tober JC, et al: Magnetic resonance angiography in the preoperative evaluation of abdominal aortic aneurysms. Am J Surg 166:173–178, 1993.
38. Fillinger MF, Raghavan ML, Marra SP, et al: In vivo analysis of mechanical wall stress and abdominal aortic aneurysm rupture risk. J Vasc Surg 36:589–597, 2002.
39. Fillinger MF, Marra SP, Raghavan ML, et al: Prediction of rupture risk in abdominal aortic aneurysm during observation: Wall stress versus diameter. J Vasc Surg 37:724–732, 2003.
40. Raghavan ML, Vorp DA, Federle MP, et al: Wall stress distribution on three-dimensionally reconstructed models of human abdominal aortic aneurysm. J Vasc Surg 31:760–769, 2000.
41. Vorp DA: Association of intraluminal thrombus in abdominal aortic aneurysm with local hypoxia and wall weakening. J Vasc Surg 34:291–299, 2001.

Chapter 38

Preoperative Imaging for Endovascular Grafts: CT Angiography

M. ASHRAF MANSOUR • KIM J. HODGSON

The management of abdominal aortic aneurysms (AAAs) has evolved dramatically over the last century, from a mandatory laparotomy to a condition now often amenable to less invasive endoluminal repair. It is interesting to note that some of the first efforts to repair AAAs were endoluminal in nature. In 1864, an English surgeon placed 75 feet of wire in an AAA to induce thrombosis. Fifteen years later, an Italian physician attempted coagulation of an AAA by passing an electrical current through a wire inserted in it.[1] In the ensuing decades, a variety of ill-fated attempts were reported, but it was not until Dubost, in 1951, described the successful technique of aortic replacement that routine repair of AAAs became possible.[2] Although initial open repairs were done with aortic homograft (a material seldom used anymore outside of infected beds), nowadays fabric grafts made of Dacron or polytetrafluoroethylene (PTFE) are used almost exclusively. In large series of open AAA repairs from centers of excellence, the hospital mortality for AAA repair was reduced to around 3% in the 1990s.[2] The vast majority of these patients are properly screened and medically managed before elective operation. In contrast, the mortality from emergent AAA repair remains largely unchanged, ranging from 50% to 90%.[2,3]

Recent efforts to reduce perioperative morbidity and mortality, as well as to extend treatment to include higher surgical risk patients, centered on devising a lesser invasive method for AAA repair.[4] It was Parodi's pioneering animal experiments, begun in 1976, that led in 1990 to the first successful endograft implantation in a patient with an AAA.[5,6] His novel concept of replacing the conduit from inside the vessel led to a wave of innovation in endograft design. Over the ensuing decade, numerous investigators using many different graft designs have shown that endovascular AAA repair

TABLE 38-1. Indications for Preoperative Angiography in AAA Patients

- Juxtarenal or suprarenal AAA

- Suspected renal artery stenosis (renovascular hypertension)

- Congenital renal anomalies (horseshoe, ectopic, pancake kidney)

- Renal transplantation

- Suspected visceral artery stenosis

- Iliofemoral occlusive disease

- Previous colon resection

- Reoperative surgery

TABLE 38-2. Desirable Inclusion Criteria for EVAR

Proximal neck
- Diameter: 18 to 26 mm*
- Length: 15 mm†
- Shape: cylindrical
- Morphology: absence of circumferential thrombus or calcification

Distal landing zone (common or external iliac)
- Diameter: 8 to 13
- Length: 10 mm
- Shape: nonaneurysmal‡
- Morphology: absence of severe tortuosity and calcification

Access site
- Patent femoral or iliac artery
- Vessel diameter greater than 7 mm

Renal function
- Serum creatinine less than 2.5 mg/L
- Renal failure on hemodialysis

Cooperative patient who can tolerate local anesthesia

EVAR = endovascular AAA repair
*Some grafts (Zenith) allow for a neck diameter less than 28 mm, and custom-made grafts can accommodate larger necks.
†Some investigators require only 10 mm of neck length.
‡For aneurysmal iliac arteries, adjunctive techniques such as bell-bottom or custom-made grafts can be used.

is both feasible and safe.[7-13] The purpose of this chapter is to review the role of CT angiography in the preoperative planning for such endovascular AAA repair (EVAR).

Open Versus Endovascular AAA Repair

Before EVAR, good surgical risk patients presenting with an AAA greater than 5 cm in maximal diameter were advised to undergo open repair, either transperitoneally or using the retroperitoneal approach. In more than 80% of elective cases, a preoperative CT scan was all that was needed to plan surgical repair. In the remaining patients, an additional angiographic investigation was necessary. The indications for preoperative angiography are listed in Table 38-1.

However, the preoperative evaluation of patients being considered for EVAR differs from open repair because of the nuances of the technique. Because most available endografts are inserted via the femoral or iliac approach, certain criteria relevant to these vessels need to be met before considering patients for EVAR[7-13] (Table 38-2). Similarly, all available endografts rely on friction for fixation to the nonaneurysmal aorta and iliac arteries, friction created or enhanced by barbs, hooks, or a self-expanding design.[14] All commercially available endografts have specific sizing recommendations that should be followed diligently to avoid problems with insertion or deployment. Therefore, it is of utmost importance to obtain adequate preoperative imaging studies to plan EVAR.

Spiral (Helical) Computed Tomography

The older generation of conventional CT scanners acquired images by moving the patient on a table in a step-wise fashion through a stationary radiographic gantry. Newer generation CT scanners have a slip-ring coupling that allows 360-degree gantry rotation and continuous scanning of a specific area while the patient is transported on the moving table.[15-20] Thus, with a single breath-hold of 25 to 30 seconds it is possible to acquire a large amount of data that can be reconstructed later into three-dimensional pictures using specialized software. Various programs are available commercially (e.g., Preview, Medical Media Systems MMS, West Lebanon, NH) (Fig. 38-1).

Compared with conventional CT scans, spiral CT scan resolution is essentially identical in the XY plane, on the order of 1 mm. The speed of movement of the table, the z-axis dimension, determines the volume that is imaged in the 30-second scan period. Therefore, resolution and scan coverage along the z-axis are inversely related. Higher resolution is achieved by decreasing the collimator width (slice thickness); however, it is important that collimation not be less than half of the table travel.[15-20]

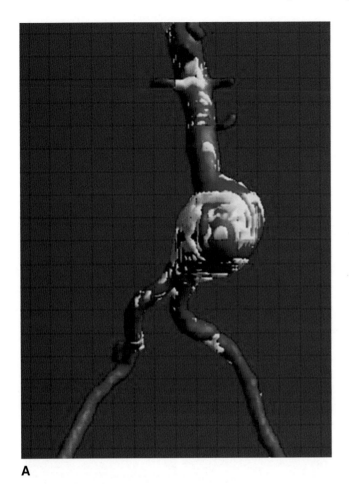

A

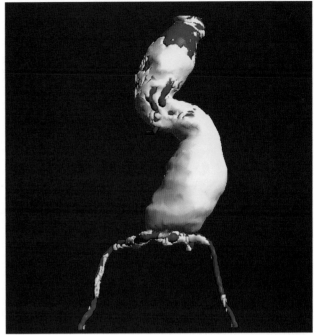

B

Figure 38-1. **A**, *3-D reconstruction of spiral CT scan showing an infrarenal AAA. Note that the proximal neck dimensions, as well as the distal extent and iliac arteries, can be clearly evaluated.* **B**, *3-D reconstruction of spiral CT scan showing an infrarenal AAA. Note the proximal neck tortuosity that exclude this patient from EVAR. (Software: Preview, Medical Media System MMS, West Lebanon, NH; photos courtesy of Medtronic-AVE, USA.)*

The use of intravenous contrast allows for opacification of vascular structures (Fig. 38-2). A bolus of 120 to 150 mL of intravenous contrast is either manually or mechanically injected. The scan should be started 20 to 30 seconds after injection to coincide with the midarterial phase. Typically, for AAA evaluation, collimation (slice thickness) is set for 2 to 5 mm, table speed at 1× to 2× collimation (in mm/sec), IV contrast bolus injection of 120 mL at 2 to 5 mL/sec, 30 to 50 seconds continuous scan time, and x-ray source rotating 360 degrees per second while breath is being held. These settings should allow acquisition of raw data over a linear distance of 9 to 50 cm. Actual scan time with the spiral technique is markedly reduced because data acquisition is continuous. This usually allows complete imaging while the patient is holding his or her breath, which eliminates motion artifacts related to breathing.[15–20]

With specialized software, reformatting into sagittal, coronal, or arbitrary planes is possible (see Fig. 38-2; Figs. 38-3 through 38-6). The ability to obtain 3-D and what are essentially 360-degree structural images allows for comprehensive evaluation of visceral and renal arteries, as well as the AAA and its proximal and distal aspects (Figs. 38-7 through 38-9). The combination of spiral CT and multiplanar reformatting is termed *CT angiography*.

Preoperative Evaluation

In considering whether or not to employ EVAR, complete evaluation of the AAA and its proximal and distal extents is needed.[20] Because the grafts are usually inserted via the femoral artery, either percutaneously or with a cutdown, the femoral (access vessel) artery must also be evaluated. The length, diameter, and shape of the proximal neck aids in the selection of graft type and size (see Fig. 38-1). Similarly, the presence or absence of tortuosity in the proximal neck or iliac arteries may modify the approach used in repair.[20–22] The characteristics that are evaluated to aid in patient selection for EVAR are listed in Table 38-2. Depending on the availability of specialized or custom-made grafts, and also the experience of the surgeon, some of the criteria for EVAR can be more permissive.

Proximal Neck

Evaluation of the proximal neck is one of the most important aspects of the preoperative evaluation. Much

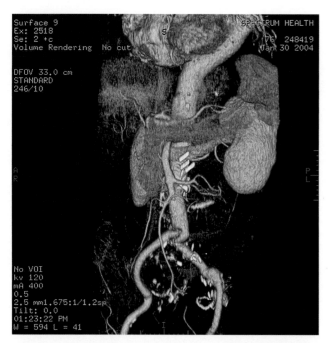

Figure 38-2. *3-D reconstruction of aorta and iliacs in a patient who had open AAA repair. In this projection, the left kidney and spleen are easily seen. The bright white marks are surgical clips. Note that the iliac aneurysms cannot be clearly seen on this projection. (Software: Soma™ Corporation, Rosemount, MN.)*

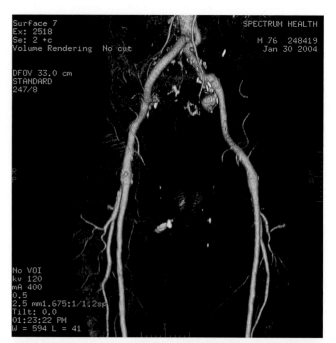

A

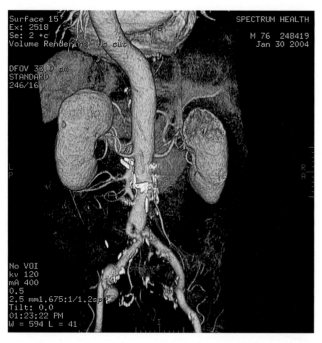

Figure 38-3. *3-D reconstruction of the patient in Figure 38-2; this picture is rotated so that one is looking from the back, and the spleen is on the opposite side. Additional surgical clips can be seen. Now, the right common iliac and hypogastric aneurysms can be seen. The reference points are noted on the picture and designated as R and L (for right and left of patient) and A and P (for anterior and posterior).*

B

Figure 38-4. *A, B, 3-D reconstruction of the patient in Figures 38-2 and 38-3, now focusing on the iliacs and femorals. These two projections clearly show that there is a right iliac aneurysm.*

of this information has been facilitated by spiral CT with 3-D reconstruction. At the outset, the accurate measurement of neck length and diameter are essential. Most aortic necks are elliptical in shape, at least in traditional axial CT images, making it difficult to measure their true diameters. This may be the true aortic configuration or may be caused by aortic angulation viewed on standard

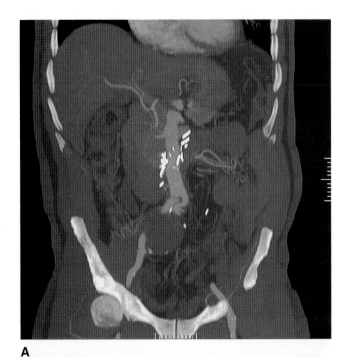

A

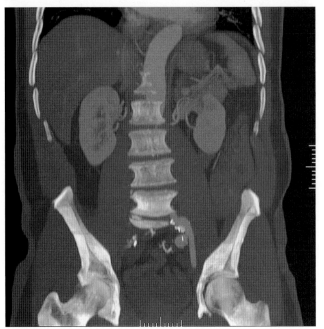

B

Figure 38-5. ***A***, ***B***, *Coronal slices of patient showing the right iliac aneurysm; surgical clips seen most clearly in* ***A***. *As the slices are reconstructed more posteriorly, the bony structures of the spine begin to appear, and now the kidneys are better defined as well as a small left hypogastric aneurysm.*

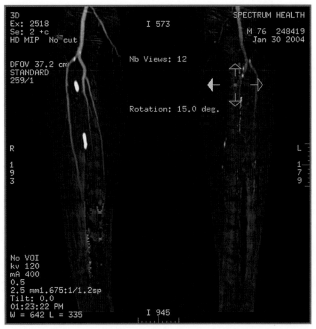

Figure 38-6. *CT angiography of the legs showing a nice trifurcation on the right, less defined on the left.*

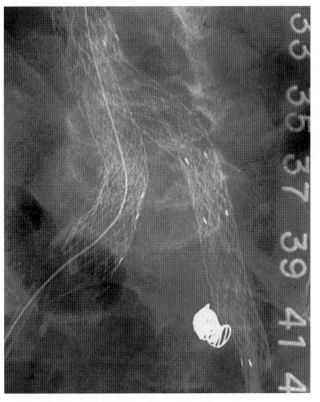

Figure 38-7. *AneuRx graft in a patient who underwent successful EVAR. Note that the right common iliac artery is ectatic and was treated with the bell-bottom technique, whereas the left hypogastric was coiled and the origin of the vessel covered with the stent graft.*

axial CT slicing. Without the benefit of 3-D reconstruction, most surgeons base their measurements on the shortest distance, assuming that angulation is responsible for the elliptical configuration; this leads to oversizing in 14% and undersizing in 5% of patients.[23] Proper assessment of the neck diameter is greatly facilitated by

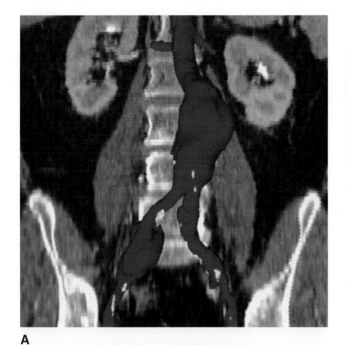

A

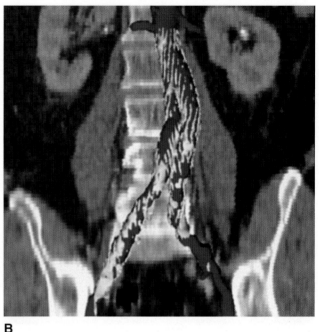

B

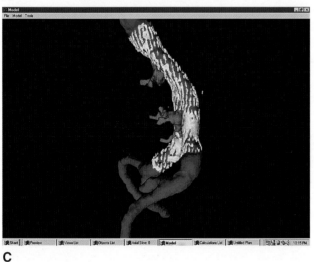

C

*Figure 38-8. **A**, 3-D reconstruction of AAA showing single renal arteries, a slightly tortuous neck but suitable for repair. **B**, 3-D reconstruction of the aorta in the same patient after successful EVAR showing satisfactory exclusion of the AAA. **C**, Spiral CT in the lateral projection showing the vessel tortuosity and good graft apposition after EVAR.*

spiral CT with 3-D reconstruction, which allows reconfiguration of the images to correspond to aortic centerline projections, largely negating the effect of tortuosity (see Fig. 38-1 and Fig. 38-8, *A*).

Whereas angulation of the neck may compromise both endograft fixation and fabric-wall apposition, other factors can also be problematic. The presence of circumferential calcification or thrombus may present a problem for EVAR because it can compromise the proximal fixation of the graft and lead to a type I endoleak. Calcification may prevent optimal endograft wall contact, and therefore may compromise attainment of a hemostatic seal; however, the problem with thrombus, or "soft plaque," that cannot be distinguished by CT, is whether to size the endograft for the inner or outer diameter measured. As previously mentioned, it is recommended that the diameter of the graft be 20% greater than the diameter of the neck to

achieve stable fixation and a hemostatic seal. These recommendations are for average aortic necks, and may require adjustment in other situations. Following EVAR, some patients develop gradual neck dilatation that may lead to graft slippage, endoleak, and possible AAA rupture after initial successful repair.[24,25] It is for this reason that lifelong CT scan follow-up is presently recommended for EVAR patients.

Visceral Vessels

Patients with a history of poorly controlled hypertension or who have symptoms suggestive of mesenteric ischemia merit complete evaluation of the visceral arteries before EVAR. Before the availability of 3-D reconstructed

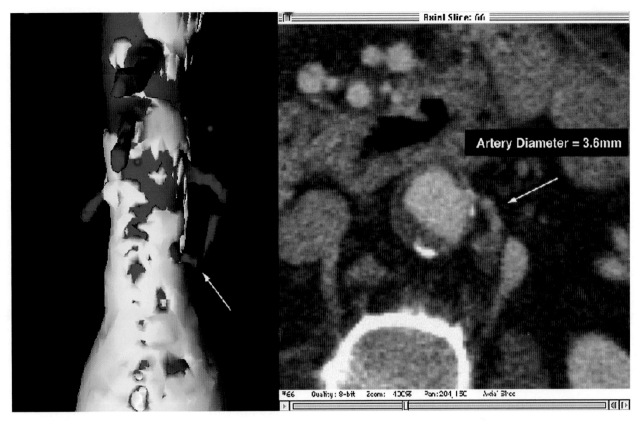

Figure 38-9. *Spiral CT focusing on the neck of the aneurysm and showing the presence of a smaller left accessory renal artery. (Software: Preview, Medical Media System MMS, West Lebanon, NH; picture courtesy of Medtronic-AVE, USA.)*

spiral CT scans, angiography was required to achieve this. However, several investigators have shown that spiral CT scans are nearly as accurate as angiography in detecting renal and mesenteric stenosis.[18-20] When detected preoperatively, some vascular surgeons prefer to address these lesions before EVAR; others advocate addressing them several months after EVAR. Pre-EVAR treatment is generally indicated if there are critical stenoses that might complicate the patient's tolerance of intravascular contrast administration, or if there is significant mesenteric disease and EVAR will be removing collateral vessels (e.g., the inferior mesenteric artery or one or more hypogastric arteries) from circulation. The delayed approach, on the other hand, is a particular consideration in patients with ostial renal or mesenteric stenoses, where projection of any stent into the aortic lumen, as is typical, could lead to stent dislodgement at the time of EVAR.

Renal and Venous Anomalies

The presence of an ectopic or horseshoe kidney may complicate EVAR because the renal arteries may arise directly from the aneurysm. Similarly, if a lower pole accessory renal artery is present, the exact location of this vessel and its contribution to overall renal perfusion needs to be determined preoperatively, with the latter typically requiring angiographic evaluation (see Fig. 38-9, A). It has been the authors' practice to cover accessory renal arteries with the endograft, if needed, to achieve adequate fixation and seal, as long as they contribute to no more than 25% of a kidney's parenchymal perfusion.

Venous anomalies (e.g., retroaortic left renal vein or a duplicated inferior vena cava) are worth noting. Although these anomalies may not impact EVAR, knowledge of their presence may avert intraoperative mishaps in case of an open conversion. A small number of ruptured AAAs with aortocaval fistula may be best treated by EVAR.[26]

Iliac Arteries

As with the proximal neck imaging, it is essential to fully evaluate the iliac arteries, including the status of the hypogastric arteries. The preferred landing zone or distal extent of the endograft is the common iliac artery; however, if the common iliac is aneurysmal or ectatic, an alternative approach has to be chosen. In some cases, it is feasible to extend the endograft into the external iliac artery with or without preoperative embolization of the ipsilateral hypogastric artery (see Fig. 38-7). If the hypogastric artery is patent, most authors advise pre-EVAR embolization to prevent a late type II endoleak. A means to accommodate ectatic, but nonaneurysmal iliac arteries is the so-called "bell-bottom" technique. This technique consists of deploying a proximal aortic cuff, which come in sizes of 20 to 28 mm, in the common iliac artery to provide adequate sealing and avoid covering the hypogastric artery[27–29] (see Fig. 38-7). The authors prefer to limit this approach to common iliac arteries no more than 2 cm in diameter and free of significant wall thrombus. The bell-bottom approach often allows the sparing of one hypogastric artery, whereas the other is sacrificed by endografting into the external iliac artery on that side after coil embolizing the hypogastric artery. This is because most patients with iliac involvement have it bilaterally.

Conversely, the presence of significant occlusive disease in the iliac vessels may need to be addressed before EVAR. This usually consists of balloon angioplasty to permit passage of the device, with any necessary stenting being deferred until the end of the procedure to avoid subsequent stent dislodgement. Some authors prefer to address significant occlusive lesions 4 to 6 weeks before EVAR to be confident in their access and to allow time for any stent to fully incorporate. In the currently available endografts, the smallest size for the main body is an 18 Fr sheath (7 mm in outer diameter); therefore, if the femoral or external iliac arteries are less than 7 mm, an alternative approach has to be contemplated (e.g., a retroperitoneal iliac artery exposure) for access into this larger vessel.

Finally, tortuous iliac arteries may be a barrier to EVAR. Because most devices are fairly stiff, it is essential that the iliac arteries be straightened out to permit passage of the endograft. Often the iliac tortuosity can be dealt with by use of stiff wires at the time of EVAR. These anatomic challenges can be easily predicted by inspection of the preoperative 3-D spiral CT scan.

Postoperative Follow-Up

Spiral CT scans play an important role in the postoperative surveillance of patients who had an ostensibly successful endovascular repair of AAA. Soon after the first endografts were implanted, several authors presented case reports of patients having sudden AAA rupture.[25] Because of numerous factors related to graft-vessel wall interaction, graft component fatigue, aneurysm expansion, and other forces, patients should be followed diligently after EVAR. Ideally, noninvasive methods should be chosen. Spiral CT is ideal for sequential comparisons, monitoring aneurysm behavior (growth vs. shrinkage), and graft position relative to a fixed reference point.[30–32]

Conclusions

Spiral CT scanning is a relatively new technique that has proven to be invaluable in the evaluation of patients being considered for EVAR because its rapid image acquisition provides high-resolution imaging. With the development of new software, it is possible to obtain 3-D reconstruction of the aorta and its major branches. Proper CT imaging of the AAA, including the proximal neck and iliac arteries, has become a requirement for all patients undergoing evaluation for possible EVAR. The availability of spiral CT with 3-D reconstruction can decrease the need for preoperative angiography in patients being considered for EVAR and can aid in procedural planning, which may minimize the number of endograft components utilized to effect the EVAR.

KEY POINTS

- Spiral CT scan with 3-D reconstruction is an excellent method to evaluate patients for possible endovascular abdominal aortic aneurysm repair.

- The ability to reconstruct images of the aorta and its branches can effectively supplant angiography.

- In patient selection for EVAR, the dimensions of the proximal neck are often the principal determinant of procedure eligibility.

- With spiral CT, accurate information about the visceral vessels and iliacs is easily obtained.

- Spiral CT is also very helpful in evaluating patients after EVAR to look for satisfactory aneurysm exclusion.

REFERENCES

1. Lazarus HM: Endovascular grafting for the treatment of abdominal aortic aneurysms. Surg Clin North Am 72:959–968, 1992.
2. Ernst CB: Abdominal aortic aneurysm. N Engl J Med 328:1167–1172, 1993.
3. Katz DJ, Stanley JC, Zelenock GB: Operative mortality rates for intact and ruptured abdominal aortic aneurysms in Michigan: An 11-year statewide experience. J Vasc Surg 19:804–817, 1994.
4. Volodos NL, Karpovich IP, Troyan VI, et al: Clinical experience of the use of self-fixing synthetic prostheses for remote endoprosthetics of the thoracic and abdominal aorta and iliac arteries through the femoral artery and as intraoperative endoprosthesis for aorta reconstruction. Vasa Suppl 33:93–95, 1991.
5. Parodi JC, Palmaz JC, Barone HD: Transfemoral intraluminal graft implantation for abdominal aortic aneurysms. Ann Vasc Surg 5:491–499, 1991.
6. Parodi JC: Endovascular repair of abdominal aortic aneurysms and other arterial lesions. J Vasc Surg 21:549–557, 1995.
7. Moore WS, Vescera CL: Repair of abdominal aortic aneurysm by transfemoral endovascular graft placement. Ann Surg 220:331–341, 1994.
8. Moore WS, Rutherford RB, for the EVT Investigators: Transfemoral endovascular repair of abdominal aortic aneurysm: Results of the North American EVT phase I trial. J Vasc Surg 23(4):543–553, 1996.

9. White RA, Donayre CE, Walot I, et al: Modular bifurcated endoprosthesis for treatment of abdominal aortic aneurysms. Ann Surg 226:381–391, 1997.

10. Blum U, Voschage G, Lammer J, et al: Endoluminal stent-grafts for infrarenal abdominal aortic aneurysms. N Engl J Med 336:13–20, 1997.

11. Chuter TAM: The bifurcated endovascular prosthesis. Adv Vasc Surg 4:37–51, 1996.

12. Zarins CK, White RA, Schwarten D, et al: AneuRx stent graft versus open surgical repair of abdominal aortic aneurysms: Multicenter prospective clinical trial. J Vasc Surg 29:292–308, 1999.

13. Ouriel K, Greenberg RK, Clair DG: Endovascular treatment of aortic aneurysms. Curr Prob Surg 39:233–348, 2002.

14. Malina M, Lindblad B, Ivancev K, et al: Endovascular AAA exclusion: Will stents with hooks and barbs prevent stent-graft migration? J Endovasc Surg 5:310–317, 1998.

15. Kalender WA, Seissler W, Klotz E, et al: Spiral volumetric CT with single-breath-hold technique, continuous transport, and continuous scanner rotation. Radiology 176:181–190, 1990.

16. Rubin GD, Walker PJ, Dake MD, et al: Three-dimensional spiral computed tomographic angiography: An alternative imaging modality for the abdominal aorta and its branches. J Vasc Surg 18:656–665, 1993.

17. Balm R, Eikelboom BC, van Leeuwen MS, et al: Spiral CT-angiography of the aorta. Eur J Vasc Surg 8:544–551, 1194.

18. Cikrit DF, Harris VJ, Hemmer CG, et al: Comparison of spiral CT scan and arteriography for evaluation of renal and visceral arteries. Ann Vasc Surg 10:109–116, 1996.

19. Fillinger MF: Spiral Computed Tomography and 3-D reconstruction Prior to Open or Endovascular Abdominal Aortic Aneurysm Repair. In Yao JST, Pearce WH (eds): Modern Vascular Surgery. New York, NY: McGraw-Hill, 2000.

20. Wyers MC, Fillinger MF, Schermerhorn ML, et al: Endovascular repair of abdominal aortic aneurysm without preoperative arteriography. J Vasc Surg 28:730–738, 2003.

21. Beebe HG, Kritpracha B, Serres S, et al: Endograft planning without preoperative arteriography: A clinical feasibility study. J Endovasc Ther 7:8–15, 2000.

22. Bayle O, Branchereau A, Rosset E, et al: Morphologic assessment of abdominal aortic aneurysms by spiral computed tomographic scanning. J Vasc Surg 26:238–246, 1997.

23. Broeders IA, Blankensteijn JD, Olree M, et al: Preoperative sizing of grafts for transfemoral endovascular aneurysm management: A prospective comparative study of spiral CT angiography, arteriography, and conventional CT imaging. J Endovasc Surg 4:252–261, 1997.

24. Matsumura JS, Chaikof EL: Continued expansion of aortic necks after endovascular repair of abdominal aortic aneurysms. J Vasc Surg 28:422–431, 1998.

25. Bernhard VM, Mitchell RS, Matsumura JS, et al: Ruptured abdominal aortic aneurysm after endovascular repair. J Vasc Surg 35:1155–1162, 2002.

26. Lau LL, O'Reilly MJG, Johnston LC, et al: Endovascular stent-graft repair of primary aortocaval fistula with an abdominal aortoiliac aneurysm. J Vasc Surg 33:425–428, 2001.

27. Kritparcha B, Pigott JP, Russell TE, et al: Bell-bottom aortoiliac endografts: An alternative that preserves pelvic bloodflow. J Vasc Surg 35:874–881, 2002.

28. Ayerdi J, McLafferty RB, Markwell SJ, et al: Indications and outcomes of AneuRx Phase III trial versus use of commercial AneuRx stent graft. J Vasc Surg 37:739–743, 2003.

29. Karch LA, Hodgson KJ, Mattos MA, et al: Management of ectatic, nonaneurysmal iliac arteries during endoluminal aortic aneurysm repair. J Vasc Surg 33:33–38, 2001.

30. May J, White GH, Yu W, et al: Endoluminal repair of abdominal aortic aneurysms: Strengths and weakness of various prostheses observed in a 4.5-year period. J Endovasc Surg 4:147–151, 1997.

31. White RA, Donayre CE, Walot I, et al: Computed tomography assessment of abdominal aortic aneurysm morphology after endograft exclusion. J Vasc Surg 33:S1–S10, 2001.

32. Yeung KK, van der Laan MJ, Wever JJ, et al: New post-imaging software provides fast and accurate volume data from CTA surveillance after endovascular aneurysm repair. J Endovasc Ther 10:887–893, 2003.

Chapter 39

Imaging Modalities for the Diagnosis of Endoleak

JAMES MAY • JOHN PRESTON HARRIS • JENIFER KIDD
• GEOFFREY H. WHITE

▬ Terminology

▬ Classification of Endoleak

▬ Modalities for Imaging Endoleak

The endoluminal method of aneurysm repair has proven to be a much less invasive method than is the conventional open operation. Blood loss at operation, the need for postoperative intensive care, and length of hospital stay are significantly less with the endoluminal technique.[1]

Failure to isolate the aneurysm from the general circulation, however, remains a cause for concern. Such failure is likely to result in further expansion of the aneurysm sac with the potential for rupture.

Terminology

Failure to isolate the aneurysm from the circulation may be detected by angiography, computed tomography (CT), or by duplex ultrasound imaging. This phenomenon had been described in the early literature on endoluminal aneurysm repair as a *leak*. This term, however, was confusing because it has been common practice to use the word *leak* to refer to extravasation of blood outside the aorta associated with aneurysm rupture. The authors proposed that a more specific term for failure to exclude the aneurysm from the circulation would be *endoleak*.[2] This term would be unique to endoluminal grafts because the leak of blood remains within the confines of the vessel but external to the endoluminal graft. The authors suggested the following definition of endoleak:

> Endoleak is a condition associated with endoluminal vascular grafts, defined by the persistence of bloodflow outside the lumen of the endoluminal graft but within an aneurysm sac or adjacent vascular segment being treated by the graft. Endoleak is caused by incomplete sealing or exclusion of the aneurysm sac or vessel segment as evidenced by imaging studies such as contrast-enhanced CT, ultrasonography, or angiography.[3]

The authors further proposed that a clear distinction should be made between endoleak related to the graft device itself and endoleak associated with flow from collateral arterial branches.[4] The authors proposed that these be identified as being Type I or Type II endoleak, respectively:

- Type I endoleak occurs when a persistent channel of bloodflow develops because of an inadequate or ineffective seal at the graft ends.

- Type II endoleak occurs when there is persistent collateral bloodflow into the aneurysm sac flowing retrogradely from patent lumbar arteries, the inferior mesenteric artery, the intercostals arteries (in thoracic aneurysm), or other collateral vessels. In this situation there is usually a complete seal around the graft attachment zones so that the complication is not related directly to the graft itself.

The authors subsequently proposed that the term *Type III endoleak* be introduced for leakage through a defect in the graft fabric or between segments of a modular endograft.[5] In the same paper, the authors suggested that bloodflow through an intact but porous fabric should be termed *Type IV endoleak*.

Classification of Endoleak

Endoleak may be classified by time of occurrence relative to the operation or by site of origin.

Time of Occurrence

An endoleak first detected during the perioperative (30 days or less) period is defined as a primary endoleak. Those detected after this period are termed *secondary endoleaks*. The occurrence of an endoleak after successful intervention or spontaneous resolution is referred to as a *recurrent endoleak*.

Site

The Ad Hoc Committee on Reporting Standards for Endovascular Aortic Aneurysm Repair has recommended

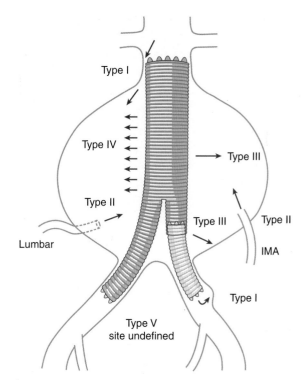

Figure 39-1. *Diagrammatic representation of sites of origin of endoleaks. Types I, III, and IV are endograft-related while Type II are collateral-related*

a classification of endoleak by site of origin.[6] Table 39-1 is a modification of this classification, and Figure 39-1 is a diagrammatic representation of the various types of endoleak. A Type I endoleak results in perigraft bloodflow caused by an inadequate or ineffective seal at either the proximal or distal graft attachment zones. Subscripts a or b indicate Type I endoleak at the proximal or distal ends of the endograft, respectively. Aortouniiliac endografts require an occluder plug in the contralateral common iliac artery to prevent retrograde flow into the abdominal aortic aneurysm (AAA) sac. Subscript c indicates bloodflow around just such an iliac occluder plug. Type II endoleak results from retrograde flow from lumbar arteries, the inferior mesenteric artery (IMA), or other collateral arteries. Type II endoleaks may be further defined by their origin and outflow sources (e.g., lumbar-lumbar, lumbar-IMA, accessory renal-lumbar/IMA, hyporgastric-lumbar/IMA, or unable to be defined). A Type III endoleak may result from any of the following:

- Fabric tears
- Dislocation between component parts of modular grafts
- Inadequate seal between component parts of modular grafts
- Dislocation, inadequate seal between component parts, and fabric tear may be distinguished by subscripts a, b, and c, respectively

TABLE 39-1. **Classification of Endoleak**

Type	Cause of Perigraft Flow
I	Inadequate seal at proximal end of endograft Inadequate seal at distal end of endograft Inadequate seal at iliac occluder plug
II	Flow from collateral vessel (lumbar, IMA, accessory renal, hypogastric) without attachment site connection
III	Flow from modular disconnection Flow from inadequate seal at modular junction Flow from fabric disruption
IV	Flow from porous fabric (less than 30 days after graft placement)
V	Flow visualized but source unidentified

Modified from Chaikof EL, Blankensteijn JD, Harris PL, et al for the Ad Hoc Committee for Standardized Reporting Practices in Vascular Surgery of the Society for Vascular Surgery/American Association for Vascular Surgery: Reporting standards for endovascular aortic aneurysm repair. J Vasc Surg 35:1048–1060, 2002.

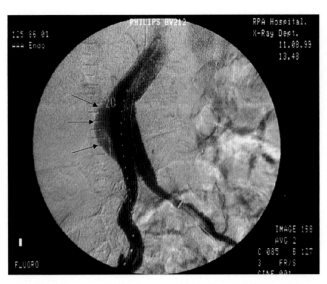

Figure 39-2. *Intraoperative completion arteriogram demonstrating Type IV endoleak due to graft fabric porosity (arrows). CT 48 hours later showed no evidence of endoleak.*

Type IV endoleak results from bloodflow through intact but porous fabric during the perioperative (30-day) period (Fig. 39-2). If a Type IV endoleak persists beyond 30 days, it must be reclassified as a Type III (fabric defect).

Type V endoleaks are those in which bloodflow can be visualized within the aneurysm sac but the source cannot be identified.

Microleaks

Matsumura and colleagues reported a failure mode after endovascular AAA repair not previously recognized.[7] They termed this a *transgraft microleak*, determining that it resulted from a fabric defect at the site of suture holes leading to a persistent Type III endoleak for up to 2½ years after operation. The study authors have emphasized that they are not describing previously unrecognized endoleaks but rather endoleaks that had been seen on standard contrast CT without the exact site of origin being identified. The authors describe a number of special maneuvers that allow the site of these small Type III endoleaks to be identified. These included "directed" angiography with balloon occlusion of the iliac limbs, and careful color-flow duplex ultrasound scanning by skilled sonographers (Fig. 39-3).

Intermittent Endoleak

The authors have recently become aware of the intermittent nature of some endoleaks. A 65-year-old male patient was shown on color duplex ultrasound and CT to have a Type I distal iliac endoleak. He was admitted

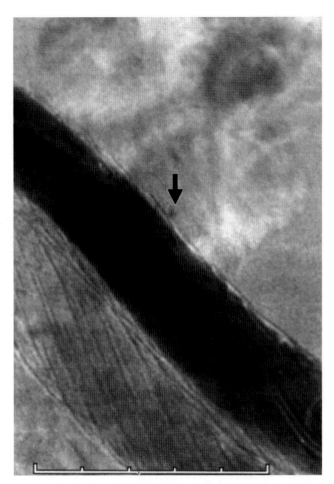

Figure 39-3. *"Directed" arteriogram of one limb of a bifurcated endograft with special tangential view to demonstrate a transgraft "microleak."*

for an aortogram and subsequent secondary extension graft to the culprit iliac limb. Following bedrest in the hospital, however, no leak could be detected despite careful and detailed angiography. Subsequent outpatient investigation by color duplex ultrasound and contrast CT demonstrated the Type I endoleak at the original site. Since managing this patient the authors have become aware of similar anecdotal experiences from colleagues.

Endotension

Endotension has been defined as aneurysm enlargement after endovascular repair in the absence of a detectable endoleak (Fig. 39-4). Explanations for persistent or recurrent pressurization of the aneurysm sac include bloodflow in the sac that is below the sensitivity limits for detection with current imaging technology[5,8,9]; and pressure transmission through thrombus[10,11] or the endograft fabric. The aneurysm may be pulsatile on physical examination, and intrasac pressure measurement may be in the near systemic range.

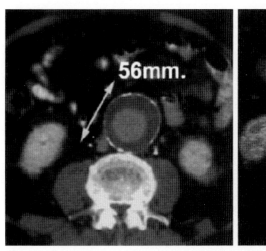
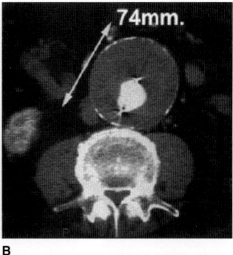

A   B

Figure 39-4. **A,** *Preoperative CT scan.* **B,** *CT scan at 24-month follow-up, showing aneurysm enlargement caused by endotension without evidence of endoleak.*

Modalities for Imaging Endoleak

The imaging of endoleak may be considered during the operative period and in the postoperative period.

Intraoperative Diagnosis of Endoleak

When primary endoleak occurs it will often be detected during the operative procedure by completion angiography. At other times primary endoleak may not be diagnosed until the early postoperative studies (e.g., CT scan or color duplex ultrasound scan) are performed.

All cases of endoleak detected within the perioperative period should be classified as primary endoleak. The cause of these early cases will usually be related to problems in the case selection, design/sizing of a particular graft, or technical problems encountered during the graft implantation. Although an endovascular graft may appear to be sealed at the time of completion angiography, and then develop an endoleak at the time of perioperative imaging, it seems more likely that this is, in fact, a primary endoleak that went undetected initially.

Intraoperative Angiography

Angiograms are usually done at intervals during the implantation procedure and upon its completion. Endoleak is diagnosed by the presence of contrast media outside of the graft lumen, filling completely or partially the lumen of the aneurysm sac. In patients with a large amount of laminated thrombus within the aneurysm, the residual lumen may be reduced to such an extent that contrast outside the graft lumen may be missed. Completion angiography should be performed using a power injector in a precise manner at several sites along the graft length. A pig-tail catheter with multiple holes in the tail is preferred to deliver a large quantity of contrast at one level. Angiography may also be performed via the side ports by introducing sheaths in the common femoral arteries bilaterally. This serves to check for perigraft reflux that has not been detected on previous films. Cine-loop angiography (set at two to four frames per second) with the capability for digital subtraction and frame-by-frame replay is essential.

Some graft fabrics being used in endografts are porous, and completion angiography may demonstrate contrast outside the endograft lumen. This may present a diagnostic dilemma. Contrast in the sac because of the porosity usually appears late during the digital subtraction angiogram (DSA) and is usually generalized along the length of the graft (see Fig. 39-2). By contrast, Type I endoleaks appear early and are localized.

Postoperative Diagnosis of Endoleak

The modalities for postoperative imaging of endoleak may be surrogate or direct.

Surrogate Modalities

Because the majority of endografts have a radio-opaque metallic frame, a plain abdominal x-ray is a useful investigation (Fig. 39-5). It may demonstrate faulty fixation more clearly and earlier than contrast CT, and it may lead to the detection of endoleak.[12] The accuracy of detecting migration can be improved by following a protocol of performing A-P, lateral, and oblique views at the level of the umbilicus.

Studies have confirmed that the presence of endoleak is usually associated with an increase in the size of the

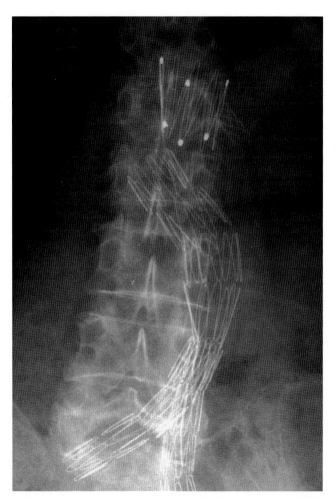

Figure 39-5. Plain x-ray of the abdomen demonstrating separation of the body of the endograft from the anchoring suprarenal uncovered stent.

aneurysm sac.[13,14] Measurement of AAA diameter by B-mode ultrasound can therefore be used as a surrogate method of detecting endoleak. CT may also be used for a similar purpose, with the option of monitoring an increase in volume of the sac in addition to the diameter of the sac.

Direct Modalities for Imaging Endoleaks

The direct methods of imaging for endoleak include color duplex ultrasound, contrast-enhanced CT, and angiography. Contrast-enhanced CT has been accepted as the gold standard for detecting the presence of an endoleak. Once an endoleak has been detected, however, carefully planned arteriography is more useful in characterizing the origin and nature of the endoleak. Color duplex ultrasound has the advantage of imaging Type II endoleaks in real time, as distinct from contrast CT and arteriography, both of which have to rely on accurate timing to image the contrast arriving in the sac via collateral circulation.

Color Duplex Ultrasound

From the beginning of the endoluminal method of treating abdominal aortic aneurysm, CT scanning has been considered the optimal diagnostic method to monitor patients after endoluminal repair. More recently, color duplex ultrasound (CDU) has emerged as an important alternative imaging modality.[15] CDU, with its advantages of low cost and low risk, can accurately monitor aneurysm size, detect endoleak, and provide dynamic and hemodynamic information not available with other testing methods (Fig. 39-6). However, the technique is operator dependent, can be time consuming, and certain aspects of device failure (i.e., wire fracture) cannot be detected.[16]

Duplex Ultrasound Evaluation of Aortic Endografts

Technique

- The patient should fast overnight to minimize intestinal gas; schedule the study for a morning appointment. The examination will take approximately 1 hour.

- Obtain operative information before the examination on what type of endograft has been used because there are three basic types and some designs feature bare stents that extend above the renal arteries

- Use a high-resolution color duplex ultrasound system with pulsed Doppler transducers ranging in frequency from 2.25 MHz to 5.0 MHz, allowing adequate depth penetration.

- Perform the examination with the patient in the supine position with the head slightly elevated. Also use the left lateral decubitus position for imaging the proximal and distal extent of the aortic graft. For the obese patient or the patient with excessive bowel gas, the examiner may have to place the

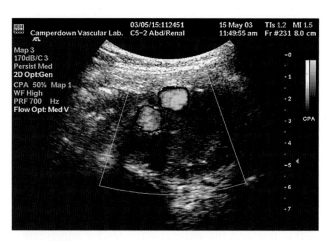

Figure 39-6. Transverse B-mode and power Doppler image of normal bifurcated endoluminal graft.

patient in various positions using other windows to visualize the endograft.

- Commence the study using B-mode imaging in the transverse plane. Identify the aorta at the level of the superior mesenteric artery. Look for the reflective metal struts of the aortic stent graft, which in some grafts can be visualized above the level of the renal arteries. The proximal extent of the graft (material) is seen as a hyperechoic signal along the aortic lumen; it can be visualized just below the level of the renal arteries. This is the superior attachment site. If the stent graft is uni-iliac or a bifurcated graft, then the inferior attachment site(s) would be the native common or external iliac artery.

- In the transverse plane, take maximum diameter measurements of the aneurysm sac. Over time there should be a decrease in the size of the residual sac. Any increase in size suggests flow to the sac and therefore a continued risk of rupture.

- Confirm patency of the renal arteries with spectral Doppler, and measure the distance of the superior attachment in relation to the renal level for possible graft migration. Then scan from the superior attachment to the inferior attachment site(s) in both transverse and sagittal planes in B-mode. The addition of harmonic imaging improves image quality and contrast resolution and will aid in diagnostic accuracy.

- Using color and spectral Doppler, assess the stent graft, looking for any perigraft flow, graft stenosis, thrombosis, or kinking, and record flow velocities throughout the body of the graft and graft limb(s). Optimize color settings so that color completely fills the graft lumen, avoiding excessive artifact. The examiner should be confident in differentiating between a true endoleak and a color artifact. The addition of power Doppler may be useful in detecting perigraft leak. Assess the patency of the native iliac and femoral arteries beyond the endograft and perform spectral Doppler analysis.

- It is important to be aware of potential sites of perigraft leak. A true leak will have reproducible arterial waveforms with different spectral Doppler characteristics, compared with flow within the aortic endograft. Try to determine the source of leak and direction of flow.

Color duplex ultrasound imaging is an accurate modality to detect early and late endoleak and device complications after endoluminal aortic surgery. The test is emerging as the diagnostic test of first choice for surveillance, allowing CT scanning and aortography to be used more selectively to plan secondary intervention. Further investigation is required to confirm the accuracy of this test and the optimal intervals for surveillance programs.

Aneurysm Diameter

Increasing diameter of an aneurysm after endoluminal grafting may indicate significant endoleak. This parameter can be accurately measured with ultrasound, and then can be used to monitor changes in aneurysm size. Raman and colleagues,[17] in a comparative study of 495 same-day CT and ultrasound examinations in 281 patients, found close correlation in aneurysm transverse diameter as measured by ultrasound and CT scans. No significant difference was found in measurement with either modality of those aneurysms that changed size.

Detection of Endoleak

The reported accuracy of ultrasound in detecting endoleak is variable, and few comparative studies have been done. Sato and colleagues,[18] in a review of the Endovascular Aneurysm Clinical Trial core laboratory records, compared 117 concurrent color duplex ultrasound and CT studies performed in 79 patients. The sensitivity, specificity, positive and negative predictive values, and accuracy of ultrasound compared to CT was 97%, 74%, 66%, 98%, and 82%, respectively.

Other authors have reported lower sensitivity, probably reflecting the critical importance of operator skill in deriving the full potential of color duplex imaging.[19]

The sensitivity of color duplex imaging in the detection of the presence and type of an endoleak may be increased when used with an intravenously administered ultrasound scan contrast agent; this may also overcome some of the problems encountered with technically difficult patients.[20]

The authors' experience has been favorable to date: a total of 113 patients (101 men, 12 women, mean age 72 years) who had color duplex imaging and CT scans after endoluminal aortic grafting were reviewed. Early endoleaks were demonstrated in 19 (17%) of the 113 patients (Fig. 39-7); 12 from the proximal graft; 3 from the distal portion of the endograft; 3 because of retrograde flow from the inferior mesenteric artery; and 1 from a lumbar artery (Fig. 39-8), all of which could be identified on the duplex scan. Six other patients, who did not have endoleak detected on their initial scan, were shown to have developed late endoleak on a subsequent duplex scan (at 24, 43, 48 months, and 3 years). Endoleaks were observed with all types of endograft devices, and were most commonly seen within the first 3 months of follow-up (Fig. 39-9).

Although an increase in diameter of an aneurysm after endoluminal grafting is said to be suggestive of endoleak, an increase in aneurysm size was observed in only 2 (10%) of the 19 patients with endoleaks in this series. Graft limb occlusion was demonstrated in 3 (2.65%), graft limb stenosis in 1 (0.88%), and a distal graft kink in 2 (1%) of the 113 patients. In comparison with CT scanning, the sensitivity of color duplex scan-

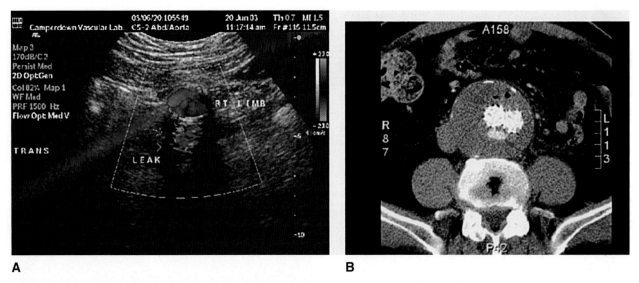

Figure 39-7. **A**, Transverse color duplex image of Type 1 distal right attachment site leak. **B**, CT confirmation of Type I endoleak from right distal attachment site.

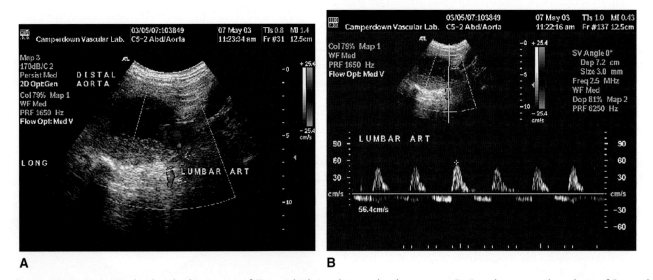

Figure 39-8. **A**, Sagittal color duplex image of Type II leak involving a lumbar artery. **B**, Doppler spectral analysis of "to and fro" flow in the lumbar artery.

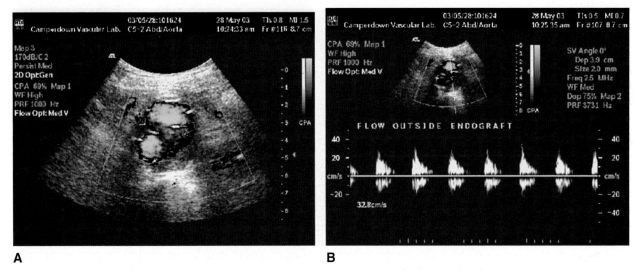

Figure 39-9. **A**, Transverse B mode and power Doppler Type III endoleak. **B**, Doppler spectral analysis Type III endoleak.

ning was 89%, specificity was 100%, PPV was 100%, NPV was 98%, and overall accuracy was 98%.

There were only two patients with an endoleak seen on duplex and not confirmed on CT scanning. In both patients there was a delay between the two tests, and spontaneous seal was considered the most likely explanation for the discrepancy.

The authors therefore use color duplex imaging as an integral part of the surveillance program after endovascular repair of abdominal aortic aneurysms.

Contrast-Enhanced CT

The timing of contrast-enhanced CT in the postoperative period is important. There is general agreement that this should be done within 30 days to establish a baseline and confirm the absence of Type I or Type III endoleak. Subsequent contrast-enhanced CT should be performed at 6 months, 12 months from operation, and annually thereafter. A noncontrast-scan should be performed before the contrast-enhanced scan. This enables pre-existing radio-opacities within the sac to be detected and distinguished from contrast medium that indicates an endoleak. Helical CT is considered preferable to conventional CT for vascular imaging. These scans are rapidly acquired, allowing uniform vascular enhancement at peak intensity with the same or a lower load of contrast material.

Endoleak is diagnosed by the presence of contrast outside the lumen of the endograft but within the lumen of the aneurysm sac. Even when significant endoleak is present, usually at least part of the aneurysm sac thromboses so that the region filling with contrast will give clues as to the site of the leak. For example, accumulation of most of the contrast in the area of the proximal implant zone is highly suggestive of proximal Type I endoleak (Fig. 39-10), whereas a small amount of contrast near the entry of a patent lumbar artery or IMA suggests retrograde flow from a Type II endoleak (Fig. 39-11).

The size of the aneurysm sac and the distance between the upper end of the endograft and lowermost renal artery should be noted and referenced to the first postoperative enhanced CT. An increase in diameter or volume of the aneurysm sac or migration of the endograft is a precursor to the development of an endoleak.

Postoperative Arteriography

Postoperative arteriography is not performed routinely. It is indicated in the following circumstances:

1. When an endoleak has been demonstrated by contrast CT or color duplex ultrasound, but its source has not been identified.

2. In patients with suspected endotension where the size of the aneurysm sac has increased but

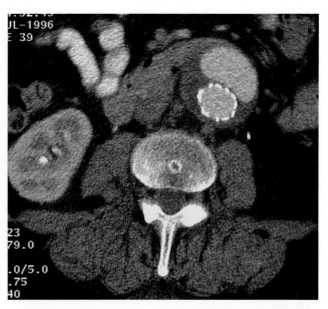

Figure 39-10. *Contrast CT of proximal Type I endoleak immediately below the AAA proximal neck.*

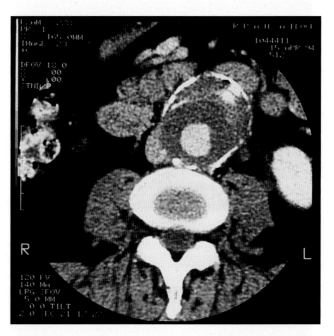

Figure 39-11. *Contrast CT suggestive of but not diagnostic of Type II endoleak emanating from the IMA.*

contrast CT and color duplex ultrasound have not detected an endoleak. Arteriography in this situation may include maneuvers recommended by Matsumura to detect microleak.

3. As a preliminary to a therapeutic intervention for a previously diagnosed endoleak.

Type I endoleak at the proximal or distal anchor zones of an endograft may be detected in the manner described under intraoperative imaging. A Type I endoleak may also be imaged by selective catheterization of the endoleak channel (Fig. 39-12). Type II endoleaks may be detected by midstream injection, with careful attention to obtaining delayed images to capture contrast arriving in the aneurysm sac via collateral circulation. Alternatively, Type II endoleaks may be imaged by selective catheterization. Lumbar endoleaks may be imaged by selective catheterization of the ascending iliolumbar artery via the internal iliac artery. In this situation, the endoleak has usually resulted from the development of a good collateral pathway between this artery and the lumbar artery responsible for the endoleak. A microcatheter can be advanced into the ipsilateral lumbar artery, then into the aneurysm sac, and finally into the corresponding contralateral lumbar artery (Fig. 39-13). This procedure enables not only the demonstration of the presence of lumbar endoleak but also therapeutic embolization to treat the endoleak. IMA endoleak may be demonstrated by selective sequential catheterization of the superior mesenteric artery, the middle colic artery, and the marginal colonic artery, leading to retrograde positioning in the inferior mesenteric artery origin (Fig. 39-14). Type II endoleaks may also be imaged by direct puncture of the sac via the lumbar route. Type IIIa (modular disconnection) and Type IIIb (incomplete seal at a modular junction) may be demonstrated by careful midstream injection at the appropriate level with attention to the appropriate degree of obliquity (Fig. 39-15).

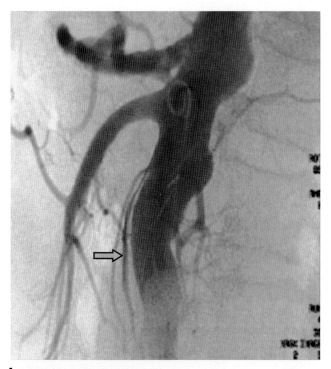

A

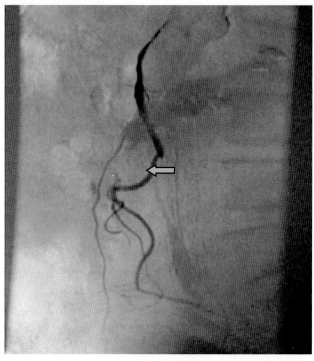

B

Figure 39-12. **A**, *Postoperative lateral aortogram demonstrating endoleak (arrow) originating from the AAA proximal neck.* **B**, *Later selective arteriogram demonstrating the same endoleak exiting the sac via the IMA (arrow).* **C**, *Coil embolization of IMA (arrow).*

C

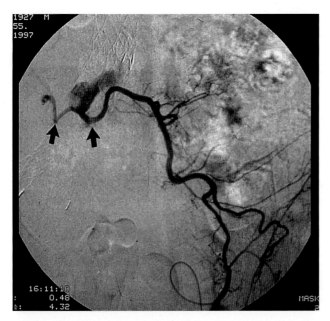

Figure 39-13. *Selective arteriogram via left internal iliac and ascending iliolumbar artery, demonstrating Type II endoleak from left fourth lumbar artery. Note the right fourth lumbar artery has also been catheterized (arrows).*

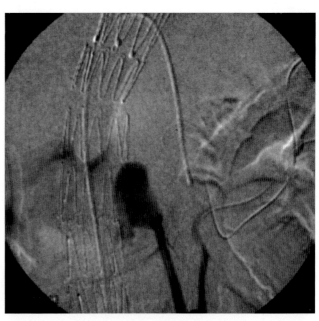

Figure 39-14. *Selective arteriogram via the superior mesenteric, middle colic, and marginal colonic arteries to demonstrate a Type II endoleak from the inferior mesenteric artery. Note the tortuous course of the catheter through the colonic arteries.*

Algorithm

An algorithm for diagnosis and management of endoleak is recommended (Fig. 39-16). Contrast CT and color duplex ultrasound are seen as complementary not alter-native investigations. Arteriography is used selectively when there is doubt regarding the source of the endoleak or as a preliminary to supplementary endovascular inter-vention for a previously diagnosed endoleak.

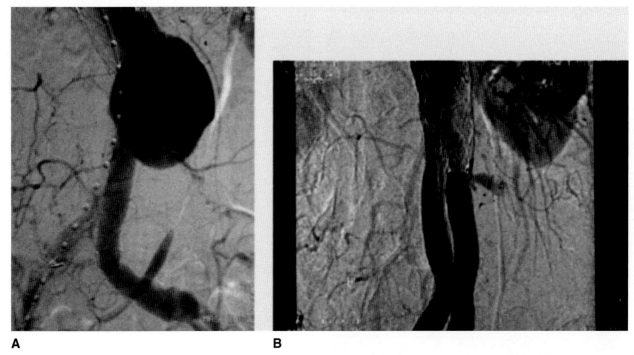

A

B

Figure 39-15. A, *Aortogram demonstrating a Type IIIa endoleak resulting from modular disconnection between the contralateral stump and contralateral limb.* **B,** *Aortogram demonstrating a Type IIIb endoleak resulting from incomplete seal between the contralateral stump and contralateral limb*

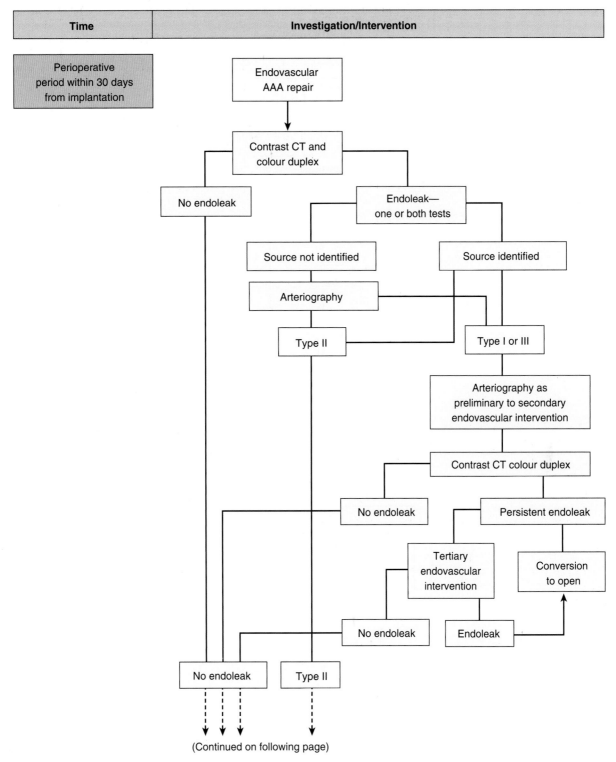

Figure 39-16. *Algorithm for diagnosis of endoleak (in two parts).*

Algorithm for Diagnosis of Endoleak

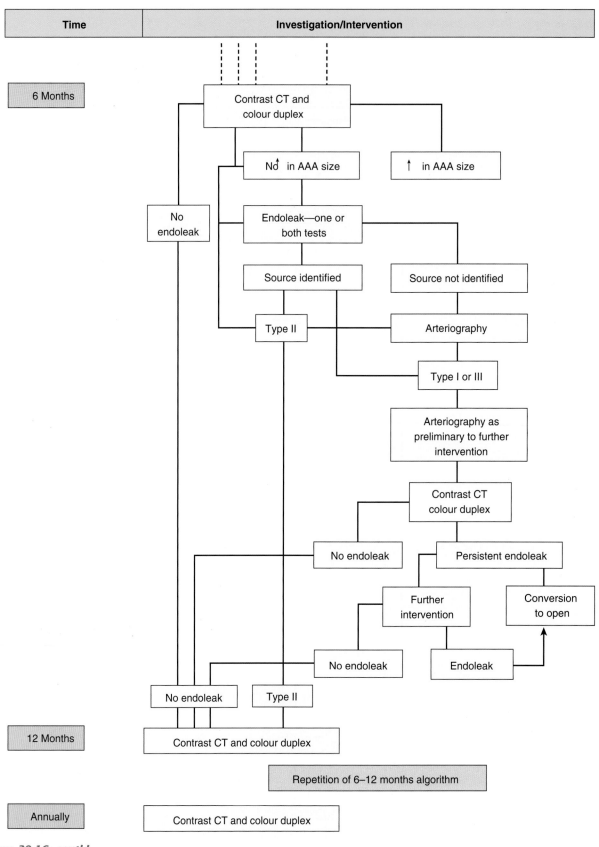

Figure 39-16, cont'd.

REFERENCES

1. May J, White GH, Yu W, et al: Concurrent comparison of endoluminal versus open repair in the treatment of abdominal aortic aneurysms: Analysis of 303 patients by life table method. J Vasc Surg 27:213–222, 1998.

2. White GH, Yu W, May J: "Endoleak": A proposed new terminology to describe incomplete aneurysm exclusion by an endoluminal graft (letter). J Endovasc Surg 3:124–125, 1996.

3. White GH, Yu W, May J, et al: Endoleak as a complication of endoluminal grafting of abdominal aortic aneurysms: Classification, incidence, diagnosis, and management. J Endovasc Surg 4:152–168, 1997.

4. White GH, May J, Waugh RC, et al: Type I and Type II endoleak: A more useful classification for reporting results of endoluminal repair of AAA (letter). J Endovasc Surg 5:189–191, 1998.

5. White GH, May J, Petrasek P, et al: Type III and type IV endoleak: Toward a complete definition of bloodflow in the sac after endoluminal repair of AAA. J Endovasc Surg 5:305–309, 1998.

6. Chaikof EL, Blankensteijn JD, Harris PL, et al for the Ad Hoc Committee for Standardized Reporting Practices in Vascular Surgery of the Society for Vascular Surgery/American Association for Vascular Surgery: Reporting standards for endovascular aortic aneurysm repair. J Vasc Surg 35:1048–1060, 2002.

7. Matsumura JS, Ryu RK, Ourier K: Identification and implications of transgraft microleaks after endovascular repair of aortic aneurysms. J Vasc Surg 34:190–197, 2001.

8. White GH, May J, Petrasek P, et al: Endotension: An explanation for continued AAA growth after successful endoluminal repair. J Endovasc Surg 6:308–315, 1999.

9. Schurink GW, Aarts NJ, Wilde J, et al: Endoleakage after stent-graft treatment of abdominal aneurysms: Implications on pressure and imaging: An in-vitro study. J Vasc Surg 28:234–241, 1998.

10. Faries PL, Sanchez LA, Marin ML, et al: An experimental model for the acute and chronic evaluation of intra-aneurysmal pressure. J Endovasc Surg 4:290–297, 1997.

11. Schurink GW, van Baalen JM, Visser MJ, et al: Thrombus within an aortic aneurysm does not reduce pressure on the aneurismal wall. J Vasc Surg 31:501–506, 2000.

12. May J, White GH, Yu W, et al: Importance of plain x-ray in endoluminal aortic graft surveillance. Eur J Vasc Endovasc Surg 13:202–206, 1997.

13. May J, White GH, Yu W, et al: A prospective study of changes in morphology and dimensions of abdominal aortic aneurysm following endoluminal repair: Preliminary report. J Endovasc Surg 2(4):343–347, 1995.

14. May J, White GH, Yu W, et al: A prospective study of anatomico-pathological changes in abdominal aortic aneurysms following endoluminal repair: Is the aneurysmal process reversed? Eur J Vasc Endovasc Surg 12:11–17, 1996.

15. Thurnher S, Cejna M: Imaging of aortic stent-grafts and endoleaks. Radiol Clin North Am 40:799–833, 2002.

16. Carter KA, Gayle RG, DeMasi RJ, et al: The incidence and natural history of Type I and II endoleak: A 5-year follow-up assessment with color duplex ultrasound scan. J Vasc Surg 35:595–597, 2003.

17. Raman KG, Missig-Carroll N, Richardson T, et al: Color-flow duplex ultrasound scan versus computed tomographic scan in the surveillance of endovascular aneurysm repair. J Vasc Surg 38:645–651, 2003.

18. Sato DT, Goff CD, Gregory RT, et al: Endoleak after aortic stent graft repair: Diagnosis by color duplex ultrasound scan versus computed tomography scan. J Vasc Surg 28(4):657–663, 1998.

19. Zannetti S, De Rango P, Parente B, et al: Role of duplex scan in endoleak detection after endoluminal abdominal aortic aneurysm repair. Eur J Vasc Endovasc Surg 19:531–535, 2000.

20. Bendick PJ, Bove PG, Long GW, et al: Efficacy of ultrasound scan contrast agents in the noninvasive follow-up of aortic stent grafts. J Vasc Surg 37(2):381–385, 2003.

Postoperative Surveillance After Endovascular Repair

DIANA EASTRIDGE • JON S. MATSUMURA

Introduction

There are four endovascular stent graft systems now approved by the Federal Drug Administration (FDA) for abdominal aortic aneurysm repair. There is an increasing awareness of this technology, both among physicians and the public. The matter of postoperative surveillance after endovascular repair of abdominal aortic aneurysm (AAA) is of increasing importance as more patients are treated with these devices. Although many medical centers are implanting devices, an even larger number of clinicians and diagnostic imaging facilities are involved in the care of this rapidly growing group of patients. Because these patients all need surveillance, and some require reintervention, it is imperative to establish a means of follow-up for these patients just as it is necessary to develop the technical skills to implant the devices.[1-3]

Follow-Up Protocols

Endovascular repair of AAA is a new technology, and long-term durability of the grafts has not yet been established. Data collected from a number of studies show that there are significant problems and rare catastrophic failures with all devices. In order to try to reduce the risk of aneurysm rupture, periodic imaging following endograft placement has been recommended.[4-11]

A protocol by which to follow these patients has been established at the authors' institution. Figure 40-1 is a flow chart that depicts the decision process for patient imaging and possible reintervention with angiography or additional endovascular procedures. Imaging in the year following implantation of the endograft is most often done at 1 month, 6 months, and at 1 year unless problems are identified. Following the initial year, annual imaging is required for life. The time frame may be tailored to fit an individual patient's success postrepair and the specific type of graft that has been implanted. The clinical scenarios for safe modification of follow-up intervals are continuing to evolve.

Although not the primary topic of this chapter, imaging follow-up is also recommended after standard open repair.

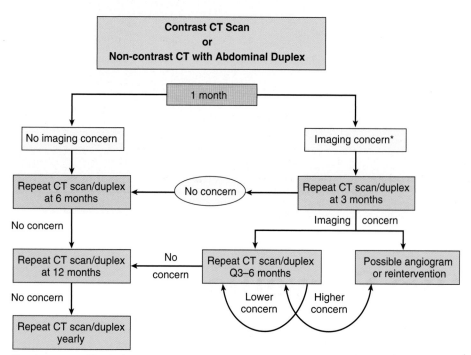

Figure 40-1. Flow chart illustrating patient follow-up after endovascular AAA repair.

*Imaging concern: Material failure, aneurysm expansion, large endoleak, poor seal zone, graft migration

The authors have recommended computed tomographic (CT) scan follow-up in the first year after emergent treatment of patients, and every 5 years for all patients having open repair. Radiographic findings include subsequent aneurysm formation, pseudoaneurysm, and abdominal wall defects.[12–14]

Imaging Modalities

Fine-cut contrast-enhanced CT scans (with precontrast, dynamic, and delayed images) allow for the measurement of the aneurysm sac and an evaluation for endoleak; seal zone (i.e., length of aorta covered by the graft before the aorta becomes aneurysmal); graft migration; and arterial patency (Figs. 40-2, 40-3, and 40-4). Measurements taken at the proximal and distal implantation sites allow for evaluation for dilation of the proximal neck of the aneurysm and of the iliac arteries. Recording of this data in an easily accessible manner allows for a quick comparison to earlier results and a means to track existing and potential problems. The record-keeping system should allow quick comparison to the most recent study, and also comparison to the initial baseline study. This is because some events, such as migration, occur over a long period of observation in small increments, and may only be noted when compared over intervals as long as 2 or 3 years.

Four-view abdominal x-rays offer additional information about the stent structure and intercomponent migration. A baseline film should always be obtained at the time of graft implantation. These x-rays allow visualization of the graft components and are used to check for breaks in the wire skeletons, separation of attachment systems, the relative movement of modular graft pieces, and kinking or compression of graft limbs. Abdominal x-rays offer less information in single-piece grafts that are not at risk for intercomponent migration, and may be obtained less commonly with these grafts, thus avoiding additional expense and exposure to radiation. In addition, abdominal films may be obtained less commonly in selected patients that have endografts with very low incidence of any migration and in those without clinically significant fractures.[1,3]

Certain patients may not be able to undergo contrast-enhanced CT scans because of severe right heart failure or radiocontrast dye allergies. There are also concerns about exposing patients to ionizing radiation and repeat exposure to potentially nephrotoxic contrast dyes.[15] The use of contrast dyes usually requires both a blood draw to check the patient's renal function and the establishment of an intravenous access during the CT scan, either of which can be burdensome and uncomfortable for the patient.

Color duplex ultrasound scan, when it is performed by experienced registered vascular technologists or dedicated physicians, has been shown by some researchers to be an acceptable alternative to evaluate endografts postoperatively.[11] However, other authors have reported less than optimal correlation with CT scanning. In addition, the patient's body habitus, patient movement, and the presence of bowel gas may influence the results of these ultrasound scans. Combining color duplex ultra-

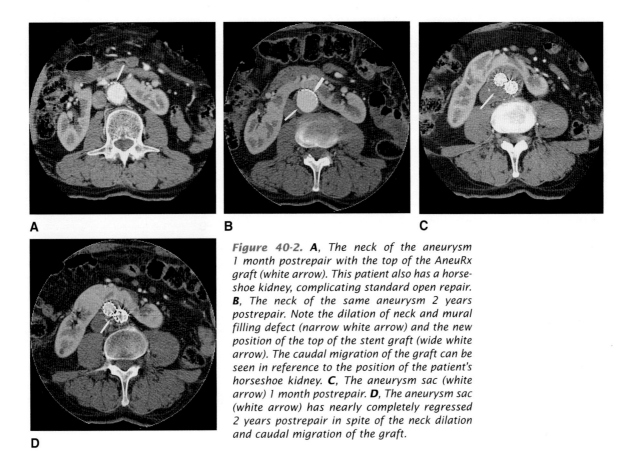

Figure 40-2. A, The neck of the aneurysm 1 month postrepair with the top of the AneuRx graft (white arrow). This patient also has a horseshoe kidney, complicating standard open repair. **B,** The neck of the same aneurysm 2 years postrepair. Note the dilation of neck and mural filling defect (narrow white arrow) and the new position of the top of the stent graft (wide white arrow). The caudal migration of the graft can be seen in reference to the position of the patient's horseshoe kidney. **C,** The aneurysm sac (white arrow) 1 month postrepair. **D,** The aneurysm sac (white arrow) has nearly completely regressed 2 years postrepair in spite of the neck dilation and caudal migration of the graft.

sound scan with a noncontrast CT and abdominal x-ray is a useful strategy in patients who cannot have radiocontrast. Using both tests permits assessment about endoleaks along with aneurysm size, seal zone, and possible graft migration.

Several specific measurements and observations are made at each subsequent patient visit. These are listed in Table 40-1 along with the imaging test(s) that are used to monitor the parameter. Some grafts are not considered safe for magnetic resonance imaging (MRI). Further testing with arteriography or interventional options is

considered based on individual patient status and the specific characteristics of each device.

Alternative Strategies for Follow-Up

In an optimal situation, the patient would return to the institution where the device was implanted for follow-up examinations. However, this is not always possible

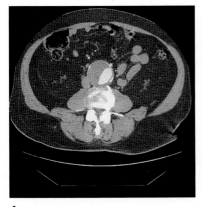
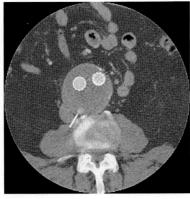

Figure 40-3. A, A 5.8-cm AAA prerepair. **B,** The aneurysm sac has enlarged to 6.7 cm 2 years postrepair with the endovascular stent graft. A Type 2 endoleak (white arrow) has contributed to the sac enlargement.

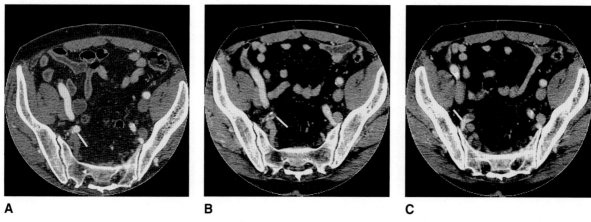

Figure 40-4. A, *A patent right hypogastric artery (white arrow) pre-endovascular repair. The right hypogastric artery (white arrow) is occluded on the postrepair image (**B**) but reconstitutes distally (**C**). The patient initially had buttock claudication that had resolved by his 6-month follow-up visit.*

because of the age and comorbidities of the patient and the travel distance. Alternative strategies may have to be developed in order to provide follow-up imaging for some patients. The availability of multidetector row CT scans is increasing, and it is helpful to establish contacts with other institutions where these scans can be performed. The films can then be sent to the original institution, where they can be reviewed by the surgeon and staff. An experienced clinical team often is helpful in reviewing imaging of complicated cases, and a multidisciplinary group composed of nurses, vascular surgeons, interventionalists, body CT radiologists, and CT technologists has been meeting monthly in the authors' institution.

These efforts will allow continued surveillance of patients who might otherwise be lost to follow-up. If significant problems are identified, efforts must be made to have the patient return for possible reintervention.

Patient Education

It is imperative to stress the importance of follow-up and the necessary requirements before implantation of the endovascular device. Establishing an early relationship with patients is beneficial when coordinating future care. Preoperative teaching and listening to the concerns of both the patient and their families can help improve long-term follow-up compliance. Establishing an individual as a contact person for each patient assists in efficiently and effectively responding to family concerns and helps reduce the chance that patients are lost to follow-up.

TABLE 40-1. Parameters and Tests After Endovascular Repair

Parameter	Primary test	Alternative test
Aneurysm sac size	CT (diameter)	CT (volume, US, MRI) Physical examination
Endoleak	CT (pre-, dynamic, and delayed contrast)	Duplex, MR (contrast agents may be used)
Neck diameters	CT	MRI
Migration relative to arterial landmarks	CT (thin cuts)	CTA, MRI
Intercomponent migration	Abdominal films	
Device fracture/suture pops	Abdominal films	
Device compression/kinking	Abdominal films	
Limb patency	Physical examination	Duplex, ABI, CT

CT, computed tomography; US, ultrasound; MRI, magnetic resonance imaging; CTA, computed tomographic angiography; ABI, ankle-brachial index.

Establishing a Database

An important component of postoperative surveillance is keeping a database with the details of subsequent examinations and imaging results. A schedule for future follow-up examinations should be included in this record as a reminder tool. Accurate reporting and recording of many parameters helps to assess the successes and failures; it is also a significant time-consuming responsibility for those involved in the care of patients after endovascular AAA repair. Unfortunately, despite these efforts, patient factors often prevent complete or ideal follow-up in this elderly and debilitated patient group. After a few years without any symptoms, many patients decide on their own not to continue with follow-up even after extensive physician counseling.

Conclusions

Endovascular repair of AAA remains an evolving technology with many unanswered questions and uncertain outcomes. Long-term follow-up is not available to assess how these patients will fare in a time frame of 10 years or greater. With FDA approval of endografts, surveillance has passed from the hands of a few research institutions into the hands of many clinicians. Because of the possibility of a catastrophic outcome for a patient whose endovascular repair fails, clinical and imaging follow-up is an important component of the care of patients treated with this technology.

REFERENCES

1. Makaroun MS, Chaikof E, Naslund T, et al for the EVT Investigators: Efficacy of a bifurcated endograft versus open repair of abdominal aortic aneurysms: A reappraisal. J Vasc Surg 35:203–210, 2002.

2. Zarins CK, White RA, Schwarten D, et al for the Investigators of the Medtronic AneuRx Multicenter Clinical Trial: AneuRx stent graft vs. open surgical repair of abdominal aortic aneurysms: Multicenter prospective clinical trial. J Vasc Surg 29:292–308, 1999.

3. Matsumura JS, Brewster DC, Makaroun MS, et al: A multicenter controlled clinical trial of open versus endovascular treatment of abdominal aortic aneurysm. J Vasc Surg 37(2):262–271, 2003.

4. Resch T, Ivancev K, Brunkwall J, et al: Distal migration of stent-grafts after endovascular repair of abdominal aortic aneurysms. J Vasc Interv Radiol 10:257–266, 1999.

5. Eskandari MK, Yao JST, Pearce WH, et al: Surveillance after endoluminal repair of abdominal aortic aneurysms. Cardiovasc Surg 9(5):469–471, 2001.

6. Ebaugh JL, Eskandari MK, Finkelstein A, et al: Caudal migration of endoprostheses after treatment of abdominal aortic aneurysms. J Surg Res 107:14–17, 2002.

7. White GH, Yu W, May J, et al: Endoleak as a complication of endoluminal grafting of abdominal aortic aneurysms: Classification, incidence, diagnosis and management. J Endovasc Surg 4:152–168, 1997.

8. Bernhard VM, Mitchell RS, Matsumura JS, et al: Ruptured abdominal aortic aneurysm associated with endovascular repair. J Vasc Surg 35(6):1155–1162, 2002.

9. Politz JK, Newman VS, Stewart MT: Late abdominal aortic aneurysm rupture after AneuRx repair: A report of three cases. J Vasc Surg 31:599–606, 2000.

10. Schurink GW, Aarts NJ, Van Bockel JH: Endoleak after stent-graft treatment of abdominal aortic aneurysm: A meta-analysis of clinical studies. Br J Surg 86:581–587, 1999.

11. Veith FJ, Baum RA, Ohki T, et al: Nature and significance of endoleaks and endotension: Summary of opinions expressed at an international conference. J Vasc Surg 35:1029–1035, 2002.

12. Edwards J, Teefey S, Zierler R, et al: Intra-abdominal para-anastomotic aneurysms after aortic bypass grafting. J Vasc Surg 15:344–353, 1992.

13. Matsumura JS, Pearce WH, Cabellon A, et al: Reoperative aortic surgery. Cardiovasc Surg 7:614–621, 1999.

14. Rodriguez HE, Matsumura JS, Morasch MD, et al: Abdominal wall hernias after open abdominal aortic aneurysm repair: Prospective radiographic detection and clinical implications. Vasc and Endovasc Surg 38:237–240, 2004.

15. Waybill MM, Waybill PN: Contrast media-induced nephrotoxicity: Identification of patients at risk and algorithms for prevention. J Vasc Inter Radiol 12:3–9, 2001.

VENOUS

Chapter 41

Vascular Diagnosis of Venous Thrombosis

NICOS LABROPOULOS • APOSTOLOS K. TASSIOPOULOS

Introduction

The venous system is a common site for thrombus formation. Deep vein thrombosis (DVT) is most often seen in hospitalized patients and is associated with significant morbidity and mortality. The precise incidence of DVT remains elusive because a large number of thrombi are silent and the autopsy rate in most countries is low. In a recent systematic review of nine large population studies, the incidence of DVT was calculated to be 5 per 10,000 people per year (weighted mean value).[1] The incidence is much lower in younger people (2 per 10,000 per year, age 30 to 49 years) and higher in the elderly (20 per 10,000 per year, age 70 to 79 years).[1] DVT and pulmonary embolism together are responsible for a large number of hospitalizations and over 50,000 deaths yearly, but the precise number is unknown.[2] If one also considers the late sequelae of DVT, it is clearly a significant problem that requires prompt diagnosis, aggressive treatment, and close follow-up.

Clinical evaluation, including assessment of risk factors, is essential in the diagnosis of venous thrombosis. In the past, phlebography was the preferred diagnostic test, but it has been replaced in the last two decades by duplex scanning (DS) ultrasound. DS is fast, reproducible, and has excellent diagnostic accuracy; therefore, it has become the method of choice for the diagnosis of acute and chronic venous disorders.

Pathophysiology and Clinical Characteristics of Venous Thrombosis

Virchow in the mid-1800s suggested that three factors are primarily responsible for the development of venous thrombosis: (1) blood abnormalities (hypercoagulability); (2) abnormalities in bloodflow (stasis); and (3) vascular trauma. The etiology of venous thrombosis is usually multifactorial, and each component of this triad has a variable impact on individual patients.

Blood abnormalities can affect both the coagulation and fibrinolytic systems. Deficiency of naturally occurring anticoagulants (e.g., antithrombin, proteins C and S, and mutations of factor V and prothrombin gene) are more prevalent in patients with spontaneous venous thrombosis.[3] The use of oral contraceptives, pregnancy, and malignancies also predispose to venous thrombosis in part by altering the properties of the coagulation system.[3]

Stasis determines the localization of venous thrombosis and is probably the most important etiologic factor in postoperative and post-trauma patients whose activity is limited. Large varicose veins in the lower extremities with sluggish bloodflow are a common site for spontaneous thrombus formation. In immobilized patients, there is prolonged blood stasis in the calf veins. Not surprisingly, several studies have suggested that DVT usually originates in these veins and then propagates proximally.[4,5]

The most common presentation of superficial vein thrombosis (SVT) is a tender cord along the course of a superficial vein associated with local inflammatory changes and ecchymosis. Thrombi in the superficial and deep veins can coexist without being contiguous. Likewise, thrombus progression can occur from superficial to deep veins or from deep to superficial veins. The saphenofemoral junction is the most common route by which a thrombus extends from superficial to deep veins.[6,7]

In the deep venous system, when the original thrombus extends and occupies the entire lumen of the affected venous segment, it causes interruption of flow followed by both ante- and retrograde thromboses. This results in development of edema within the deep muscular fascia that causes pain. Edema and pain of the affected limb are the most common presenting symptoms of DVT. In cases of extensive DVT, a characteristic clinical picture consisting of severe pitting edema of the extremity, pain and blanching (phlegmasia alba dolens) is seen. Further progression may lead to impedance of venous return from that limb, venous congestion, and finally cessation of the arterial bloodflow in the limb (phlegmasia cerulea dolens). These patients are at risk of limb loss. Occasionally the original thrombus may not involve the entire lumen and may propagate without interrupting flow, developing a long, floating tail that may detach from the venous wall and cause pulmonary embolism in the absence of previous signs of DVT. Some early thrombi developing in the valve sinusoids do not propagate: They are subsequently dissolved by the intrinsic fibrinolytic system and may appear as endothelialized fibrin segments within the valve pockets.

Duplex Scanning Ultrasound Examination

The introduction of DS in the 1980s was a major advance in the diagnosis of venous thrombosis. The Doppler mode gives functional information about spontaneous and phasic venous flow and about the function of the venous valves. The B-mode offers real-time anatomic images of the vein wall and lumen, and it can visualize intraluminal thrombus. Evaluation of the thrombus includes its anatomic location and extent. When pressure is applied by the probe, normal veins are easily compressed and collapse. Resistance to compression is seen when thrombus is present, and it increases with the age of the thrombus.

Color-flow scanning is performed using medium frequency linear array transducers of 4 to 7 MHz. In obese patients, lower frequency transducers at 2 to 3.5 MHz may be used to allow imaging at deeper sites. The examination starts with the patient in the supine position. The patient is instructed to shift his or her weight slightly on the contralateral hip. This takes pressure off of the examined limb when compressions are being done and is more comfortable for the patient. On the examined limb, the leg should be externally rotated with the knee slightly bent.

The probe is first placed just below the inguinal ligament. Examination of the deep veins begins with a transverse view of the common femoral vein (CFV). The confluence of the great saphenous vein (GSV) and the CFV (saphenofemoral junction) is also seen in this view. The CFV is compressed by exerting light pressure over the area with the transducer. The vein should be easily collapsed, and compressions should be made every 3 to 5 cm. If the applied pressure is not adequate to fully collapse the vein, then more pressure can be applied until the adjacent artery diameter is reduced. This will ensure that there is adequate pressure at the level of the vein. The compressions continue into the femoral vein (FV) from the proximal thigh to the distal thigh (adductor or Hunter's canal). Characterization of flow is being done in the longitudinal view (Fig. 41-1). The Doppler cursor is placed in the center of the vessel, and spontaneous and phasic flow is observed. This is followed by evaluation of distal augmentation using the following maneuver: With the color mode on, the CFV is identified and a longitudinal view is obtained with the Doppler cursor in the center of the vessel. With the other hand, the thigh below the probe or the calf is squeezed; the vessels examined should fill with color wall to wall. The maneuver is repeated with the Doppler on, and augmentation on the tracing is recorded.

After completing compressions and documenting flow in the CFV and FV, the popliteal and calf veins should be examined. The popliteal vein (POPV) is located behind the knee in the popliteal fossa. This can be seen with the patient keeping the leg externally rotated. Once the POPV is visualized, transverse compressions and augmentation of flow with color and Doppler are performed. Care should be taken to perform transverse compressions in the proximal and distal segments of the popliteal vein until the tibial-peroneal trunk. Next, the entire popliteal

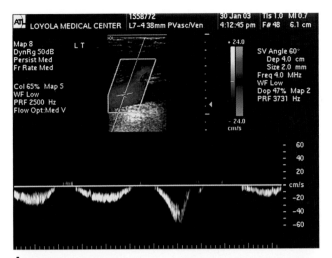

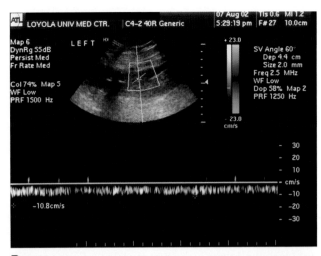

A

B

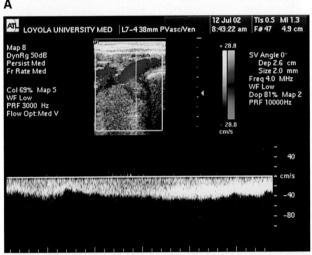

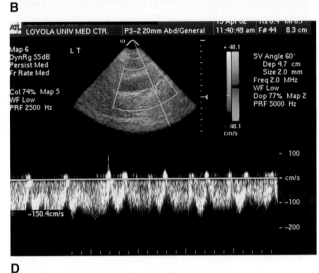

C

D

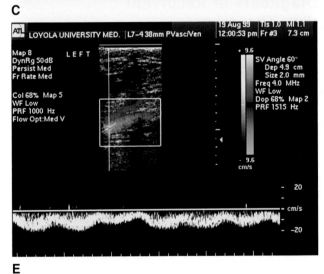

E

Figure 41-1. *Normal and abnormal vein flow characteristics.* ***A***, *Normal flow in the CFV just above the saphenofemoral junction. It is spontaneous, phasic (right atrial pressure and respiration), and has a good augmentation (velocity was increased from 25 to 55 cm/sec during mild manual compression of the distal thigh).* ***B***, *Low amplitude, nonphasic flow and without augmentation during distal compression in the proximal CFV of a male patient with iliac vein thrombosis.* ***C***, *Increased flow in a collateral (deep external pudendal vein) in a female patient with iliofemoral thrombosis. The flow is diverted from the CFV to the collateral because the proximal CFV is completely occluded.* ***D***, *Very high velocity in the saphenofemoral junction of a male patient caused by extrinsic compression from a hematoma after cardiac catheterization through the left common femoral artery.* ***E***, *Spontaneous continuous flow in the left popliteal and medial gastrocnemial veins of a male patient with acute cellulitis.*

fossa should be examined to rule out the presence of Baker's cyst or a hematoma as the cause of symptoms.

For the examination of the calf veins, the patient may remain in the supine position or sit up (if patient condition permits) with the legs hanging over the side of the bed. The examination starts at the ankle, initially visu-

alizing the posterior tibial and peroneal veins. The posterior tibial veins are found posterior to the tibia; the peroneal veins can be seen in the same view, directly medial to the fibula. The peroneal veins can also be imaged from the posterolateral aspect of the calf behind the fibula when the medial approach is not adequate.

Once compressions are completed, flow can be demonstrated in both sets of veins with color and/or Doppler. The anterior tibial veins are evaluated through the anterior tibialis muscle in the anterior-lateral aspect of the calf. These are examined only in the presence of local trauma or symptoms because the prevalence of thrombosis is less than 1%.[8]

The soleal sinus and gastrocnemius veins of the calf are imaged next. The gastrocnemius veins are first identified near their confluence with the popliteal vein at the popliteal skin crease and are followed within the muscle belly (first muscle under the fascia) down to the calf. Compression maneuvers in both the medial and lateral gastrocnemius veins are performed. The soleal veins are found first just below the sural triangle (at this level, the soleus is the first muscle under the fascia) and are followed up in both directions. They can be traced to either the posterior tibial and/or peroneal veins. The veins are compressed against the tibia and the fibula to make sure that they collapse. If compression is inadequate or not possible, then color imaging with low flow settings (PRF less than 1500 Hz) and distal augmentation is performed. Color imaging is also performed after a negative compression test to increase the confidence of diagnosis. This method is useful in identifying small nonocclusive thrombi and recanalized veins from an old thrombosis. When imaging of the calf veins is not optimal in the supine position, the examination is performed with the leg in the dependent position.

Finally, the great and small saphenous veins need to be examined. Transverse compressions of the GSV from the groin to the ankle should be documented. The small saphenous vein (SSV) can be visualized from its junction to the POPV in the popliteal fossa (saphenopopliteal junction) to the ankle. Transverse compressions should be performed throughout its length.

Diagnostic Criteria

The test is negative when any one of the following criteria is present:

- Complete approximation of the near and far vein wall during compression without any space seen other than the walls
- Complete color filling of the lumen without any defects

DVT is diagnosed when any one of the following criteria is present:

- Partially compressible or noncompressible vein
- Echogenic material within the vein
- Filling defect on color imaging
- Absence of Doppler signal

DS can assist in estimating the age of the venous thrombus. In chronic DVT the following characteristics may be present:

- The thrombosed venous segments can be contracted and sometimes unable to be traced by DS throughout their length.
- Bright echoes are often seen within the lumen because of the old thrombus and/or the scar tissue.
- Partial recanalization with filling defects and reflux may also be detected.
- In fully recanalized veins, wall thickening with luminal reduction may be seen.
- Collateral veins are usually found around the obstructed segments.

In patients with acute DVT the thrombus and venous wall characteristics are different:

- The vein is distended.
- The lumen is partially compressible or noncompressible.
- The lumen is usually echolucent or has an intermediate echogenicity, but the brightness is much less than the surrounding tissues.
- The vein wall is thin and smooth.
- Large collateral veins are not usually seen.

Figure 41-2, *A* through *G* shows the characteristics described above.

Diagnosis of Recurrent Vein Thrombosis

The diagnosis of recurrent vein thrombosis is similar to the one described above for a first episode. Diagnosis of recurrent SVT is rather easy because the presence of signs and symptoms at the site of thrombosis indicate a new event. On the other hand, the diagnosis of recurrent DVT is more difficult because the presence of old thrombus complicates the interpretation of ultrasound or phlebography.[9] In addition, a validated clinical model that would allow clear diagnosis of recurrent DVT does not exist. The diagnosis is easier if the recurrent thrombosis occurs in the contralateral extremity, which was not affected in the first episode; or if the new thrombus occurs in a location that was not previously involved. Often, however, thrombi reoccur in previously thrombosed vein segments. The presence of either a filling defect on color mode, or of a noncompressible vein indicates thrombosis. Establishing the diagnosis of recurrent DVT, however, requires comparison of the location and size of this thrombus to those seen in a previous DS examination. An increase of greater than 2 mm in the compressed diameter of a previously thrombosed venous segment has been reported to be diagnostic of recurrent DVT.[10,11]

These results come from a single center that has performed this study in the femoral and popliteal veins only; therefore these results need further confirmation from other centers before widespread acceptance. Following the diagnosis of a first episode of DVT, serial examina-

tions are not usually performed because there is no reimbursement in the absence of symptoms and there is no evidence that routine examinations are either necessary or cost-effective. Figure 41-3 shows an example of a recurrent DVT.

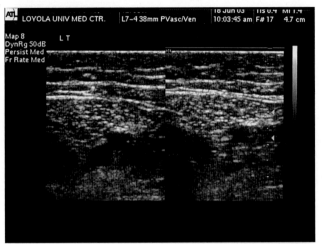

A

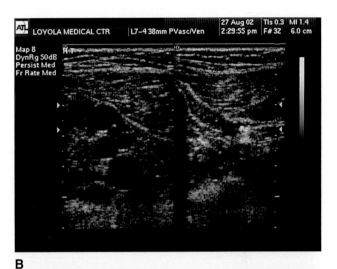

B

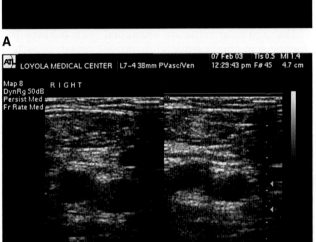

C

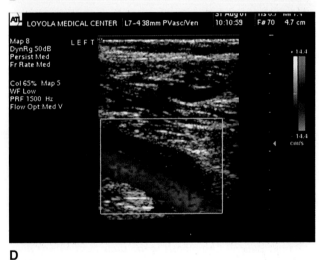

D

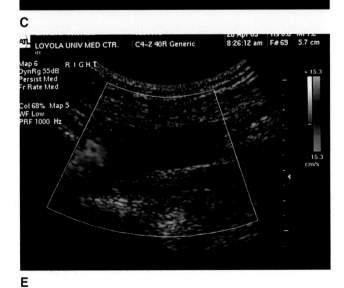

E

Figure 41-2. Acute and chronic deep vein thrombosis. *A, Split screen showing complete compression of the left femoral vein in the middle thigh of a female patient; and B, complete compression of posterior tibial and peroneal veins in the right middle calf of a male patient. In both pictures only the accompanying arteries are seen during the compression. C, Acute thrombosis of the right CFV in a male patient 2 weeks after total knee replacement. The vein is distended, contains echolucent material, and is noncompressible. D, Acute thrombosis of the left popliteal vein in a male patient with symptoms of pulmonary embolism and a high probability ventilation-perfusion lung scanning. There is no color filling, and the lumen is echolucent and less bright than the surrounding tissues. The popliteal artery is normal. E, Partial filling defect in the right CFV of male heart transplant patient after cardiac catheterization. It is likely that the vein was injured during the arterial cannulation. The filling defect is at the near wall (anterior) of the vein, which is the area to be injured by the catheter.*

Continued

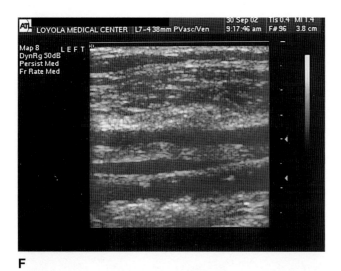

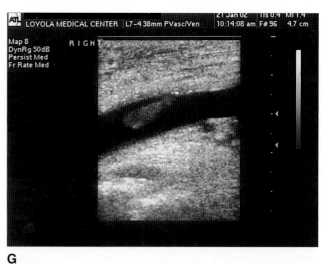

F

G

*Figure 41-2, cont'd. **F**, Chronic thrombosis of the left popliteal vein in a male patient with known previous femoropopliteal thrombosis. The thrombus is echogenic and has similar brightness with surrounding extraluminal tissues. **G**, Localized free-floating thrombus in the right common femoral vein of a male patient 3 days after total hip replacement. All free-floating thrombi are acute and, in contrast to old beliefs, are not more dangerous than the acute adherent thrombi.*

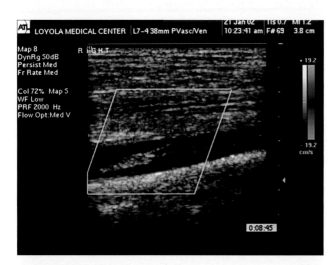

Figure 41-3. Recurrent thrombosis in the right peroneal vein of a male patient. Thrombosis in the same location was diagnosed 2 years ago. This patient presented with calf tenderness. The peroneal vein is distended with old echogenic material in the center and echolucent (recent) material around it. There is no color filling during distal augmentation.

Inferior Vena Cava and Iliac Veins

The iliac veins and inferior vena cava (IVC) should be examined selectively. Example of situations requiring imaging of these vessels include: continuous CFV flow with limited or no phasicity by Doppler; poor distal augmentation of the CFV; asymmetry in the CFV waveforms; and bilateral limb swelling with normal lower extremity venous duplex.

IVC and iliac veins are examined with a lower frequency transducer (phased or curved-linear array less than 4 MHz). The imaging starts with the external iliac vein at the inguinal ligament. After the CFV is identified, the color is turned on and the transducer is moved cephalad. The external iliac vein is seen diving down above the femoral head. Often the internal iliac vein is seen posteriorly, but diagnosis of thrombosis is usually not made by DS for this vein. The common iliac vein next is imaged up to its confluence with the contralateral iliac. Diagnosis of thrombosis in these veins is done by color because compression is not possible in many patients. Either absence of color or a filling defect indicates thrombosis. Similar findings can be seen when these veins are externally compressed by a mass. In this scenario, if the vein is completely occluded, the absence of thrombus near the site of compression cannot rule out thrombosis.

A vein segment with stenosis has reduced velocities proximal to it and increased velocities just distal to it. This is seen in the May-Thurner syndrome, in which the left common iliac vein is compressed by the right common iliac artery. Because of this condition, the left iliac vein should be examined more often in cases of edema associated with absence of thrombosis at the ipsilateral limb.

The iliac veins are best seen lateral to the midline following the line that connects the anterior superior iliac spine and the umbilicus. The IVC is seen to the right of the aorta, at the midline right over the spine. It is followed from the confluence of the iliac veins up to its entrance into the right atrium. The vessel is best imaged from the midline approach, but depending on the size of the abdomen, the patient may need to be turned onto the right or left side.

When compared with phlebography, duplex scanning offers several significant advantages. It is totally noninvasive, can be repeated as many times as necessary, can image all the individual vein segments and tributaries, and can differentiate between acute and chronic thrombus. These advantages have made duplex scanning the preferred diagnostic test for the diagnosis and follow-up of DVT. Figure 41-4 illustrates several examples of pathology in the pelvic veins.

Incidental Findings

The most common clinical symptoms of DVT are pain and edema of the affected extremity. The diagnosis of DVT, however, is made in less than 50% of patients presenting with such symptoms. Several other conditions that present with the same symptoms can be diagnosed with DS during examinations performed to rule out DVT.

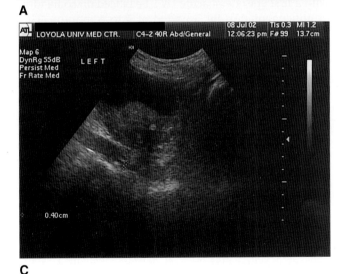

A

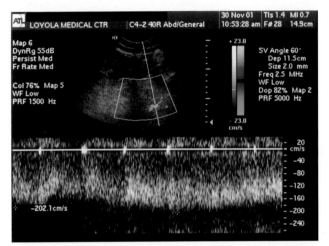

B

C

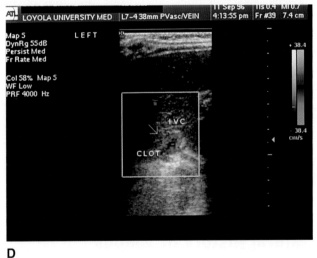

D

Figure 41-4. Pathology in the iliocaval veins. **A**, *Acute thrombosis in the right external iliac vein in a female patient 3 weeks after aortocoronary bypass. The vein is distended, has a homogenous texture, and there is absence of color medial to the external iliac artery. **B**, Compression of the left common iliac vein by the right common iliac artery in a male patient who presented with recent swelling of his left calf and thigh. This condition is known as the May-Thurner syndrome and also as the Cockett syndrome. The vein velocity is 202 cm/sec and the velocity ratio across the stenosis was 12.6 (202/16). **C**, Compression of the left common iliac vein in a female patient by a mass shown to be lymphoma on histology. The patient had worsening swelling in the left calf and thigh. The diameter of the vein was only 4 mm and was less than half the size of the adjacent common iliac artery. **D**, Acute thrombosis in the inferior vena cava of a young male patient after a major abdominal surgery. A clear filling defect is seen in the center of the cava. A linear probe was used because the patient was a child and the cava was located only 4.5 cm below the skin.*

Continued

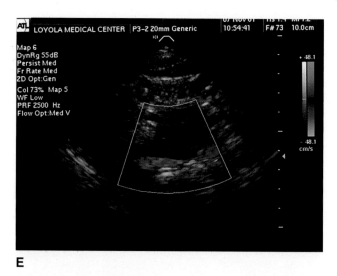

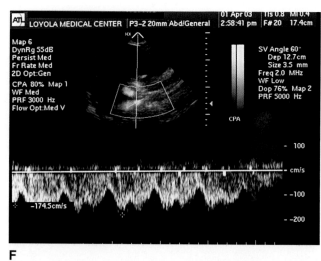

E

F

Figure 41-4, cont'd. E, Compression of the inferior vena cava in a young male patient by an adjacent tumor, which is seen as a round homogenous structure superior to the vein. He presented with bilateral lower extremity swelling. The lumen of the cava is significantly reduced at the site of the compression. The velocity ratio across the narrowing was 8.9 (98/11). F, Significant stenosis in the inferior vena cava of a male patient after liver transplant. The patient had bilateral lower extremity and scrotum swelling. The stenosis occurred at the cavocaval anastomosis. The velocity ratio across the stenosis was 10.3 (175 cm/sec/17 cm/sec).

Some of the conditions most commonly encountered include Baker's cysts, enlarged hematomas, lymph nodes, musculoskeletal injuries, aneurysms, and tumors. In addition, vascular anomalies such as duplications and aberrant anatomic patterns are not uncommon in both the superficial and deep veins. In cases of soft-tissue hematoma or of a ruptured Baker's cyst, anticoagulation is obviously contraindicated. When duplications are present, thrombus in one branch can be easily missed when the other is normal. It is very important that the person performing the DS is aware of these incidental findings and looks carefully for them when the diagnosis of DVT is not obvious.

Examples of incidental findings are presented in Figure 41-5, *A* through *D*.

Natural History of Venous Thrombosis

Thrombus in the below-knee segment of the GSV is benign unless it extends into the above-knee segment. In a recent prospective study, it was shown that 33% of patients with thrombus in the above-knee segment of GSV had a documented episode of pulmonary embolism. However, the proximity of the thrombus to the saphenofemoral junction was not associated with pulmonary embolism. The authors concluded that their findings warrant a larger prospective study.[12] Furthermore, spontaneous SVT in the absence of varicose veins has been associated with a high incidence of hypercoagulable states.[13]

Current guidelines suggest that patients diagnosed with a first episode of acute DVT be placed on some form of anticoagulation for a period of 3 to 6 months. This usually results in resolution of the acute symptoms, which is caused by recovery of the venous outflow as a result of either recanalization of the occluded segment or development of collaterals. Recanalization starts within the first week from the acute episode, and reduction in the thrombus load is most significant in the first 3 months. Approximately 56% of patients followed by serial scans appeared to have complete resolution of the thrombus.[14] It has been shown, however, that thrombus evolution after the acute event is a dynamic process, with spontaneous lysis of the original thrombus and further thrombotic events occurring as competing processes.[15] Recurrent thrombosis is a common event: its cumulative incidence has been reported to be 17% at 2 years, 25% at 5 years, and 30% at 8 years.[16,17] The risk for recurrent DVT is significantly higher in patients with cancer or hypercoagulable states, compared with those in whom the original episode was associated with surgery or recent trauma.[16]

The most feared complication of acute DVT is pulmonary embolism (PE). Untreated proximal DVT carries a 50% risk for PE with a 10% risk for fatal PE.[18,19] Appropriate anticoagulation reduces this risk to less than 5%. This risk reduction is surprisingly high considering that anticoagulation has no effect on the existing thrombus but simply prevents propagation of the existing thrombus or recurrent thrombosis.

Recanalization is associated with various degrees of venous reflux in the venous system. Following an episode of DVT, up to 79% of limbs in some studies may exhibit

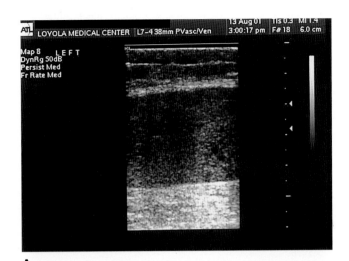

A

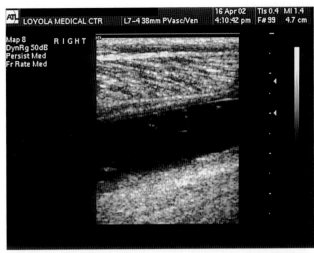

B

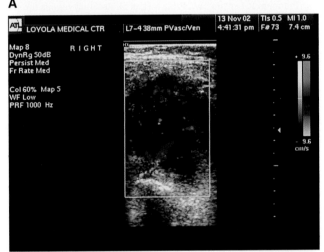

C

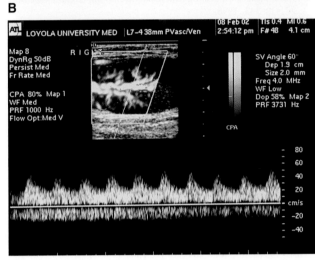

D

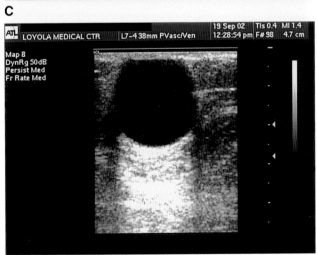

E

Figure 41-5. *Incidental findings.* **A,** *Hemorrhagic Baker's cyst extending in the posteromedial calf. The cystic content and blood has dissected between the deep fascia and the medial head of the gastrocnemius muscle. The echotexture is homogenous and the patient had pain and swelling in the calf for the last 3 days without any improvement. The cyst was excised and the hemorrhagic content in the calf was evacuated.* **B,** *Fresh hematoma dissecting between the medial gastrocnemius and soleus muscle 2 days after calf injury. The patient had calf pain and swelling that was getting worst.* **C,** *Vascular mass in the posterolateral midcalf. The patient had localized calf pain in the area of the mass. The mass was removed and it was diagnosed as lymphoma on histology.* **D,** *Large lymph node in the groin of a patient with severe inflammation caused by many episodes of cellulitis. High flow was detected in the lymph node. These patients have high arterial and venous flow as a result of the vasodilatation from the inflammation.* **E,** *Seroma in the medial aspect of the lower thigh in a patient that had a previous arterial bypass graft with great saphenous vein. This is a cystic structure with clear fluid producing significant acoustic impedance enhancement below it.*

late clinical manifestations of pain, edema, and lipodermatosclerosis and/or ulcerations, known as the postthrombotic syndrome (PTS). Persistent venous obstruction may also contribute to venous hypertension and the development of PTS but is seen less commonly than reflux. Prandoni and colleagues[16] found that after the initial episode of DVT, the incidence of PTS is 23% at 2 years, 28% at 5 years, and 29% at 8 years. The development of ipsilateral recurrent DVT was strongly associated with the risk of PTS.

REFERENCES

1. Fowkes FJ, Price JF, Fowkes FG: Incidence of diagnosed deep vein thrombosis in the general population: Systematic review. Eur J Vasc Endovasc Surg 25:1–5, 2003.
2. Peterson KL: Acute pulmonary thromboembolism: Has its evolution been redefined? Circulation 99:1280–1283, 1999.
3. Heit JA, Silverstein MD, Mohr DN, et al: The epidemiology of venous thromboembolism in the community. Thromb Haemost 86:452–463, 2001.
4. Lohr JM, Kerr TM, Lutter KS, et al: Lower extremity calf thrombosis-to treat or not to treat. J Vasc Surg 14:618–623, 1991.
5. White R, McGahan J, Daschbach M, et al: Diagnosis of deep-vein thrombosis using duplex ultrasound. Ann Intern Med 111:297–304, 1989.
6. Chengelis DL, Bendick PJ, Glover JL, et al: Progression of superficial venous thrombosis to deep vein thrombosis. J Vasc Surg 24:745–749, 1996.
7. Blumenberg RM, Barton E, Gelfand ML, et al: Occult deep venous thrombosis complicating superficial thrombophlebitis. J Vasc Surg 27:338–343, 1998.
8. Labropoulos N, Webb KM, Kang SS, et al: Patterns and distribution of isolated deep calf vein thrombosis. J Vasc Surg 30:787–793, 1999.
9. Hirsh J, Lee AY: How we diagnose and treat deep vein thrombosis. Blood 99:3102–3110, 2002.
10. Prandoni P, Lensing AW, Bernardi E, et al: DERECUS Investigators Group. The diagnostic value of compression ultrasonography in patients with suspected recurrent deep vein thrombosis. Thromb Haemost 88:402–406, 2002.
11. Prandoni P, Cogo A, Bernardi E, et al: A simple ultrasound approach for detection of recurrent proximal-vein thrombosis. Circulation 88:1730–1735, 1993.
12. Verlato F, Zucchetta P, Paolo P, et al: An unexpectedly high rate of pulmonary embolism in patients with superficial thrombophlebitis of the thigh. J Vasc Surg 30:1113–1115, 1999.
13. Lohr JM, Muck PE, Oliverio EA, et al: Superficial vein thrombophlebitis: A clinical marker for a hypercoagulable state. Presented at the 14th annual meeting of the American Venous Forum, February 21–24, 2002, La Jolla, CA.
14. Killewich LA, Macko RF, Cox K, et al: Regression of proximal deep venous thrombosis is associated with fibrinolytic enhancement. J Vasc Surg 26:861–868, 1997.
15. Meissner MH, Caps MT, Bergelin RO, et al: Propagation, rethrombosis, and new thrombus formation after acute deep vein thrombosis. J Vasc Surg 22:558–567, 1995.
16. Prandoni P, Lensing AWA, Cogo A, et al: The long-term clinical course of acute deep venous thrombosis. Ann Intern Med 125:1–7, 1996.
17. Prandoni P, Lensing AW, Prins MH, et al: Residual venous thrombosis as a predictive factor of recurrent venous thromboembolism. Ann Intern Med 17(137):955–960, 2002.
18. Barritt DW, Jordan SC: Anticoagulant drugs in the treatment of pulmonary embolism: A controlled trial. Lancet 1:1309–1312, 1960.
19. Anderson FA, Wheeler HB: Physician practices in the management of venous thromboembolism: A community-wide survey. J Vasc Surg 15:707–714, 1992.

Chapter 42

Importance of Ultrasound Follow-Up After Deep Venous Thrombosis

MARK H. MEISSNER

Because the signs and symptoms of acute deep venous thrombosis (DVT) are nonspecific, the clinical diagnosis is inaccurate and requires objective confirmation. Although contrast venography historically has been the gold standard diagnostic test for acute DVT, it has largely been replaced by venous duplex ultrasonography at most institutions. Venous ultrasonography is widely available, noninvasive, is portable, and unlike venography, has a mean sensitivity and specificity of 97% and 94%, respectively, for the detection of proximal DVT.[1] The high specificity of ultrasonography allows anticoagulation to be instituted without confirmatory venography, whereas the high sensitivity makes it possible to withhold anti-coagulation if serial examinations of the proximal veins are negative. Venous duplex ultrasonography has also been a critical tool in defining the natural history of acute DVT, allowing the course of thrombi in specific venous segments to be noninvasively followed over time. Studies employing duplex ultrasonography have shown the early natural history of acute DVT to be characterized by a balance between processes tending to restore the venous lumen (recanalization) and recurrent thrombotic events.[2,3]

Unfortunately, the accuracy and availability of duplex ultrasonography has led to its overutilization, often for indications beyond those established by prospective trials. An estimated 1 million patients annually undergo investigation for suspected acute DVT in North America[1,4] and a substantial majority of these examinations are negative. It has been estimated that approximately 7 venous duplex scans are performed for each DVT diagnosed.[5] Furthermore, increasing numbers of studies are ordered for the follow-up of an established DVT. Although such follow-up studies have been critical in establishing the natural history of DVT, their clinical utility remains poorly defined. Not only are such studies expensive and a strain on vascular lab resources, they often arise from misconceptions about the role of ultrasound in the treatment of DVT and may result in management errors. Unfortunately, there are few data regarding the utility of serial ultrasound (US) for most purposes, with the American Thoracic Society concluding "there is … no uniformly accepted standard of care for repeating US after DVT is diagnosed."[6] Potential indications for serial studies include their use in algorithms limiting examination to the proximal veins, excluding propagation of isolated calf vein thrombosis, the diagnosis of recurrent DVT, and as a guide to the duration of anticoagulation.

Diagnostic Algorithms Employing Serial Ultrasonography

Validation of any diagnostic test requires accuracy trials to establish the sensitivity and specificity in comparison to a gold standard test. This is followed by management trials in which the test is used to guide clinical care. Establishing the sensitivity and specificity of venous ultrasound requires that consecutive patients with suspected DVT prospectively undergo both ultrasonography and venography with independent blinded interpretation of the results according to explicitly defined standards.[1,7,8] As noted above, such trials have established ultrasonography to have a mean sensitivity of 97% and specificity of 94% for proximal venous thrombosis. Unfortunately, most methodologically sound accuracy trials have limited examination to the proximal veins, often with simple compression of the common femoral and popliteal veins to the level of the tibial confluence.

Management trials are required to establish the safety of treating patients or withholding anticoagulants according to the results of a diagnostic test. As 3% to 7% of proximal thromboses will have an initially negative compression ultrasound of the proximal veins, presumably because of the propagation of isolated calf vein thrombosis, serial studies are required if limited examinations are performed.[9,10] The incidence of thromboembolism within 6 months of serially negative proximal venous examinations is less than 2%,[1,10] and management trials have shown withholding anticoagulation in symptomatic patients with two negative ultrasound examinations 5 to 7 days apart to be safe.[9,11] Unfortunately, this approach requires follow-up examinations (the vast majority of which are negative) in 70% to 80% of patients.[12] Although adding a second ultrasound examination saves 0.74 lives per 1000 patients, the incremental cost is $390,000 dollars per life saved.[13]

Not only are strategies based upon serial studies of all patients with an initially negative proximal venous examination of dubious cost-effectiveness, they are inconvenient for the patient and time-consuming for the vascular laboratory. Alternative strategies have therefore been developed to limit the number of serial examinations required based upon either determination of clinical probability or D-dimer levels. Wells and colleagues[14] have developed a model that allows stratification of patients into low, moderate, and high pretest probability groups based upon eight clinical features or risk factors and the likelihood of an alternative diagnosis (Table 42-1).

TABLE 42-1. **Stratification of Pretest Probability**

Clinical Feature	Score
Active cancer (treatment ongoing or within previous 6 months or palliative)	1
Paralysis, paresis, or recent plaster immobilization of the lower extremities	1
Recently bedridden for more than 3 days or major surgery within 4 weeks	1
Localized tenderness along the distribution of the deep venous system	1
Entire leg swollen	1
Calf swelling by more than 3 cm when compared with the asymptomatic leg (measured 10 cm below tibial tuberosity)	1
Pitting edema (greater in the symptomatic leg)	1
Collateral superficial veins (nonvaricose)	1
Alternative diagnosis as likely or greater than that of deep vein thrombosis	− 2

Low probability, 0 points or less; moderate probability, 1 to 2 points; high probability, 3 points or more. (From Wells PS, Anderson DR, Bormanis J et al: Value of assessment of pretest probability of deep-vein thrombosis in clinical management. Lancet 350:1795–1798, 1997. Reproduced with permission from Elsevier.)

Because the negative predictive value of a normal ultrasound in the low probability group is high, serial scanning may be unnecessary in these patients. Strategies combining proximal venous ultrasound with clinical probability can reduce the requirement for serial examinations to 28% of outpatients and 38.7% of hospitalized patients.[15,16] Such strategies are also safe, with an incidence of thromboembolism over 3 months following a negative evaluation of only 0.6% in outpatients and 1.8% in hospitalized patients. Others have incorporated D-dimer measurements into algorithms that limit serial studies to those with a negative proximal venous ultrasound and a positive D-dimer.[17,18] Such an approach may require proximal venous ultrasound examinations to be repeated in as few as 12.8% of patients with an initially negative scan.[17]

Complete color-flow duplex evaluation of both the proximal and calf veins is an alternative to limited examination of the proximal veins. Unfortunately, strategies employing a single complete examination have not been widely accepted because of the perceived insensitivity of ultrasound for the detection of isolated calf vein thrombosis. However, limited data suggest that the sensitivity and specificity for calf vein thrombosis may be as high as 95% and 100%, respectively, for technically adequate studies. However, it is only 30% and 70%, respectively, for technically limited studies.[19] Unfortunately, as both the availability and acceptance of venography have decreased, trials evaluating the accuracy of a complete, technically adequate duplex are now difficult to perform. However, data from early management trials suggest that such an approach is likely safe. Among 1646 consecutive symptomatic patients in whom all venous segments from the groin to the ankle were evaluated, the diagnostic failure rate caused by technically inadequate studies was only 1% and the incidence of thromboembolism among the 1023 patients followed for 90 days after a negative study was only 0.3%.[20] Similarly, complete lower extremity ultrasonography was technically inadequate in 1.4% of 623 consecutive symptomatic outpatients, and among the 401 patients followed for 3 months after a negative scan, the incidence of subsequent venous thromboembolism was only 0.5%.[12]

It is important that all vascular laboratories adopt a validated algorithm for the ultrasound diagnosis of acute DVT. Optimally such protocols would be based upon methodologically rigorous accuracy and management trials. Although the use of serial scans confined to the proximal veins is safe, this approach is inconvenient, resource intensive, and of doubtful cost-effectiveness. Alternative strategies that limit the need for follow-up studies are therefore needed. Algorithms that combine proximal venous ultrasound with either clinical probability or D-dimer measurements are also safe and significantly reduce the number of required examinations. Similarly, early management trials suggest that a single, technically adequate examination from the groin to the ankle is also

safe. Although somewhat dependent on locally available resources, there is currently little need for strategies that rely on serial imaging of all patients with an initially negative scan.

Isolated Calf Vein Thrombosis

Based upon perceived differences in pathophysiology and natural history, isolated calf vein thrombosis is often considered separately from proximal venous thrombosis. Thrombi that remain confined to the calf veins are associated with fewer thrombotic risk factors, a lower prevalence of associated malignancy, and less extensive activation of coagulation.[21,22] Although associated with late manifestations of the post-thrombotic syndrome in almost one quarter of patients,[21,23] isolated calf vein thrombi are generally associated with a low risk of symptomatic pulmonary embolism. However, propagation to more proximal segments occurs in 15% to 23% of untreated limbs with thrombosis initially confined to the calf veins.[21,24-26]

Based primarily on the risk of proximal propagation, most authorities have concluded that the benefits of treatment exceed the risk and inconvenience of anticoagulation in most patients.[27] Current consensus guidelines recommend that, in the absence of contraindications, patients with isolated calf vein thrombosis receive anticoagulation for at least 6 to 12 weeks.[28] However, serial ultrasonography to exclude proximal propagation is a reasonable alternative in patients with calf vein thrombosis who are poor candidates for anticoagulation. The frequency and duration of such follow-up have not been defined by prospective studies, although testing at 2- or 3-day intervals for 10 to 14 days after presentation has been recommended.[27] Given the efficacy of anticoagulation in preventing thrombus propagation, routine follow-up studies of patients with calf vein thrombosis treated with conventional anticoagulation are not indicated.

Documenting Recurrent Thrombotic Events

Adequate anticoagulation is effective in preventing symptomatic recurrent venous thromboembolism. The incidence of recurrent thromboembolism during treatment is only 2.6%[29] to 5%[28]; however, there is a linear increase in the cumulative risk of recurrent venous thromboembolism after discontinuing anticoagulant therapy corresponding to an annual risk of 5% to 6%.[30] The long-term risk of symptomatic recurrence after a first thrombotic event may be as high as 20.8% to 24.2% after 5 years[31-33] and 30% after 8 years.[34] This risk is clearly higher among those with irreversible risk factors and idiopathic thrombosis.

Although symptoms of pain and edema are common after an episode of acute DVT, objectively documented recurrent thrombosis is present in only about one third of these patients.[35-38] Just as for the index DVT, objective verification of these events is therefore required, and recurrent lower extremity symptoms are an appropriate indication for follow-up ultrasonography. Because manifestations of the post-thrombotic syndrome may be similar to those of recurrent DVT, examination should include an evaluation of reflux as well as of residual or new venous obstruction.

Unfortunately all diagnostic tests for recurrent DVT have some limitations. Variable degrees of residual occlusion, partial recanalization, intimal thickening, and collateral formation may mask new ipsilateral filling defects on venography and limit the utility of ultrasonography in this setting. Compression ultrasound studies may remain abnormal in 50% of patients after 6 months and in 27% to 70% of patients after 1 year.[37,39-41] Incompressibility of a previously normal venous segment is diagnostic of recurrent thrombosis; however, documenting recurrent thrombosis of a previously involved segment may be more difficult. Although in vitro echogenicity correlates with organization, in vivo assessment can be subjective, and even acute thrombi may show various stages of organization.[42] Despite these limitations, color-flow ultrasonography does have some utility in the identification of recurrent DVT.[43] Ultrasound characteristics that are useful in differentiating chronic thrombosis from recurrent DVT are shown in Table 42-2. Other potentially useful strategies include an assessment of thrombus thickness when maximally compressed by the transducer. In comparison to previous examinations, an increase of 2 mm or greater in the compressed thickness of common femoral and popliteal vein thrombi has been reported to have a sensitivity and specificity of 100% for recurrent proximal venous thrombosis.[37] This approach has been proven safe, with only 1.3% of patients having a documented recurrence after serial studies showing a less than 2-mm change in maximally compressed diameter.[38] Because the positive predictive value of a 2-mm or greater increase in maximally compressed diameter is only 90%,[38] other researchers have suggested that only diameter increases of 4 mm or greater be considered diagnostic, and that increases between 1 and 4 mm only require further diagnostic testing.[44]

These considerations suggest that a baseline duplex examination after completion of anticoagulation may be appropriate in at least some patients.[37,39,41] Because recurrent thrombosis is at least as common in the contralateral extremity,[29,30,34] completion of therapy studies should include bilateral examinations. Such evaluation is likely most important in those at highest risk for recurrent thromboembolism, including those with idiopathic thrombosis, congenital or acquired thrombophilia, malignancy, a previous history of DVT, and thrombosis at a young age. Postoperative DVT and other reversible thrombotic risk factors are associated with a substantially lower risk of recurrent thrombosis.[31,33,34] The cost-effectiveness of obtaining baseline studies in those with transient, resolved risk factors is unknown and may be more difficult to justify.

Ultrasound and the Duration of Anticoagulation

The appropriate duration of anticoagulation after an episode of acute DVT has been established by randomized clinical trials in which bleeding and recurrent venous thromboembolism have been the standard primary endpoints. Such trials have established therapeutic doses of either subcutaneous low molecular weight or intravenous unfractionated heparin administered for 5 to 7 days, followed by oral anticoagulant therapy continued for at least 3 to 6 months, as the standard of care for the treatment of acute DVT.[28] The duration of anticoagulation is based on the patient's underlying risk factors. It is clear that some patients benefit from an extended course of oral anticoagulation. The risk of recurrent venous thromboembolism is significantly increased in those patients with idiopathic thrombosis or irreversible risk factors such as malignancy or antiphospholipid antibodies.[45] Most data suggest that the risk of recurrent thrombosis is minimized if patients with reversible risk factors are treated for 3 to 6 months, and patients with a first episode of idiopathic DVT or irreversible risk factors are treated for at least 6 months.[46,47] Anticoagulation

TABLE 42-2. Ultrasound Characteristics of Acute Versus Chronic Thrombus

Diagnostic Criteria	Acute Thrombus	Chronic Thrombus
Incompressibility	Spongy	Firm
Vein Diameter	Dilated	Decreased
Echogenicity	Echolucent	Echogenic
Heterogeneity	Homogenous	Heterogeneous
Luminal surface	Smooth	Irregular
Collaterals	Absent	Present
Flow channel	Confluent	Multiple
Free-floating tail	May be present	Absent

From Meissner MH: Venous Duplex Scanning. In Rutherford RB (ed): Vascular Surgery, 5th ed. Philadelphia: WB Saunders, 2000. Reproduced with permission.

for at least 12 months may be warranted in those with persistent anticardiolipin antibodies, congenital anticoagulant deficiencies, unresolved malignancy, or recurrent idiopathic venous thromboembolism.[28,47]

As implied by the endpoint of recurrent venous thromboembolism, anticoagulant treatment is directed primarily towards interrupting activated coagulation. Although the rate and degree of recanalization appear to be important determinants of the post-thrombotic syndrome, neither of these factors has been extensively evaluated as primary therapeutic endpoints. Furthermore, at least some data suggest that early termination of treatment based upon normalization of noninvasive studies is associated with a worse outcome. Early discontinuation of anticoagulation based upon normalization of impedance plethysmography at 4 weeks was associated with a significantly higher rate of recurrent thrombosis (8.6% vs. 0.9%).[48]

Unfortunately, the benefit of prolonging anticoagulation until no residual thrombus is present is not presently known. Based on observations from natural history studies, there would seem to be little benefit from such an approach. Despite the fact that a 3- to 6-month course of anticoagulation appears to be adequate for patients with reversible risk factors, thrombus resolution is incomplete in many patients after this time. Only approximately 55% of subjects will show complete recanalization within 6 to 9 months of thrombosis.[49-51]

However, there are at least some theoretical reasons why linking the duration of anticoagulation to endpoints such as complete recanalization or activated coagulation might be beneficial. Although there are other determinants (e.g., the level of fibrinolytic inhibition), the degree of activated coagulation has been related to the extent of recanalization.[51] It is possible that incomplete recanalization is a marker for ongoing activation of coagulation and that extended anticoagulation might be beneficial in such patients. It is likely that, rather than being an anatomic or hemodynamic factor, residual venous thrombosis reflects an underlying hypercoagulable state.[36] Others have shown that abnormal D-dimer levels 3 months after discontinuation of oral anticoagulants are associated with a 2.45-fold increased risk of recurrence.[45] Persistently high D-dimer levels were significantly more common in patients with idiopathic thrombosis or permanent risk factors than among those with transient risk factors.

Observational studies have additionally suggested that recurrence rates are higher among those with incomplete recanalization. Using limited examination of the femoral and popliteal veins, Piovella[52] defined normalization as residual thrombus at maximal compression occupying less than 40% of the uncompressed diameter. At 1 year, normalization had occurred in 100% of asymptomatic postoperative patients, 59% of cancer-free symptomatic patients, and only 23.3% of symptomatic patients with

cancer. The probability of recurrent DVT was 8 times higher among patients without ultrasound normalization at 6 months. Prandoni and colleagues,[36] also using an approach that evaluated only the common femoral and popliteal veins, defined complete recanalization as a compressed diameter of 2 mm or less on a single test or 3 mm or less on two consecutive tests. Limited compression ultrasound normalized in 38.8% of patients at 6 months and 73.8% of patients at 36 months. No differences in normalization were noted between those with idiopathic and secondary thrombosis; however, the hazard ratio for a recurrent event was 2.9 when residual thrombosis was present. Both of these studies suggest that residual venous thrombus is an independent risk factor for recurrent thrombotic events. Despite these findings, it must be emphasized that they were derived from very limited compression studies using somewhat arbitrary definitions that differ significantly from the thorough examinations employed by most natural history studies and many clinical vascular laboratories.

Broad guidelines for the duration of anticoagulation are based upon a patient's underlying risk factors and are supported by randomized clinical trials. Although extended anticoagulation in high-risk patients (e.g., those with idiopathic DVT) significantly reduces the rate of recurrence, it is associated with a 1% to 4% per year risk of major bleeding complications.[53] Even when the patient's clinical characteristics are considered, approximately 70% of patients with idiopathic thrombosis will not have a recurrence, whereas 10% of those having reversible risk factors will have further events.[36] More individualized approaches, based upon a patient's underlying thrombotic tendency and residual thrombus burden, are attractive because they would minimize recurrent thrombotic events in high-risk patients while minimizing exposure of lower-risk patients to potential bleeding complications.[53] Unfortunately, despite very promising observational data, such approaches are not supported by evidence from appropriately controlled management trials and cannot yet be recommended. There is, therefore, no current indication to perform follow-up ultrasonography as a guide to the duration of anticoagulation, and this practice should be discouraged pending further trials.

Other Potential Indications for Follow-Up Ultrasonography

Its widespread availability has led to the use of follow-up ultrasonography for many other indications in the absence of significant supporting evidence. Such indications have included the routine follow-up of patients with established DVT while receiving adequate anticoagulation. As noted above, prospective clinical trials have clearly established the safety of treating patients with standard anticoagulation without serial imaging studies to follow the course of the thrombus. The role of ultrasound in following thrombi with free-floating elements is somewhat more controversial, but the data are inconsistent regarding their embolic risk, and most evidence suggests little role for such studies. Although some venographic series have reported these thrombi to be associated with a 4.9-fold increased risk of pulmonary embolism despite adequate anticoagulation,[54] others[55] have demonstrated the incidence of recurrent pulmonary embolism to be similarly low among those with (3.3%) and without (3.7%) free-floating thrombi. Furthermore, it is not entirely clear that free-floating thrombi detected by ultrasonography (defined by the observation of color-flow completely surrounding a central filling defect in both longitudinal and transverse views) are analogous to those identified by venography. Although free-floating elements are seen in 10% to 18% of ultrasound documented thromboses,[56-58] retrospective series have reported the incidence of pulmonary embolism associated with such thrombi to be as low as 2.7%.[58] When followed with serial scans, most ultrasound-documented free-floating thrombi become attached rather than embolizing. Despite treatment recommendations that have included vena caval filtration[59] and bedrest until the thrombus becomes attached,[60] there are currently no prospective, controlled trials supporting routine treatment of free-floating thrombi with modalities other than anticoagulation.[61] There is therefore little indication for routine ultrasound follow-up of patients being treated with adequate anticoagulation in the absence of new symptoms.

Conclusions

The accuracy and widespread availability of venous duplex ultrasonography have led to its acceptance as the primary diagnostic test for acute DVT in many institutions. Its noninvasive nature has also made it possible to perform serial follow-up studies, an application that has allowed the natural history of acute DVT to be determined. Unfortunately, follow-up studies are increasingly being used clinically, a use that potentially strains scarce vascular laboratory resources and that can potentially lead to inappropriate patient management. Potential indications for follow-up venous examinations are shown in Table 42-3. Valid indications for follow-up studies may include those used in algorithms employing serial examinations of the proximal veins in patients with an initially negative examination. However, such algorithms should include some stratification of pretest probability or D-dimer testing to limit the need for serial examinations. Other valid indications for follow-up examinations include the serial evaluation of isolated calf vein thrombosis in the presence of contraindications to anticoagulation, documentation of recurrent thrombotic events, and as a baseline study after completion of anticoagulation in patients at significant risk for recurrence. Although some series have suggested a higher risk of recurrent thrombosis in patients with incomplete recanalization, there are not yet any controlled data to suggest that the standard duration of anticoagulation should be extended in patients with residual thrombus, and the use of ultrasound to guide the duration of anticoagulation should be discouraged for the present. Similarly, there is no evidence that, in the absence of new symptoms, serial follow-up studies are useful in the management of patients receiving adequate anticoagulation.

REFERENCES

1. Kearon C, Julian JA, Math M, et al: Noninvasive diagnosis of deep venous thrombosis. McMaster diagnostic imaging practice guidelines initiative. Ann Intern Med 128:663–677, 1998.
2. van Ramshorst B, van Bemmelen PS, Honeveld H, et al: Thrombus regression in deep venous thrombosis: Quantification of spontaneous thrombolysis with duplex scanning. Circulation 86:414–419, 1992.

TABLE 42-3. Indications for Follow-Up Venous Duplex Scanning

Indication	Valid	Comment
Proximal venous diagnostic algorithms	Yes	Algorithms using pretest probability/D-dimer most efficient
Isolated calf vein thrombosis	Yes	If anticoagulation contraindicated
Recurrent symptoms	Yes	
Completion of therapy	Yes	Baseline examination in high-risk patients
Guiding duration of anticoagulation	No	Lacking prospective, controlled trials
Follow-up in the absence of symptoms	No	
Free-floating thrombus	No	Prospective natural history data inadequate

3. Meissner MH, Caps MT, Bergelin RO, et al: Propagation, rethrombosis, and new thrombus formation after acute deep venous thrombosis. J Vasc Surg 22:558–567, 1995.

4. Strothman G, Blebea J, Fowl R: Contralateral duplex scanning for deep venous thrombosis is unnecessary in patients with symptoms. J Vasc Surg 22:543–547, 1995.

5. Criado E, Burnham C: Predictive value of clinical criteria for the diagnosis of deep-vein thrombosis. Surgery 122:578–583, 1997.

6. American Thoracic Society: The diagnostic approach to acute venous thromboembolism. Clinical practice guideline. J Respir Crit Care Med 160:1043–1066, 1999.

7. White RH, McGahan JP, Daschbach MM, et al: Diagnosis of deep-vein thrombosis using duplex ultrasound. Ann Int Med 111:297–304, 1989.

8. Wells P, Lensing A, Davidson B, et al: Accuracy of ultrasound for the diagnosis of deep venous thrombosis in asymptomatic patients after orthopedic surgery. Ann Intern Med 122:47–53, 1995.

9. Cogo A, Lensing AWA, Koopman MMW, et al: Compression ultrasonography for diagnostic management of patients with clinically suspected deep vein thrombosis: Prospective cohort study. BMJ 316:617–620, 1998.

10. Heijboer H, Buller HR, Lensing AWA, et al: A comparison of real-time compression ultrasonography with impedance plethysmography for the diagnosis of deep-vein thrombosis in symptomatic outpatients. N Engl J Med 329:1365–1369, 1993.

11. Birdwell B, Raskob G, Whitsett T, et al: The clinical validity of normal compression ultrasonography in outpatients suspected of having deep venous thrombosis. Ann Intern Med 128:1–7, 1998.

12. Elias A, Mallard L, Elias M, et al: A single complete ultrasound investigation of the venous network for the diagnostic management of patients with a clinically suspected first episode of deep venous thrombosis of the lower limbs. Thromb Haemost 89:221–227, 2003.

13. Hillner BE, Philbrick JT, Becker DM: Optimal management of suspected lower-extremity deep venous thrombosis: An evaluation with cost assessment of 24 management strategies. Arch Intern Med 152:165–175, 1992.

14. Wells PS, Hirsh J, Anderson DR, et al: A simple clinical model for the diagnosis of deep-vein thrombosis combined with impedance plethysmography: Potential for an improvement in the diagnostic process. J Intern Med 243:15–23, 1998.

15. Wells PS, Anderson DR, Bormanis J, et al: Value of assessment of pretest probability of deep-vein thrombosis in clinical management. Lancet 350:1795–1798, 1997.

16. Wells PS, Anderson DR, Bormanis J, et al: Application of a diagnostic clinical model for the management of hospitalized patients with suspected deep-vein thrombosis. Thromb Haemost 81:493–497, 1999.

17. Bernardi E, Prandoni P, Lensing AW, et al: D-dimer testing as an adjunct to ultrasonography in patients with clinically suspected deep vein thrombosis: Prospective cohort study. The Multicentre Italian D-dimer Ultrasound Study Investigators Group. BMJ 317:1037–1040, 1998.

18. Heijboer H, Ginsberg JS, Buller HR, et al: The use of the D-dimer test in combination with noninvasive testing versus serial non-invasive testing alone for the diagnosis of deep-vein thrombosis. Thromb Haemost 67:510–513, 1992.

19. Rose S, Zwiebel W, Nelson B, et al: Symptomatic lower extremity deep venous thrombosis: Accuracy, limitations, and role of color duplex flow imaging in diagnosis. Radiology 175:639–644, 1990.

20. Schellong SM, Schwarz T, Halbritter K, et al: Complete compression ultrasonography of the leg veins as a single test for the diagnosis of deep vein thrombosis. Thromb Haemost 89:228–234, 2003.

21. Meissner M, Caps M, Bergelin R, et al: Early outcome after isolated calf vein thrombosis. J Vasc Surg 26:749–756, 1997.

22. Meissner MH, Zierler BK, Bergelin RO, et al: Markers of plasma coagulation and fibrinolysis after acute deep venous thrombosis. J Vasc Surg 32:870–880, 2000.

23. Prandoni P, Villalta S, Polistena P, et al: Symptomatic deep-vein thrombosis and the post-thrombotic syndrome. Haematologica 80:42–48, 1995.

24. Kakkar VV, Flanc C, Howe CT, et al: Natural history of post-operative deep-vein thrombosis. Lancet 2:230–232, 1969.

25. Lohr J, Kerr T, Lutter K, et al: Lower extremity calf thrombosis: To treat or not to treat? J Vasc Surg 14: 618–623, 1991.

26. Lagerstedt CI, Olsson C, Fagher BO, et al: Need for long-term anticoagulant treatment in symptomatic calf vein thrombosis. Lancet 2:515–518, 1985.

27. Raskob G: Calf-Vein Thrombosis. In Hull R, Raskob G, Pineo G (eds): Venous Thromboembolism: An Evidence-Based Atlas. Armonk, NY: Futura Publishing, 1996.

28. Hyers TM, Agnelli G, Hull RD, et al: Antithrombotic therapy for venous thromboembolic disease. Chest 119:176S–193S, 2001.

29. Schulman S, Granqvist S, Holmstrom M, et al: The duration of oral anticoagulant therapy after a second episode of venous thromboembolism. The Duration of Anticoagulation Trial Study Group. N Engl J Med 336:393–398, 1997.

30. Schulman S, Rhedin A, Lindmarker P, et al: A comparison of 6 weeks with 6 months of oral anticoagulant therapy after a first episode of venous thromboembolism. N Engl J Med 332:1661–1665, 1995.

31. Hansson P-O, Sorbo J, Eriksson H: Recurrent venous thromboembolism after deep venous thrombosis: Incidence and risk factors. Arch Intern Med 160:769–774, 2000.

32. Lindmarker P, Schulman S: The risk of ipsilateral versus contralateral recurrent deep vein thrombosis in the leg. The DURAC Trial Study Group. J Intern Med 247:601–606, 2000.

33. Holmstrom M, Aberg W, Lockner D, et al: Long-term clinical follow-up in 265 patients with deep venous thrombosis initially treated with either unfractionated heparin or dalteparin: A retrospective analysis. Thromb Haemost 82:1222–1226, 1999.

34. Prandoni P, Lensing A, Cogo A, et al: The long-term clinical course of acute deep venous thrombosis. Ann Intern Med 125:1–7, 1996.

35. Hull RD, Carter CJ, Jay RM, et al: The diagnosis of acute, recurrent, deep venous thrombosis: A diagnostic challenge. Circulation 67:901–906, 1983.

36. Prandoni P, Lensing AW, Prins MH, et al: Residual venous thrombosis as a predictive factor of recurrent venous thromboembolism. Ann Intern Med 137:955–960, 2002.

37. Prandoni P, Cogo A, Bernardi E, et al: A simple ultrasound approach for detection of recurrent proximal vein thrombosis. Circulation 88:1730–1735, 1993.

38. Prandoni P, Lensing AW, Bernardi E, et al: The diagnostic value of compression ultrasonography in patients with suspected recurrent deep vein thrombosis. Thromb Haemost 88:402–406, 2002.

39. Murphy TP, Cronan JJ: Evolution of deep venous thrombosis: A prospective evaluation with US. Radiology 177:543–548, 1990.

40. Mantoni M: Deep venous thrombosis: Longitudinal study with duplex US. Radiology 179:271–273, 1991.

41. Baxter GM, Duffy P, MacKechnie S: Color Doppler ultrasound of the postphlebitic limb: Sounding a cautionary note. Clin Radiol 43:301–304, 1991.

42. O'Shaughnessy AM, Fitzgerald DE: Determining the stage of organization and natural history of venous thrombosis using computer analysis. Int Angiol 19:220–227, 2000.

43. Meissner MH: Venous Duplex Scanning. In Rutherford RB (ed): Vascular Surgery, 5th ed. Philadelphia: WB Saunders, 2000.

44. Kearon C, Ginsberg JS, Hirsh J: The role of venous ultrasonography in the diagnosis of suspected deep venous thrombosis and pulmonary embolism. Ann Intern Med 129:1044–1049, 1998.

45. Palareti G, Legnani C, Cosmi B, et al: Risk of venous thromboembolism recurrence: High negative predictive value of D-dimer performed after oral anticoagulation is stopped. Thromb Haemost 87:7–12, 2002.

46. Watzke HH: Oral anticoagulation after a first episode of venous thromboembolism: How long? How strong? Thromb Haemost 82 (Suppl 1):124–126, 1999.

47. Schulman S: Oral anticoagulation in venous thromboembolism: Decisions based on more than mere feelings. J Intern Med 245:399–403, 1999.

48. Levine MN, Hirsh J, Gent M, et al: Optimal duration of oral anticoagulant therapy: A randomized trial comparing 4 weeks with 3 months of warfarin in patients with proximal deep vein thrombosis. Thromb Haemost 74:606–611, 1995.

49. Killewich LA, Macko RF, Cox K, et al: Regression of proximal deep venous thrombosis is associated with fibrinolytic enhancement. J Vasc Surg 26:861–868, 1997.

50. Arcelus JI, Caprini JA, Hoffman KN, et al: Laboratory assays and duplex scanning outcomes after symptomatic deep vein thrombosis: Preliminary results. J Vasc Surg 23:616–621, 1996.

51. Meissner MH, Zierler BK, Chandler WL, et al: Coagulation, fibrinolysis, and recanalization after acute deep venous thrombosis. J Vasc Surg 35:278–285, 2002.

52. Piovella F, Crippa L, Barone M, et al: Normalization rates of compression ultrasonography in patients with a first episode of deep vein thrombosis of the lower limbs: Association with recurrence and new thrombosis. Haematologica 87:515–522, 2002.

53. Prins MH, Marchiori A: Risk of recurrent venous thomboembolism-expanding the frontier. Thromb Haemost 87:1–3, 2002.

54. Monreal M, Ruiz J, Salvador R, et al: Recurrent pulmonary embolism. A prospective study. Chest 95:976–979, 1989.

55. Pacouret G, Alison D, Pottier J-M, et al: Free-floating thrombus and embolic risk in patients with angiographically confirmed proximal deep venous thrombosis. Arch Intern Med 157:305–308, 1997.

56. Voet D, Afschrift M: Floating thrombi: Diagnosis and follow-up by duplex ultrasound. Brit J Radiol 64:1010–1014, 1991.

57. Berry R, George J, Shaver W: Free-floating deep venous thrombosis: A retrospective analysis. Ann Surg 211:719–723, 1990.

58. Baldridge E, Martin M, Welling R: Clinical significance of free-floating venous thrombi. J Vasc Surg 11:62–69, 1990.

59. Greenfield LJ: Free-floating thrombus and pulmonary embolism. Arch Intern Med 157:2661–2662, 1997.

60. Caprini JA, Arcelus JI, Hoffman KN, et al: Venous duplex imaging follow-up of acute symptomatic deep vein thrombosis of the leg. J Vasc Surg 21:472–476, 1995.

61. Goldhaber SZ: A free-floating approach to filters. Arch Intern Med 157:264–265, 1997.

Chapter 43

Evaluation of Chronic Venous Disease

NICOS LABROPOULOS • LUIS R. LEON JR.

Chronic venous disease (CVD) of the lower extremities is a result of venous hypertension caused by reflux, obstruction, or both.[1] Signs and symptoms may include leg-tiredness or heaviness; burning sensation; itching; aching; cramps; restless limbs; swelling; spider, reticular, and varicose veins; skin changes; atrophie blanche; and ulceration.

Most patients with CVD have a primary etiology. Many factors have been associated with the development of CVD, but for most of them the evidence is weak. These factors include physical characteristics (e.g., height, obesity, age, sex, and race); work, diet, geographical location, social class, and lifestyle; contraceptive pills and hormone replacement therapy; pregnancy and number of pregnancies; and family history of CVD. Of these factors, the strongest associations have been shown with family history and with female sex. Cornu-Thenard and colleagues[2] reported that CVD was detected in 90% of people in whom both parents had CVD. When only one parent was affected, varicose veins were present in 62% of females and 25% of males. The San Diego study showed that superficial disease is more prevalent in females, but skin damage and deep vein disease were less common.[3] The Edinburgh Vein Study[4] did not identify lifestyle risk factors for reflux, but it showed that roles may be played by previous pregnancy, lower use of oral contraceptives, obesity, and mobility at work in females; and by height and straining in males.

In the United Kingdom (UK), female sex, increased age, pregnancy, geographical site, and race were found to be risk factors for varicose veins. Obesity, family history, or occupation were not clearly related to an increased risk.[5] Those same factors were found to be significantly associated to CVD in other population groups.[6–10]

Impact of the Problem

CVD is seen in all decades of life. CVD is cause of considerable morbidity, and it represents the most prevalent vascular disease.[3] Some 27% of adults have detectable lower extremity venous disease,[11] which has a large impact on quality of life regarding pain, physical functioning, mobility, negative emotional reactions, and social isolation.[12] The prevalence of its sequelae (e.g., pigmentary changes and eczema) has been estimated between 3% and 11% of the population.[1] The prevalence of active and healed ulcers combined is around 1%[1] in the Western countries, but this increases to 4.0% in persons over the age of 65 years.[13] The treatment of venous ulcers costs more than $90 million monthly in the United States,[14] and 1.3% of the total health care budget is being spent on such treatment in the UK.[15]

The deleterious complications of CVD can be corrected, but a precise assessment is imperative to differentiate the patterns of CVD so that treatment can be tailored accordingly. Clinical diagnosis of CVD is unreliable. In addition, considerable difficulty exists with regard to which tests to use and how to read their results accurately.[1] This chapter describes the current diagnostic tools available to the vascular practitioner to obtain an accurate diagnosis and to plan a treatment modality.

Pathophysiology of Chronic Venous Disease

Development of incompetent valves has been proposed as an etiology for primary varicose veins. Vein dilation with compromise of valvular competence caused by an inherent weakness of the vein wall is another possible explanation: This currently represents the predominant theory.[16] Primary venous reflux can occur in any superficial or deep vein of the lower extremities, often at different sites. That suggests that reflux is caused by a local or multifocal process in addition to, or separate from, a retrograde process.[17] This is in contrast with the traditional assumption that hemodynamic abnormalities in CVD develop in a retrograde fashion starting at the saphenous-femoral junction (SFJ) level.[17] CVD can also be secondary to an acquired condition. Development of deep venous thrombosis (DVT) accounts for 18% to 28% of limbs with CVD.[18,19] Both primary and secondary etiologies can coexist in the same limb. Congenital etiology is rare and only accounts for 1% to 3% of cases of CVD.[18,19]

Obstruction can result from DVT in the setting of inadequate recanalization and collateralization; or, rarely, as a consequence of extrinsic venous compression or congenital abnormalities of the iliofemoral venous system.[20] Recanalization occurs in most patients with lower extremity venous occlusion after a variable period of time; the faster it happens, the higher the association with competent valves.[21] After an acute episode of DVT, lysis of the thrombus occurs at different times depending on the location of the vein and competence of the valve. The lysis time for competent segments ranges between 214 and 474 days, compared with 65 and 130 days for segments that did not develop reflux, in all locations studied except the posterior tibial vein, where the lysis times for patients with and without competent veins were not different (80 and 72 days, respectively).[22]

Analysis of venographic data in large series studying patients with DVT showed that the left limb was more commonly involved (61% vs. 39%, p < 0.01).[23] Ouriel found that proximal DVT was more commonly encountered on the left side; distal DVT occurred with a more symmetrical distribution.[24] One theoretical explanation to this fact was proposed. The left iliac vein is usually located posterior to the right iliac artery and can be compressed between the artery and the fifth lumbar vertebra. Different grades of compression may lead to different levels of venous stasis changes. McMurrich in 1908 first described the occurrence of leg swelling caused by left iliac vein compression. It was later defined anatomically by May and Thurner in 1957, and clinically by Cockett and Thomas in 1965.[25] The clinical importance of iliac vein obstruction is increasingly recognized; apparently it results in more severe clinical presentations than more distal segmental obstructions.[26] Other conditions that cause extrinsic compression of the venous system (e.g., neoplasms,[27] heterotopic bone formation,[28] retroperitoneal fibrosis,[29,30] and enlarged lymph nodes) have been related to the development of venous thrombosis.

The likelihood of developing clinical sequelae of postphlebitic syndrome has been extensively studied. Risk factors have been identified: ipsilateral recurrent DVT,[31] a combination of reflux and obstruction,[32] and popliteal vein reflux[33-35] were significantly associated with the highest incidence of skin changes and ulceration. In patients with acute DVT, reflux developed in 17% of the limbs 1 week after the initial episode, 37% developed 1 month after, and 69% developed by the end of the first year. It appears to be more prevalent in the segments previously affected with DVT.[36] Patients with signs and symptoms of postphlebitic syndrome have a 3.5 times greater chance of having combined reflux and obstruction than did patients without the syndrome.[32] Prandoni and colleagues[37] followed 355 patients after a first episode of DVT, and found a cumulative incidence of recurrent venous thromboembolism of 17.5% after 2 years, 24.6% after 5 years, and 30.3% after 8 years. The incidence of the postphlebitic syndrome was 22.8%, 28%, and 29.1% after 2, 5, and 8 years, respectively.[37,38] Ipsilateral recurrent DVT was recognized as a strong risk factor associated with development of postphlebitic syndrome, with a hazard ratio of 6.4. The 8-year survival of this cohort was 70.2%.[37,38]

Microcirculation

The most common histologic abnormalities observed in lower extremity veins and skin affected by CVD are vein wall and dermal tissue fibrosis.[39–41] The exact mechanism that results in these injuries is unknown. Venous hypertension causes macromolecules and erythrocyte extravasation; this results in skin discoloration from the hemosiderin deposition and accumulation of mast cells, macrophages, fibroblasts, and white blood cells.[39,42–44] Mast cells release histamine, which is responsible for the itching seen in about a third of patients with CVD. White blood cells stimulate the fibroblasts to produce connective tissue, which leads to lipodermatosclerosis.[39] All these factors contribute to local skin changes seen in disease progression.[45,46]

Diagnostic Methods

The diagnostic methods for evaluation of CVD can be invasive (e.g., phlebography and pressure measurements) or noninvasive (e.g., duplex ultrasound [DU] and plethysmographic tests). These tests are used for assessing reflux and chronic venous obstruction. They are important tests for studying the natural history of CVD, improving patient selection for treatment, and for determining the effect of conservative and interventional management.

Physiologic Tests

Physiologic tests provide quantitative measurements of venous hemodynamics. They include venous pressure measurements, strain-gauge plethysmography (SPG), light reflection rheography (LRR), photo plethysmography (PPG), air plethysmography (APG), and foot volumetry. Because treatment is available for CVD, evaluation with the above techniques can identify the cause and estimate the functional severity.

Venous Pressure Measurements

The most common venous pressure measurement has been the ambulatory venous pressure (AVP). It is based on the assumption that superficial veins are a single compartment, and the pressure measured in one vein is reflection of the pressure throughout the compartment. A 21-gauge butterfly needle is placed into a suitable superficial vein of the foot. This is connected to a pressure transducer, amplifier, and recorder. The patient is asked to stand still and hold on to a frame, and the resting pressure is recorded. Next, the patient is asked to do 10 tiptoe movements, one per second, while changes in venous pressure are recorded. The pressure at the end of the exercise has been defined as the AVP. The time needed for the pressure to return to the resting level is the pressure recovery time.[47] In the normal limb, each pumping cycle lowers the pressure: It takes 6 to 10 cycles to reach maximal pressure drop. When exertion stops, the pressure goes up slowly as the blood returns to the veins, until a maximum point is reached after 2 to 5 minutes. For practical reasons, the 90% recovery time is measured on occasion because it is easier to define and reproduce. An AVP greater than 30 mmHg is considered abnormal. The higher the AVP, the greater the severity of CVD. A linear relationship was found between the incidence of ulceration and AVP.[48]

Dorsal foot vein pressure measurements always decrease with exercise. This may not be true for the popliteal vein, as was demonstrated by simultaneous pressure measurements in the dorsal and the popliteal veins in 45 limbs with CVD signs and symptoms.[49] The popliteal vein pressure increased in 9 limbs (20%), decreased somewhat in 15 limbs (33%), and fell more markedly in 21 extremities (47%). It is not routinely used because of its invasive nature.

Photo Plethysmography

Photo plethysmography measures variations in light absorption in the skin to estimate changes in venous pressure. Hemoglobin is the most abundant chromophore in the skin; therefore light absorption depends on the blood volume in the skin veins.[50] PPG uses an infrared light–emitting diode; a photoelectric cell that measures light reflected from the skin is attached to the limb.[50] The erythrocyte absorbs maximum light in the sitting or standing position when the vein pressure is elevated. Absorption decreases when the pressure falls (e.g., in exertion).[1] The trace that is obtained reflects the changes in light absorption that occur when the limb is stressed (e.g., in ankle dorsiflexion) and during relaxation.[50] The trace is a reflection of the work of the muscles in emptying the veins. Venous emptying and refilling times can then be calculated. Vein reflux causes rapid venous refilling times during relaxation after exertion. A refilling time greater than 23 seconds is normal; refill time of less than 20 seconds is evidence of venous reflux.[50] False negatives can occur when there is significant arterial inflow disease or diminished ankle mobility.[51]

Light Reflection Rheography

LRR is a variation of PPG that uses infrared light and three light diodes, instead of one, to reduce the effect of external light or surface reflection.[52] Like for PPG, patients with leg edema, cellulitis, or with any foot condition that would limit dorsiflexion are not suitable candidates for LRR.

Strain-Gauge Plethysmography

Strain-gauge plethysmography, another variation of the same principle, uses wires, straps, silicon rubber, or other strain gauges to encircle the leg and to sense tension changes caused by a change in the calf diameter on exertion.[52,53] It provides quantitative information about venous emptying and reflux. Variations in the technique and exercise methods have been described,[53,54] but the preferred method involves 20 knee bends at a rate of 30 per minute. The patient stands still until vein plexus refilling occurs (normally in 1 to 2 minutes).[1] Venous refilling time and expelled volume are calculated. Then a 2.5-cm wide cuff is applied in the below-the-knee location and inflated to a pressure of 70 mmHg. If reflux is only superficial, the cuff application normalizes the venous return time.[1] It is considered to be suitable for screening to rule out CVD.[54]

Air Plethysmography

APG uses an air bladder to induce calf diameter or volume changes than can be measured. The 35 cm long, polyurethane, tubular air chamber is applied around the calf and connected to a pressure transducer, an amplifier, and a pen or computerized recorder. A 100-mL syringe is incorporated into the system for calibration to milliliters of limb volume change. It provides information on venous reflux, obstruction, and calf muscle pump function.

To evaluate reflux, the patient is placed in supine position with the legs elevated to empty the veins. Then the heels are rested on a leg support. The air bladder is inflated to 6 mmHg, the lowest value needed to keep it on the leg without compressing the veins. A 14 cm wide thigh tourniquet is applied next to the groin using 80 mmHg of pressure. The functional venous volume (VV) increases until it plateaus, at which time the tourniquet is quickly deflated. The resultant volume decrease is due to venous outflow.[55] The normal VV is 80 to 150 mL; this can rise to 400 mL in patients with CVD.[1] The venous filling index (VFI, mL/sec) is calculated by dividing 90% of VV by the time taken for 90% filling (VFT90); this expresses the average vein-filling rate. It is normally less than 2 mL/sec with slow vein filling from the arterial bed, and can be up to 30 mL/sec for severe reflux. A value of greater than 7 mL/sec has shown to correlate with skin ulcers.[56] The residual volume fraction (RVF) is calculated at the end of 10 tiptoe movements from the residual volume divided by the VV. Abnormal RVF is greater than 40%. This is a result of reflux, poor calf muscle pump performance, or a combination of the two.[57] The RVF worsens with the severity of CVD.[57] Significant proximal obstruction has shown to interfere with this measurement.[56]

The outflow fraction (OF) is calculated as a percentage, dividing the amount of blood that leaves the limb in the first second by the total VV. The procedure is repeated to calculate the OF using superficial occlusion (OFs). The prominent superficial veins are digitally occluded at the knee level just before tourniquet deflation. The digital occlusion falsely elevates the VV by 10 mL. The initial volume and not the one after digital occlusion should be used to avoid false readings.[55]

Foot Volumetry

Norgren and Thulesius introduced foot volumetry in 1973 as a noninvasive method of functional evaluation of venous insufficiency.[58] It measures changes in volume of the foot during exercise using the plethysmographic principle.[1] The volumeter uses an open box filled with water at 14 cm high. A photoelectric sensor connected to a recorder senses the water level. It quantifies the degree of venous insufficiency and differentiates superficial reflux from deep reflux or a combination of both.[1] After standardized exercise, which decreases the blood volume in the limb, the patient is asked to rest, and the volume returns to its baseline level. The experience is repeated using a tourniquet to compress the superficial system at the below-the-knee and the ankle levels to discriminate between superficial and deep insufficiency.[1] The severity of the disease is judged by the reflux time, calculated by the sum of reflux time at six levels. The venous function is globally measured with expelled volume and refilling flow (Q; mL/100 mL × min) after exercise, and expelled volume related to foot volume (EVrel; mL/100 mL).[59] The ratio Q/EVrel is calculated as well, and is useful to discriminate between normal limbs and those with CVD.[1] The severity of the venous disorder and the need for treatment are accurately judged by foot volumetry as a global measure.[59] It is also used to assess therapeutic interventions and to follow patients after they develop DVT to address the extent of valve damage.[1]

Reflux Assessment

Continuous-Wave Doppler Ultrasound

Continuous-wave Doppler ultrasound is used to detect reflux in the outpatient setting. Assessment of a vein is best performed with the patient standing still. The Doppler ultrasound probe is placed at a 45-degree angle. It is crucial to ensure that the ultrasound beam is at the same plane as the axial stream. The patient then performs a Valsalva maneuver to evaluate the groin. In the rest of the limb, thigh, or calf, compression is used to augment bloodflow, and it is followed by sudden release. In normal limbs, there will be no detectable signals during the Valsalva maneuver or during compression release. This method can detect the presence or absence of reflux but it cannot identify its extent and patterns. Therefore, its use now is very limited because most patients undergo treatment only after a duplex ultrasound examination.

Duplex Ultrasound

DU is an inexpensive, quick, and noninvasive method that enabled the authors to quantify venous reflux in individual veins.[47,60,61] Several studies have shown DU to be superior to venography, and it is now regarded as the test of choice to diagnose venous reflux and to assess recurrence.[62–65] Additionally, it has added valuable information in the understanding of the pathogenesis of CVD.[17,66]

Evaluation of the Superficial and Deep Venous Systems

The patient is asked to stand holding on to a frame. Body weight is placed on the contralateral extremity, relaxing the limb under examination, with the knee slightly flexed. Imaging is performed with a color-flow scanner using a multifrequency 4- to 7-MHz linear array transducer. When examining superficial veins found within 1 cm in the subcutaneous fat, a 10-MHz transducer is used. Veins that are found in areas deeper than 6 cm are evaluated with a 3-MHz transducer. The SFJ, common femoral, and the origin of both femoral veins are examined in the standing position. The effect of the Valsalva maneuver and of manual compression of the calf or thigh and sudden release is noted. Manual compression is sufficient to demonstrate reflux; however, when measurements are performed on flow or duration of reflux, standard compression pressures should be used. Subsequently, the femoropopliteal segment and the axial calf veins (posterior and anterior tibial, peroneal, and gastrocnemial veins) are examined in the sitting position with the patient facing the examiner and the foot resting on a stool. In this position, distal compression of the calf or foot is also undertaken. These positions ensure maximum filling of the veins and allow reflux to occur on release of the calf compression.[67] Patients often have to rotate in order to trace the veins in all aspects of the limb. This is particularly important for nonsaphenous veins that are found in many different locations.[68]

The great saphenous vein (GSV) and small saphenous vein (SSV) are examined along their whole length with intermittent calf compression and sudden release (Fig. 43-1). The GSV is identified in the saphenous eye, which is made by the fascial sheets.[69,70] If the vein is outside the saphenous eye, then it is not the GSV but an accessory saphenous or a tributary. The SSV is found within the triangular fascia, which is made by the deep fascia and the fascias of the medial and lateral heads of the gastrocnemius muscle.[71] Foot compression is used when examining the distal ends. All major tributaries, when incompetent, are followed and their course and connections are noted. The majority of patients have reflux in the GSV and its tributaries.[72] Of the tributaries, the posterior and anterior arch vein in the calf and the anterior and medial accessory veins in the thigh are most commonly incompetent.[73]

Color-flow imaging is used initially to locate the appropriate artery (red) and then the adjacent veins are identified. The color image obtained in the vein is different (blue) from that obtained in the artery, indicating that during compression the flow is in the opposite direction to that of the artery. Absence of color on release of the compression indicates absence of reflux and, by inference, competent valves. The appearance of red color in the vein on release of the compression indicates the presence of reflux. This reflux is documented by recording the Doppler waveform. Reflux in the vein under investigation is considered to be present if the duration of the reverse flow is greater than 0.5 sec. Reflux of shorter duration is considered physiologic (i.e., the reverse flow recorded just before closure of the valves).[47,60] This has been evaluated in several reports. In the largest and most recent study,[74] the following was found regarding the best cut-off values for reflux: In the superficial veins, deep femoral veins, and deep calf veins, reflux is greater than 500 ms; in the perforating veins, reflux is greater than 350 ms; and in the common femoral, femoral, and popliteal veins, reflux is greater than 1000 ms.

Reflux is separated into segmental or multisegmental. Reflux is considered to be segmental when it is confined to a single venous segment (i.e., the popliteal vein alone) and multisegmental when it is confined to more than venous segments (i.e., the popliteal vein and the common femoral vein).[75]

Anatomic variations in both the superficial and deep veins are common. Therefore, careful examination and identification of these variations is necessary. For example, the popliteal vein is duplicated in up to 40% of limbs, and pathology is most often found in one of the two veins. Duplications exist in the femoral vein in the thigh and in the GSV and SSV. Triple systems may be

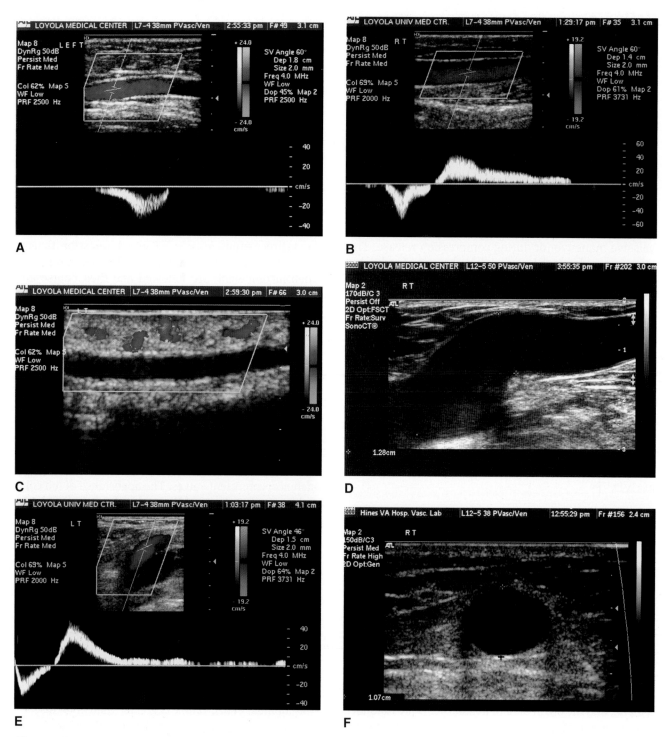

Figure 43-1. **A**, Normal GSV in the midthigh. The vein is located in the fascial compartment. It has normal size and no reflux. **B**, GSV reflux in the lower thigh in a female patient who had varicose veins. The vein is dilated and has prolonged reflux. SFJ was normal. **C**, Normal GSV in the calf. This segment of GSV is most often nonvaricose and may also be spared from reflux. It is in adhesion with the saphenous nerve and for these reasons its removal is avoided. There is reflux in tributaries, which are located superficially to GSV. **D**, Grossly dilated SFJ with spontaneous contrast from the stagnant flow in the standing position. This vein had a significant reflux from SFJ to the upper calf. **E**, Prolonged reflux in the SPJ. The popliteal vein was normal as seen by the absence of color filling after the release of the distal compression. **F**, Dilated SSV in the upper calf. This vein is found in the fascial compartment between the two heads of the gastrocnemius muscle.

seen (e.g., GSV, popliteal, and femoral), and occasionally some veins may be hypoplastic or aplastic (e.g., posterior tibial, GSV, and SSV).[76]

Evaluation of the Perforating Veins

Transverse and oblique scanning is used for the evaluation of the perforating veins because the long axis of these vessels is seen in these planes. A vein is identified as a perforator only if it pierces through the deep fascia (Fig. 43-2). The fascia is easily seen because it is made of collagen and therefore appears bright on the image. Augmentation of bloodflow by distal compression of the limb is used to determine valvular integrity. Reflux or outward flow in these veins is seen only in combination with the superficial and deep veins.[77] Bidirectional flow may be seen in some perforator veins. Only the net outward flow (from deep to superficial) is being evaluated

to determine reflux. The examination starts from the medial malleolus, following the cross-section image of the posterior arch and GSV upward to the knee region. The anterior arch is scanned only if it is varicose. The main trunk of the GSV is imaged from the knee region to the upper thigh. The anterior and posteromedial accessory veins and other thigh tributaries are followed for perforators only if they are varicose. The SSV is scanned from the lateral malleolus until its insertion in the popliteal vein. Medial and lateral varicose tributaries of this vein are also scanned. When a vessel is identified as a perforator vein, its location is recorded as above or bellow the knee. Also any area with varicose veins or a vein cluster is imaged for detecting perforator veins in that area. The above-knee perforators are further divided as upper, middle, and lower thigh. Those in the below-knee segment are divided as upper, middle, and lower thirds of the calf of the GSV and SSV.[75]

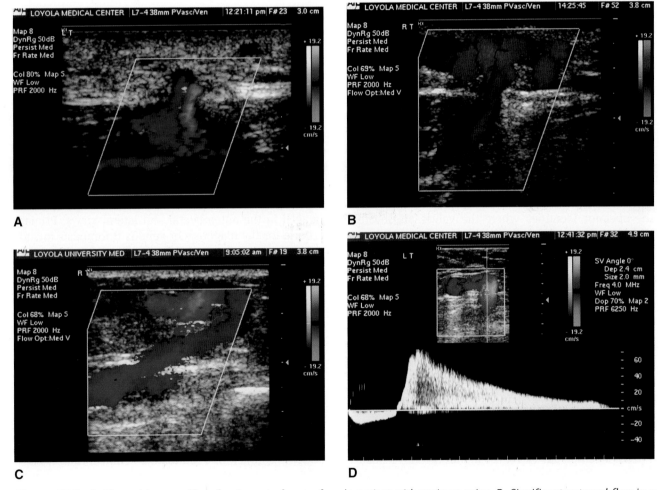

A   **B**

C   **D**

Figure 43-2. A, *Normal lower calf perforator vein from a female patient with varicose veins.* **B,** *Significant outward flow in a lower calf perforator from a male patient with a venous ulcer in the medial malleolus. The vein is dilated even at the fascial level. The refluxing blood is emptying in local tributaries and not in the GSV.* **C,** *Dilated posterior midcalf perforator vein in a female patient with skin changes. She had significant reflux in SSV, segmental reflux in GSV, and marked reflux in the posterior arch vein.* **D,** *Significant high velocity reflux in a midthigh perforator vein. This patient had GSV reflux from SFJ to knee.*

Evaluation of the Ulcer Bed

The veins of the ulcerated area are defined as those passing through the ulcer or within 2 cm from the periphery of the ulcer. In ulcers found over the medial malleolus, the veins are the GSV, the posterior arch, the posterior tibial vein, and the peroneal vein. In ulcers found on the lateral malleolus, the veins are the SSV, with its tributaries; and the peroneal veins. In the ulcers found on the anterior aspect of the leg, the veins are the anterior arch of the GSV and the anterior tibial veins. The relative perforating veins are also assessed by this technique. These veins are imaged by a sterile technique that has been described previously.[78,79] Briefly, the entire surface of the ulcer is covered with a sterile transparent surgical dressing; or, alternatively, the scanhead is covered with a sterile surgical glove that is filled with ultrasonic gel. This technique allows excellent transmission of the ultrasound beam to image the veins, and the ulcer is still protected from additional bacterial contamination. Detection of reflux in these veins is determined by manual compression of the foot and sudden release.

Descending Venography

Descending venography was first done at the Straub Clinic in 1968.[80] It is best done with the patient in a steep, semi-erect position, with a Valsalva maneuver to show functional valve integrity. Dynamic filming using fluoroscopy is needed to demonstrate the function of individual valves. A catheter is introduced percutaneously into the common femoral view (CFV).

When contrast material refluxes distally, one may see valve stations in specific locations. If the proximal valve is competent, distal valves will not be seen. In this manner, the operator identifies where the valves are located. Knowing that, contrast injection is repeated while the patient performs a Valsalva maneuver, and the previously identified valves are observed under stress. If the contrast medium refluxes in any of these tributaries, the distal extent of flow is noted. Because the density of contrast is greater than that of blood, one can observe the heavier contrast settle into the valve cusps of a slowly flowing or static blood column under fluoroscopic monitoring.[80] If the proximal valves are competent, reflux in more distal levels can be missed. Therefore the catheter is advanced to the popliteal vein to assess competency distally.

The normal valve closes completely without any leakage when facing proximal resistance. The harder the push against a competent valve, the tighter the valve closure becomes, whereas the harder the push against an incompetent valve, the greater the reflux that is elicited. Individual valves are categorized as normal or with minimal, moderate, or severe leakage, and five grades of reflux were described (0 to 4).[80]

Tests for Chronic Venous Obstruction

DVT is the most important cause of venous outflow obstruction.[81] There are interventions available to improve venous function. Proper patient selection requires quantitative measurements of insufficiency because venous bypass is contraindicated in severe cases.[82] Evidence to support this was shown previously. Some 68 limbs with obstructed deep veins were studied hemodynamically; 62% were found to have significant insufficiency, but this was detected by contrast venography in only 14.3% of cases.[82]

The tests in this category include contrast ascending venography, contrast descending venography, DU, femoral vein pressures, magnetic resonance venography (MRV), arm/foot pressure differential, and venous obstruction resistance.

Ascending Venography

Ascending venography has been considered the gold standard for assessment of vein patency, vein anatomy, and to investigate the etiology of CVD.[1,83] Radio-opaque contrast material is injected into a dorsal foot vein in the 60-degree erect position. This may be somewhat difficult because of foot edema caused by the very medical condition that requires venography to be performed. An ankle tourniquet inflated to 120 to 140 mmHg is used to direct the contrast into the deep veins. The semierect position or a second midthigh cuff is used to prolong the contrast time. Each leg is examined separately. The table is tilted 20 to 60 degrees downward, and internal rotation of the foot and ankle is performed to separate the images of the tibia and fibula. The calf deep veins are imaged in the anterolateral and lateral views. Primary criteria for the diagnosis of venous thrombosis include an obvious intraluminal thrombus, nonvisualization of named deep veins despite adequate venous filling, or eccentric luminal filling defects seen in more than one projection.[84] Secondary criteria include a paucity of vessels with adequate filling of named deep veins; a persistent, concentric focal luminal narrowing; extensive collateral formation around a focal, nonvisualized area; and obvious recanalization, indicating chronic thrombosis.[84] If the visualization of the iliac veins and IVC is not satisfactory, contrast is injected through the CFV.

Venography poses important clinical and methodologic limitations. It is invasive and has significant morbidity, particularly in the setting of systematic screening for patients enrolled in a randomized clinical trial. It has a 1.3% risk of developing DVT.[85] In addition, venography cannot provide hemodynamic information about the severity of CVD.[1] The development of alternative safer and noninvasive methods has significantly reduced its use.[1]

Duplex Ultrasound

DU is also used to evaluate venous inflow and outflow. The veins are examined with patients in the reverse Trendelenburg position for both acute and chronic thrombosis. The latter is characterized by complete or partial luminal obstruction (Fig. 43-3). The lumen may be reduced in size, and the walls can be thickened. In patients with partial recanalization, flow channels are seen and usually have reflux. Around the area of obstruction, collateral veins may be seen depending on its severity. Endoluminal echoes are echogenic because the thrombus remodels into the fibrous tissue. DU can identify flow in individual veins and can assess their flow characteristics, but it cannot quantify the hemodynamic significance of the obstruction. It is also limited by its field of view, imaging multiple areas and collateral pathways at one ultrasonic slice. Therefore other methods such as venography and MRV are necessary if interventional treatment is planned.

Femoral Vein Pressures

Femoral vein pressure addresses the degree of venous flow obstruction by measuring the pressure elevation and pressure gradient after exertion and the time for these parameters to return to resting levels.[86] This adds useful information to the morphologic assessment of contrast venography. Absolute pressure values during rest and exercise are less reliable indicators. Exercise is usually induced with 10 foot dorsiflexions or 20 calf muscle contractions.[1] Good correlation was found between femoral vein pressures and the severity of post-thrombotic iliocaval obstruction.[86] Even though no set standards are available for this test,[1] a pressure gradient cutoff set up at 5 mmHg, and doubled resting femoral pressure values after exercise, have been suggested to justify venous bypass.[87] In cases of ipsilateral iliac thrombosis, and in the absence of IVC involvement, the contralateral femoral has lower pressure. This asymmetry can further substantiate the significance of the obstruction.

Magnetic Resonance Venography

Improvements in magnetic resonance technology have allowed an increasing role for this modality in CVD diagnosis. It is able to identify vein wall inflammatory changes, to differentiate acute from chronic thrombi, to distinguish patent from occluded veins, and to provide information about neighboring soft tissues.[88] MRV offers several advantages over venography. It is noninvasive, and contrast material is not needed. A computer-generated venous roadmap is produced that can be rotated in innumerable views without the need for additional

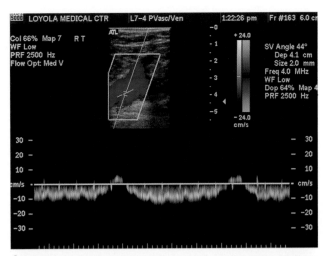

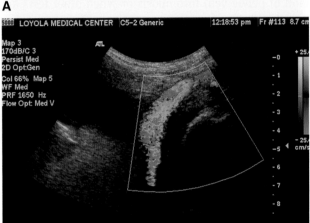

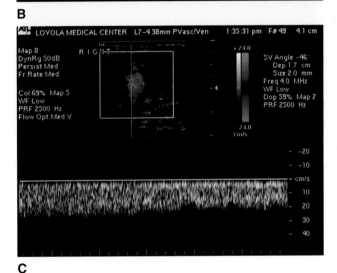

Figure 43-3. **A**, *Normal common femoral vein with spontaneous and phasic flow. In quiet breathing the phasicity is largely caused by changes in the right atrial pressure and not by respiration.* **B**. *Chronic obstruction of the left iliac and femoral veins in a patient with pain and swelling after a DVT that never recanalized.* **C**, *High flow in venous collaterals of the deep external pudendal vein from a patient with chronic iliofemoral obstruction.*

contrast.[88] It allows investigation of congenital malformations.[89] In addition, review of axial images is possible, allowing venous cross-section analysis to detect subtle defects that can be missed in two-dimensional views. It has some drawbacks, such as an inability to be used with claustrophobic or noncooperative patients or in patients with non-MRV compatible metallic implants, and it has a higher cost.[88] When compared with venography, it has shown comparable sensitivity and specificity.[88] It has been shown to detect flow in the internal iliac vein and its tributaries, an area not well visualized by venography.[90,91]

Magnetic resonance imaging can be used as a definitive examination when initial screening studies are unclear, or as a first-line methodology if there is suspicion of pelvic vein thrombosis or when other tests are unavailable.[92]

Arm/Foot Pressure Differential

This technique is based on the principle that an arm/foot venous pressure differential occurs with venous obstruction, and that collateralization or recanalization can be assessed by monitoring venous pressure changes in the leg after inducing hyperemia.[93] With the patient supine, 21-gauge butterfly needles are placed simultaneously into a dorsal foot vein and into a dorsal vein of the hand. Both needles are connected to a pressure transducer for continuous pressure recording before and after reactive hyperemia of the foot. Hyperemia is induced by thigh occlusion, using a tourniquet for 3 minutes; or by papaverine.[81,94] Outflow obstruction is classified in four grades, 1 to 4, from fully compensated to fully decompensated, depending on the pressure differential at rest and during hyperemia. This test is clinically used to choose the appropriate individualized intervention for venous reconstruction (e.g., performance of venous bypass rather than valve transposition or repair). A bypass is indicated when a grade 3 or 4 obstruction is diagnosed.[1]

This technique proved to be reliable and easily accomplished in combination with AVP measurements.[93] The combination of this technique and the foot vein pressure elevation after induced hyperemia are a reliable way to diagnose and grade global chronic obstruction.[95]

Venous Obstruction Resistance

Venous obstruction resistance (VOR) is calculated from simultaneous recordings of volume and pressure outflow curves. The pressure outflow curve is obtained by placing a 21-gauge butterfly needle in a vein in the dorsum of the foot while the volume outflow curves are simultaneously recorded. Pressure outflow curves are obtained using APG as described above. The volume outflow curves are obtained with and without superficial vein occlusion. The latter allows the clinician to predict the flow by drawing a tangent at any point of the curve. Therefore the resistance can be calculated by dividing the corresponding pressure from the venous outflow curve by the flow.[81] A sharp increase in the VOR occurs with venous outflow pressures below 20 mmHg, likely because of a smaller cross-sectional area from vessel collapse at low pressures.[81]

VOR measurements correlate with arm/foot pressure differential recordings and can be used reliably to determine the magnitude of the venous obstruction.[81] They also correlate well with the level and severity of obstruction.[81]

Intramuscular Pressures

The wick catheter technique was described in 1968 for measurement of subcutaneous pressure. It has been modified for intramuscular insertion and monitoring of interstitial fluid pressures. The technique was shown to be accurate and reproducible in animal studies. Its main clinical application has been in the diagnosis and treatment of compartment syndrome.[96] It has been also used to assess the influence of DVT on intramuscular pressure.[96,97] This is particularly useful in the identification of patients with venous claudication in the presence of chronic venous obstruction. In an acute setting, it can be used to determine if fasciotomy is needed.[96] The catheter is placed in the anterior tibial and the deep posterior compartments of the affected leg. The normal pressure is usually less than 15 mmHg, and it is higher in the anterior compartment.[98] Patients experience symptoms when the pressure is greater than 30 mmHg.[98,99] Increased intramuscular pressure reduces bloodflow and can cause ischemia. The intramuscular pressure is higher in the thrombosed leg than in the contralateral leg, and the difference is proportional to the extension of the thrombus.[98,99] Iliofemoral thrombosis causes a significantly higher pressure than calf thrombosis.

Technetium 99M-Sulfur Colloid Lymphoscintigraphy

Technetium 99M-sulfur colloid lymphoscintigraphy (TCL) is used to diagnose lymphedema. Raju and colleagues[100] observed that in several cases, TCL improved or normalized after stent placement for a coexisting iliac venous stenosis, suggesting that the abnormality may represent a correctable condition rather than lymphedema. Technetium 99M-sulfur colloid is administered through an intradermal and subcutaneous injection into the first web space. Leg and pelvis images are obtained using a gamma camera at different times. Patients walk before and in between the imaging. Results are called normal when the radioactive material flows symmetrically with the opposite limb in a cephalad direction, and when nodes are visualized as early as 10 minutes and well developed 20 minutes afterward. Results are abnormal if nodal visualization is faint or delayed beyond 30 minutes. When nodal visualization fails to occur at 60 minutes, lymphatic activity is called absent. Treatment of venous obstruction may improve the lymph transport mechanism; it also seems to improve after reflux treatment with venous valve reconstruction. Aggressive investigation for a venous basis of edema in these patients is suggested; if found and corrected, significant clinical improvement in limb swelling and pain may be achieved in many patients.[100]

Intravascular Ultrasound

Intravascular ultrasound (IVUS) is characterized by the ability to show tomographic sections of the lumen and wall of blood vessels. It provides in vivo assessment of the luminal area and the analysis of the vessel three-layer wall. IVUS-generated results correlated well with histology and angioscopy in in vitro studies.[101] It compares favorably with standard venography. It is superior for the estimation of the degree of iliac vein stenosis. Venography underestimates the degree of stenosis by 30%, and it was shown to be inaccurate in detecting obstructions greater than 70%. IVUS is also superior when choosing the length and size of stents to be used during interventional procedures. IVUS-guided therapeutic interventions have shown good ulcer healing rates, edema resolution, and pain relief.[26]

The concept of a significant obstruction being a stenosis of greater than 70% to 80% came from arterial studies. It may not hold true for veins because of important hemodynamic and anatomic differences.[36] Hence, it is unclear when a stenosis should be considered significant. At this time, IVUS appears to be the best test available for its diagnosis.

The CEAP Classification System

In February 1994, an international committee of the American Venous Forum, led by Andrew Nicolaides at a meeting organized by the Straub Foundation in Hawaii, adopted a single classification system for CVD: the CEAP classification.[102] A consensus document was produced based on clinical manifestations (C), etiology (E), anatomic distribution of involvement (A), and pathophysiologic findings (P). It was published in 25 journals and books in eight languages,[102] and currently most published papers on venous disease quote the CEAP classification.[102] It is useful for both clinical and research purposes.

Clinical Grading

The clinical section of CEAP grades the severity of CVD in seven classes (0 to 6). It was designed as a framework of classes with ascending severity. Limbs can be further characterized as symptomatic (s) or asymptomatic (a) in each class.[103] Overall, approximately 75% are symptomatic limbs. No association between the CEAP class and the presence of symptoms can be found, but the severity of symptoms appears to be related to the stage of the disease.[104] An increasing mean value of each severity index tested correlates with increasing C classes in prior studies.[103] Varicose veins are the most common sign, and several signs from one or more of the classes can be present in a single limb.[104] Figure 43-4 shows the prevalence of signs in CVD, taking into account the worst class only. Clearly, when all signs are considered, the overall prevalence of telangiectasias and varicose veins is greater than 80%. Skin changes are found in 20% to 25% of limbs. Approximately 7.5% to 14% of patients with CVD have healed or active venous ulcers.[1,14,105]

In a multicenter study in Europe, data from 872 patients were analyzed regarding the clinical definition of each CEAP class. A significant association has been shown between ascending severity and risk factors, including age of the patient, history of previous DVT, the diameter of the most dilated varicose vein, venous symptomatology, and the presence of a corona phlebectatica.[106] The intraobserver reproducibility was good but the interobserver reproducibility was poor.[106] That prompted an effort to increase the accuracy of "C" in CEAP. Precise definitions of clinical items and detailed explanations for the individual classes were produced in a recent paper.[38]

Etiology

The etiology of CVD can be primary, secondary, or congenital.[104] Primary etiology accounts for the largest number of patients, and it is most often confined to the superficial venous system.[66] It has been shown to be the cause in about two thirds of the limbs studied (see Fig. 43-4).[18,19,104] It denotes an unknown etiology, and includes all cases of reflux but the post-thrombotic.[18] The secondary problems have a known cause (e.g., post-thrombotic or post-traumatic occlusions or reflux) when they have been proved by objective tests.[18] They are present in 18% to 28% of limbs with CVD. The congenital problems account for 1% to 3% of cases and include birth defects (e.g., Klippel-Trenaunay syndrome[18]) and valve aplasia.[107] They may be recognized at birth or later in life.

Anatomic Distribution

The anatomic distribution in all clinical classes is based on 1000 consecutive limbs with CVD evaluated in the authors' center. Superficial veins are affected in the vast majority of limbs with CVD, with a 90% superficial vein involvement, compared with 30% of deep vein and 20% of perforator vein involvement.[18,19,104] Reflux confined

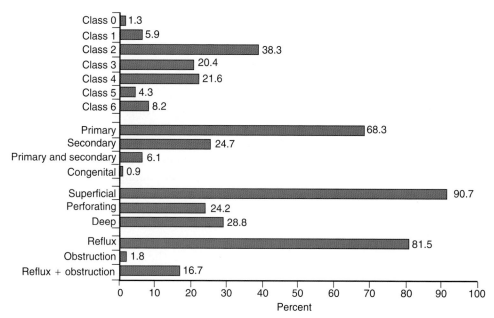

Figure 43-4. *This chart shows data from 1000 consecutive limbs with CVD using the CEAP classification. These are taken from a large prospective study in which the first author is the principal investigator. In the anatomic classification only the overall involvement of each venous system is shown.*

to the superficial veins only is responsible for 17% to 54% of CEAP classes 5 and 6.[18,57,66,72,78,79] About 80% to 90% of limbs in these classes have incompetent superficial veins.[18,57,66,104] Reflux in the saphenous veins and their tributaries has the highest prevalence.[17] Isolated deep vein reflux is a rare occurrence, being present in less than 10% of patients with venous ulcers.[57,66] Most limbs in the low clinical classes have reflux limited to the superficial system only, whereas those with CVD classes 4 to 6 have a complex reflux pattern and involve deep and perforator veins commonly.[103,108]

Pathophysiology

Present data suggest that abnormalities in the venous endothelium and smooth muscle cells result in vein wall dilatation with resultant valve incompetence and venous reflux.[108] Vein reflux alone is present in about 80% of limbs, obstruction alone is found in 2%, and a combination of the two in 17% of cases (see Fig. 43-4).[18,103] The latter is most commonly seen in higher clinical classes, and it carries a worse prognosis for skin damage and ulceration than either reflux or obstruction separately.[32] The prevalence of DVT increases with higher clinical classes, and this can explain the higher prevalence of deep vein involvement. The E, A, and P are not widely employed. Apparently easily used by some and cumbersome to others, refinements have been suggested to make these more universally user-friendly.[109]

Severity Scoring

In the year 2000, a new venous clinical severity scoring system (VCSS) was developed.[110] Clinical features of CVD are graded from 0 to 3 as absent, mild, moderate,

and severe. Points from 0 to 3 are added to address the impact of conservative therapy (compression and elevation). A maximum of 30 points can be reached. Another score was designed, the Venous Segmental Disease Score (VSDS), in which 11 venous segments are categorized according to presence of reflux and/or obstruction based on imaging studies alone. A maximum score of 10 can be reached.[110] In addition, the pre-existing CEAP disability score was modified (venous disability score, VDS), substituting the reference to work and an 8-hour working day with the patient's prior normal activities.

These new scoring schemes complement the current CEAP system.[110] An observational study was recently designed to validate this scoring system. They demonstrated good correlation with anatomic extent. VCSS and CEAP were equally sensitive and significantly superior for measuring outcomes after superficial venous surgery.[111] Although CEAP alone is good for the routine clinical use, the VSDS and VCSS provide better measuring standards for evaluating outcome.

Conclusions

Detection of reflux and obstruction and evaluation of the calf muscle pump can be done with the current methods. Significant improvement has occurred in the pathophysiology and management of CVD through these tests. When necessary, a combination of imaging and physiologic tests provide a more complete assessment. Far from being perfect tools, there is significant room for improvement in many areas. Statistical validation of tests needs to be rigorous to improve accuracy.

REFERENCES

1. Nicolaides AN: Investigation of chronic venous insufficiency: A consensus statement. Circulation 102:E126–E163, 2000.
2. Cornu-Thenard A, Boivin P, Baud JM, et al: Importance of familial factor in varicose disease. J Dermatol Surg Oncol 20:318–326, 1994.
3. Criqui MH, Jamosmos M, Fronek A, et al: Chronic venous disease in an ethnically diverse population: The San Diego Population Study. Am J Epidemiol 158:448–456, 2003.
4. Fowkes FG, Lee AJ, Evans CJ, et al: Lifestyle risk factors for lower limb venous reflux in the general population: Edinburgh Vein Study. Int J Epidemiol 30:846–852, 2001.
5. Callam MJ: Epidemiology of varicose veins. Br J Surg 81:167–173, 1994.
6. Tovalin Ahumada H, Lazcano Ramirez F: Health status of urban passenger transportation conductors in Mexico City. Bol Oficina Sanit Panam 111:324–332, 1991.
7. Brand FN, Dannenberg AL, Abbott RD, et al: The epidemiology of varicose veins: The Framingham Study. Am J Prev Med 4:96–101, 1988.
8. Abramson JH, Hopp C, Epstein LM: The epidemiology of varicose veins. A survey in western Jerusalem. J Epidemiol Community Health 35:213–217, 1981.
9. Beaglehole R, Salmond CE, Prior IAM: Varicose veins in New Zealand: Prevalence and severity. NZ Med J 84:396–399, 1976.
10. Seidell JC, Bakx KC, Deurenberg P, et al: Overweight and chronic illness: A retrospective cohort study, with a follow-up of 6 to 17 years, in men and women of initially 20 to 50 years of age. J Chron Dis 39:585–593, 1986.
11. Moneta GL, Nehler MR, Porter JM: Pathophysiology of Chronic Venous Insufficiency. In Rutherford RB (ed): Vascular Surgery, 5th ed. Philadelphia: WB Saunders, 2000.
12. van Korlaar I, Vossen C, Rosendaal F, et al: Quality of life in venous disease. Thromb Haemost 90:27–35, 2003.
13. Callam M: Prevalence of chronic leg ulceration and severe chronic venous disease in western countries. Phlebology (Suppl.) 1:6–12, 1992.
14. Hume M: A venous renaissance? J Vasc Surg 15:947–951, 1992.
15. Office of Health Economics: Chronic Venous Disease of the Leg. Report 108. London: Office of Health Economics, 1992.
16. Turton EP, Scott DJ, Richards SP, et al: Duplex-derived evidence of reflux after varicose vein surgery: Neo-reflux or neovascularization? Eur J Vasc Endovasc Surg 17:230–233, 1999.
17. Labropoulos N, Giannoukas AD, Delis K, et al: Where does venous reflux start? J Vasc Surg 26:736–742, 1997.
18. Kistner RL, Eklof B, Masuda EM: Diagnosis of chronic venous disease of the lower extremities: The "CEAP" classification. Mayo Clin Proc 71:338–345, 1996.
19. Labropoulos N: CEAP in clinical practice. Vasc Surg 31:224–225, 1997.
20. Gloviczki P, Stanson AW, Stickler GB, et al: Klippel-Trenaunay syndrome: The risks and benefits of vascular interventions. Surgery 110:469–479, 1991.
21. Killewich LA, Bedford GR, Beach KW, et al: Spontaneous lysis of deep venous thrombi: Rate and outcome. J Vasc Surg 9:89–97, 1989.
22. Meissner MH, Manzo RA, Bergelin RO, et al: Deep venous insufficiency: The relationship between lysis and subsequent reflux. J Vasc Surg 18:596–605; discussion 606–608, 1993.
23. Mewissen MW, Seabrook GR, Meissner MH, et al: Catheter-directed thrombolysis for lower extremity deep venous thrombosis: Report of a national multicenter registry. Radiology 211:39–49, 1999.
24. Ouriel K, Green RM, Greenberg RK, et al: The anatomy of deep venous thrombosis of the lower extremity. J Vasc Surg 31:895–900, 2000.
25. Wolpert LM, Rahmani O, Stein B, et al: Magnetic resonance venography in the diagnosis and management of May-Thurner syndrome. Vasc Endovascular Surg 36:51–57, 2002.
26. Neglen P, Raju S: Proximal lower extremity chronic venous outflow obstruction: Recognition and treatment. Semin Vasc Surg 15:57–64, 2002.
27. Viselli AL, Feuer GA, Granai CO: Lower limb ischemic venous thrombosis in patients with advanced ovarian carcinoma. Gynecol Oncol 49:262–265, 1993.
28. Orzel JA, Rudd TG, Nelp WB: Heterotopic bone formation (myositis ossificans) and lower-extremity swelling mimicking deep-venous disease. J Nucl Med 25:1105–1107, 1984.
29. Mathew CV, Shanabo A, Zyka I, et al: Retroperitoneal fibrosis with large-vessel obstruction: An uncommon vascular disorder. Acta Chir Scand 151:475–480, 1985.
30. Rhee RY, Gloviczki P, Luthra HS, et al: Iliocaval complications of retroperitoneal fibrosis. Am J Surg 168:179–183, 1994.
31. Ziegler S, Schillinger M, Maca TH, et al: Post-thrombotic syndrome after primary event of deep venous thrombosis 10 to 20 years ago. Thromb Res 101:23–33, 2001.
32. Johnson BF, Manzo RA, Bergelin RO, et al: Relationship between changes in the deep venous system and the development of the postthrombotic syndrome after an acute episode of lower limb deep vein thrombosis: A 1- to 6-year follow-up. J Vasc Surg 21:307–12; discussion 313, 1995.
33. Shull KC, Nicolaides AN, Fernandes e Fernandes J, et al: Significance of popliteal reflux in relation to ambulatory venous pressure and ulceration. Arch Surg 114:1304–1306, 1979.
34. Brittenden J, Bradbury AW, Allan PL, et al: Popliteal vein reflux reduces the healing of chronic venous ulcer. Br J Surg 85:60–62, 1998.
35. Saarinen JP, Domonyi K, Zeitlin R, et al: Postthrombotic syndrome after isolated calf deep venous thrombosis: The role of popliteal reflux. J Vasc Surg 36:959–964, 2002.
36. Markel A, Manzo RA, Bergelin RO, et al: Valvular reflux after deep vein thrombosis: Incidence and time of occurrence. J Vasc Surg 15:377–382, 1992.
37. Prandoni P, Lensing AW, Cogo A, et al: The long-term clinical course of acute deep venous thrombosis. Ann Intern Med 125:1–7, 1996.
38. Prandoni P: Long-term clinical course of proximal deep venous thrombosis and detection of recurrent thrombosis. Semin Thromb Hemost 27:9–13, 2001.
39. Pappas PJ, You R, Rameshwar P, et al: Dermal tissue fibrosis in patients with chronic venous insufficiency is associated with increased transforming growth factor-beta 1 gene expression and protein production. J Vasc Surg 30:1129–1145, 1999.
40. Pappas PJ, DeFouw DO, Venezio LM, et al: Morphometric assessment of the dermal microcirculation in patients with chronic venous insufficiency. J Vasc Surg 26:784–795, 1997.
41. Pappas PJ, Gwertzman GA, DeFouw DO, et al: Retinoblastoma protein: A molecular regulator of chronic venous insufficiency. J Surg Res 76:149–153, 1998.
42. Rook A, Wilkinson DS, Ebling FJG, et al (eds): Textbook of Dermatology, 4th ed. Oxford: Blackwell Scientific, 1986.
43. Scott HJ, Coleridge Smith PD, Scurr JH: Histological study of white blood cells and their association with lipodermatosclerosis and venous ulceration. Br J Surg 78:210–211, 1991.
44. Matic M, Duran V, Ivkov-Simic M, et al: Microcirculatory changes in chronic venous insufficiency. Med Pregl 53:579–583, 2000.
45. Leu AJ, Leu HJ, Franzeck UK, et al: Microvascular changes in chronic venous insufficiency: A review. Cardiovasc Surg 3:237–245, 1995.
46. Duran W, Pappas PJ, Schmid-Schonbein GW: Microcirculatory inflammation in chronic venous insufficiency: Current status and future directions. Microcirculation 7(6 Pt 2):S49–S58, 2000.
47. Vasdekis SN, Clarke GH, Nicolaides AN: Quantification of venous reflux by means of DU. J Vasc Surg 10:670–677, 1989.
48. Nicolaides AN, Hussein MK, Szendro G, et al: The relation of venous ulceration with ambulatory venous pressure measurements. J Vasc Surg 17:414–419, 1993.

49. Neglen P, Raju S: Ambulatory venous pressure revisited. J Vasc Surg 31:1206–1213, 2000.
50. Sarin S, Shields DA, Scurr JH, et al: Photoplethysmography: A valuable noninvasive tool in the assessment of venous dysfunction? J Vasc Surg 16:154–162, 1992.
51. Schroeder PJ, Dunn E: Mechanical plethysmography and Doppler ultrasound. Diagnosis of deep-venous thrombosis. Arch Surg 117:300–303, 1982.
52. Physiologic and Other Tests for Venous Evaluation. In Weiss RA, Feied C, Weiss MA (eds): Vein Diagnosis and Treatment: A Comprehensive Approach. New York: McGraw-Hill, 2001.
53. Mason R, Giron F: Noninvasive evaluation of venous function in chronic venous disease. Surgery 91:312–317, 1982.
54. Struckmann J, Mathiesen F: A noninvasive plethysmographic method for evaluation of the musculovenous pump in the lower extremities. Acta Chir Scand 151:235–240, 1985.
55. Kalodiki E, Calahoras LS, Delis KT, et al: Air plethysmography: The answer in detecting past deep venous thrombosis. J Vasc Surg 33:715–720, 2001.
56. Harada RN, Katz ML, Comerota A: A noninvasive screening test to detect "critical" deep venous reflux. J Vasc Surg 22:532–537, 1995.
57. Labropoulos N, Giannoukas AD, Nicolaides AN, et al: The role of venous reflux and calf muscle pump function in nonthrombotic chronic venous insufficiency. Correlation with severity of signs and symptoms. Arch Surg 131:403–406, 1996.
58. Brudin LH, Landgren IM, Bengtsson M, et al: A modified method of curve analysis in foot volumetry and its reference values. Clin Physiol 9:189–197, 1989.
59. Danielsson G, Norgren L, Jungbeck C, et al: Global venous function correlates better than duplex derived reflux to clinical class in the evaluation of chronic venous disease. Int Angiol 22:177–181, 2003.
60. van Bemmelen PS, Bedford G, Beach K, et al: Quantitative segmental evaluation of venous valvular reflux with duplex ultrasound scanning. J Vasc Surg 10:425–431, 1989.
61. Szendro G, Nicolaides AN, Zukowski AJ, et al: DU in the assessment of deep venous incompetence. J Vasc Surg 4:237–242, 1986.
62. Labropoulos N, Touloupakis E, Giannoukas AD, et al: Recurrent varicose veins: Investigation of the pattern and extent of reflux with color-flow duplex imaging. Surgery 119:406–409, 1996.
63. Neglen P, Raju S: A comparison between descending phlebography and duplex Doppler investigation in the evaluation of reflux in chronic venous insufficiency: A challenge to phlebography as the gold standard. J Vasc Surg 16:687–693, 1992.
64. Welch HJ, Faliakou EC, McLaughlin RL, et al: Comparison of descending phlebography with quantitative photoplethysmography, air plethysmography, and duplex quantitative valve closure time in assessing deep venous reflux. J Vasc Surg 16:913–920, 1992.
65. Valentin LI, Valentin WH, Mercado S, et al: Venous reflux localization: Comparative study of venography and DU. Phlebology 8:124–127, 1993.
66. Labropoulos N, Delis K, Nicolaides AN, et al: The role of the distribution and anatomic extent of reflux in the development of signs and symptoms in chronic venous insufficiency. J Vasc Surg 23:504–510, 1996.
67. Labropoulos N, Leon M, Nicolaides AN, et al: Venous reflux in patients with previous deep venous thrombosis: Correlation with ulceration and other symptoms. J Vasc Surg 20:20–26, 1994.
68. Labropoulos N, Tiongson J, Pryor L, et al: Nonsaphenous superficial vein reflux. J Vasc Surg 34:872–877, 2001.
69. Caggiati A: Fascial relationships of the long saphenous vein. Circulation 100:2547–2549, 1999.
70. Caggiati A, Bergan JJ, Gloviczki P, et al: International Interdisciplinary Consensus Committee on Venous Anatomical Terminology. Nomenclature of the veins of the lower limbs: An international interdisciplinary consensus statement. J Vasc Surg 36:416–622, 2002.
71. Caggiati A: Fascial relationships of the short saphenous vein. J Vasc Surg 34:241–246, 2001.
72. Labropoulos N, Leon M, Geroulakos G, et al: Venous haemodynamic abnormalities in patients with leg ulceration. Am J Surg 169:572–574, 1995.
73. Labropoulos N, Mansour MA, Kang SS, et al: Primary superficial vein reflux with competent saphenous trunk. Eur J Vasc Endovasc Surg 18:201–206, 1999.
74. Labropoulos N, Tiongson J, Landon P, et al: Definition of venous reflux in lower extremity veins. J Vasc Surg 38:793–798, 2003.
75. Labropoulos N, Delis K, Nicolaides AN, et al: The role of the distribution and anatomic extent of reflux in the development of signs and symptoms in chronic venous insufficiency. J Vasc Surg 23:504–510, 1996.
76. Caggiati A, Ricci S: The caliber of the human long saphenous vein and its congenital variations. Anat Anz 182:195–201, 2000.
77. Labropoulos N, Mansour MA, Kang SS, et al: New insights into perforator vein incompetence. Eur J Vasc Endovasc Surg 18:228–234, 1999.
78. Hanrahan LM, Araki CT, Rodriguez AA, et al: Distribution of valvular incompetence in patients with venous stasis ulceration. J Vasc Surg 13:805–812, 1991.
79. Labropoulos N, Giannoukas AD, Nicolaides AN, et al: New insights into the pathophysiologic condition of venous ulceration with color-flow duplex imaging: Implications for treatment? J Vasc Surg 22:45–50, 1995.
80. Kistner RL, Ferris EB, Randhawa G, et al: A method of performing descending venography. J Vasc Surg 4:464–468, 1986.
81. Labropoulos N, Volteas N, Leon M, et al: The role of venous outflow obstruction in patients with chronic venous dysfunction. Arch Surg 132:46–51, 1997.
82. Schanzer H, Younis C, Train J, et al: Therapeutic implications of venographic obstruction in chronic venous stasis. J Cardiovasc Surg (Torino) 31:173–177, 1990.
83. Leizorovicz A, Kassai B, Becker F, et al: The assessment of deep vein thromboses for therapeutic trials. Angiology 54:19–24, 2003.
84. Patterson RB, Fowl RJ, Keller JD, et al: The limitations of impedance plethysmography in the diagnosis of acute deep venous thrombosis. J Vasc Surg 9:725–729, 1989.
85. Hull R, Hirsh J, Sackett DL, et al: Clinical validity of a negative venogram in patients with clinically suspected venous thrombosis. Circulation 64:622–625, 1981.
86. Albrechtsson U, Einarsson E, Eklof B: Femoral vein pressure measurements for evaluation of venous function in patients with postthrombotic iliac veins. Cardiovasc Intervent Radiol 4:43–50, 1981.
87. Gloviczki P, Pairolero PC, Cherry KJ, et al: Reconstruction of the vena cava and of its primary tributaries: A preliminary report. J Vasc Surg 11:373–381, 1990.
88. Carpenter JP, Holland GA, Baum RA, et al: Magnetic resonance venography for the detection of deep venous thrombosis: Comparison with contrast venography and duplex Doppler ultrasonography. J Vasc Surg 18:734–741, 1993.
89. Huch Boni RA, Brunner U, Bollinger A, et al: Management of congenital angiodysplasia of the lower limb: Magnetic resonance imaging and angiography versus conventional angiography. Br J Radiol 68:1308–1315, 1995.
90. Laissy JP, Cinqualbre A, Loshkajian A, et al: Assessment of deep venous thrombosis in the lower limbs and pelvis: MR venography versus duplex Doppler sonography. Am J Roentgenol 167:971–975, 1996.
91. Dupas B, el Kouri D, Curtet C, et al: Angiomagnetic resonance imaging of iliofemorocaval venous thrombosis. Lancet 346:17–19, 1995.

92. Erdman WA, Jayson HT, Redman HC, et al: Deep venous thrombosis of extremities: Role of MR imaging in the diagnosis. Radiology 174:425–431, 1990.

93. Raju S, Fredericks R: Venous obstruction: An analysis of 137 cases with hemodynamic, venographic, and clinical correlations. J Vasc Surg 14:305–313, 1991.

94. Illig KA, Ouriel K, DeWeese JA, et al: Increasing the sensitivity of the diagnosis of chronic venous obstruction. J Vasc Surg 24:176–178, 1996.

95. Neglen P, Raju S: Detection of outflow obstruction in chronic venous insufficiency. J Vasc Surg 17:583–589, 1993.

96. Mubarak SJ, Hargens AR, Owen CA, et al: The wick catheter technique for measurement of intramuscular pressure: A new research and clinical tool. J Bone Joint Surg Am 58:1016–1020, 1976.

97. Saffle JR, Maxwell JG, Warden GD, et al: Measurement of intramuscular pressure in the management of massive venous occlusion. Surgery 89:394–397, 1981.

98. Qvarfordt P, Eklof B, Ohlin P, et al: Intramuscular pressure, bloodflow, and skeletal muscle metabolism in patients with venous claudication. Surgery 95:191–195, 1984.

99. Qvarfordt P, Eklof B, Ohlin P: Reference values for intramuscular pressure in the lower leg in man. Clin Physiol 2:427–434, 1982.

100. Raju S, Owen S Jr., Neglen P: Reversal of abnormal lymphoscintigraphy after placement of venous stents for correction of associated venous obstruction. J Vasc Surg 34:779–784, 2001.

101. Chrzanowski L, Jedrzejewski K: Intravascular ultrasound assessment of blood vessel morphology. Folia Morphol (Warsz) 61:309–312, 2002.

102. Allegra C, Antignani PL, Bergan JJ, et al: International Union of Phlebology Working Group. The "C" of CEAP: Suggested definitions and refinements: An International Union of Phlebology conference of experts. J Vasc Surg 37:129–131, 2003.

103. Porter JM, Moneta GL: Reporting standards in venous disease: An update. International Consensus Committee on Chronic Venous Disease. J Vasc Surg 21:635–645, 1995.

104. Labropoulos N: Hemodynamic changes according to the CEAP classification. Phlebolymphology 40:130–136, 2003.

105. Ioannou CV, Giannoukas AD, Kostas T, et al: Patterns of venous reflux in limbs with venous ulcers. Implications for treatment. Int Angiol 22:182–187, 2003.

106. Carpentier PH, Cornu-Thenard A, Uhl JF, et al: Societe Francaise de Medecine Vasculaire; European Working Group on the Clinical Characterization of Venous Disorders. Appraisal of the information content of the C classes of CEAP clinical classification of chronic venous disorders: A multicenter evaluation of 872 patients. J Vasc Surg 37:827–833, 2003.

107. Plate G, Brudin L, Eklof B, et al: Physiologic and therapeutic aspects in congenital vein valve aplasia of the lower limb. Ann Surg 198:229–233, 1983.

108. Giannoukas AD, Tsetis D, Ioannou C, et al: Clinical presentation and anatomic distribution of chronic venous insufficiency of the lower limb in a typical Mediterranean population. Int Angiol 21:187–192, 2002.

109. Moneta GL: Regarding the "C" of CEAP: Suggested definitions and refinements: An International Union of Phlebology conference of experts. J Vasc Surg 37:224–225, 2003.

110. Rutherford RB, Padberg FT Jr, Comerota AJ, et al: Venous severity scoring: An adjunct to venous outcome assessment. J Vasc Surg 31:1307–1312, 2000.

111. Kakkos SK, Rivera MA, Matsagas MI, et al: Validation of the new venous severity scoring system in varicose vein surgery. J Vasc Surg 38:224–228, 2003.

Chapter 44

Screening and Surveillance for DVT in High-Risk Patients

ROBERT F. CUFF

■ Venography

■ Fibrinogen Scans

■ Impedance Plethysmography

■ Wells' Pretest Probability Criteria

■ D-Dimer Testing

■ Venous Duplex Ultrasound

■ Computed Tomography Scan

■ Magnetic Resonance Imaging

■ Surveillance Programs

■ Conclusions

Deep venous thrombosis (DVT) and subsequent venous thromboembolic events remain a significant cause of death and morbidity in hospitalized patients. Stratification of patients into risk groups based on commonly known risk factors has been well described.[1] The rate of DVT ranges from 9% to as high as 80% in hospitalized patients without prophylaxis.[2] The patients at highest risk for DVT include those over the age of 40 years who have a past history of DVT, cancer, or hypercoaguable state; and those who have undergone a major trauma, orthopedic surgery, or have a spinal cord injury. These groups have a risk of proximal or calf DVT as high as 20% and 80%, respectively.[1,3]

With appropriate use of prophylactic therapy (including mechanical devices, low-molecular-weight heparins, and unfractionated heparin), the risk of DVT can be reduced by as much as 88%.[1] Although prophylaxis remains the cornerstone of management for DVT, some authors have found up to a 23% risk of DVT and subsequent thromboembolic events even with appropriate therapy in ventilated intensive care unit (ICU) patients.[4]

The goal of a screening or surveillance program is to identify the presence of DVT before a life-threatening thromboembolic event. A high level of suspicion based on the patient's clinical situation remains the key component of any screening or surveillance program. The ideal screening test would have a high sensitivity, be cost-effective, be applicable to all high-risk patients, and be noninvasive. At this time the ideal test does not exist. Which screening and surveillance test is the most appropriate will depend on the individual characteristics of a particular patient.

Venous duplex ultrasound, D-dimer levels, fibrinogen scans, impedance plethysmography, computed tomography scans, magnetic resonance scans, and venography have all been employed for screening; all have their limitations (Table 44-1).

Venography

Often considered the gold standard for DVT detection, ascending venography is rarely used today for screening. Its invasive nature, limited availability, and potential for inducing venous thrombosis have relegated this test to use as a confirmatory examination in limited cases.

Fibrinogen Scans

Iodine labeled-fibrinogen uptake studies ([125] I-fibrinogen) were first used clinically in 1970.[5] After receiving a dose of iodide to block thyroid uptake of the tracer, a patient is given the radioactive tracer. Four hours later, scanning is performed and subsequently repeated every 24 hours. Radioactive readings are compared to the precordium and are considered positive if activity in the vein is 20% higher than the precordium over 24 hours. The sensitivity of this study is between 49% and 81%.[5] Disadvantages include the long delay to diagnosis, poor sensitivity compared to other methods, poor detection of pelvic and proximal thigh thrombus, and patient exposure to radioactivity.

Impedance Plethysmography

By temporarily obstructing the venous outflow from a limb and then recording the change in volume with release of the cuff, an estimate of the volume of blood return can be obtained. This can then be evaluated to determine whether the vein is patent. Impedance plethysmography was shown to be effective in identifying occlusive proximal thrombus in symptomatic patients, but unfortunately it cannot be used in many high-risk patients because of bandages or extremity trauma, and it will often not detect nonocclusive thrombus. Its estimated sensitivity as a surveillance test is only 33%.[5]

Wells' Pretest Probability Criteria

In 1997, Wells and colleagues proposed and validated a set of parameters to screen patients for DVT based on their medical history and physical examination findings (Fig. 44-1).[6] These parameters were found to be very accurate in dividing patients into two categories: (1) those likely to have DVT; and (2) those not likely to have DVT. The main focus of this work was to safely decrease the number of patients who required ultrasound screening. By combining the pretest parameters with D-dimer assays, the researchers were able to decrease the number of duplex ultrasound studies by 42% overall.[6] In addition,

TABLE 44-1. **Screening Tests for DVT**

Test	Accuracy	Limitations
Venography	Sensitivity: 100%* Specificity: 100%*	Invasive; risk of inducing DVT; 5% to 15% indeterminate
Impedance Plethysmography	Sensitivity: 73% to 96%† Specificity: 83% to 95%†	Poor for nonocclusive thrombus
Fibrinogen scanning	Sensitivity: 49% to 81%	Radiation exposure and long delay to diagnosis
Duplex ultrasound	Sensitivity: 93% to 100%‡ Specificity: 97% to 100%‡	Time consuming, user dependent
D-dimer assay	NPV: 89% to 99%	Only accurate for excluding DVT, limited evaluation in inpatient population
Computed tomography	Sensitivity: 93% to 100% Specificity: 100%	Radiation exposure, expensive
Magnetic resonance imaging	Sensitivity: 87% to 100% Specificity: 95% to 100%	Expensive, limited availability

*Excluding 5% to 15% of tests that are considered indeterminate.
†In symptomatic patients. Sensitivity is only 19% to 33% in asymptomatic patients.
‡For proximal DVT only.
For whole blood agglutination study in combination with clinical predictive parameters.
For calf and proximal DVT.

Clinical Characteristic	Score
Active cancer (patient receiving treatment for cancer within the previous 6 months or currently receiving palliative treatment)	1
Paralysis, paresis, or recent plaster immobilization of the lower extremity	1
Recently bedridden for 3 days or more, or major surgery within the previous 12 wks requiring general or regional anesthetic	1
Localized tenderness along the distribution of the deep venous system	1
Entire leg swollen	1
Calf swelling at least 3 cm larger than on the asymptomatic side (measured 10 cm below the tibial tuberosity)	1
Pitting edema confined to the symptomatic leg	1
Collateral superficial veins (nonvaricose)	1
Previously documented DVT	1
Alternative diagnosis at least as likely as DVT	–2

Figure 44-1. Wells' clinical model for pretest probability of DVT. A score of 2 or higher indicates that the probability of DVT is likely; a score of less than 2 indicates that the probability of DVT is unlikely.

only 38% of patients felt to be unlikely to have DVT required any duplex scanning. In follow-up, only 0.4% of patients initially ruled out for DVT developed venous thromboembolism.[6] How well this protocol can be applied to inpatients has yet to be determined.

D-Dimer Testing

Several serum or whole blood D-dimer assays are available. The most accurate (but also most expensive and time-consuming) is the enzyme-linked immunosorbent assay (ELISA). The most widely studied is the rapid whole blood agglutination (SimpliRed). The combination of whole blood agglutination D-dimer assay and clinical evaluation has been shown to be an effective method of screening patients in an outpatient setting.[6–8] A recent randomized study by Wells and colleagues showed promising results for this combined approach for ruling out DVT in emergency department patients.[6] The D-Dimer test had a negative predicted value of 99.1% in patients who were felt to be at low-risk for DVT based on clinical parameters, and it had a negative predictive value of 89% in patients felt to be likely to have a DVT. Wells and colleagues showed a significant decrease in the need to perform venous duplex in this study. Unfortunately, the patients at highest risk for DVT often have conditions such as recent trauma, surgery, arterial thrombosis, pneumonia, myocardial infarction, or disseminated intravascular coagulation (DIC), all of which will elevate D-dimer levels independent of DVT.

The effectiveness of D-dimer testing in critically ill hospital patients has been debated.[9,10] A study by Owings and colleagues showed elevated D-dimer in severely injured patients for 48 hours, making D-dimer assays of little value during that period. They concluded that D-dimer levels could be used to exclude thromboembolism in severely injured patients, with a negative predictive value of 100%; and that assays may be of value for screening during prolonged hospitalizations.[9]

Venous Duplex Ultrasound

Advantages of venous duplex ultrasound (DU) include being noninvasive, portable, and relatively inexpensive; and its ability to differentiate acute from chronic thrombus. The technique for venous duplex scanning has been well described by many authors. Several variables can be evaluated to determine the presence of acute thrombus. These include vein incompressibility, visualization of thrombus, absence of spontaneous flow, and absence of phasic flow with respiration. When a combination of these diagnostic variables is used, a sensitivity of 95% can be obtained.[11] Disadvantages include its inability to scan patients with extremity trauma and inaccessible extremities, its poor visualization of pelvic and proximal thrombus, the user-dependent accuracy, and its time-consuming examinations. Despite these limitations, venous duplex scanning has become the most commonly used test for DVT screening and surveillance.

Computed Tomography Scan

Computed tomography (CT) is increasingly being used to detect pulmonary embolism, and it has been recently evaluated as a screening test for DVT.[12–14] The reported sensitivity ranged from 93% to 100%, with a specificity of 100% for femoropopliteal thrombus. The accuracy of the test was comparable to duplex ultrasound, and CT had the advantage of being able to evaluate the iliac and inferior vena cava systems. Loud and colleagues found combined CT venography and CT pulmonary angiography to be an accurate and efficient evaluation for a patient with suspected PE.[14] The disadvantage of CT is its cost and its radiation exposure when compared with sonography.

Magnetic Resonance Imaging

Magnetic resonance (MR) imaging of the lower extremities is noninvasive and very accurate. The sensitivity is

87%, 100%, and 100%, respectively, for calf, thigh, and pelvic DVT with correstponding specificities of 97%, 100%, and 95%.[15] In addition, MR can be used safely in pregnant women, can differentiate between acute and chronic DVT, and may provide information regarding potential pelvic disease as the etiology for the DVT. MR scanning is mainly used as a confirmatory test or to evaluate the proximal venous systems because its cost and limited availability make it a poor screening test.

the incidence of silent DVT is significant enough to warrant some form of surveillance. Until randomized studies are completed comparing duplex ultrasound, D-dimer testing, and prophylaxis alone, weekly screening ultrasound studies are recommended in high-risk patients with prolonged hospitalizations. CT or MRI scans in patients with a history of pelvic surgery, trauma, cancer, or a history of previous pelvic DVT is a noninvasive method to evaluate the iliac and vena cava circulation for DVT.

Surveillance Programs

The routine duplex ultrasound screening of trauma patients for DVT to prevent thromboembolism during a prolonged hospitalization has been met with mixed reviews. When used, duplex ultrasound screening is usually performed on a semiweekly or weekly basis. Some studies found little evidence that it is either cost-effective or prevented thromboembolism.[16,17] Overall, DVT was found in only 2.5% of patients, and only 5 of 21 duplex scans were positive in patients with pulmonary embolism.[11] However, in selected high-risk populations,

Conclusions

For outpatient screening, a combination of clinical predictive parameters and D-dimer testing is an effective method of identifying patients for venous duplex scan. For the highest-risk patients, venous duplex scan remains the most effective screening method (Fig. 44-2). For patients who have prolonged hospitalization, initiating appropriate prophylactic therapy and venous duplex scanning of symptomatic patients is recommended (Fig. 44-3). Further studies need to be conducted to evaluate the use of D-dimer assays in hospitalized, high-risk patients.

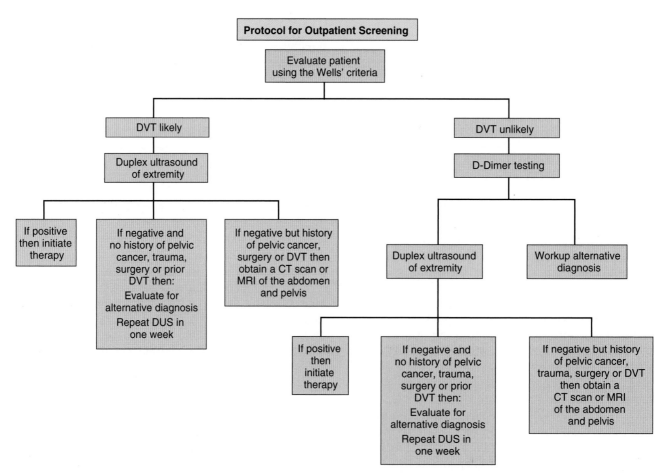

Figure 44-2. Protocol for outpatient screening.

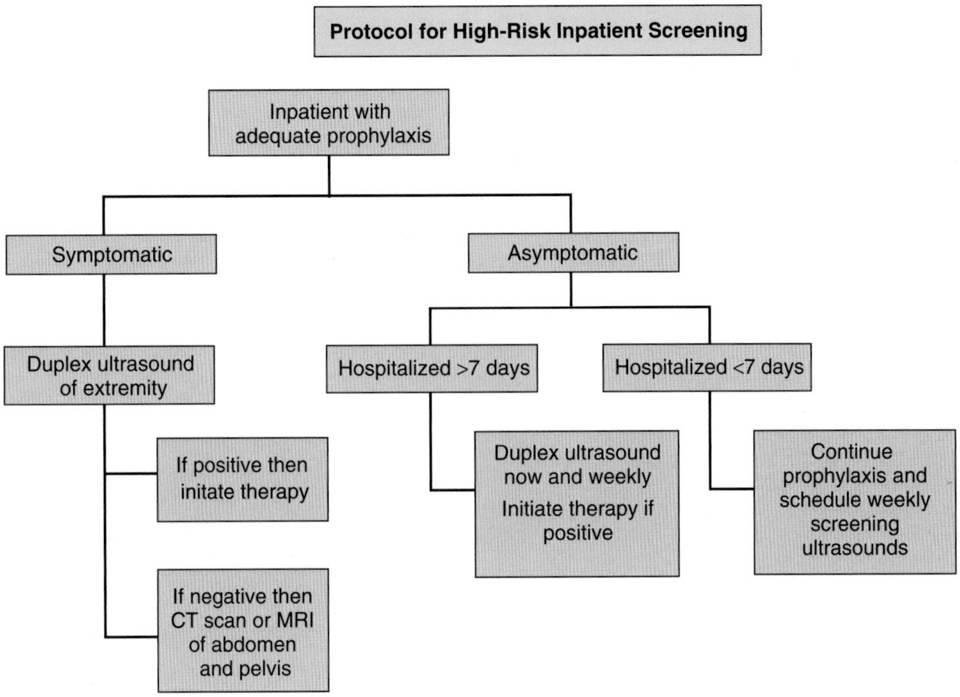

Figure 44-3. Protocol for high-risk inpatient screening.

REFERENCES

1. Geerts WH, Heit J, Clagett GP, et al: Prevention of venous thromboembolism. Chest 119(1 Supp):132S–175S, 2001.
2. Rocha AT, Tapson VF: Venous thrombosis in intensive care patients. Clin Chest Med 24(1):103–122, 2003.
3. Kelsey LJ, Fry DM, VanderKolk WE: Thrombosis risk in the trauma patient. Heme/Onc Clinics 14(2):417–430, 2000.
4. Ibrahim, EH, Iregui M, Prentice D, et al: Deep vein thrombosis during prolonged mechanical ventilation despite prophylaxis. Crit Care Med 30(4):771–774, 2002.
5. Criado E, Passman MA: Physiologic Assessment of the Venous System. In Rutherford RB (ed): Vascular Surgery, 5th ed. Philadelphia: WB Saunders, 2000.
6. Wells PS, Anderson DR, Rodger M, et al: Evaluation of D-dimer in the diagnosis of suspected deep-vein thrombosis. N Engl J Med 349:1227–1235, 2003.
7. Dryjski M, O'Brien-Irr MS, Harris LM, et al: Evaluation of a screening protocol to exclude the diagnosis of deep venous thrombosis among emergency department patients. J Vasc Surg 34(6):1010–1015, 2001.
8. Tick LW, Ton E, van Voorthuizen T, et al: Practical diagnostic management of patients with clinically suspected deep vein thrombosis by clinical probability test, compression ultrasonography and D-dimer test. Am J Med 113(8):630–635, 2002.
9. Owings JT, Gosselin RC, Anderson JT, et al: Practical utility of the D-dimer assay for excluding thromboembolism in severely injured trauma patients. J Trauma 51(3):425–429, 2001.
10. Brotman DJ, Segal JB, Jani JT: Limitations of D-dimer testing in unselected patients with suspected venous thromboembolism. Am J Med 114(4):276–282, 2003.
11. Meissner MH: Venous Duplex Scanning. In Rutherford RB (ed): Vascular Surgery, 5th ed. Philadelphia: WB Saunders, 2000.
12. Monnin-Delhom ED, Gallix BP, Achard C: High resolution unenhanced computed tomography in patients with swollen legs. Lymphology 35(3):121–128, 2002.
13. Yoshida S, Akiba H, Tamakawa M, et al: Spiral CT venography of the lower extremities by injection via an arm vein in patients with leg swelling. Br J Radiol 74(887):1013–1016, 2001.
14. Loud PA, Katz DS, Klippenstein DL, et al: Combined CT venography and pulmonary angiography in suspected thromboembolic disease: Diagnostic accuracy for deep venous evaluation. Am J Roentgenol 174(1):61–65, 2000.
15. Rosen CL, Tracy JA: The diagnosis of lower extremity deep venous thrombosis. Emer Med Clin 19(4):895–912, 2001.
16. Cipolle MD, Wojcik R, Seislove E, et al: The role of surveillance duplex screening in preventing venous thromboembolism in trauma patients. J Trauma 52(3):453–462, 2002.
17. Spain DA: Venous thromboembolism in the high-risk trauma patient: Do the risks justify aggressive screening and pro-phylaxis? J Trauma 42(3):463–467; discussion 467–469, 1997.

Chapter 45

Upper Extremity Venous Duplex Imaging

JOANN LOHR

- Introduction
- Technique
- Duplex Findings

Introduction

The number of patients who come into the vascular laboratory for evaluation of upper extremity problems is far smaller than the number who come for lower extremity testing. However, this number recently has grown, accompanying the increase in radial artery harvesting for coronary bypass grafting and the Dialysis Outcomes Quality Initiatives (DOQI) recommendations for increased establishment of arteriovenous fistula (AVF).[1] Preoperative vein mapping for dialysis access has had a significant impact on the use of the vascular laboratory. Unfortunately, the ability of the vascular laboratory to provide information is limited by reimbursement issues, scheduling problems, and technologist

availability. The data presented in this chapter summarize the experience of upper extremity duplex imaging in an Intrasocietal Commission for Accreditation of Vascular Laboratory (ICAVL)–accredited vascular laboratory. Upper extremity evaluations have increased to 13.9% of all studies performed annually in this vascular laboratory, up from 4.8% only 5 years ago.[2] Table 45-1 lists the indications for upper extremity scans conducted over the previous 12 months. Only 43% (191/442) of the upper extremity evaluations were done to rule out thrombosis.

All patients who had an upper extremity duplex scan were included in this study. Hospital charts were reviewed and medical history, risk factors, hospital course, demographic information, treatment, and follow-up data were collected and entered into a vascular registry. Variables collected include signs and symptoms; duration; admitting diagnosis; possible hypercoagulable states; presence, type, and extent of existing neoplasia; presence and type of peripheral or central venous access; type of venous catheter (e.g., single-lumen, triple-lumen, or Swan-Ganz); and site of placement and duration. Also recorded were the presence of pacemakers and defibrillators, IV fluids administered, and whether the patient was receiving total parental nutrition (TPN). Diagnostic tests and location of thrombi were reviewed, as were type of anticoagulant or lytic therapy.

A total of 701 upper extremity venous duplex scans to rule out thrombosis were analyzed. Some 38% were

The authors acknowledge the invaluable assistance of the John J. Cranley Vascular Laboratory staff; Wendy Thompson and the staff of the E. Kenneth Hatton MD Institute for Education and Research for data management and manuscript preparation; and Two Herons for editorial review.

TABLE 45-1. **Indications for Upper Extremity Scans**

Indications	Number
Upper extremity venous duplex to rule out thrombosis	191
Upper extremity dialysis evaluations	142
Upper extremity radial artery bypass harvest	16
Upper extremity graft surveillance	35
Evaluation for line placement	9
Upper extremity arterial duplex	8
Upper extremity symptoms with/without cold challenge	35
Thoracic outlet evaluation	6
Total	442

TABLE 45-2. **Veins Involved by Thrombosis***

Veins Involved	Total
Subclavian	103
Cephalic	99
Internal jugular	78
Axillary	59
Brachial	56
Basilic	61
External jugular	19
Radial	6
Antecubital	8
Ulnar	3
Total	492

*Several patients had multiple vein segments involved.

positive for thrombosis, and isolated superficial venous thrombosis was identified in 85 patients. Distribution and sites of veins are presented in Table 45-2.

Technique

A scanning protocol was followed for each duplex scanning session. The upper extremity examination begins with a detailed assessment of signs, symptoms, past medical history, and risk factor analysis. The patient then is placed in a supine position, and the radial vein is visualized from the wrist to the brachial vein. Next, the ulnar vein is followed from the wrist to the antecubital fossa, where the ulnar and radial veins form the brachial vein; the brachial vein is followed into the upper arm. At the junction of the basilic and brachial veins, the axillary vein is formed. The axillary vein is followed under the shoulder in the direction of the clavicle. The junction of the cephalic and axillary veins forms the subclavian vein. The junction of the subclavian and jugular veins originating at the innominate vein is not visualized routinely because of its depth; however, Doppler signals analyzed in this area provide indirect information about the patency of the central veins, and newer color scanners have increased the ability to image them. Doppler signals of the subclavian vein are assessed: Normally, the flow is spontaneous and phasic with augmentation, and no reflux is identified. The internal jugular vein is examined from the clavicle cephalad until it dives under the mandible. Doppler signals of the internal jugular vein also are

obtained to assess spontaneous and phasic flow. Finally, the superficial veins are assessed by following the basilic vein along the ulna until it joins the brachial vein. The largest-diameter antecubital vein connects the basilic and cephalic systems at the antecubital fossa. The antecubital perforator also is seen connecting the cephalic and brachial veins. The cephalic vein is traced along the radius and up the arm, where it joins with the axillary vein.

For reporting convenience and ease of communication, the upper extremity is divided into zones (Fig. 45-1). In each examination, the position of the probe and localizing abnormal findings are reported. Each zone covers approximately 10 cm in length. Zone 1 is located at the suprasternal notch, Zone 3 at the acromial clavicular process, Zone 5 at the anticubital fossa, and Zone 8 at the wrist.

When a visible intraluminal thrombus is identified, several of its characteristics are assessed to determine its relative age; these characteristics include clot occlusiveness, clot retraction, clot distention, vein compressions, echogenicity and homogeneity, the development of collateral venous channels, and recanalization. The clot may be partially or totally occluding (Figs. 45-2 and 45-3). A totally occluding clot indicates an acute process. Free-floating thrombi actually are tethered distally but extend cephalad in the vein without a more proximal attachment to the vessel wall. These free-floating thrombus tails exhibit a side-to-side waving in the venous lumen that can be induced by gently bouncing the probe on the skin or with respiration (Fig. 45-4). Free-floating tails usually become attached to the venous wall within 1 to 2 weeks.

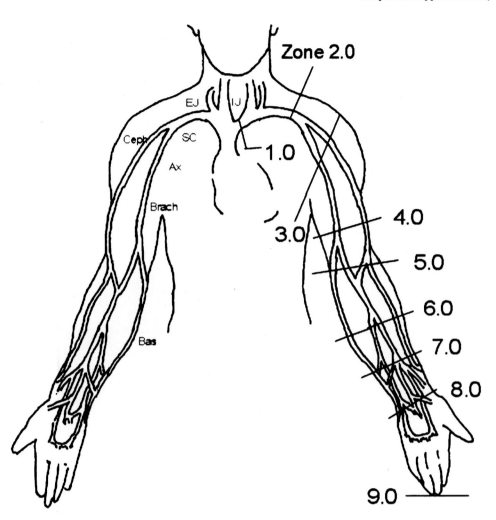

Zone 2.0

EJ IJ

Ceph SC

Ax

Brach

Bas

1.0

3.0

4.0

5.0

6.0

7.0

8.0

9.0

Figure 45-1. Zones of reference for upper extremity venous scanning: midline = 1.0, acromion = 3.0, elbow = 5.0, wrist = 8.0, and fingertip = 9.0. (Reprinted with permission from Elsevier Science.)

Duplex Findings

Venous Abnormalities

Clot retraction is defined as the concentric separation of the thrombus from the vein walls; there appears to be a very thin gap between the thrombus and the circumference of the venous wall. Retraction is thought to occur within a few hours of thrombus formation through clot contraction of the platelet fibrin mesh formation and extrusion of serum. Clot retraction usually lasts only 1 to 2 weeks, and then the clot becomes adherent to the vein wall.

Clot distention occurs when the vein is dilated to a larger-than-normal diameter by a thrombus in a cross-sectional area. In this context, clot distention differs from venous distention caused by obstruction or by venous hypertension in the absence of an intraluminal thrombus. In the latter, it is possible to completely collapse the wall

of the vein with the pressure of the probe and receive a Doppler signal. Veins exhibiting clot distention gradually shrink over several weeks to months.

An acutely thrombosed vein may be partially compressible. Unlike a chronically thrombosed vein, acute thrombi can be deformed by only light probe pressure. When viewed transversely, the round vein appears oblong (Fig. 45-5). A thrombus remains soft for approximately 24 hours after formation. The clot surface may be smooth or irregular; this usually is best assessed by a longitudinal view of the thrombus tip. Acute thrombi tend to have smooth, rounded tips because of continued surrounding flow.

Echogenicity is defined as the overall brightness of the clot compared with the surrounding tissues. Brightly echogenic thrombi tend to be chronic because serum resorption makes them denser. Apparent changes in echogenicity may be influenced by electrical gains of the instruments, depth of the structure being assessed,

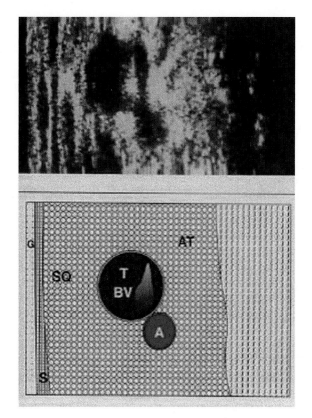

Figure 45-2. *Acute thrombosis of the brachial vein: G = gel, S = skin, SQ = subcutaneous tissue, AT = areolar tissue, T = totally occluding acute thrombus, BV = brachial vein, A = brachial artery. (Reprinted with permission from Elsevier Science.)*

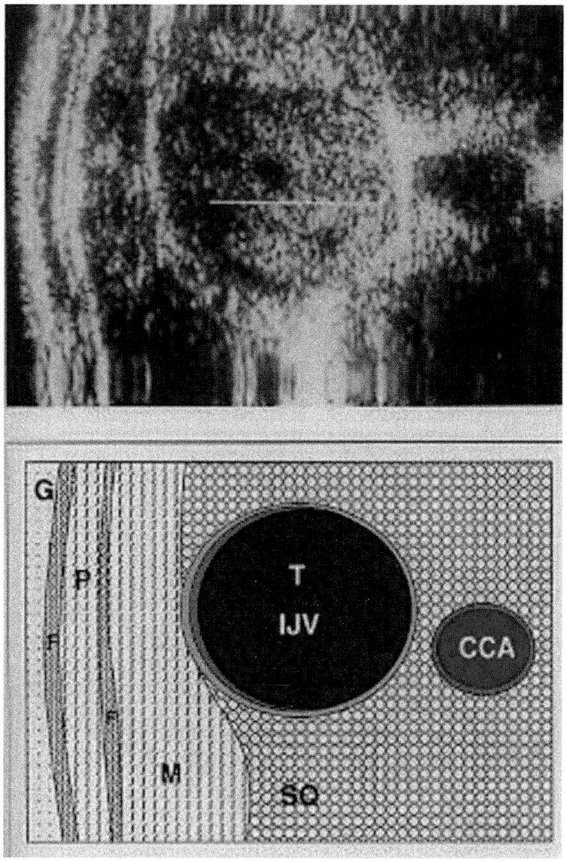

Figure 45-3. *Acute thrombus of the internal jugular vein: G = gel, SQ = subcutaneous tissue, P = platysma muscle, F = fascia, M = sternocleidomastoid muscle, IJV = internal jugular vein, T = acute thrombus, CCA = common carotid artery. (Reprinted with permission from Elsevier Science.)*

and acoustic shadow of the overlying tissues, making echogenicity a somewhat subjective finding. Homogeneity also is assessed. Acute thrombi tend to be homogeneous, whereas chronic thrombi tend to be heterogeneous.

Development of collateral venous channels is an absolute sign of chronic thrombosis. These channels are very small, lie parallel to the main vein trunk, and do not contain valves. Normal venous tributaries are larger, enter the main venous channel at an acute angle, and contain valves. Collateral venous channels are best visualized in a transverse field and may be seen as early as 1 to 2 weeks after initial thrombosis; however, they usually are not visible for a month or more after venous occlusion.

Recanalization is evidenced by an open, collapsible channel that runs through a thrombus. The recanalized channel, which is surrounded entirely by a clot, tends to occur rather late.

Using the aforementioned characteristics, thrombi were classified as acute, chronic, or indeterminate (Table 45-3). Classification must be based on the characteristics of the entire thrombus rather than on an isolated segment because the deep venous thrombosis is a continuing process. For this reason, a single thrombus may manifest various aging characteristics in different regions. Repeat duplex scans often are necessary, and commonly show the evolution of characteristics that are equivocal with the initial scans.

Soft-tissue Abnormalities

Some scans may be performed to evaluate soft-tissue abnormalities, which can be differentiated by their characteristics. The topic of pulsatile groin masses in patients with a history of femoral trauma was reviewed by Montefusco.[3] The study indicates that features of pseudoaneurysm include visible intraluminal swirling and turbulent Doppler spectra. Further, common associated findings include a centrifugal thrombus with a superimposed arterial spectrum and a visible arterial laceration.

Abscesses, on the other hand, have hyperechoic contents, give off no Doppler signal, have inducible eddy motions, and often have an echo-dense capsule. Commonly associated findings include regional solidification.

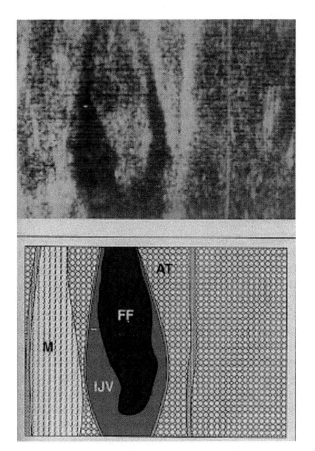

Figure 45-4. Free-floating thrombus in the internal jugular vein: M = sternocleidomastoid muscle, AT = areolar tissue, IJV = internal jugular vein, FF = free-floating thrombus. (Reprinted with permission from Elsevier Science.)

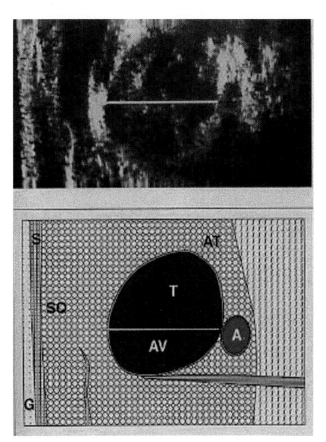

Figure 45-5. Acute thrombus in the axillary vein: G = gel, S = skin, SQ = subcutaneous tissue, T = totally occluding acute thrombus, AV = axillary vein, A = axillary artery, AT = areolar tissue. (Reprinted with permission from Elsevier Science.)

TABLE 45-3. Clot Characteristics: Relative Value in Clot Aging†

Characteristic	Acute Value		Chronic Value	
Degree of occlusion	Total	**	Partial	**
Free-floating	Free	****	Stationary	**
Clot retraction	Retracted	***	Adherent	***
Clot distention	Distended	***	Contracted	**
Clot compressibility	Soft	****	Firm	*
Surface character	Smooth	**	Irregular	**
Echogenicity	Faint	*	Bright	*
Homogeneity	Homogeneous	**	Heterogeneous	**
Collaterals	Absent	*	Present	****
Recanalization	Absent	*	Present	****

†Four asterisks indicate a diagnostic level; three asterisks, good; two asterisks, fair; and one asterisk, poor (nondiagnostic). Each asterisk indicates the relative value to be given to each criterion in interpretation of clot age. Many criteria are valuable only when present, and the overall decision represents a weighted average. (Reprinted with permission from Elsevier Science.)

Hematomas exhibit a variable echo density, are non-compressible, have no fluid movements or clear margins, and give off no Doppler signal. If hematomas are less than 12 hours old, they may be hypoechoic with focal liquefaction. If they are more than 2 weeks old, dissection through the soft tissues commonly is seen.

Edema fluid is radiolucent, follows tissue planes, and is not compressible. Lymph nodes are spherical and encapsulated with a mixed internal echogenicity and are noncompressible. Small lymph nodes may be invisible or difficult to see. Large lymph nodes, of course, are seen in the presence of infection, cellulitis, or tumors. In fact, the duplex scan image of large, swollen lymph nodes shows an architecture strikingly similar to the cross-section of a lymph node that is depicted in pathology textbooks.

Cysts are slightly echogenic and are best seen in a transverse view, where they can be distinguished from the surrounding tissue structures. Cysts may be partially compressible and, at times, may compress an artery or vein, causing an increase in peak velocity signals.

Duplex scanning holds special value for the evaluation of aneurysms, pseudoaneurysms, and for the surveillance of grafts. In the past 5 years there has been rapid expansion in the use of duplex imaging for the diagnosis and evaluation of upper extremity venous thrombosis, arterial suitability, and soft-tissue abnormalities, and for the evaluation of grafts. Requests for examination of the upper extremity have increased, and this area of clinical interest likely will continue to expand.

A multicenter collaborative study that assessed the accuracy of lower extremity duplex scanning reported that the procedure was 97% sensitive in extremities with positive phlebograms.[4] However, the phlebogram was negative in 191 extremities and was considered to be incorrect in 6 instances. Thus the phlebogram was not a perfect standard when negative, and the duplex scan was slightly more accurate.[5,6]

It has not been possible to generate similar data for the upper extremity because there is a blind area behind the clavicle (Fig. 45-6). Thus a negative duplex scan does not absolutely rule out thrombosis of the subclavian vein. In the author's study, a phlebogram was requested when there was doubt; unfortunately, only 10 were obtained. Although all were confirmatory, it is possible that some subclavian vein thromboses were missed. In most cases, however, a negative duplex scan and normal Doppler signals in the subclavian vein were accepted as evidence of normal venous flow. Rapid-sequence spiral CT scanning offers another modality to evaluate this area.

In the author's vascular laboratory, all scans are performed with commercially available high-resolution duplex instrumentation. Both black-and-white and color

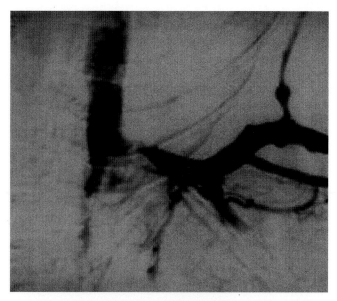

Figure 45-6. *Innominate vein occlusion. (Reprinted with permission from Elsevier Science.)*

scanners are used. The interpreting physician grades all scans for quality using a three-part system:

- *Poor* indicates that a portion of the scan was not interpretable or a segment of the extremity was not visualized.
- *Fair* indicates that diagnosis could be made but the entire extremity was not well visualized.
- *Good* indicates that all structures were well visualized.

Because duplex scanning has become the standard of practice to evaluate extremity veins, grading and assessment are an important means to ensuring the accuracy and reliability of a vascular laboratory.

To perform at the level required for ICAVL certification, a vascular laboratory must conduct phlebography in less than 10% of patients. Because duplex scanning is significantly dependent on the technologist's skill, quality control issues are central to continuing validation of this test. Formal comparison with phlebography is no longer available in this laboratory. When possible, blinded duplicate scanning programs by different technologists are used as a method to document quality control and improve test reliability. Further, physicians who are responsible for interpreting findings and overseeing the vascular laboratory must be personally skilled in the techniques of venous duplex imaging and the use of equipment. Finally, better scanner resolution also has improved the results of venous duplex imaging.[7-12]

Unfortunately, symptoms of deep vein thrombosis of the upper extremity are not diagnostic, especially for acute thrombosis. The author's study demonstrated that

TRIHEALTH - GOOD SAMARITAN HOSPITAL
JOHN J. CRANLEY VASCULAR LABORATORY

DIALYSIS ACCESS, DUPLEX ARTERIAL AND VENOUS MAPPING
TECHNICAL WORKSHEET

Patient Name:		Date:	
Tech:	Tape:	Meter:	
Planned Procedure:			

Brachial Blood Pressure	Right	Left

DOMINANT HAND: RIGHT ☐ LEFT ☐

ARM STUDIED R L	VEIN		VEIN	
LOCATION	Pre	Post	Pre	Post
1				
1.5				
2				
2.5				
3				
3.5				
4				
4.5				
5				
5.5				
6				
6.5				
7				
7.5				
8				

	Velocity	Diameter
Brachial Artery		
Proximal		
Mid		
Distal		
Radial Artery		
Proximal		
Mid		
Distal		

BRV	NV	N	TA	PA	TI	PI	TC	PC
CEPH	NV	N	TA	PA	TI	PI	TC	PC
BAS	NV	N	TA	PA	TI	PI	TC	PC
IJ	NV	N	TA	PA	TI	PI	TC	PC
SCV	NV	N	TA	PA	TI	PI	TC	PC

SPA	Velocities		
Baseline		Radial Dom	☐
Radial Comp		Ulnar Dom	☐
Ulnar Comp		Mixed	☐

COMMENTS:

Figure 45-7. Evaluation of the arteries and veins protocol.

of those scans performed to rule out venous thrombosis, 75% did not identify a thrombus. All of these patients, however, were referred to the vascular laboratory because they had symptoms, the most common being pain, tenderness, and swelling. Pain and tenderness were as common in the extremities that proved to have venous thrombosis as in those that were negative. Swelling was more common in the extremities with a confirmed thrombosis, but this finding did not achieve statistical significance.

Catheter-induced thrombosis is an increasingly common event because the central veins are used more often for access, nutrition, chemotherapy, and monitoring. In the author's study, the most common associated risk factor for upper extremity thrombosis was a central or peripheral venous catheter. Indwelling catheters and malignancy were the most commonly combined risk factors; however, no identifiable risk factors were present in 10% (11/107) of patients with thrombosis. Hyperalimentation (TPN) was infused in 27% of patients with thrombosis. Further, screening and venography demonstrate that 30% to 60% of patients with central venous catheters will have a thrombus in the axillary subclavian venous segment, and 3% of these patients will develop clinically symptomatic subclavian vein thrombosis. Pulmonary emboli have been reported in 5% to 12% of a series of upper extremity thrombosis, and it is estimated that 1% of these patients will die. Major vein thrombosis in the upper extremities, much like that in the lower extremities, may spread from a superficial vein into the deep system; therefore, upper extremity surveillance of isolated superficial vein thrombosis (SVT) is recommended.[13,14]

Proximal Upper Extremity DVT

Spontaneous axillary-subclavian vein thrombosis tends to occur in younger males who have an employment history of over-the-head activity. Similarly, primary effort vein thrombosis affects males more often than females and has an approximate right arm–to–left arm ratio of 2:1. Peak age of occurrence is 28 years (see Figs. 45-5 and 45-6). Primary vein thrombosis presents with a more characteristic pattern than does spontaneous axillary-subclavian vein thrombosis, often in the right arm of a male patient or in a left-handed patient who has exerted his extremity in an unusual way. The arm often is swollen and may be purplish. Superficial veins may be more prominent, and a visible collateral network may be identified. Swelling, followed by pain and cyanosis, and prominent collateral veins are the most common presenting findings for primary effort vein thrombosis. Secondary thrombosis, however, can be defined and categorized into those associated with hyperalimentation, dialysis, chemotherapy catheters, local tumor radiation, hypertonic or sclerotic solutions, or hypercoagulability.[15]

In the instance of dialysis access, upper extremity evaluations increasingly are being requested before placement. Preoperative evaluation of dysfunctional dialysis grafts allows operative planning.[16] Vein mapping improves graft durability in patients with disadvantaged outflow, and vein size and continuity can be established. The protocol implemented in the author's vascular laboratory evaluates both veins and arteries (Fig. 45-7). Bloodflow in the superficial palmar arch is assessed at baseline with radial and ulnar comparison. In addition, calcifications and aberrant arterial anatomy are identified. Veins are evaluated using tourniquet distention if less than 3 mm at rest.

The growing number of uses for duplex imaging for upper extremity veins and arteries has expanded the indications and frequency of the application.[17] Currently, upper extremity venous imaging and duplex scans are used to assist peripherally inserted central catheter (PICC) line and central line insertion. Duplex imaging also can facilitate access to central veins for lytic treatment. Increasingly, upper extremity venous imaging is moving not only from the diagnostic realm but also into that of therapeutics and treatment.

Duplex imaging is a practical method of diagnosis for upper extremity venous thrombosis. The small mass of the upper extremity, as compared to the lower extremity, makes scanning easier and more likely to be accurate. Upper extremity venous imaging can effectively assist in the diagnosis of a spectrum of conditions including aneurysms, cysts, hemorrhages, and thrombosis of grafts. Although the blind area behind the clavicle requires careful insonation, the area may be decreased by recent color-flow imaging. Still, thorough evaluation of the Doppler signal in this area is important in preventing false-negative interpretations of central vein thrombosis. The use of duplex scanning is growing to include the evaluation of upper extremity abnormalities and arterial anomalies; this growth is expected to increase as venous imaging proves useful in diagnostic as well as therapeutic and treatment situations.

REFERENCES

1. Kidney Disease Outcomes Quality Initiative (K/DOQI). NFK K/DOQI Guidelines. Available at: www.kidney.org/professionals/doqi/index.cfm. Accessed 24 July 2003.
2. Lohr J, et al: Upper extremity venous imaging with duplex scanning. In Bernstein E (ed): Vascular Diagnosis, 4th ed. Mosby-Year Book, 1993.
3. Montefusco C, et al: The role of duplex ultrasonography in the differentiation of pseudoaneurysm, hematoma, and access. J Vasc Tech 14:11–17, 1990.
4. Cranley JJ, et al: Near parity in the final diagnosis of deep venous thrombosis by duplex scan and phlebography. Phlebology 4:71–74, 1989.
5. Cranley JJ: Seeing is believing: A clot is a clot, on a duplex scan or phlebogram. Echocardiography 4:423 (editorial), 1987.
6. Cranley JJ: Diagnosis of deep venous thrombosis. In Bernstein EF (ed): Recent Advances in Noninvasive Diagnostic Techniques in Vascular Disease. St Louis: Mosby, 1990.

7. Flannagan LD, Sullivan ED, Cranley JJ: Venous imaging of the extremities using real-time B-mode ultrasound. In Bergan JJ, Yao JST (eds): Surgery of the Veins. Orlando, FL: Grune & Stratton, 1984.

8. Karkow WS, Ruoff BA, Cranley JJ: B-mode venous imaging. In Kempezinski RF, Yao JST (eds): Practical Noninvasive Vascular Diagnosis. Chicago: Mosby, 1987.

9. Kerr TM, et al: Analysis of 1084 consecutive lower extremities involved with acute venous thrombosis diagnosed by duplex scanning. Surgery 108:520–527, 1990.

10. Kerr TM, et al: Upper extremity venous thromboses diagnosed by duplex scanning. Am J Surg 160:202–206, 1990.

11. Sullivan ED, Peter DJ, Cranley JJ: Real-time B-mode venous ultrasound. J Vasc Surg 1:465–471, 1984.

12. Talbot SR: Use of real-time imaging in identifying deep venous obstruction: A preliminary report. Bruit 6:41–42, 1982.

13. Lutter KS, et al: Superficial thrombophlebitis diagnosed by duplex scanning. Surgery 110:42–46, 1991.

14. Gloviczki P, Kazmier FJ, Hollier LH: Axillary-subclavian venous occlusion: The morbidity of a nonlethal disease. J Vasc Surg 4:333–337, 1986.

15. Donayre CE, White GH, Mehringer SM, Wilson SE: Pathogenesis determines late morbidity of axillo-subclavian vein thrombosis. Am J Surg 152:179–184, 1986.

16. Wladis AR, et al: Improving longevity of prosthetic dialysis grafts in patients with disadvantaged venous outflow. J Vasc Surg 32:997–1005, 2000.

17. Lohr JM, et al: Upper extremity hemodynamic changes after radial artery harvest for coronary artery bypass grafting. Ann Vasc Surg 14:56–62, 2000.

Chapter 46

Ultrasound-Guided Filter Placement

VASANA CHEANVECHAI • BRIAN G. HALLORAN • MARSHALL
E. BENJAMIN

- Ultrasound-Guided Filter Placement
- Technique for Duplex-Guided Filter Insertion
- Clinical Experience
- Follow-Up
- Cost
- Conclusions

Ultrasound-Guided Filter Placement

Venous thromboembolism remains a challenging and somewhat enigmatic problem for practitioners of virtually all specialties, but is particularly so for those in the surgical specialties. The pathophysiologic risk factors for development of deep venous thrombosis (DVT) are well known, and countless well-designed studies have clearly defined patient groups at high risk for DVT and pulmonary embolism (PE). One large patient population is the critically ill/multitrauma patient. There are well-recognized and well-validated pharmacologic and physiomechanical techniques for prophylaxis to reduce the incidence of DVT and fatal PE in these high-risk patient groups. Nevertheless, there remain over 500,000 DVTs

that occur in the United States each year, and more than 100,000 deaths caused by PEs. Despite our awareness of this problem, many physicians still consider PE deaths to be the single most preventable cause of death among adult patients.

Review of the relative risk levels suggested by meta-analysis of reported studies allows one to appreciate the complex clinical realities of venous thromboembolism. Consensus studies[1] have defined high-risk patient groups as having a 4% to 8% incidence of proximal DVT, associated with a 0.5% to 1% incidence of fatal PE. The very high-risk patient groups have had an observed incidence of proximal DVT of more than 8%, associated with a 1% to 5% incidence of fatal PE. The unprecedented study of Geerts and colleagues[2] observed that proximal DVT occurred in 18% of multitrauma patients when no DVT prophylaxis was used. Despite a clear understanding of the efficacy and an aggressive use of all effective methods of DVT prophylaxis, fatal PE remains a critical problem in trauma/critical care patients. This becomes particularly disturbing when one considers that many of these (typically younger) trauma patients would have a normal life expectancy if they recovered from their traumatic injuries.

The consideration of venous thromboembolism in the multitrauma patient is further complicated by clinical compromises in the application of available DVT prophylaxis. Patients with closed head injuries or other significant neurospinal trauma, multiorgan trauma, or other potential hemodynamic instability may not be candidates for antithrombotic prophylaxis with low-dose or low-molecular-weight heparin. Furthermore, in patients with significant extremity trauma that requires skeletal fixation, intermittent mechanical compression devices may not be fully functional or even feasible. Unlike the patient presenting for an elective colon resection where risk can be clearly assessed and DVT prophylaxis thoughtfully employed, multitrauma patients appear with unpredictable combinations and permutations of injuries and risk, making prevention of venous thromboembolism a continuing dilemma.

From a practical standpoint, the prevention of fatal PE is straightforward:

1. Prevent DVT: Formation of major, proximal DVT can be prevented using pharmacologic and mechanical techniques. However, in some cases DVT prophylaxis cannot be used, and in others, even the most "effective" prophylaxis does not guarantee a clinically acceptable risk reduction of subsequent fatal pulmonary embolism.

2. Detect proximal DVT that are not prevented before they embolize: Venous duplex ultrasound scanning has been used in programs of routine interval DVT surveillance for high-risk patient groups. These examinations can be performed at the bedside in virtually all clinical settings without risk or discomfort to the patient. In the largest study of DVT surveillance reported to date,[3] this strategy was effective in nearly eliminating fatal PE in a high-risk neurosurgical population. Despite the use of "effective" DVT prophylaxis in all patients, proximal DVT was diagnosed by surveillance duplex scan in 5% of cases. Furthermore, 80% of proximal DVT were asymptomatic at the time of diagnosis. Earlier diagnosis of these DVT by surveillance duplex scan allowed definitive treatment, and fatal PE occurred in only 0.07% of more than 2500 patients studied.

3. Ignore DVT altogether: Prevent migration of proximal DVT by empiric or prophylactic placement of a vena caval filter. In neurosurgical patients discovered to have proximal DVT by surveillance duplex scan, inferior vena cava (IVC) filters were placed to prevent PE because standard anticoagulant treatment was contraindicated.[4] This treatment plan effectively eliminated fatal PE in these patients. As noted previously, multitrauma and critical care patients often remain in the high-risk or very high-risk categories for fatal PE, even when multimodality DVT prophylaxis is used. This has led some physicians to recommend prophylactic placement of IVC filters in selected patients with the presumption that this may be the only effective means of preventing fatal pulmonary embolism.

There has been a great liberalization of the indications for placement of an IVC filter to prevent PE. The above discussion lends credence to these expanded indications, including even prophylactic IVC filter placement in the absence of documented DVT or PE for selected high-risk patients. The development of percutaneous techniques for filter placement has simplified the procedure; however, despite the routine use of percutaneous venous access, filter insertion has required fluoroscopic guidance, which in most institutions requires transport of the patient to the operating room (OR) or to an interventional suite. Multitrauma patients may have closed head or neurospinal injuries in association with major pelvic or long bone fractures, and many (during their high-risk period) require inotropic or ventilatory support. Transportation of these patients often requires additional medical, nursing, and paramedical staff and can be cumbersome and/or hazardous.

Advancing technology with duplex ultrasound scanning has allowed routine diagnostic evaluation of deep abdominal vascular structures including the aorta, portal veins, renal and visceral vessels, and the inferior vena cava. The authors' own experience[5,6] indicated that IVC filters could be routinely imaged after placement, and thrombotic complications of these procedures could be documented. This experience, combined with the increasing portability of the ultrasound units, made it logical to consider bedside, duplex-scan–guided filter insertion (DGFI) as an alternative technique for placement of an IVC filter in critically ill or multitrauma patients. This technique would avoid the need for transport of patients out of critical-care units and thus greatly simplify their management. In 1997, Nunn and colleagues[7] from Vanderbilt University were the first to publish their experience with ultrasound-guided filter placement. They successfully inserted Greenfield filters in 49 out of 55 trauma patients. Soon after, Sato and colleagues[8] from Eastern Virginia Medical School reported their experience with DGFI using the Vena Tech filter in 53 multitrauma patients. The vast majority of complications in these studies involved the failure to adequately visualize the landmark anatomy with ultrasound. Others have reported successful placement of filters using intravascular ultrasound (IVUS).[9]

The mandatory use of fluoroscopic guidance for IVC filter placement in the past has been based on several presumed requirements. However, most of these presumptions are seriously flawed or clinically unimportant, including the following:

1. Vena cavagram is necessary for precise placement of the IVC filter below the renal veins: The left renal vein is an easily identifiable ultrasonographic anatomic landmark and is the lower of the renal veins. Furthermore, the right renal artery is easily visualized by duplex scan (in patients suitable for deep scanning), passing posterior to the IVC

at the level of the renal veins. An IVC filter placed below the level of either of these vessels will be appropriate and effective. Finally, concern about the absolute need for placement of modern IVC filters in precise approximation to the renal veins is generally overstated. The original concern arose from the fact that older devices (IVC clips and umbrellas) were associated with IVC thrombosis in 50% to 60% of cases. It was thought that the vena cava above the clip (but below the renal veins) would be an area of stasis where thrombus would form and could embolize. This anecdotal concern seems to have persisted despite the fact that IVC thrombosis occurs in only 3% to 12% of cases with modern IVC filters. Concern about thrombosis following placement of an IVC filter above the renal veins would be reasonable because acute right renal vein thrombosis is clearly associated with renal dysfunction. However, well-documented experience with modern IVC filters placed intentionally above the renal veins indicates that this technique can be safely performed and is effective for PE prevention.[10] Any suggestion that a modern IVC filter (e.g., the Greenfield filter) must be placed in a precise, venographically controlled relationship to the renal veins is clearly a therapeutic overstatement.

2. Vena cavagram is essential to measure the diameter of the IVC: Because the diameter of modern (conical) IVC filters is no more than 28 mm, when the diameter of the IVC was greater 28 mm by cavagram, it was believed that conical devices could not engage the wall of the IVC and might migrate cephalad. In such cases of "mega-cava," an alternative device (e.g., the bird's-nest filter) would be necessary. The accuracy of ultrasound for diameter measurement of vascular structures (e.g., abdominal aortic aneurysm) has been well documented. Furthermore, during DGFI, both saggital and short-axis duplex ultrasound imaging of the IVC is routine. Interestingly, most IVC (particularly in critically ill patients who may be hypovolemic) are elliptical rather than cylindrical, with a reduced AP diameter compared to transverse. Cavagrams performed exclusively in an AP projection would thus routinely overestimate the diameter of the IVC. In addition, vast clinical experience to date suggests that acute IVC filter migration during placement is rare and has happened even when a vena cavagram had been performed.

3. The vena cavagram will identify venous anomalies such as a duplicated, or left-sided IVC: Routine saggital and transverse ultrasound imaging of the IVC can accurately identify most clinically relevant, major IVC anomalies. These anatomic variants

occur quite rarely and, as above, could hardly justify the performance of a contrast study in every patient having placement of an IVC filter.

Technique for Duplex-Guided Filter Insertion

All procedures are performed at the patient's bedside in the intensive care unit by a vascular surgeon, with ultrasound imaging performed by a vascular technologist experienced with deep abdominal scanning (Fig. 46-1). Before the procedure, each patient undergoes a complete lower extremity venous duplex ultrasound scan.

- Lower extremity veins: Patients with established acute DVT undergo lower extremity venous duplex scans for diagnosis. In addition, patency of the common femoral and iliac veins is confirmed. The right common femoral vein is favored for IVC filter insertion, but if thrombus is present, the left femoral may be used. Rarely, bilateral iliac or common femoral DVT may be present. In such cases, internal jugular vein access would be required for filter insertion. Most critical care areas are designed to have the majority of monitoring and support equipment at the head of the bed, making bedside DGFI using the jugular vein approach unnecessarily complex. Filter placement in such cases should be performed under fluoroscopic guidance.

- Inferior vena cava: Imaging of the IVC is performed with a commercially available color Doppler duplex ultrasound scanner using a low-frequency, deep abdominal scan head. A subxiphoid or subcostal approach is typically employed, but a right flank approach may also be useful. Because it is desirable to place the IVC filter below the renal veins, one anatomic landmark is the confluence of the left renal vein with the IVC. The vena cava diameter is measured in both the long and short axes in this area. Imaging at this level will also identify major anatomic anomalies of the vena cava. Long-axis imaging of the vena cava allows visualization of the right renal artery, seen end-on as it passes behind the IVC (Fig. 46-2A). Additionally, identification of the right renal artery can be confirmed by Doppler spectral waveform analysis (Fig. 46-2B). Placement of the filter at this level ensures appropriate position below the renal veins, and an attempt is made to maintain this anatomic localization throughout the procedure. In every case, preliminary IVC scan must ensure adequate visualization of the aforementioned structures. If these anatomic landmarks cannot be visualized, the filter is placed using fluoroscopic guidance; or, more recently, with the assistance of IVUS.

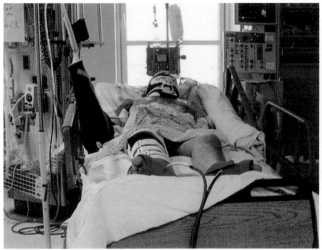 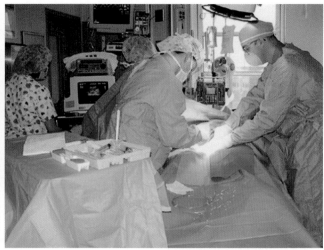

A   B

Figure 46-1. The set-up for DGFI. **A,** A typical multitrauma patient in the intensive care unit intubated with neurospinal and long bone fractures, invasive monitoring, and several intravenous drips. **B,** Note the vascular technologists at the head of the bed with the ultrasound screen in full view of both the technologists and the surgeon.

Transfemoral venous catheterization is performed, and the filter carrier is advanced until it can be visualized at the level of the right renal artery (as described above). Filter insertion can be observed in real time. Direct visualization of the wire and filter carrier within the vena cava is maintained throughout the procedure, and once infrarenal positioning of the carrier is confirmed, the filter is deployed (see Fig. 46-2C). Following insertion, accurate deployment in the IVC is documented with both longitudinal and cross-sectional imaging (see Fig. 46-2D).

Following successful filter placement, duplex ultrasound scanning of the IVC and the femoral vein insertion site is performed 5 to 7 days after the procedure, or before discharge. This initial follow-up scan is performed primarily to diagnose IVC thrombosis or thrombosis at the insertion site, but it also confirms the anatomic location of the filter.

Clinical Experience

Bedside DGFI has been performed in 67 multitrauma patients at the authors' institution. This group was typical of a trauma population with a predominance of young men, and included 50 men and 17 women with a mean age of 43 years. The indication for IVC filter placement was acute, proximal DVT in eight cases (12%); the other 59 patients had filters placed purely for PE prophylaxis. Some form of DVT prophylaxis had been used in 60 patients (i.e., intermittent pneumatic compression in 50, low-dose heparin in 10). DVT prophylaxis was not possible or was contraindicated in seven cases (Table 46-1).

When ultrasound visualization of anatomic landmarks was successful, no conversions to fluoroscopic guidance were required in these 67 cases. Vena caval filter placement was performed through the right common femoral vein in 59 cases and via the left common femoral vein in 8 patients. All patients had Greenfield IVC filters placed; 60 had titanium filters and 7 had stainless steel filters. The authors favor the titanium Greenfield filter for DGFI because the metal carrier of the titanium filter is more echogenic and thus easier to visualize in the IVC than is the plastic carrier used with the newer "over-the-wire" stainless steel filters.

As noted above, all patients had postinsertion duplex scans of the IVC and femoral vein insertion site approximately 1 week after the procedure. No patient had early insertion site thrombosis or IVC thrombosis. Suprarenal placement was recognized in one case; this was felt to represent an error in interpretation of the ultrasound during placement of the filter early in the authors' experience. The postprocedural scan noted that the filter was circumferentially engaged in the IVC wall with no evidence of tilt, and no further treatment was required.

There were no deaths caused by PE in this series, and no patient suffered a documented nonfatal PE. Five patients died from their traumatic injuries (7.2% mortality). There were no serious complications directly associated with filter insertion.

Follow-Up

Follow-up IVC and lower extremity venous duplex scans have been performed in 40 patients (65% of survivors)

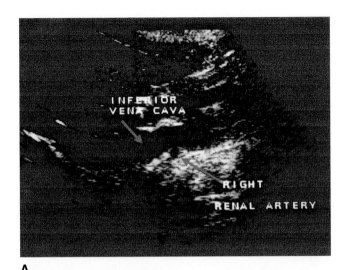

A

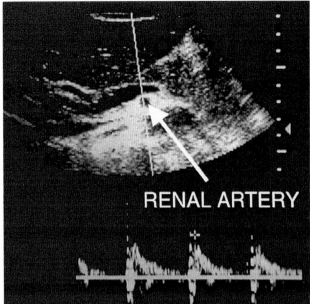

B

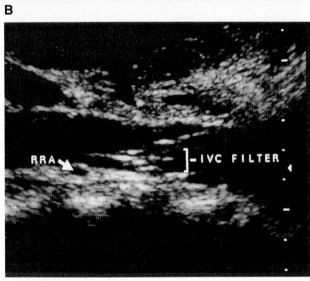

C

D

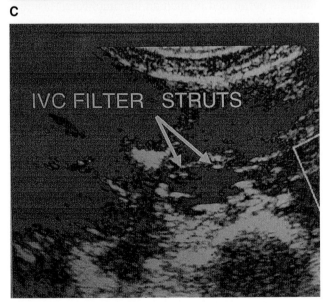

E

Figure 46-2. **A,** *Longitudinal image of the IVC and the right renal artery end-on.* **B,** *The right renal artery identified with Doppler spectral waveform analysis.* **C,** *Direct visualization of the guide wire and filter carrier within the vena cava.* **D,** *Post-deployment longitudinal scan confirming infrarenal positioning.* **E,** *Postdeployment cross-sectional scan showing filter struts engaged in the caval wall.*

TABLE 46-1. Patient Demographics and Methods of DVT Prophylaxis

Bedside Duplex-Guided Filter Insertion in Multitrauma Patients (n = 67)	Prophylaxis (n = 59)	Established DVT (n = 8)
Demographics		
Male	46	4
Female	13	4
Mean age	35	58
DVT Prophylaxis		
Mechanical compression	47	3
Low-dose heparin	9	1
None	3	4

from 1 to 18 months (mean of 5 months) following DGFI. One patient had a nonocclusive thrombus visualized in the filter 3 weeks after insertion, but the IVC remained patent on further follow-up. An additional patient developed insertion site thrombosis and IVC thrombosis at 1 month. These findings resolved by the 6-month follow-up study. The patient did not suffer a PE or have any postphlebitic changes. Longer follow-up revealed 1 (new) acute DVT in the 40 patients studied. Additionally, there was evidence of filter migration in one patient.

Extended follow-up study of any multitrauma patient population has generally been compromised in the past both by patient mortality and patient reliability. Nevertheless, in this experience with follow-up in nearly 70% of cases, the incidence of thrombotic complications (i.e., IVC thrombosis and insertion site thrombosis) appears significantly lower than previously observed in the overall population of patients with IVC filters at the authors' institution. Aswad and colleagues[5] performed routine follow-up duplex scan on 174 patients having IVC filter placement and observed IVC thrombosis in 12% of cases and insertion site thrombosis in nearly 25% of cases. However, no patient having prophylactic IVC filter placement in that original series was observed to have IVC thrombosis. Similarly, IVC thrombosis has been observed following DGFI in only one case (1.5%). Some of the reasons for this difference are self-evident. The overall hospital group includes elderly patients with more complex multisystemic medical comorbidities (including, not infrequently, disseminated malignancies with active thromboembolic disease) as an indication for treatment. This difference in the risk of IVC thrombosis is very clinically relevant. One of the major concerns regarding prophylactic IVC filter placement has been the long-term sequelae of these devices in a younger patient population. At present it appears that the risk of thrombotic complications of this procedure is acceptably low, at least in the early follow-up period.

Cost

The cost of (or charges for) materials and professional activities involved in placement of an IVC filter would not be expected to be significantly different for bedside placement compared with traditional placement in the OR or in an interventional suite. Generally however, the OR/interventional radiology (IR) suites involve facility fees that may be considerable. Perhaps most important are the intangible costs of the time and additional personnel routinely required to transport and attend these critically ill patients throughout the procedure. In this regard, bedside DGFI should offer considerable savings in terms of the expenditure of critical medical care resources. In the authors' experience, the physician and nursing staffs caring for these patients have uniformly expressed their appreciation that IVC filter insertion could be performed in such an uncomplicated fashion.

Conclusions

Bedside DGFI is a safe, reliable, and effective method of filter insertion and PE prevention in carefully selected, high-risk, multitrauma, or critical-care patients. Bedside filter placement was associated with a lower incidence of thrombotic complications, and early and intermediate follow-up have revealed no untoward sequelae from these procedures. Under optimal circumstances, this technique greatly simplifies management of patients judged to be at high risk from the complications of venous thromboembolism. Our experience suggests that this technique can be safely applied, more broadly, to patients in critical-care areas who might require an IVC filter. Bedside DGFI should be considered in complex, high-risk patients in whom other forms of DVT prophylaxis are ineffective or unavailable.

REFERENCES

1. Clagett GP, Anderson FA Jr, Geerts W, et al: Prevention of venous thromboembolism. Chest 114(5 Suppl):531S–560S, 1998.
2. Geerts WH, Jay RM, Chen E, et al: A prospective study of venous thromboembolism after major trauma. N Engl J Med 331:1601–1606, 1994.
3. Flinn WR, Sandager GP, Silva MB, et al: Prospective surveillance for perioperative venous thrombosis. Arch Surgery 131:472–480, 1996.
4. Swann KW, Black PM, Baker MF: Management of symptomatic deep venous thrombosis and pulmonary embolism on a neurosurgical service. J Neurosurg 64(4):563–567, 1986.
5. Aswad MA, Sandager G, Pias O, et al: Early duplex scan evaluation of four vena caval interruption devices. J Vasc Surg 24(5):809–818, 1996.
6. Sandager GP, Zimmer S, Silva MB, et al: Ultrasonographic characteristics of transvenous vena caval interruption devices. J Vasc Technol 16:17–21, 1992.
7. Nunn CR, Neuzil D, Naslund T, et al: Cost-effective method for bedside insertion of vena caval filters in trauma patients (see comments). J Trauma-Injury Infect Crit Care 43(5):752–758, 1997.
8. Sato DT, Robinson KD, Gregory RT, et al: Duplex directed caval filter insertion in multitrauma and critically ill patients. Ann Vasc Surg 13(4):365–371, 1999.
9. Oppat WF, Chiou AC, Matsumura JS: Intravascular ultrasound-guided vena cava filter placement. J Endovasc Surg 6(3):285–287, 1999.
10. Greenfield LJ, Proctor MC: Suprarenal filter placement. J Vasc Surg 28(3):432–438, discussion 438, 1998.

Part Three

Miscellaneous

Chapter 47

Evaluation of the Hepatoportal Circulation

ALGIRDAS EDVARDAS TAMOSIUNAS • NICOS LABROPOULOS

- Indications
- Examination Technique
- Anatomy
- Portal Hypertension
- Role of Doppler US in Surgical Planning and Surveillance
- Miscellaneous

Indications

Routine abdominal ultrasound usually relies on B-mode imaging. The use of Doppler is limited to differentiate vascular from nonvascular structures.[1]

Main indications to perform vascular Doppler examination of the hepatoportal system are:

1. Examination for portal hypertension
   - Patients with acute and chronic diseases of the liver
   - To rule out portal hypertension in patients presenting with gastroesophageal varices and/or bleeding; ascites
   - Evaluation of the effects of the medical treatment of portal hypertension and pathophysiology of portal hypertension[2,3]

2. Differentiation of the focal liver diseases
3. Evaluation of the hepatoportal vasculature before surgical procedures and surveillance after:
   - Liver resection
   - Surgical portosystemic shunts and transjugular intrahepatic portosystemic shunts (TIPS)
   - Liver transplantation

Examination Technique

In the diagnosis of hepatoportal system pathology B-mode scanning, pulsed wave (spectral) Doppler (PWD), color Doppler imaging (CDI), and power Doppler imaging are most common ultrasound (US) scanning modalities.[4-7] Other modalities include endoscopic ultrasound for evaluation of gastroesophageal varices and azygos vein bloodflow. Application of ultrasound contrast agents is not common, and their exact place in clinical diagnosis needs further evaluation.[8-11] Three-dimensional reconstruction could facilitate perception of liver vasculature anatomy, but it is difficult to perform in deep structures and is very time-consuming.[12]

For the deep abdominal ultrasound scanning, multifrequency curved linear array and phased array sector transducers with a mean frequency of 2 to 5 MHz are usually employed. Tissue harmonics and high-frequency

(5- to 7-MHz) transducers with elevation beam focusing that is able to provide good penetration are of value to get better spatial resolution. High-frequency 5- to 14-MHz linear arrays may be useful in characterizing the contour of the liver and superficial portosystemic collaterals (see Fig. 47-12), and in pediatric patients.

Patients are examined in basal fasting condition in the morning after assuming a relaxed supine position. Ultrasound examination starts with the B-mode evaluation of the liver. Intrahepatic vessels and spleen are best seen from intercostal and subcostal approaches. Left and right anterior oblique, and semierect positions are used in the phase of deep inspiration for optimal imaging. After gray scale imaging, all vasculature related to the liver is located with CDI, and PWD is used to obtain quantitative flow characteristics. Examination of the extrahepatic portal vein (PV) and tributaries starts by placing the transducer in the epigastrium to obtain good quality axial view of the main PV and surrounding structures (e.g., the common bile duct and hepatic artery). The measurements of the PV with respiratory variations are obtained, and Doppler imaging is performed. After the imaging of the main PV, splenic vein, superior mesenteric vein, and inferior mesenteric vein are imaged. The characteristic sonographic changes to diagnose portal hypertension (PH) are presented in Table 47-1.[4-16]

Doppler Imaging

The parameters used to characterize bloodflow in arteries are peak systolic velocity, end-diastolic velocity, and mean and time-averaged maximum velocities. For the characterization of the arterial bloodflow, two indexes are employed: (1) resistance (Pourcelot) index (RI), which is systolic velocity minus end-diastolic velocity divided by systolic velocity; and (2) the pulsatility (Gosling) index (PI), which is systolic velocity minus end-diastolic velocity divided by mean velocity.[17] The resistance index is usually employed for characterization of bloodflow in arteries feeding low resistance areas, as in the parenchymal organs (i.e., liver, kidney, and spleen). The pulsatility index is more common to characterize bloodflow in arteries feeding higher resistance vascular beds such as the fasting intestinal tract.[13,17] Temporal parameters such as hepatic artery (HA) acceleration time and acceleration index are not common; nevertheless, they recently were shown to correlate with portal vein pressure.[18]

For the characterization of bloodflow in veins, the maximal velocity and mean velocity are used. For description of the bloodflow in veins, qualitative characteristics such as direction and phasicity are employed.[16] Duplex ultrasound provides mean flow velocity, and the cross-sectional area of the vessel and volume bloodflow can be calculated in both arteries and veins. It was shown that portal flow quantitative Doppler measurements could be reproducible if operators receive appropriate training.[19] Congestion index of the PV, introduced by Moriyasu in 1986,[20] is the ratio between the cross-sectional area and the bloodflow velocity of the portal vein; it shows weak correlation with the portal vein pressure and severity of the liver cirrhosis.[18,21] Doppler perfusion index is the ratio of hepatic artery to total liver bloodflow. It may be

TABLE 47-1. Ultrasound Findings Consistent With Chronic Liver Diseases and PH on Different Ultrasound Scanning Modes

B-Mode	Doppler US	
	PWD	*CDI*
Chronic liver diseases and cirrhosis (predispose to PH): • Nodularity of HV and intrahepatic PV contour • Splenomegaly • Hypertrophy of the HA • Congestive splenomegaly • Ascites • Hypertrophy of the caudate lobe • Increased diameters of PV and tributaries	• Decreased bloodflow velocity in PV • Loss of respiratory variations of bloodflow in PV • Presence of hepatofugal flow in PV • Hepatofugal flow in PC • Decreased pulsatility in hepatic veins • Decreased pulsatility in SMA • Increased pulsatility in hepatic arteries	• Flow direction in PV, branches, and tributaries • Location and size of PC • Thrombosis of the hepatic vessels
Portal hypertension: • Lack of respiratory variations of PV • Presence of PC—thrombosis of the PV • Portal hypertensive gastropathy		

PH, portal hypertension; HV, hepatic vein; PV, portal vein; HA, hepatic artery; PC, portosystemic collaterals; US, ultrasound; PWD, pulsed wave Doppler; SMA, superior mesenteric artery; CDI, color Doppler imaging.

used for detection of liver metastases as the arterial component increases in metastatic liver disease.[22]

In the liver, Doppler US largely has been used in order to establish the volume and direction of portal flow; the character of flow in tumors; and the patency and stenoses of the native and transplant hepatic artery, portal vein, and hepatic veins. Investigators have recently expanded the use of duplex imaging in evaluation of liver disease.

CDI is based on the same duplex imaging principles, employing multiple Doppler gates to cover certain anatomic areas. It provides combination of cross-section anatomy and functional imaging. This method identifies blood vessels not seen on conventional B-mode scanning, and depicts their lumens with color-coded information about the direction and speed of bloodflow.[23] In theory, power Doppler imaging is up to three times more sensitive to the slow flow and may be used for initial evaluation of the regions in which portosystemic collaterals are suspected.[6,24] It does not provide directional information, so either the CDI or pulsed wave Doppler should be used further to certify hepatofugal flow.

Anatomy

The liver has a unique double blood supply: Approximately 70% to 75% of the blood comes from the portal vein and the remaining 25% to 30% from the hepatic artery.[25]

Branches of the portal vein, hepatic artery, bile ducts, lymphatics, and nerves are surrounded by connective tissue and enter the porta hepatis and branch further throughout the liver in the portal tracts. The portal triad includes the artery, vein, and bile duct. There are few anastomoses between intrahepatic portal vein branches; most of them are less than 2 mm in diameter, whereas the hepatic arteries and their branches typically do not anastomose beyond the liver porta.[26] The interlobular veins and arteries branch around the periphery of the hepatic lobule and then end in the hepatic sinusoids. The hepatic sinusoids empty into the central veins; they leave the hepatic lobule and fuse to form larger hepatic veins that eventually drain into the inferior vena cava.[25-27]

Arterial Supply

The liver receives its entire arterial blood supply from the common HA that begins from the celiac artery. The celiac artery originates from the aorta above the pancreatic neck; after a short 1 to 2 cm anterior course, it gives three branches: the left gastric, the splenic, and the common hepatic artery. The latter courses to the right and gives off the gastroduodenal artery. Beyond this level, the common HA is called the proper hepatic artery; it travels with the main portal vein and common bile duct in the hepatogastric ligament toward the porta

hepatis. On ultrasound scans, the proper hepatic artery typically projects above the main PV and common bile duct (Fig. 47-1, A). The proper HA approaches the liver porta and branches into the right and left hepatic arteries. The middle HA usually originates from the left HA and feeds the quadrate lobe of the liver, but its origin from the right HA is also common. Analysis of the blood supply of the liver by Michels showed that the conventional celiac artery textbook anatomy occurs only in about 55% of the population. Almost half of all patients have either a replaced or an accessory right, left, or common hepatic artery.[28] All the possible anatomic variations must be kept in mind when the examiner is facing difficulties in locating the HA or in differentiating between various arteries in the hepatopancreatic zone.

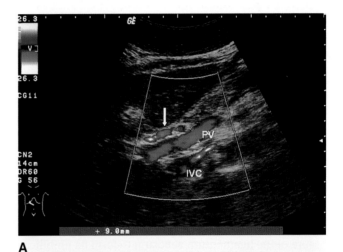

A

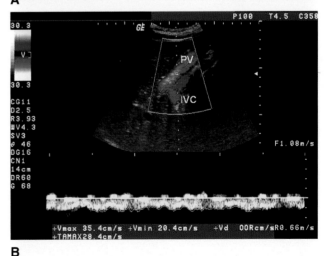

B

*Figure 47-1. Normal portal vein. **A**, Oblique sagital view of the main portal vein measuring 9 mm in diameter. Common hepatic artery (white arrow) projects just above the main portal vein (PV). Note the proximity of the PV to the inferior vena cava (IVC). **B**, Triplex scan of the normal portal vein. Continuous hepatopetal flow measuring time averaged maximum velocity of 28 cm/sec, which equals the mean velocity of 16 cm/sec. Small flow components above the baseline are produced because of helical (spiral) flow pattern in the PV.*

Portal Vein and Tributaries

The PV develops from the umbilical and the vitelline veins, and it measures 6 to 8 cm in length. Various congenital abnormalities of the PV (e.g., duplication, aneurysm, anomalous pulmonary venous drainage, and abnormal ventral position) have been described. Agenesis of the right or left portal vein is the most commonly reported congenital anomaly.[29-31]

The PV is formed behind the neck of the pancreas by the confluence of the splenic and superior mesenteric veins. In about a half of the population, the inferior mesenteric vein enters the splenic vein; in the remainder it either joins the junction of the splenic and superior mesenteric veins or joins the superior mesenteric vein.[27] As the PV enters the lesser omentum it receives the left gastric (former called the coronary) vein, the right gastric vein, and the superior pancreaticoduodenal vein. The normal upper diameter limit of the PV, based on US studies, is considered to be less than 13 mm (see Fig. 47-1, *A*). A diameter greater than 20 mm is consistent with PV aneurysm.[32,33] Normal diameters of splenic, superior mesenteric, and inferior mesenteric veins are up to 10, 13, and 8 mm, respectively.[34]

The PV is the largest-caliber intrahepatic vessel, making it the easiest to identify by ultrasound and to trace up to the third order branches. As the PV enters the liver at the porta hepatis, it divides into right and left portal veins. The right PV, which varies from 0 to 3 cm in length, usually receives the cystic vein of the gallbladder before dividing into anterior and posterior segmental branches (Fig. 47-2). The left PV goes horizontally to the left as its transverse part. It then turns directly forward to the fissure of the ligamentum venosum to form its umbilical portion near the ligamentum teres (Fig. 47-3). In approximately 20% of the population, internal PV branching pattern is not as described, with the trifurcation of the portal vein been the most common variation.[30]

Hepatic Veins

The three major hepatic veins run along planes that separate each of the four major liver segments (Fig. 47-4, *A*). The left HV courses in the intersegmental plane between the medial and lateral segments and drains the lateral segment and a small part of the medial segment. The middle HV goes through the interlobar plane and divides the liver into the left and right lobes. In about 85% of patients, the middle HV joins the left HV before the latter reaches the inferior vena cava (IVC). In the other 15%, the middle HV enters independently into the IVC.[35] The right HV courses between the anterior and posterior segments of the right lobe between the bifurcation of the right PV into its anterior and posterior segmental branches.

Lymphatics

The liver has the largest lymphatic drainage of any body organ.[26] It begins in the space of Disse and then communicates with the interlobular lymphatics, which join together to form the large lymphatics that drain from the porta of the liver to the celiac lymph nodes. Substantially less developed lymphatics follow the HV and IVC into the posterior mediastinum. Inflammatory abdominal conditions and chronic liver lymphadenopathy are characterized by enlarged regional lymph nodes with

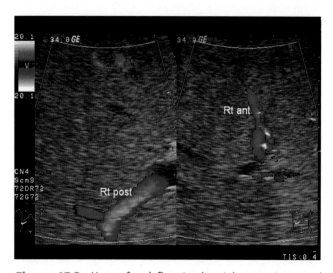

Figure 47-2. Hepatofugal flow in the right anterior portal vein branch. Right anterior branch of the hepatic artery flow direction is opposite to the portal vein. Normal hepatopetal flow in right posterior PV branch is still preserved.

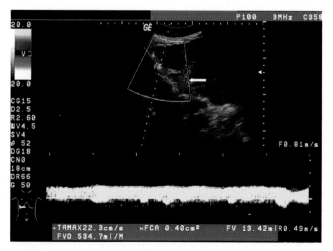

Figure 47-3. Group 5 portosystemic collaterals. Prominent paraumbilical vein starting off the umbilical portion of the left portal vein (arrow). Volume flow in the shunt is calculated and equals 534 mL/min.

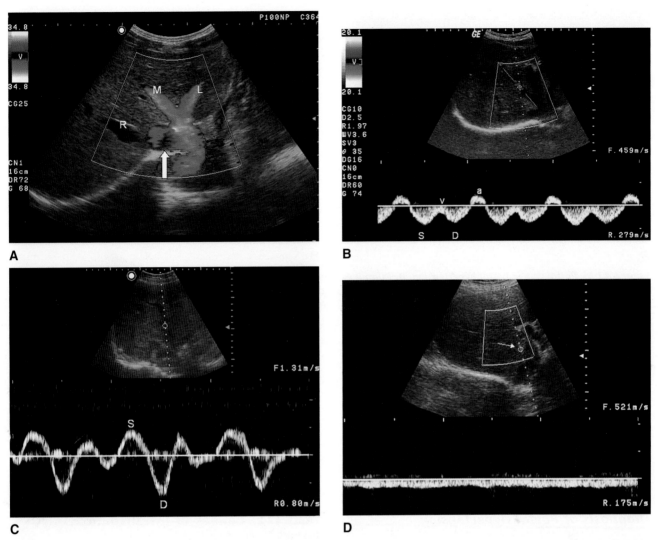

Figure 47-4. *Hepatic veins.* **A,** *Transverse view of the three main hepatic veins and IVC (white arrow). Right (R), middle (M), and left (L) veins are seen as "bunny" on color Doppler imaging points to the IVC. The right hepatic vein is not filled with color because of perpendicular incidence of the Doppler beam.* **B,** *Normal highly pulsatile Doppler waveform in the middle hepatic vein. Two prominent antegrade waves: systolic (S) and diastolic (D) interchange with two small antegrade waves a and v.* **C,** *Hepatic veins in posthepatic portal hypertension. Reversed systolic wave (S) caused by right heart failure and tricuspid valve regurgitation.* **D,** *Hepatic veins in advanced cirrhosis. Hepatic veins are small caliber, and abnormal nonpulsatile dampened Doppler waveform in middle hepatic vein is present.*

an anteroposterior diameter exceeding 1.0 cm. Cassani and colleagues found this condition present in up to 57% of cases in chronic liver diseases.[36] Common sites are the liver hilum and hepatoduodenal ligament going to the celiac axis (Fig. 47-5). Other regions are much less common.

Portal Hypertension

Portal hypertension is a common syndrome characterized by an increase of the pressure gradient between the PV and the IVC above the normal range of 2 to 6 mmHg.[37] A pressure gradient of more than 6 mmHg is abnormal,

and a pressure gradient above 10 mmHg is consistent with clinically significant portal hypertension and high risk of variceal bleeding.[2,3] With an IVC pressure in healthy individuals of up to 8 mmHg, the mean portal blood pressure should be less than 10 to 12 mmHg.[37-39]

PH is the consequence of increased portal resistance and increased blood inflow. Under normal conditions the main source of resistance is the liver, but the normal liver resistance to portal bloodflow is very low. When the resistance is increased, a bigger pressure gradient is needed to maintain the same bloodflow, and therefore PH develops. In that case, excess blood inflow from PV tributaries (caused by visceral vasodilatation and splenomegaly) is harmful because it contributes to further increase of the pressure gradient.[37,40,41]

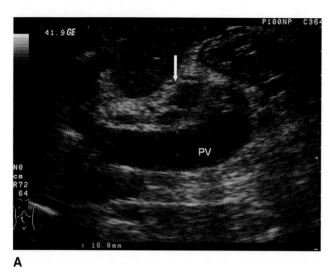

A

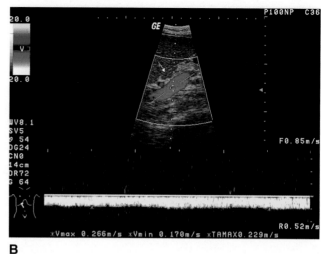

B

*Figure 47-5. Portal vein in portal hypertension. **A**, Dilated main portal vein measuring almost 17 mm diameter. Enlarged lymph nodes are seen above the PV (arrow). **B**, Continuous slow hepatopetal flow in the main PV (mean velocity 13 cm/sec) in liver cirrhosis patient consistent with portal hypertension. Note enlarged lymph nodes (arrow) in the hepatoduodenal ligament.*

Classification of PH is based on the anatomic location of obstruction to the PV flow. Depending on the site of the increased resistance, PH is classified as prehepatic, when the obstruction is somewhere in the portal vein or its tributaries; intrahepatic, when the obstruction is located somewhere in the liver; and posthepatic, when the obstruction is in the liver veins, IVC, or even further because of increased blood pressure in the right heart.[39]

Diagnosis of Portal Hypertension

Many modalities are in use to diagnose PH, but no one method seems to be ideal. Laboratory tests are of little value. Instrumental investigations are applied to get functional information (e.g., to measure portal and variceal pressure), anatomic information (e.g., the presence and location of portosystemic collaterals), or both.[42–46] These are based on imaging and may be invasive or noninvasive. Noninvasive diagnostic modalities are ultrasound, computed tomography (CT), magnetic resonance imaging (MRI), and radionuclide scanning. Invasive diagnostic modalities are the angiographic procedures. During the last decade, the use of angiography declined with the advent of Doppler ultrasound, CT, and MR. Nevertheless, it remains the gold standard for preoperative imaging of the portal venous system.[2,3,44,46]

Intrahepatic Portal Hypertension

Chronic liver diseases change function and structure of the liver and eventually result in liver cirrhosis (LC). The etiological factors leading to LC and portal hypertension in order of prevalence are listed in Table 47-2. In LC the micro- and macro-architecture of the liver is distorted, leading to an increased resistance to bloodflow.[47] The

causes of increased hepatic resistance to bloodflow may be classified as (1) structural, related to distorted architecture, and basically irreversible; or (2) functional, related to changes in venous and endothelial cell tone, which are rapidly reversible and can be modulated pharmacologically.[47–50]

TABLE 47-2. Causes of Intrahepatic Portal Hypertension

Chronic Liver Disease	Other
Viral hepatitis B and C	Liver tumors
Alcoholic liver disease	Idiopathic portal hypertension
Autoimmune hepatitis	Shistosomatosis
Primary biliary cirrhosis	Radiation
Primary sclerosing cholangitis	
Drug induced (toxic) hepatitis	
Hemochromatosis	
Wilson's disease	
Extrahepatic cholestasis	
Posthepatic venous congestion (as a cause of LC)	
Hypervitaminosis A	

LC, liver cirrhosis.

Clinical manifestations of LC include ascites; hepatic encephalopathy; variceal bleeding; spontaneous bacterial peritonitis; hematologic changes; jaundice; hyperdynamic circulation; splenomegaly; portal hypertensive gastropathy; and hepatopulmonary, portopulmonary, and hepatorenal syndromes.[40,41,51,52] All these appear to be direct manifestations of hepatocellular insufficiency and portal hypertension syndromes.[41] Some complications (e.g., variceal bleeding) are predominantly defined by portal hypertension, whereas others (e.g., hepatic encephalopathy and hepatic failure) result from both.

Portal Vein System and Portal Systemic Collaterals

In liver cirrhosis, when PH is present, the PV trunk and its tributaries usually become dilated (see Fig. 47-5, *A*). Absolute diameters of the PV and its branches are the first markers of PH described back in 1982 by Bolondi.[16] The cut-off of upper PV diameter of 13 mm seems to be specific but not sensitive enough to rely on.[7] The intrahepatic portion of the PV and its branches may be compressed by regenerative nodules.[5] In advanced LC and/or with the presence of hypercoagulable states, the PV may become thrombosed and then partially recanalized (Fig. 47-6, *A* through *C*), presenting as "cavernous transformation."[7,53]

Normal PV flow in healthy individuals is characterized by continuous laminar hepatopetal flow with low respiratory, cardiac cycle, and posture-related variations. Increased PV pulsatility occasionally could be present in the normal population.[54] Mean PV flow velocity is reported to be around 15 to 18 cm/sec[55] and should not be confused with time averaged maximum velocity (see Fig. 47-1, *B*). With the progression of PH flow, velocities decrease (see Fig. 47-5, *B*), and it was shown that PV blood velocity less than 10 cm/sec correlates with poor prognosis in LC patients.[55]

The portal vein and its tributaries typically have no valves to prevent reverse flow. When resistance to bloodflow is increased, it cannot handle the same portal bloodflow without an elevated portal-systemic pressure gradient. Many of PV tributaries establish anastomotic connections with the inferior and superior vena cava

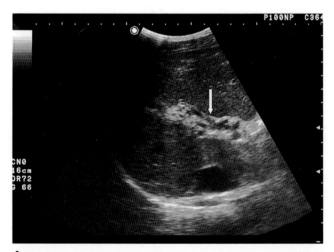

A

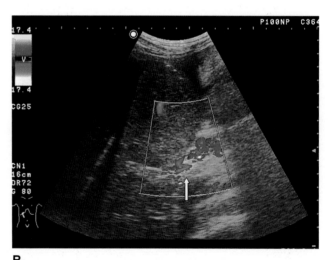

B

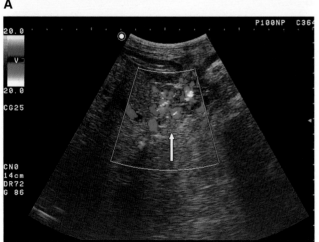

C

Figure 47-6. Chronic portal vein thrombosis. Cavernous transformation of the left portal vein on (**A**) B-mode and (**B**) color Doppler imaging c (arrow). **C**, Prominent multiple collateral veins (arrow) where main portal vein should be located.

and shunt blood around a portal vein obstruction or the diseased liver. In this case, portosystemic collaterals (PC) develop as flow in some bigger veins changes its direction from normal hepatopetal (toward the liver) into hepatofugal (away from the liver) (Fig. 47-7, *A*), and small venules enlarge and serve as significant shunts.[27] The diameter of the portal vein may decrease to normal limits with development of PC.[5] Presence of hepatofugal flow in PV system and PC are diagnostic for PH and may alter therapeutic management of LC patients.[37] Intrahepatic to extrahepatic collateral veins may preserve hepatopetal flow in the intrahepatic PV branch drained by the collateral or even in the main PV. This is a common finding in the left branch of the portal vein when the prominent paraumbilical collaterals are present.

It must be emphasized that the presence of PC does not always mean that the patient has PH; this is especially true considering prehepatic blockade. In the case of acute PV obstruction, which is later relieved by intervention, PC may stay big enough to be visualized by ultrasound. However, hepatofugal flow in those may be absent, and PV pressures may be normal. On the other

hand, PH may manifest clinically after stress (e.g., blood volume overload) when portal pressure is within the normal range under the usual investigative fasting conditions.[56,57] Normal liver functioning at low PV pressures switches to the "portal circulatory dysfunction" state in early liver disease, with normal pressures but abnormal responses to the circulatory stress.[56,58] Hepatofugal flow in patients with chronic liver disease usually develops gradually: At first it appears in one or several segmental PV branches as reversed flow component with respiratory variations (see Fig. 47-2). Eventually, with the progression of the underlying liver disease, fully reversed PV flow may develop. Reversal flow component with every cardiac cycle is characteristic to posthepatic PH (Fig. 47-8, *A*, *B*).

The statement that PC are present is based on following gray scale and Doppler imaging criteria:

1. Abnormal hypoechoic tortuous tubular or oval cystic structures (varices) on B-mode

2. Varices demonstrated by CDI

3. Presence of hepatofugal flow in PV tributaries

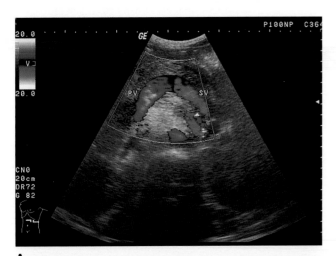

A

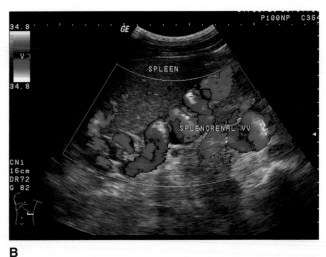

B

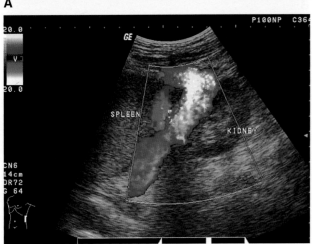

C

Figure 47-7. Group 3 portosystemic collaterals. ***A***, *Reversed (hepatofugal) flow in the main portal vein.* ***B***, *Splenic vein (SV) feeding large splenorenal collaterals (varices).* ***C***, *Large collateral vein between the right kidney and the lower pole of the spleen shunting blood from the splenic hilum to the lumbar and epigastric veins.*

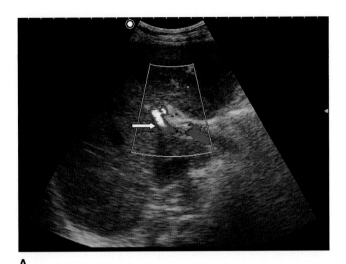

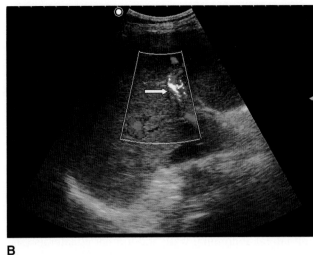

A   **B**

Figure 47-8. *To and fro flow in posthepatic portal hypertension.* ***A,*** *Color Doppler imaging shows hepatopetal flow direction in the left portal vein (arrow) interchanging with (**B**) hepatofugal flow in the same left portal vein.*

Five major anatomic areas should be meticulously examined to locate PC.

Group 1. Collaterals posterior to the left lobe of the liver from the confluence of the PV to the gastroesophageal (GE) junction: left gastric vein (LGV) collaterals and GE varices (Fig. 47-9, *A* and *B*). Doppler imaging of the GE collaterals is usually affected by motion artifacts caused by the pulsations transmitted from the heart; nevertheless, sensitivity of the CDI diagnosing GE varices may be as high as 80%.[59]

The left gastric vein (former called the coronary gastric vein) is a direct tributary of the portal vein. It drains the abdominal part of the esophagus, where it usually anastomoses through the submucosal esophageal plexus with tributaries of the azygos venous system that drain

the thoracic esophagus into the superior vena cava. PH causes a considerable distention of these submucosal veins, producing esophageal varices.[37] The right gastric vein is small and does not seem to become a large collateral route. Occasionally, a distinct vein is seen in PH along the splenic vein and is considered one of the multiple LGV. In most cases it drains to the GE junction like the typical LGV.[60] Other routes (e.g., the so-called paraesophageal collaterals, draining directly to the left subclavian vein, to the portopulmonary by way of a pulmonary vein, and to the left renal vein) have been reported but are much less common and are usually impossible to visualize by ultrasound.[60–62]

Group 2. Collaterals from the anteromedial side of the spleen to the splenic hilum, where gastrosplenic liga-

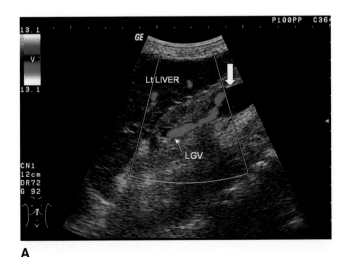

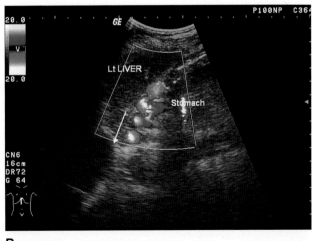

A   **B**

Figure 47-9. *Group 1 portosystemic collaterals.* ***A,*** *Left gastric vein (small arrow) originating from the confluence of the portal vein (large arrow).* ***B,*** *Varicosity posterior to the left liver lobe extending toward the gastroesophageal junction (arrow) in the sagital plane.*

ment is situated; and the short gastric veins collaterals (Fig. 47-10, *A* and *B*). These collaterals generally are easier to image by ultrasonography than are the left gastric vein and esophageal varices because of their proximity to the abdominal wall.

The short gastric veins usually supply gastric fundal varices when esophageal varices are supplied usually by LGV.[63] The presence of the fundal varices and short gastric veins correlates with lower portal pressures, rather than when esophageal/cardiac varices, which supplied by LGV, are present.[64]

Group 3. Collaterals around the upper pole of the left kidney, left kidney vein, and splenic hilum; splenorenal collaterals (see Fig. 47-7, *B*) and lower pole of the spleen and lateral abdominal wall; and lumbar collaterals (see Fig. 47-7, *C*).

The splenic vein is located very close to the left renal vein. In PH, splenorenal collaterals can be formed with the left renal vein or communicate in the retroperitoneal fat around the kidney with veins of both the renal and lumbar tributaries of the inferior vena cava and hemiazygos vein.[42,43,60,61,65] Reversed flow in the splenic vein should prompt the investigator that these PC are present.

The other possibility for the splenic vein is to form collaterals through the short gastric veins toward the left gastric vein and the GE junction.[42,43] In this case, depending on whether the communications with the left renal vein are present, it can either feed the GE varices or, by contrast, drain them to the left renal vein.

Group 4. Collaterals fed by superior mesenteric vein or inferior mesenteric vein when hepatofugal flow in those veins is present (Fig. 47-11, *A* and *B*). These are varices in the retroperitoneum around the IVC, posterior and inferior to the pancreas, that drain the superior mesenteric vein and inferior mesenteric vein to IVC collaterals.

Superior mesenteric vein branches in the mesenterium can form direct communications with the IVC and hemiazygos vein. These communications are called the veins of Retzius.[60,61]

Inferior mesenteric vein forms anastomoses with the hemorrhoidal plexuses and can anastomose with the left testicular (ovarian) vein, which drains into the IVC.[40,66,67]

Group 5. The region from the umbilical portion of the left PV to the anterior abdominal wall and diaphragm for the paraumbilical vein, and the coronary ligament of the liver collaterals (see Fig. 47-3).

Paraumbilical Veins. There are small veins around the ligamentum teres that communicate with the umbilical portion of the left branch of portal vein. The original umbilical vein is occluded after birth with dense connective tissue and cannot be reopened. In PH, usually only one vein becomes considerably distended and communicates at the umbilicus with superficial abdominal veins to produce the classical caput medusae appearance. These superficial veins can drain either superiorly into the superior vena cava through the axillary-subclavian system, or inferiorly into the inferior vena cava through the femoral-iliac system.[68-72] Slow hepatofugal flow (less than 5 cm/sec) may be detected in healthy people in umbilical ligament fissure as well, when the pressures in the portal system are normal.[73]

Other PC. Omental veins and varices occasionally can be fed by short gastric veins and are more common when portal vein thrombosis is present (Fig. 47-12). Gallbladder varices have been reported in patients with portal hypertension.[43,61,74]

Direct intrahepatic communications can form between the portal and hepatic veins (Fig. 47-13, *A* and *B*). They probably represent dilated sinusoids and are found rarely in advanced cirrhosis.[27,31,75]

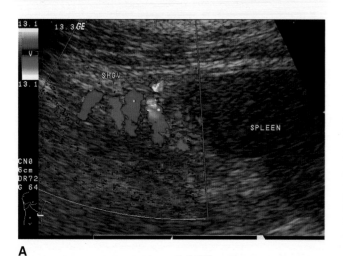

A

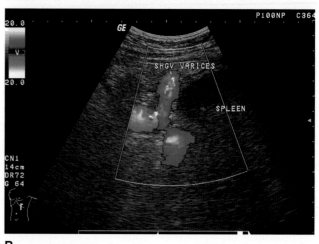

B

Figure 47-10. *Group 2 portosystemic collaterals.* **A,** *Short gastric veins are visualized around the anteromedial margin of the spleen.* **B,** *Large portosystemic shunt draining blood from the gastrosplenic ligament to the superior epigastric veins.*

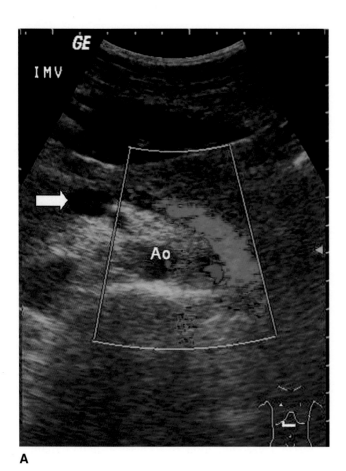

A

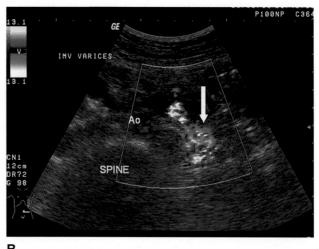

B

Figure 47-11. Group 4 portosystemic collaterals. **A**, Hepatofugal flow direction in the inferior mesenteric vein originating from the portal vein confluence (arrow). **B**, The mesenterium varicose veins (arrow) in the left lower abdominal quadrant are seen on color Doppler imaging in the same patient.

Rarely, intrahepatic branches of the left portal vein can form significant transhepatic collaterals (see Fig. 47-16, *B*) with the extrahepatic veins coursing to the esophagus or IVC.[61,76] In patients who have had prior abdominal surgery, peristomal collaterals may develop at the peris-

tomal mucocutaneous junction or at the peristomal adhesions.[61]

The presence of PC contributes to two major problems: development of portal-systemic encephalopathy, caused by shunting of intestinal blood directly into the systemic circulation; and formation of varices and variceal bleeding. The varices are usually formed in locations where significant amount of shunting to the systemic circulation is present. Clinically, the most important site of PC varices is the gastroesophageal junction, because bleeding from these appears to be a primary direct cause of mortality among LC patients.[3,77,78] Bleeding from other than GE varices (e.g., mesenteric and hemorrhoid plexus) appears to be rare and is not a significant problem (less than 7%).[43] It is solely caused by PH, and strongly correlates with the pressure in the PV system. The bleeding does not occur when the pressure is below 12 mmHg.[2,3,47,79] PV congestion index and HA acceleration index correlate with portal pressures; however, Doppler US does not provide reliable pressure measurements.[17,19] The primary feeding collateral for GE varices is LGV. The paraumbilical vein, fundal varices, and short gastric veins with splenorenal collaterals appear to be beneficial in reducing incidence of variceal bleeding because they divert bloodflow from the GE varices and decompress the PV system.[5,43]

Figure 47-12. Other portosystemic collaterals. Omental varices just beneath the abdominal wall (arrow) imaged with linear array 7-MHz transducer.

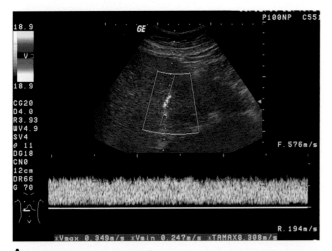

A

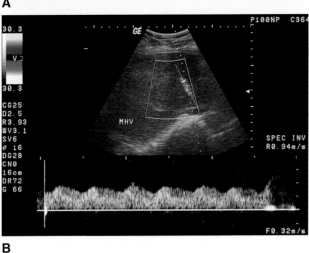

B

*Figure 47-13. Spontaneous intrahepatic portosystemic shunt. **A**, Continuous flow in the prominent intrahepatic shunt connecting the right anterior branch of the portal vein and the middle hepatic vein. **B**, Middle hepatic vein outflow is markedly increased with loss of the characteristic waveform pattern in the same patient.*

Arterial Changes in Portal Hypertension

In LC, portal blood inflow to the liver decreases and hepatic arteries become unique blood provider to the liver. The hepatic artery hypertrophies and becomes markedly dilated in its intra- and extrahepatic course. Dilated branches, displaced by regenerative nodules within the liver and shortened because of loss of liver parenchyma, are very tortuous, presenting as a "corkscrew" on imaging studies.[4,5] Normal HA flow is low resistance (RI less than 0.7) compared with parenchymal organs (Fig. 47-14). The increase in hepatic artery RI was shown to correlate with severity of LC.[5,11,80] Lafortune and colleagues[80] demonstrated a normal increase in hepatic artery RI in healthy subjects shortly after a meal; this increase was not observed in patients with cirrhosis.

In advanced cirrhosis, HA form direct communications with the PV and contribute in the increase of PV

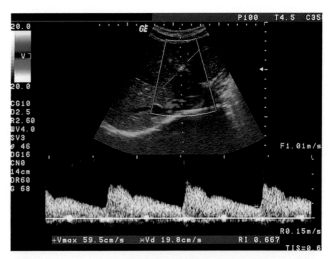

Figure 47-14. Normal hepatic artery. Normal low resistance Doppler waveform (RI-0.67) in the left hepatic artery.

pressure; this is also typical for Osler-Rendu-Weber disease (Fig. 47-15).[5] In those branches of the HA where direct shunting to lower-pressure portal or hepatic venous systems is present, the RI decreases dramatically; at the same time, RI values in other segments may be within normal limits.

Visceral vasodilatation is a classical hemodynamic feature in LC. It contributes to increased portal blood-flow to the diseased liver and maintains increased portal pressure.[37-39] Alvarez and colleagues in 1991 first reported that the superior mesenteric artery (SMA) pulsatility index was reduced in LC.[81] The SMA is indirectly responsible for at least half of portal vein inflow, and it plays an important role in visceral vasodilatation and portal hypertension.[82,83]

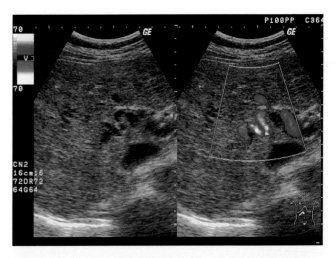

Figure 47-15. Rendu-Osler-Weber disease. Prominent tortuous right hepatic artery branch, with high velocity A-V flow to the hepatic veins. Note the high color Doppler scale (70 cm/sec), indicating high velocities characteristic for arteriovenous shunting.

Hepatic Veins in Portal Hypertension

Normal HV have a pulsatile multiphasic flow pattern comparable to IVC (see Fig. 47-4, *B*). Any changes in the IVC flow waveforms will change HV flow accordingly, provided that HV are patent (see Fig. 47-4, *C*). In LC, hepatic veins become narrowed and the contour of the walls is irregular because of external compression from regenerative cirrhotic nodules.[84,85] Pulsatility in the HV may become damped by the rigid fibrous liver parenchyma (see Fig. 47-4, *D*). Development of the direct shunting from the PV or HA also could change normal flow patterns in the HV (see Fig. 47-13, *B*). Occlusion of the hepatic veins or Budd-Chiari syndrome may occur in late stages of LC, with development of hepatocellular carcinoma (Fig. 47-16, *A* and *C*).[86,87]

Prehepatic Portal Hypertension

The main cause of prehepatic PH is thrombosis of the PV, splenic vein, and mesenteric veins. Extrinsic compression by nearby masses and congenital anomalies of the portal system are much less common.[7] The main causes of PV thrombosis in the adult population are considered to be malignancy caused by invasion, external compression of the venous structures, and LC.[88,89] Inflammatory conditions in the abdominal cavity predispose to portal vein thrombosis, which is more common in pediatric patients. Omphalitis, pylephlebitis after umbilical vein catheterization, appendicitis, typhlitis, sepsis, and dehydration could cause acute PV thrombosis in neonates.[90] It is relatively easy to identify by ultrasound because of proximity of the vasculature of the liver. Surgical manipulations in the abdominal cavity, trauma, and pancreatitis are other identifiable causes of PV thrombosis. The coagulation disorders are found in as high as 69% of cases of mesenteric thrombosis, and it appears to be that PV thrombosis is usually caused by multiple factors.[88,91] On the other hand, in patients with antiphospholipid antibody syndrome, mesenteric vein thrombosis was found in 5.1% of patients.[89] The clinical picture is usually determined by the location and extent of the thrombus, and it varies from symptom-free to acute life-threatening complications.

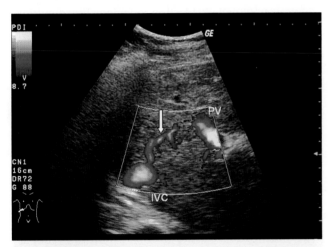

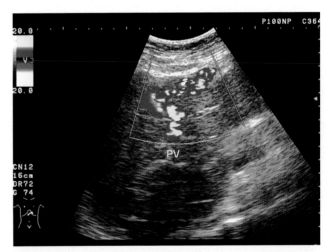

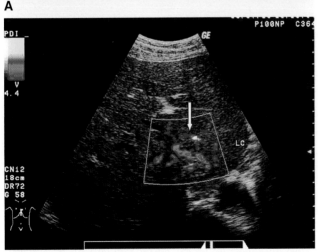

Figure 47-16. Budd-Chiari syndrome. *A*, Hepatic veins are impossible to visualize on B-mode. Small collateral vein (arrow) directly connecting the left portal vein and the inferior vena cava. *B*, Other prominent transhepatic collateral connecting the left portal vein with the diaphragmatic and superior epigastric veins. *C*, Multiple "spider" veins in the area of the caudate lobe of the liver (arrow).

The main characteristics of thrombosis are failure to identify flow in the PV or its branches by CDI (Fig. 47-17, *A*) or flow around the thrombus with focal color filling defects in the nonocclusive thrombosis are; these should be confirmed by PWD. Acute thrombosis of the portal vein and branches could be difficult to access on B-mode scan if the thrombus is hypoechoic. The investigator must be aware that in patients with acute or chronic liver disease, flow velocities in the intrahepatic PV could be very low or even undetectable (stagnant). This could be misinterpreted as PV thrombosis; therefore, the Doppler scale and wall filter settings should be as low as possible. In case of malignant thrombosis, intrathrombus flow can be detected (Fig. 47-17, *B*) and flow in unaffected PV areas may be well preserved. In chronic stage of thrombosis, the thrombus becomes more hyperechoic, retracts, and the so-called "cavernous transformation" of the PV may develop[53] (see Fig. 47-6, *A* through *C*). Multiple tubular serpiginous channels overtaking the place of the normal PV characterize cavernous transformation. Bloodflow is readily identified by CDI in those periportal collaterals and in the partially recanalized thrombus. Registering hepatopetal flow direction and velocities may be confusing because of tortuosity of the vessels. In some areas affected by thrombosis, partial or complete lysis of thrombus may be seen with patent lumen and markedly thickened hyperechoic walls of the PV.

Thrombosis of the PV can produce any of the PC described earlier. For the isolated SV thrombosis when the main PV is patent, the anterior gastric vein often serves as a main collateral, connecting splenic hilum with the distal PV; this is well visualized on transverse plane by CDI just below the abdominal wall.[92] Congestive splenomegaly is a common finding in SV thrombosis, but it may be absent when thrombosis is proximal, develops gradually, and good collateral outflow is present.[4-7]

Posthepatic Portal Hypertension

Increased blood pressure in IVC because of severe coronary heart disease, cardiomyopathy, constrictive pericarditis, or valvular heart disease will increase the pressures in the portal system. Any increase of the mean blood pressure in IVC above 10 mmHg should result in a mean PV blood pressure well above 10 mmHg, which is consistent with PH. Nevertheless, the hepatoportal pressure gradient remains normal as long as the liver is intact. The hepatic veins are dilated on B-mode scan, and the right HV exceeds 0.9 to 1.0 cm in diameter with abnormal waveform present.[7] PV Doppler waveform may be pulsatile with short flow reversal component (to and fro flow pattern) present during every cardiac cycle (see Fig. 47-8, *A* and *B*).

These patients may exhibit a clinical picure called Budd-Chiari syndrome; it is similar to IVC or major HV thrombosis. It is characterized by hepatomegaly, ascites, and right upper abdominal quadrant pain. The Budd-Chiari syndrome first described by Budd in 1849 was attributed to thrombosis of the HV. Later it became synonymous with any obstruction to venous blood outflow from the liver.[93]

The term *veno-oclusive disease* of the liver is usually reserved to the nonthrombotic occlusion of small branches of hepatic veins when the major HV remain patent and normal flow patterns are preserved. It is most commonly caused in the United States and Europe by chemotherapy and radiotherapy before bone marrow transplantation.[94]

Classic Budd-Chiari syndrome caused by hypercoagulable states is common in Western countries, whereas

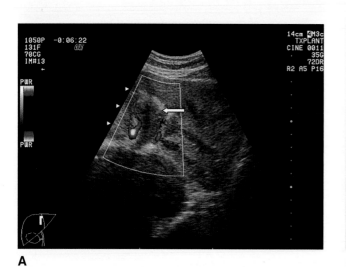

A

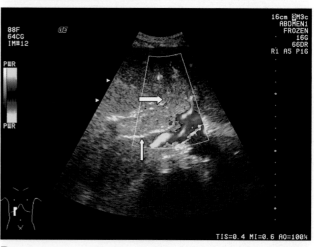

B

Figure 47-17. Acute portal vein thrombosis. **A,** Blank iso-hypo echoic thrombus in the left portal vein (arrow). **B,** Isoechoic thrombus in the left portal vein with internal flow (vertical arrow) characteristic for malignancy.

the majority of cases in the Far East and in South African blacks are caused by membranous obstruction and primary thrombosis of the IVC. Clinically, obstruction of the IVC is less severe than is thrombosis of the main hepatic veins until it involves hepatic veins.[93,95]

Budd-Chiari syndrome sonographically is characterized by thrombus in one or more hepatic veins. In chronic stage it is often difficult to see the thrombus in the HV. Failure to visualize HV and stenosis of the HV followed by prestenotic dilatation and thickening of the walls are the most common B-mode findings (see Fig. 47-16, A). When the thrombus is confined to one of the HV, clinical symptoms may be absent, and it could be just an incidental finding. When all three main HV are involved, the classic triad described by Chiari is seen. Doppler facilitates evaluation of the affected veins by demonstrating reversed flow, lack of pulsatility, and absence of flow in the presence of complete thrombosis.[86,87] The collateral pattern identified by CDI differs depending on the site and magnitude of the obstruction. When the thrombosis is inside the HV, intrahepatic collaterals to the PV branches and systemic veins around the confluence of the HV and enlarged caudate lobe "spider web" are seen (see Fig. 47-16, C). When primarily the IVC is involved, lumbar veins serve as collaterals bypassing the obstructed IVC. Portal bloodflow may be affected: Flow velocities are reduced, to and fro flow pattern is common, and PS described previously may develop. Hepatic artery resistance index is also increased because venous outflow is compromised.[7,84–87]

Role of Doppler US in Surgical Planning and Surveillance

US is widely used in the management of patients suffering from diseases of the hepatoportal system. It is a good tool for patient selection and surveillance after surgical procedures and drug treatment.[96,97] It has minimal discomfort, and lowers the cost compared with other imaging methods. The portal flow velocity, volume flow, and congestion index of the main PV are the most common measurements used to evaluate effectiveness of different drugs (e.g., beta blockers and nitrates) in lowering portal pressure and prevent GE bleeding.[96] However, there is no good correlation between those parameters and pressures in the PV system.[98] Evaluation of the SMA flow, to assess changes of the blood inflow that contribute to portal pressure elevation, is also helpful.[82,83] Doppler US can also be used to monitor the effects of the thrombolysis and anticoagulation of hepatoportal thrombosis.

Most often Doppler US is used for the planning and surveillance of surgical procedures (e.g., percutaneous and endovascular treatment of the hepatic tumors, resection of the liver, surgical portal systemic shunts, trans-

jugular intrahepatic portosystemic shunts, and liver transplantation). The preoperative Doppler evaluation is very important because it helps to choose the proper procedure, and it enables the operator to have a reference point to evaluate the effect of the treatment.[99] The main objectives to be achieved by ultrasound imaging before any surgical interventions on hepatoportal vasculature are:

- Anatomic characteristics and measurements of the portal vein, hepatic veins, and hepatic artery (in combination with CT and MRI)
- Patency (thrombosis, external compression) of those vascular structures; proximity and involvement with tumors, if any
- Flow patterns: phasicity in hepatic veins, direction and velocities in the portal vein, velocities and resistance index of the hepatic artery for comparison after interventions
- Presence, location, and size of PC

Surgical Portosystemic Shunts

Most common surgical portosystemic shunts to reduce PV pressure are small-bore H-graft interposition portocaval, side-to-side portocaval, mesocaval, and distal splenorenal shunts.[90] Mesoatrial shunts are used to control Budd-Chiari syndrome when it is causing PH. The major reason to use the Doppler ultrasound is to determine the patency of the shunt. Flow in the anastomosis or interposition prosthetic shunt is usually turbulent, and velocities vary in large extent depending on the bore diameter (Fig. 47-18). Currently there are no established velocity criteria for surgical shunt stenoses. Imaging of the region of anastomosis with CDI is usually possible in proximal surgically created shunts; failure by a skilled sonographer to visualize the functioning anastomosis is usually consistent with the shunt occlusion. Doppler US depicts changes in intra- and extrahepatic portal vein bloodflow. After the creation of the portosystemic shunt, flow directions in the intrahepatic PV branches and main PV depend on the location of the shunt (proximal or distal) and diameter of the anastomosis.[57,100] If the main goal of the operation is to reduce portal pressure to a maximum, as happens with the large diameter side-to-side portosystemic shunt, intrahepatic PV branches will exhibit full hepapatofugal flow, whereas preanastomotic PV tributaries will have vigorous hepatopetal flow. Hyperdynamic high velocity inflow from the dilated hepatic artery becomes prominent in the first week after surgery and compensates for the loss of portal flow (known as hepatic buffer response).[101]

A well-functioning distal splenorenal shunt causes hepatofugal flow in the splenic vein, shunting part of the portal inflow away from the liver to the left renal vein. Flow velocities in the main portal vein are reduced. When the anastomosis fails, flow direction in the splenic vein

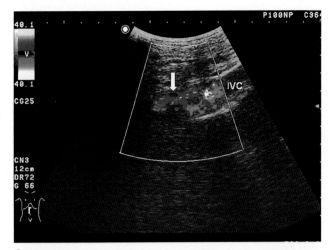

A

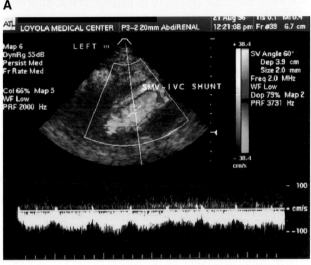

B

*Figure 47-18. Surgical mesocaval portosystemic shunt. **A**, Patent mesocaval shunt from the superior mesenteric vein (arrow) to the inferior vena cava. **B**, The pattern of flow velocity is very high and continuous; this picture is from a different patient.*

returns to hepatopetal. Small diameter side-to-side portal vein, mesocaval, and H-graft interposition shunts are created to preserve adequate liver perfusion by the PV. The expected reduction in portal pressures may prevent or reduce GE bleeding. Flow directions in the main PV and the intrahepatic PV branches are supposed to be hepatopetal.[100]

However, visualization of the anastomosis is much more complicated in distal splenorenal shunts; therefore, indirect characteristics related to flow in the PV tributaries should be used. Evaluation of the flow patterns shortly after surgery is useful for the follow-up.

TIPS

During the last 10 years there has been a dramatic decrease in open surgery–created shunts because of the advent of the transjugular intrahepatic portosystemic shunts (TIPS) procedure. During this procedure, the right portal vein usually is connected with the right or middle hepatic vein using a stent or a stent-graft.[102–104] Main indications for TIPS are to control the GE bleeding and refractory ascites. Most recently, TIPS has been shown to improve renal function in hepatorenal syndrome.[105] However, it appears that neither TIPS nor surgically created shunts improve survival of the patients.[106] Surgically created partial and selective shunts seem to be preferred over TIPS in patients with well-preserved liver function. The continuous surveillance after this procedure is especially important because shunt failure rates caused by stenosis and occlusion are reported to be 25% to 50% in 1 year.[103] Visualization of the TIPS is usually easy because the liver serves as a nice acoustic window. The material of the shunt itself may affect intraluminal flow visualization and flow measurements. Imaging modalities and protocols to assess patency of the TIPS are different from center to center. The most common Doppler parameters to diagnose hemodynamically significant TIPS stenosis are as follows:

1. Maximum shunt velocity below 50 to 60 cm/sec, or higher than 200 to 250 cm/sec[107–109]

2. Decrease of shunt velocity by 50 cm/sec and change of flow direction in portal vein branches in comparison with the examination performed just after the shunt placement[109,110]

3. Inability to obtain Doppler signal in the shunt is consistent with shunt occlusion[107,108,110,111] (Fig. 47-19)

Using these parameters, sensitivity and specificity approaches 100% in some references, and in most centers, exceeds 90%.[112,113] Another report has shown poor results

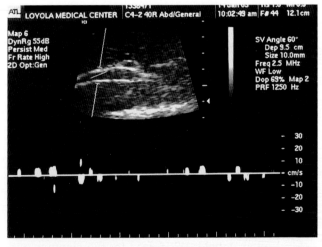

Figure 47-19. Thrombosis of a portosystemic shunt few months after its insertion. The shunt contains homogenous material and there is absence of Doppler signal. The patient subsequently underwent a successful liver transplantation.

(sensitivity 35%, specificity 83%), suggesting that Doppler ultrasound should be replaced by venography for the TIPS surveillance.[114]

Liver Transplantation

Since 1968, when Starzl performed first liver transplantation, this has become a widely used, common surgical procedure for treatment of end-stage liver diseases (and, occasionally, for hepatic malignancy).[115] About 5000 transplantations were performed in the United States in 2001, with a 5-year survival in selected centers approaching 90%.[116,117]

The most common technique is orthotropic liver transplantation of the whole cadaver liver. Because of a shortage of the liver donors, other techniques are being increasingly employed. These include split liver transplantation, in which one liver is divided to treat two patients; living donor left lobe (usually two and three segments) for pediatric patients; and right lobe living donor transplantation in adults. Living donor transplantation of the left hepatic lobe in adults is common in Asian countries where cadaver transplantation is problematic because of cultural and religious beliefs. Marginal liver and domino transplantations are performed as well to deal with extreme organ shortage.[117]

During orthotropic liver transplantation, the recipient's liver is removed and all three donor liver vascular systems and the bile duct are connected to the recipient, creating at least four vascular anastomoses. The hepatic portion of the IVC of the donor is connected to the recipient's, creating two end-to-end anastomoses: (1) proximal (suprahepatic or cranial); and (2) distal (infrahepatic or caudal). The recipient hepatic part of the IVC is removed with the diseased liver. If there is a large mismatch between the IVC diameters of the donor and recipient, a "piggyback" technique may be used in which the proximal part of the donor IVC is anastomosed end-to-side to the recipient's spared IVC, and the distal part of the donor's IVC is closed. When only the right hepatic lobe is transplanted, the right hepatic vein is connected end-to-end to the recipient's right hepatic vein or directly to the IVC. In the left lobe transplantation, left hepatic vein anastomosis is performed accordingly.

Donor portal vein typically is connected end-to-end to the recipient's PV. If this anastomosis is impossible because of congenital abnormalities, or because of thrombosis of the main PV, the anastomosis may be created to another patent portal tributary, usually the superior mesenteric vein. In transplantation of one lobe of the liver, the donor right or left portal vein is connected to the recipient's main portal vein.

The donor hepatic artery is usually mobilized in its maximum length (including celiac artery and small aortic patch) to connect it to the recipient's common hepatic artery. As mentioned previously, anatomic variations of the liver arteries are very common, hence additional anastomoses and interposition grafts may be employed in connecting donor and recipient arterial systems.

Biliary anastomosis is performed end-to-end on a T-tube catheter, which is left in place for a couple of weeks. When the bile duct length is insufficient, which happens when only one lobe of the liver is transplanted from a living donor, an anastomosis is performed to the Roux-en-Y jejunal loop. Bile ducts of the transplanted liver are supplied solely by the transplanted artery. Arterial collaterals are absent in early stages after transplantation, so the patency of the arterial system is crucial for the biliary system.[118,119]

Ultrasound evaluation before transplantation must follow the same common rules discussed above for any surgical intervention on the hepatoportal vasculature. The documentation of large PC collaterals is very important because if those are not ligated, portal perfusion of the transplanted liver may be compromised after transplantation. Ultrasound is helpful to exclude diffuse and focal liver diseases in living donors and for the follow-up after removal of one of the liver lobes.

Unfortunately, is not possible to plan a liver transplantation and rely solely on ultrasound imaging. The combination of different imaging modalities used in transplantation protocols varies from center to center. Plain angiography, CT, CT angiography, MRI, and MR angiography are usually employed to check vascular anatomy and obtain volumetric data.[118,119]

Post-transplantation Doppler ultrasound is primarily employed to evaluate the patency of the surgically created anastomoses between the donor liver and the recipient's vasculature. A detailed description of the operation performed, preferentially with schematic drawings, will make the examination much faster (easier) and more reliable. In the early postoperative period examination is commonly performed as a bedside procedure. Bandages and drain tubes make it difficult to get a good acoustic window for the vascular structures, so removal of some bandages is usually necessary.

The examination of the transplanted liver vasculature is best started from the portal system. Ultrasound examination is started from the B-mode imaging to evaluate changes in liver parenchyma (focal liver lesions) and perihepatic fluid collections. Any infrahepatic fluid collection in the porta hepatis area should be differentiated from possible portal vein and hepatic artery aneurysms using Doppler (CDI). Flow patterns in the main portal vein, intrahepatic branches, and extrahepatic tributaries are documented to exclude acute portal vein thrombosis. Flow velocities in the anastomosis area and proximal and distal portal vein should be recorded to serve as a reference for future examinations. Increased velocities and disturbed flow on CDI in the anastomotic area are a common finding, usually caused by the discrepancy of portal vein sizes in the donor and recipient, and by some angulations (kinking) of the anastomosed portal vein. Size discrepancies are especially common in pediatric patients with biliary atresia treated by the Kasai procedure.[120,121] Significant kinking demonstrated by CDI may occur if the length of the portal vein is excessive. There are no published criteria to classify portal vein stenosis. The authors think that an increase in blood velocities by up to two times is acceptable, whereas an increase of more than three times should be evaluated with angiographic imaging modalities.

The most common vascular complications are stenosis and occlusion of the hepatic artery, reported to be as high as 25% to 30% in living donor pediatric patients[116,118]; however, the introduction of microsurgery techniques has reduced the incidence to below 5%. In adult cadaveric liver transplantation it varies from 1.5% to 9%.[116-122]

Early occlusion results in loss of the transplant (and retransplantation) if revascularization procedures are not performed in time. Doppler US performed in asymptomatic post-transplant patients in the first days after transplantation could detect hepatic artery thrombosis and save the transplanted liver.[118,119,121] The examination of the hepatic artery should start from the documentation of its patency. Failure to visualize a transplanted artery in its usual course does not necessarily mean that the artery is occluded because the location could be significantly altered during surgery. Visualization of normal flow in the intrahepatic branches may suggest that the common HA is patent, and an attempt to trace it by CDI in retrograde fashion should be made. When the main artery is identified and confirmed to be patent, the region of the anastomosis should be interrogated with PWD to rule out stenosis. Velocities higher than 200 cm/sec are consistent with hemodynamically significant hepatic artery stenosis.[119] If there is history of multiple anastomoses, all those areas should be meticulously examined. During the first days after transplantation the arterial waveform is usually high resistance, probably because of postoperative liver edema. At the end of the first week, resistance gradually decreases to normal values (RI less than 0.7).[118] An increase in HA resistance in the late post-transplantation period may be caused by the rejection or by the recurrence of chronic liver disease. Those findings are unspecific, however, and diagnosis of the rejection should rely on liver biopsy.

When the area of anastomosis is impossible to visualize, and low resistance dampened poststenotic arterial waveform in intrahepatic branches is present, stenosis in the common hepatic artery must be suspected and angiography should be considered. Hepatofugal direction of the bloodflow in some intrahepatic arteries may be observed because the liver receives transcapsular collaterals from the diaphragmatic surface[57] in the presence of proximal HA occlusion.

A pseudoaneurysm of the hepatic artery is one of the possible rare arterial complications and should be differentiated from the subhepatic fluid collections by CDI. A-V

fistulas and arteriobiliary fistula have been reported via anecdotal data in post-transplant patients.[120,121]

Finally, hepatic veins and the IVC are examined for patency. Complications such as thrombosis of the hepatic veins and IVC or stenosis of the anastomosis are very rare.[122] The transplanted liver hepatic veins exhibit the same phasic flow characteristic as in the normal liver. Loss of the phasicity and development of the continuous monophasic flow distal to the interrogation point may be caused by IVC stenosis or obstruction. Such stenosis usually develops in the anastomotic area (Fig. 47-20). Intraoperative US is widely used in many medical centers to confirm patency of the arterial and venous anastomoses in the operating room. In living donors it is used to identify the plane of resection, anatomic variations of the hepatic veins, and hepatic artery and portal vein branching.[123]

Miscellaneous

Contrast Agents

Ultrasound contrast agents (USCA) are very small gas bubbles ranging from 1 to 10 µm in diameter. This size allows them to cross the pulmonary barrier and enter the arterial circulation when injected intravenously. They increase acoustic backscatter and Doppler signal from blood pool up to 30 dB and can be detected by B-mode imaging in large vessels and by Doppler in smaller vessels.

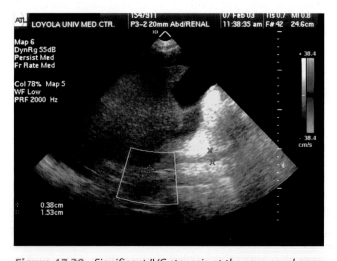

Figure 47-20. *Significant IVC stenosis at the cavo-caval anastomosis. The patient presented with abdominal pain and bilateral lower extremity swelling. The diameter of the IVC was reduced to 3.8 mm at the area of stenosis, and it was significantly smaller than the distal diameter at 15.3 mm. The diameter stenosis was estimated to be around 75%. The peak vein velocity before and after the stenosis was 191 cm/sec and 16 cm/sec, giving a post- to prestenotic velocity ratio of 12.*

Some of them, because of their nonlinear behavior, emit second harmonic frequencies. Others break, emitting high-intensity harmonic signals under the influence of high acoustic energy transmitted from ultrasound scanhead; these can be imaged by B-mode harmonic scanning, CDI, and power Doppler harmonic imaging.[12,124–126] Different chemical substances stabilize the microbubbles so they are in the bloodstream from seconds to an hour. USCA can be used to facilitate examination in several ways:

- Help to visualize patency of deep-lying hepatic vessels in technically difficult patients
- Improve detection of TIPS and surgical portosystemic shunt stenosis
- Enhance arterial and venous imaging in liver transplant
- Depict vascularization patterns and improve early detection and differentiation of hepatic neoplasms, especially those that are small and deep
- Evaluate perfusion parameters and opacification patterns because US contrast transit time in liver parenchyma and tumors is similar to that used in contrast-enhanced CT of the liver

Other USCA, which are still experimental and are not available for clinical practice, include tissue specific agents that are taken up selectively by the reticuloendothelial system (RES). These could be used to differentiate normal tissue of the liver and spleen from tumors lacking an RES. Another type that could be used to evaluate fresh thrombus in early stages is aerosomes with a ligand to activated platelets.[127–131]

USCA are currently under intense investigation for many clinical applications; however, their use for routine US examinations is under question because it significantly increases examination costs and time.

Doppler Characteristics of Benign and Malignant Liver Tumors

Liver masses are found as an incidental finding on any imaging modality, or when there is an examination to rule out malignancy in the presence of symptoms and risk factors (Table 47-3). The use of Doppler ultrasound in combination with other imaging modalities such as CT and MRI could facilitate the differentiation of tumors from other lesions by the presence or absence of flow and distinctive vascularisation patterns (e.g., size and number of identifiable vessels, type of vessels [arteries or veins], and central or peripheral branching). When vessels are present, the quantitative characteristics of flow velocities, resistance index in intratumor arteries, and velocity ratios of tumor to normal hepatic arteries may be used.[132] However, Doppler characteristics are influenced by many factors (e.g., size of the lesion, proximity to US transducer, quality of US equipment, and operator skills). It cannot replace biopsy for definite diagnosis.[126,133–136]

Currently, hepatocellular carcinoma (HCC) is the most common primary malignant hepatic tumor. Main risk factors in the United States and Europe are infection with hepatitis virus B and C and alcoholic liver cirrhosis, whereas the primary risk factor in Asia and Africa aree exposure to carcinogens. In its natural course, LC regenerative nodules progress into low-grade dysplastic nodules, then into high-grade dysplastic nodules, and eventually turn into HCC.[134,135] Ultrasound differentiation between these is often impossible, and even guided liver biopsy findings are not reliable.[137,138] HCC

TABLE 47-3. Most Common Focal Liver Lesions Identifiable by Ultrasound

Benign Tumors	Malignant Tumors	Focal Nontumorous Lesions
Cavernous and capillary hemangioma	HCC	Abscess
Simple biliary cyst	Cholangiocarcinoma Lymphoma	Echinococus
Biliary cystadenoma	Cystadenocarcinoma	Hematoma
Focal nodular hyperplasia (FNH)	Angiosarcoma	HA aneurysm
Hepatadenoma regenerative (dysplastic) cirrhotic nodules	Kaposi sarcoma	Infarction
Hamartoma	Metastases	Peliosis hepatis
Lipoma		Focal fatty infiltration (sparing)
Pediatric	**Pediatric**	**Connective tissue (ligament and**
Hemangioendothelioma	Hepatoblastoma	diaphragmatic) interpositions

HCC, hepatocellular carcinoma; HA, hepatic artery.

is a hypervascular tumor with a typical "basket" flow pattern (Fig. 47-21) identifiable in larger masses.[137] High velocity arterial flow is characteristic to HCC and has been described to be greater than 90 cm/sec.[138]

Doppler US is particularly useful in evaluating the involvement of neighboring vascular structures (e.g., extrinsic compression or invasion by the tumor). Doppler US was shown in studies to be equal to MRI in preoperative evaluation of the vascular involvement by the HCC.[123,139] Involvement of vascular structures is typical for HCC, and both portal and hepatic veins may be invaded. Malignant thrombus close to PV bifurcation, invading proximal hepatic veins and the IVC, makes liver resection impossible. If the thrombus is confined to one of the liver lobes, resection can still be performed.[115]

The most common benign liver tumor is cavernous hemangioma: It is a well-demarcated, homogenous, hyperechoic mass. Internal vessels usually are not seen in small tumors. Color flash or diffuse blush in the hemangiomas may be seen by power Doppler imaging or when USCA are employed, but they are not characteristic to the lesion.[132,133]

The liver is the second-most common site of metastasis (after regional lymph nodes) for many malignant tumors. Metastases from the different sites have different echo patterns and different vascularization. It is very difficult to differentiate primary malignant and benign liver tumors from the metastases.[136] Peak flow arterial velocities above 40 cm/sec were shown to be characteristic to malignant liver tumors.[132] The presence of internal flow is more characteristic to HCC than to metastatic tumors. Internal flow was shown to be present in 33% of liver metastases, compared with 75% of detectable intratumor flow in HCC.[138] In the presence of diffuse small-liver metastases, measurement of Doppler perfusion index may be of value.[22]

Liver Infarction

Because of its unique dual blood supply, infarction of the liver is rare when the normal ratio of arterial to portal bloodflow is preserved. When the arterial part of bloodflow becomes more important (e.g., in liver cirrhosis or transplanted liver), the occlusion of the hepatic artery or its branches results in liver infarction. It may be a wedge-shaped peripheral lesion or a rounded, centrally located mass, usually hypoechoic on B-mode. In immunocompromised patients, abscess formation may be observed in the infarcted area. It is difficult to differentiate hepatic infarction from the other focal liver lesions. When hepatic artery occlusion is present, and a new intrahepatic mass develops shortly after, liver infarction should be suspected.[120,121]

Aneurysms and Arteriovenous Fistulae

Aneurysms and pseudoaneurysms of the hepatic artery are second (after splenic) among the visceral aneurysms. Hepatic artery true aneurysms are usually extrahepatic and are located in the common hepatic artery; they may be congenital or caused by atherosclerosis, vasculitis, or infection.[31] Intrahepatic pseudoaneurysms are usually traumatic and caused by liver biopsy. Extrahepatic pseudoaneurysms are most common after liver transplantation.[121,140,141] A characteristic swirling flow pattern in the aneurysm sack is visualized by CDI and recorded by PWD (Fig. 47-22). The neck of the pseudoaneurysm may be identified with flow to and from the pseudoaneurysm sack.

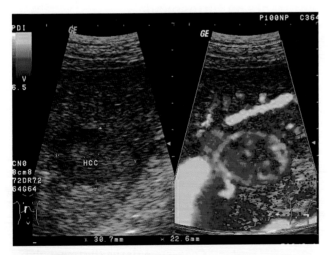

Figure 47-21. *Hepatocellular carcinoma. Solid isoechoic liver mass with hypoechoic halo on B-mode measuring 3 cm in diameter. On the right, split-screen power Doppler imaging depicts the characteristic hypervascular "basket" pattern.*

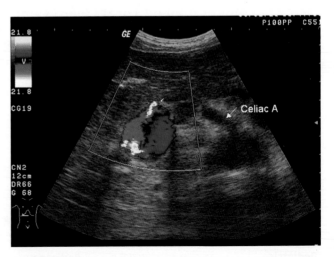

Figure 47-22. *Hepatic artery aneurysm. Extrahepatic sacular hepatic artery aneurysm (large arrow).*

An intrahepatic arteriovenous fistula between the PV and hepatic artery is usually caused by trauma and rupture of the hepatic artery pseudoaneurysm after liver biopsy or therapeutic intravascular interventions. Large arteriovenous fistulas may cause severe portal hypertension, rapid development of PC, and bleeding from GE varices.[140-142] High-intensity signal with intense aliasing is detected by CDI. Spectral Doppler shows high-velocity, very low-resistance, turbulent flow typical for A-V fistula. Small A-V connections between the hepatic artery and portal system, as well as between hepatic artery and hepatic veins, may form in advanced LC, Rendu-Osler-Weber disease (see Fig. 47-15), large HCC, and hemangiomas.[140]

Gas in the Portal System

Portal venous gas is characterized by small, hyperechoic, freely moving reflectors that sometimes produce reverberation artifact in the portal system. Inflammatory bowel diseases, abscesses, ileus, and abdominal trauma usually causes it.[31] The intrahepatic pattern closely resembles the one observed in aerobilia; therefore, visualization of the gas in extrahepatic PV helps to make the correct diagnosis.

REFERENCES

1. AIUM standard for the performance of an ultrasound examination of the abdomen or retroperitoneum. American Institute of Ultrasound in Medicine. J Ultrasound Med 21(10):1182–1187, 2002.
2. de Franchis R: Developing consensus in portal hypertension. J Hepatol 25(3):390–394, 1996.
3. de Franchis R: Updating consensus in portal hypertension: Report of the Baveno III Consensus Workshop on definitions, methodology, and therapeutic strategies in portal hypertension. J Hepatol 33(5):846–852, 2000.
4. Ralls PW: Color Doppler sonography of the hepatic artery and portal venous system. Am J Roentgenol 155:943–950, 1990.
5. Shapiro RS, Stancato-Pasik A, Glajchen N, et al: Color Doppler applications in hepatic imaging. Clin Imaging 22:272–279, 1998.
6. Rubin JM, Bude RO, Carson PL, et al: Power Doppler US: A potential useful alternative to mean frequency-based color Doppler US. Radiology 190:853–856, 1994.
7. Zwiebel WJ: Sonographic diagnosis of hepatic vascular disorders. Semin Ultrasound CT MRI 16:8–48, 1995.
8. Liu JB, Goldberg BB: Endoluminal Ultrasound. In Goldberg B, Pettersson H (eds): Ultrasonography. Oslo: The Nicer Institute ISIS Medical Media, 1996.
9. Liu JB, Miller LS, Feld RI, et al: Gastric and oesophageal varices: 20 Mhz transnasal endoluminal US. Radiology 187:363–366, 1993.
10. Caletti GC, Brocchi E, Baraldini M, et al: Assessment of portal hypertension by endoscopic ultrasonography. Gastrointest Endosc 36:21–27, 1990.
11. Bolondi L, Gaiani S, Zironi G, et al: Color Doppler endosonography in the study of portal hypertension. In Heyder N, Hahn EG, Goldberg BB (eds): Innovations in Abdominal Ultrasound. Heidelberg: Springer-Verlag, 1992.
12. Forsberg F, Goldberg BB: Contrasts Agents and 3-D Ultrasound. In Goldberg B, Pettersson H (eds): Ultrasonography. Oslo: The Nicer Institute ISIS Medical Media, 1996.
13. Patriqiun H, Lafortune M, Burns PN, et al: Duplex Doppler examination in portal hypertension: Technique and anatomy. Am J Roentgenol 149:71–76, 1987.
14. Giorgio A, Francica G, de Stefano G, et al: Sonographic recognition of intraparenchymal regenerating nodules using high-frequency transducers in patients with cirrhosis. J Ultrasound Med 10:355–359, 1991.
15. Awaya H, Mitchell DG, Kamishima T, et al: Cirrhosis: Modified caudate-right lobe ratio. Radiology 224(3):769–774, 2002.
16. Bolondi L, Gandolfi L, Arienti V, et al: Ultrasonography in the diagnosis of portal hypertension. Radiology 142:167–172, 1982.
17. Taylor KJW: Gastrointestinal Doppler Ultrasound. In Taylor KJW, Burns PN, Wells PNT (eds): Clinical Applications of Doppler Ultrasound. New York: Raven Press, 1988.
18. Tasu JP, Rocher L, Peletier G, et al: Hepatic venous pressure gradients measured by duplex ultrasound. Clin Radiol 57(8):746–752, 2002.
19. Sacerdoti D, Gaiani S, Buonamico P, et al: Interobserver and interequipment variability of hepatic, splenic, and renal arterial Doppler resistance indices in normal subjects and patients with cirrhosis. J Hepatol 27(6):986–992, 1997.
20. Moriyasu F, Nishida O, Ban N, et al: "Congestion index" of the portal vein. Am J Roentgenol 146(4):735–739, 1986.
21. Aoki H, Hasumi A, Hashizume M, et al: Hemodynamic analysis of findings in patients with portal hypertension: Multicenter analysis in Japan. Japan Portal Hypertension Study Group. Hepatogastroenterology 42(6):1030–1038, 1995.
22. Leen E, Angerson WJ, Wotherspoon H, et al: Detection of colorectal liver metastases: Comparison of laparotomy, CT, US, and Doppler perfusion index and evaluation of postoperative follow-up results. Radiology 195(1):113–116, 1995.
23. Wells PNT: Ultrasonic colour-flow imaging. Phys Med Biol 39:2113–2145, 1994.
24. Burns PN, Powers JE, Hope-Simpson D, et al: Power Doppler imaging combined with contrast-enhancing harmonic Doppler: A new method for small-vessel imaging. Radiology 193(p):366, 1994.
25. Cormack DH: Ham's Histology. Philadelphia: JB Lippincott, 1987.
26. Kelly DE, Wood RL, Enders AC: Bailey's Textbook of Microscopic Anatomy. Baltimore: Williams & Wilkins, 1984.
27. Schneck CD: Embryology, Histology, Gross Anatomy, and Normal Imaging Anatomy of the Liver. In Friedman AC, Dachman AH (eds): Radiology of the Liver, Biliary Tract, and Pancreas. St. Louis: Mosby, 1994.
28. Michels NA: Newer anatomy of the liver and its variant blood supply and collateral circulation. Am J Surg 112:337–347, 1966.
29. Gray SM, Skandalakis JE: Embryology for Surgeons. Philadelphia: WB Saunders, 1972.
30. Vine H, Sequeira J, Widrich W, et al: Portal vein aneurysm. Am J Radiol 132:557–560, 1979.
31. Gallego C, Velasco M, Marcuello P, et al: Congenital and acquired anomalies of the portal venous system. Radiographics 22(1):141–159, 2002.
32. Ohnishi K, Nakayama T, Saito M, et al: Aneurysm of the intrahepatic branch of the portal vein. Gastroenterology 86:169–173, 1984.
33. Kim EE, Romero J, Kim CG: Portal venous aneurysm demonstrated by magnetic resonance imaging. Clin Imaging 22:360–363, 1998.
34. Ohnishi K, Sato S, Pugliese D, et al: Changes of splanchnic circulation with progression of chronic liver disease studied by echo-Doppler flowmetry. Am J Gastroenterol 82:507–511, 1987.
35. Nakamura S, Tsuzuki T: Surgical anatomy of the hepatic veins and the inferior vena cava. Surg Gynecol Obstet 152:43–50, 1981.

36. Cassani F, Valentini P, Cataleta M, et al: Ultrasound-detected abdominal lymphadenopathy in chronic hepatitis C: High frequency and relationship with viremia. J Hepatol 26:479–483, 1997.

37. Bosch J, Groszman RJ: Portal Hypertension: Pathophysiology and Treatment. Oxford: Blackwell, 1994.

38. Bosch J, Garcia-Pagan JC, Feu F, et al: Portal Hypertension: Clinical Pathobiology. In Arias IM, Boyer JL, Fausto N, et al (eds): The Liver: Biology and Pathobiology. New York: Raven Press, 1994.

39. Groszman RJ, Atterbury CE: The pathophysiology of portal hypertension: A basis for classification. Semin Liver Dis 2:177–186, 1982.

40. Henriksen JH: Cirrhosis: Ascites and hepatorenal syndrome. Recent advances in pathogenesis. J Hepatol 23(Suppl)25–30, 1995.

41. Zimmerman HJ, Lewis JH, Kassianides: Cirrhosis. In Okuda K, Benhamou JP (eds): Portal Hypertension. Clinical and Physiological Aspects. Tokyo, Berlin, Heidelberg, New York, London, Paris, Hong Kong, Barcelona: Springer-Verlag, 1991.

42. Watanabe K, Kimura K, Matsusani S, et al: Portal hemodynamics in patients with gastric varices. A study in 230 patients with esophageal and/or gastric varices using portal vein catheterization. Gastroenterology 95:434–440, 1988.

43. Ahn J, Cooper JM, Silberzweig JE, et al: Venographic appearance of portosystemic collateral pathways. Brit J Radiol 70:1302–1306, 1997.

44. Okuda K, Takayasu K, Matsusani S: Angiography in portal hypertension. Gastroenterol Clin North Am 21:61–83, 1992.

45. Bolondi L, Piscaglia F, Siringo S, et al: Imaging Techniques and Haemodynamic Measurements in Portal Hypertension. In de Franchis R (ed): Portal Hypertension, 2nd ed. Blackwell Science, 1996.

46. Pieters PC, Miller WJ, DeMeo JH: Evaluation of the portal venous system: Complementary roles of invasive and noninvasive imaging strategies. Radiographics 17:879–895, 1997.

47. Rockey D: The cellular pathogenesis of portal hypertension: Stellate cell contractility, endothelin, and nitric oxide. Hepatology 25:2–5, 1997.

48. Lautt WW, Greenway CV, Legare DJ, et al: Localization of intrahepatic portal vascular resistance. Am J Physiol 251:375–381, 1986.

49. Zhang JX, Bauer M, Clemens MG: Vessel- and target cell-special actions of endothelin-1 and endothelin-3 in rat liver. Am J Physiol 269:269–277, 1995.

50. McCuskey RS: A dynamic and static study of hepatic arterioles and hepatic sphincters. Am J Anat 119:455–478, 1966.

51. Krowka MJ: Hepatopulmonary syndrome versus portopulmonary hypertension: Didtinctions and dilemmas. Hepatology 25:1282–1284, 1997.

52. Battista S, Bar F, Mengozzi G, et al: Hyperdynamic circulation in patients with cirrhosis: Direct measurement of nitric oxide levels in hepatic and portal veins. J Hepatol 26:75–80, 1997.

53. De Gaetano AM, Lafortune M, Patriquin H, et al: Cavernous transformation of the portal vein: Patterns of intrahepatic and splanchnic collateral circulation detected with Doppler sonography. Am J Roentgenol 165:1151–1155, 1995.

54. Gallix BP, Taourel P, Dauzat M, et al: Flow pulsatility in the portal venous system: A study of Doppler sonography in healthy adults. Am J Roentgenol 169(1):141–144, 1997.

55. Zoli M, Iervese T, Merkel C, et al: Prognostic significance of portal hemodynamics in patients with compensated cirrhosis. J Hepatol 17(1):56–61, 1993.

56. Zimmon DS: Pumping portal blood for therapy and knowledge. J Hepatol 25:106–108, 1996.

57. Wachsberg RH, Bahramipour P, Sofocleous CT, et al: Hepatofugal flow in the portal venous system: Pathophysiology, imaging findings, and diagnostic pitfalls. Radiographics 22(1):123–140, 2002.

58. Bernadich C, Fernandez M, Bandi J, et al: Mechanical pumping of portal blood to the liver: Hemodynamic effects of a new experimental treatment for portal hypertension. J Hepatol 25:98–15, 1996.

59. Tamosiunas AE, Speiciene D, Irnius A: Application of color Doppler ultrasound for diagnosis of liver cirrhosis gastroesophageal varices. Med Sci Monit 5(5):966–969, 1999.

60. Kimura K, Ohto M, Matsusani S, et al: Relative frequency of portal-systemic pathways trough the "posterior" gastric vein. Portographic study in 460 patients. Hepatology 12:725–728, 1990.

61. Okuda K, Matsutani S: Portal-systemic collaterals: Anatomy and Clinical Implications. In Okuda K, Benhamou JP (eds): Portal Hypertension. Clinical and Physiological Aspects. Tokyo, Berlin, Heidelberg, New York, London, Paris, Hong Kong, Barcelona, Springer-Verlag, 1991.

62. Hoevels J, Joelsson B: A comparative study of oesophageal varices by endoscopy and percutaneous transhepatic esophageal phlebography. Gastrointest Radiol 4:323–329, 1979.

63. Hashizume M, Sugimachi K: Classification of gastric lesions associated with portal hypertension. J Clin Gastroent Hepatol 10:339–343, 1995.

64. D'Amico G, Montalbano L, Pagliaro L, et al: Natural history of congestive gastropathy in cirrhosis. Gastroenterology 99:1558–1564, 1990.

65. Sie A, Johnson MB, Lee KP, et al: Color Doppler sonography in spontaneous splenorenal portosystemic shunts. J Ultrasound Med 10:167–169, 1991.

66. Hosking SW, Smart HL, Johnson AG, et al: Anorectal varices, hemorrhoids, and portal hypertension. Lancet 1:349–352, 1989.

67. Naveau S, Poznard T, Pauphilet C, et al: Rectal and colonic varices in cirrhosis (letter). Lancet 1:349–352, 1989.

68. Mostbeck GH, Wittrich GR, Horold G, et al: Hemodynamic significance of the paraumbilical vein in portal hypertension: Assessment with duplex US. Radiology 170:339–342, 1989.

69. Sugiura N, Karasawa E, Saotome N, et al: Portosystemic collateral shunts originating from the left portal veins in portal hypertension: Demonstration by color Doppler flow imaging. J Clin Ultrasound 20:427–432, 1992.

70. Gibson PR, Gibson RN, Ditchfield MR, et al: A comparison of duplex Doppler sonography of the ligamentum teres and portal vein with endoscopic demonstration of gastroesophageal varices in patients with chronic liver disease or portal hypertension, or both. J Ultrasound Med 11:327–331, 1991.

71. Lafortune M, Constantin A, Breton G, et al: The recanalized umbilical vein in portal hypertension: A myth. Am J Roentgenol 144:549–553, 1985.

72. Gibson RN, Gibson PR, Donlan JD, et al: Identification of a patent paraumbilical vein by using Doppler sonography: Importance in the diagnosis of portal hypertension. Am J Roentgenol 153:513–516, 1989.

73. Wachsberg RH, Obolevich AT: Bloodflow characteristics of vessels in the ligamentum teres fissure at color Doppler sonography: Findings in healthy volunteers and in patients with portal hypertension. Am J Roentgenol 164(6):1403–1405, 1995.

74. Chawla A, Dewan R, Sarin SK: The frequency and influence of gallbladder varices on gallbladder functions in patients with portal hypertension. Am J Gastroenterol 90:2010–2014, 1995.

75. Mori H, Hayashi K, Fukuda T, et al: Intrahepatic portosystemic venous shunt: Occurrence in patients with and without liver cirrhosis. Am J Roentgenol 149:711–714, 1987.

76. Popper H, Elias H, Petty DE: Vascular pattern of the cirrhotic liver. Am J Clin Pathol 22:717–729, 1952.

77. The North Italian Endoscopic Club for the Study and Treatment of Esophageal Varices: Prediction of the first variceal hemorrhage in patients with cirrhosis of the liver and esophageal varices: A prospective multicenter study. N Engl J Med 319:983–989, 1988.

78. Merkel C, Bolognesi M, Bellon S, et al: Prognostic usefulness of hepatic vein catheterisation in patients with cirrhosis and esophageal varices. Gastroenterology 102:973–979, 1991.

79. Nevens F, Fevery J: Measurement of variceal pressure and its clinical implications. Scand J Gastroenterol 29:6–10, 1994.

80. Lafortune M, Dauzat M, Pomier-Layrargues G, et al: Hepatic artery: Effect of a meal in healthy persons and transplant recipients. Radiology 187(2):391–394, 1993.

81. Alvarez D, Mastai R, Lennie A, et al: Noninvasive measurement of portal venous flow in patients with cirrhosis: Effects of physiological and pharmacological stimuli. Dig Dis Sci 36:82, 1991.

82. Taourel P, Perney P, Dauzat M, et al: Doppler study of fasting and postprandial resistance indices in the superior mesenteric artery in healthy subjects and patients with cirrhosis. J Clin Ultrasound 26:131–136, 1998.

83. Piscaglia F, Gaiani S, Gramantieri L, et al: Superior mesenteric artery impedance in chronic liver diseases: Relationship with disease severity and portal circulation. Am J Gastroenterol 93(10):1925–1930, 1998.

84. Menu Y, Alison D, Lorphelin JM, et al: Budd-Chiari syndrome: US evaluation. Radiology 157:761–764, 1985.

85. Bolondi L, Li Bassi S, Gaiani S, et al: Liver cirrhosis: Changes of Doppler wave-form of hepatic veins. Radiology 178:513–516, 1991.

86. Bellin MF, Challier E, Valla D, et al: Budd-Chiari syndrome: Value of duplex sonography and colour Doppler imaging for diagnosis and follow-up. Eur Radiol 5:379–386, 1995.

87. Millener P, Grant EG, Rose S, et al: Color Doppler imaging findings in patients with Budd-Chiari syndrome: Correlation with venographics findings. Am J Roentgenol 161:307–312, 1993.

88. Sobhonslidsuk A, Reddy KR: Portal vein thrombosis: A concise review. Am J Gastroenterol 97(3):535–541, 2002.

89. Kumar S, Sarr MG, Kamath PS: Mesenteric venous thrombosis. N Engl J Med 345(23):1683–1688, 2001.

90. Orloff MJ, Orloff MS, Girard B, et al: Bleeding esophagogastric varices from extrahepatic portal hypertension: 40 years' experience with portal-systemic shunt. J Am Coll Surg 194(6):717–728, 2002.

91. Fisher NC, Wilde JT, Roper J, et al: Deficiency of natural anticoagulant proteins C, S, and antithrombin in portal vein thrombosis: A secondary phenomenon? Gut 46(4):534–539, 2000.

92. Okuda K, Ohnishi K, Kimura K, et al: Incidence of portal vein thrombosis in liver cirrhosis: A angiographic study in 708 patients. Gastroenterol 89:279–286, 1985.

93. Okuda K: Inferior vena cava thrombosis at its hepatic portion (obliterative hepatocavopathy). Semin Liver Dis 22(1):15–26, 2002.

94. Shen-Gunther J, Walker JL, Johnson GA, et al: Hepatic venoocclusive disease as a complication of whole abdominopelvic irradiation and treatment with the transjugular intrahepatic portosystemic shunt: Case report and literature review. Gynecol Oncol 61(2):282–286, 1996.

95. Okuda K, Kage M, Shrestha SM: Proposal of a new nomenclature for Budd-Chiari syndrome: Hepatic vein thrombosis versus thrombosis of the inferior vena cava at its hepatic portion. Hepatology 28(5):1191–1198, 1998.

96. Piscaglia F, Gaiani S, Donati G, et al: Doppler evaluation of the effects of pharmacological treatment of portal hypertension. Ultrasound Med Biol 25(6):923–932, 1999.

97. Rice S, Lee KP, Johnson MB, et al: Portal venous system after portosystemic shunts or endoscopic sclerotherapy: Evaluation with Doppler sonography. Am J Roentgenol 156:85–89, 1991.

98. Merkel C, Sacerdoti D, Bolognesi M, et al: Doppler sonography and hepatic vein catheterization in portal hypertension: Assessment of agreement in evaluating severity and response to treatment. J Hepatol 28(4):622–630, 1998.

99. Marshall MM, Beese RC, Muiesan P, et al: Assessment of portal venous system patency in the liver transplant candidate: A prospective study comparing ultrasound, microbubble-enhanced, colour Doppler ultrasound with arteriography and surgery. Clin Radiol 57(5):377–383, 2002.

100. Zervos EE, Goode SE, Rosemurgy AS: Small-diameter H-graft portacaval shunt reduces portal flow yet maintains effective hepatic bloodflow. Am Surg 64(1):71–75; discussion 75–76, 1998.

101. Gulberg V, Haag K, Rossle M, et al: Hepatic arterial buffer response in patients with advanced cirrhosis. Hepatology 35(3):630–634, 2002.

102. Cejna M, Peck-Radosavljevic M, Thurnher SA, et al: Lammer creation of transjugular intrahepatic portosystemic shunts with stent-grafts: Initial experiences with a polytetrafluoroethylene-covered nitinol endoprosthesis. Radiology 221:437–446, 2001.

103. Haskal ZJ: Improved patency of transjugular intrahepatic portosystemic shunts in humans: Creation and revision with PTFE stent-grafts. Radiology 213:759–766, 1999.

104. Otal P, Smayra T, Bureau C, et al: Preliminary results of a new expanded-polytetrafluoroethylene-covered stent-graft for transjugular intrahepatic portosystemic shunt procedures. Am J Roentgenol 178(1):141–147, 2002.

105. Arroyo V, Guevara M, Gines P: Hepatorenal syndrome in cirrhosis: Pathogenesis and treatment. Gastroenterology 122(6):1658–1676, 2002.

106. Boyer TD: Is transjugular intrahepatic portosystemic shunt a panacea for the complications of portal hypertension? Hepatology 28(2):590–592, 1998.

107. Murphy TP, Beecham RP, Kim HM, et al: Long-term follow-up after TIPS: Use of Doppler velocity criteria for detecting elevation of the portosystemic gradient. JVIR 9:275–281, 1998.

108. Feldstein VA, Patel MD, LaBerge JM: Transjugular intrahepatic portosystemic shunt: Accuracy of Doppler US in determination of patency and detection of stenoses. Radiology 201:141–147, 1996.

109. Dodd GD III, Zajko AB, Orons PD, et al: Detection of transjugular intrahepatic portosystemic shunt dysfunction: Value of duplex Doppler sonography. Am J Roentgenol 164(5):1119–1124, 1995.

110. Lafortune M, Martinet JP, Denys A, et al: Short- and long-term hemodynamic effects of transjugular intrahepatic portosystemic shunts: A Doppler/manometric correlative study. Am J Roentgenol 164:997–1002, 1995.

111. Zizka J, Elias P, Krajina A, et al: Value of Doppler sonography in revealing transjugular intrahepatic portosystemic shunt malfunction: A 5-year experience in 216 patients. Am J Roentgenol 175(1):141–148, 2000.

112. Menzel J: Duplex ultrasonography of TIPS: How useful is it? Gastroenterology 116(5):1272–1273, 1999.

113. Foshager MC, Ferral H, Nazarian GK, et al: Duplex sonography after transjugular intrahepatic portosystemic shunts (TIPS): Normal hemodynamic findings and efficacy in predicting shunt patency and stenosis. Am J Roentgenol 165:1–7, 1995.

114. Owens CA, Bartolone C, Warner DL, et al: The inaccuracy of duplex ultrasonography in predicting patency of transjugular intrahepatic portosystemic shunts. Gastroenterology 114(5):975–980, 1998.

115. Choti MA: Surgical management of hepatocellular carcinoma: Resection and ablation. J Vasc Interv Radiol 13(9 Pt 2):S197–S203, 2002.

116. Samstein B, Emond J: Liver transplants from living related donors. Ann Rev Med 52:147–160, 2001.

117. Trotter JF, Wachs M, Everson GT, et al: Adult-to-adult transplantation of the right hepatic lobe from a living donor. N Engl J Med 346(14):1074–1082, 2002.

118. Garcia-Criado A, Gilabert R, Nicolau C, et al: Early detection of hepatic artery thrombosis after liver transplantation by Doppler ultrasonography: Prognostic implications. J Ultrasound Med 20(1):51–58, 2001.

119. Dodd GD III, Memel DS, Zajko AB, et al: Hepatic artery stenosis and thrombosis in transplant recipients: Doppler diagnosis with resistive index and systolic acceleration time. Radiology 192(3):657–661, 1994.

120. Langnas AN, Marujo W, Srtatta RJ, et al: Vascular complications after orthotopic liver transplantation. Am J Surg 161:76–83, 1991.

121. Nghiem HV: Imaging of hepatic transplantation. Radiol Clin North Am 36:429–443, 1998.

122. Hellinger A, Roll C, Stracke A, et al: Impact of colour Doppler sonography on detection of thrombosis of the hepatic artery and the portal vein after liver transplantation. Langenbecks Arch Chir 381(3):182–185, 1996.

123. Jarnagin WR, Bach AM, Winston CB, et al: What is the yield of intraoperative ultrasonography during partial hepatectomy for malignant disease? J Am Coll Surg 192(5):577–583, 2001.

124. Forsberg F, Goldberg BB, Liu JB, et al: Tissue-specific US contrast agent for evaluation of hepatic and splenic parenchyma. Radiology 210(1):125–132, 1999.

125. Shi WT, Forsberg F: Ultrasonic characterization of the non-linear properties of contrast microbubbles. Ultrasound Med Biol 26(1):93–104, 2000.

126. Wilson SR, Burns PN, Muradali D, et al: Harmonic hepatic US with microbubble contrast agent: Initial experience showing improved characterization of hemangioma, hepatocellular carcinoma, and metastasis. Radiology 215(1):153–161, 2000.

127. Strobel D, Krodel U, Martus P, et al: Clinical evaluation of contrast-enhanced color Doppler sonography in the differential diagnosis of liver tumors. J Clin Ultrasound 28(1):1–13, 2000.

128. Kono Y, Moriyasu F, Nada T, et al: Ultrasonographic arterial portography with second harmonic imaging: Evaluation of hepatic parenchymal enhancement with portal venous flow. J Ultrasound Med 18(6):395–402, 1999.

129. von Herbay A, Vogt C, Haussinger D: Pulse inversion sonography in the early phase of the sonographic contrast agent Levovist: Differentiation between benign and malignant focal liver lesions. J Ultrasound Med 21(11):1191–1200, 2002.

130. Bernatik T, Strobel D, Hahn EG, et al: Detection of liver metastases: Comparison of contrast-enhanced wide-band harmonic imaging with conventional ultrasonography. J Ultrasound Med 20(5):509–515, 2001.

131. Wilson SR, Burns PN: Liver mass evaluation with ultrasound: The impact of microbubble contrast agents and pulse inversion imaging. Semin Liver Dis 21(2):147–159, 2001.

132. Numata K, Tanaka K, Kiba T, et al: Use of hepatic tumor index on color Doppler sonography for differentiating large hepatic tumors. Am J Roentgenol 168:991–995, 1997.

133. Gaiani S, Volpe L, Piscaglia F, et al: Vascularity of liver tumours and recent advances in Doppler ultrasound. J Hepatol 34(3):474–482, 2001.

134. Okuda K: Hepatocellular carcinoma-history, current status, and perspectives. Dig Liver Dis 34(9):613–616, 2002.

135. El-Serag HB: Hepatocellular carcinoma and hepatitis C in the United States. Hepatology 36(5 Suppl 1):S74–S83, 2002.

136. Gaiani S, Casali A, Serra C, et al: Assessment of vascular patterns of small liver mass lesions: Value and limitation of the different Doppler ultrasound modalities. Am J Gastroenterol 95(12):3537–3546, 2000.

137. Tanaka S, Kitamura T, Fujita M, et al: Color Doppler flow imaging of liver tumors. Am J Roentgenol 154(3):509–514, 1990.

138. Nino-Murcia M, Ralls PW, Jeffrey RB Jr, et al: Color-flow Doppler characterization of focal hepatic lesions. Am J Roentgenol 159(6):1195–1197, 1992.

139. Hann LE, Schwartz LH, Panicek DM, et al: Tumor involvement in hepatic veins: Comparison of MR imaging and US for preoperative assessment. Radiology 206(3):651–656, 1998.

140. Bodner G, Peer S, Karner M, et al: Nontumorous vascular malformations in the liver: Color Doppler ultrasonographic findings. J Ultrasound Med 21(2):187–197, 2002.

141. Bolognesi M, Sacerdoti D, Bombonato G, et al: Arterioportal fistulas in patients with liver cirrhosis: Usefulness of color Doppler US for screening. Radiology 216(3):738–743, 2000.

142. Okuda K, Musha H, Nakajima Y, et al: Frequency of intra-hepatic arteriovenous fistula as a sequela to percutaneous needle puncture of the liver. Gastroenterology 74:1204–1207, 1978.

Chapter 48

Evaluation of the Extremity Before Hemodialysis Access and Postoperative Surveillance

JOAQUIM J. CERVEIRA • BRAJESH K. LAL • PETER J. PAPPAS

- ▰ Introduction
- ▰ Preoperative Evaluation
- ▰ Postoperative Evaluation
- ▰ Conclusions

Introduction

Vascular access procedures and their subsequent complications represent a major cause of morbidity, hospitalization, and cost for chronic hemodialysis patients.[1-3] According to the The National Kidney Foundation Dialysis Outcomes Quality Initiative (DOQI) Clinical Practice Guidelines for Vascular Access, the ideal dialysis access graft would prove durable, provide superior hemodialysis, demonstrate a low incidence of infection, and require few interventions to maintain patency. This document suggests that autogenous arteriovenous fistulae (AVFs) approximate the ideal access graft. As a result, its authors recommend that "primary AV fistulae should be constructed in at least 50% of all new kidney failure patients electing to receive hemodialysis as their initial form of renal replacement therapy. Ultimately, 40% of prevalent patients should have a native (arteriovenous) AV fistula."[4] Despite these national recommendations, only about 30% of patients beginning hemodialysis in the United States currently have an autogenous AVF as their primary dialysis access site.[5]

Multiple studies have demonstrated that autogenous AVFs demonstrate superior overall patency and lower revision rates when compared with prosthetic grafts.[6-8] Autogenous fistulae are less prone to recurrent stenoses, thrombosis, or infection.[9] However, some investigators have reported that if failure to mature is included in assessing autogenous fistulae patency, there are no differences in access rates and overall function when compared with prosthetic grafts.[10,11] Demographic factors that decrease fistula maturation include advanced age, female sex, African American race, diabetes mellitus, and obesity. All these factors are associated with small vessels with diminished bloodflow.[12]

Some 350,000 end-stage renal disease (ESRD) patients were receiving hemodialysis in the United States in 1999 according to the U.S. Renal Data System.[13] Presently, the incidence of new hemodialysis patients is increasing at an average rate of 6% per year, with concurrent increases in patient age and comorbidities. Currently, over 70% of patients beginning dialysis have three or more comorbid conditions.[14]

Preoperative Evaluation

It is clear from previous reports that fistula creation without some form of preoperative evaluation is associated with a high failure-to-mature rate and, subsequently, an inability to successfully access the fistula for hemodialysis.[11] Therefore, in order to increase the proportion of functional autogenous fistulae, the authors' group has proposed and evaluated the utility of preoperative noninvasive assessment of the upper extremity arterial and venous anatomy before dialysis access surgery.

Over the past 30 years, ultrasound has played an increasing role in the evaluation of vascular pathology. In the 1980s, mobile systems and higher-frequency transducers became available, allowing better imaging, with direct application for vascular access evaluation. By the 1990s, the ability to diagnose stenotic lesions and predict access failure was well reported.[15,16] With these improvements, as well as the favorable experience with lower extremity Doppler ultrasound (DU) vein mapping for distal revascularization, the authors began to utilize routine preoperative noninvasive imaging of the upper extremity to enhance the ability to identify suitable arteries and veins for hemodialysis access.

Since 1994, the authors' group at the University of Medicine and Dentistry of New Jersey–New Jersey Medical School (UMDNJ-NJMS) has utilized the noninvasive vascular laboratory to assess the arterial and venous anatomy of the upper extremity. Based on the anatomic criteria identified in the vascular laboratory, the optimal type of dialysis access as well as the anatomic site were determined for each individual patient. Utilizing this approach, the number of autogenous AVFs increased from 14% to 63%, whereas the number of prosthetic grafts placed decreased from 38% to 8.3%.[17] In addition, preoperative physical examination alone was found to be insufficient for identifying suitable veins for autogenous access in 54% of patients.

Since the publication of this initial experience, other investigators have reported a similar experience.[12,18-20] Allon and colleagues[12] reported a significant increase in the placement of autogenous AVF (from 34% to 64%) after preoperative vascular mapping was implemented. Although primary access failure was higher for fistulas than for prosthetic grafts (46% vs. 21%), the subsequent long-term failure rate was significantly higher for bridge grafts than for AVF. Likewise, Robbin and colleagues[20] reported an increase in autogenous fistula creation (from 32% to 58%) with preoperative ultrasound vascular mapping.

Patient Assessment

Evaluation of the patient's general medical condition includes a careful review of cardiovascular factors such as the presence of atherosclerotic risk factors (e.g., diabetes, hypertension, hyperlipidemia, coronary artery disease, and cigarette smoking) that may severely impact both inflow and outflow vessels.

A review of prior dialysis procedures is essential because it may reveal potential difficulties in establishing suitable access. Of particular concern is the central venous system because previous central venous catheters can lead to unrecognized outflow obstruction in up to 30% of patients.[21]

In addition, prior prosthetic graft placement does not preclude future AVF creation. A review of patients with failed prosthetic AV grafts referred to UMDNJ-NJMS from outside institutions indicated that over 40% of these patients were candidates for autogenous AVFs. Of these patients, 25% had suitable veins ipsilateral to the failed prosthetic AV graft.

Patient Examination

The examination of the patient undergoing evaluation for dialysis access should focus on the adequacy of the inflow artery and outflow vein. The inflow artery must be capable of providing adequate and reliable flow while not compromising distal perfusion to the hand. Brachial, radial, and ulnar pulses should be noted, and the Allen test, with a subsequent waveform analysis in the vascular laboratory, should be performed to confirm collateral patency of the palmar arch.

Adequacy of the venous outflow vein is also critical. Application of a tourniquet may enable veins to dilate and identify accessory veins that may impair AVF maturation. Evidence of central vein stenosis should also be sought. Specific signs of central vein stenosis (e.g., swollen arm, shoulder, or breast, or dilated collateral veins) are easily recognizable but are generally absent unless the stenosis is severe or acute.

Although the physical examination is a key component of preoperative access planning, it is often inadequate in obese patients and is limited in assessing deeper veins such as the basilic vein. In addition, physical examination is unlikely to identify areas of stenosis, postphlebitic vein wall fibrosis, or nonocclusive thrombosis of veins from previous venopuncture.

Noninvasive Vascular Imaging

The authors' protocol for the noninvasive imaging of the upper extremity includes DU visualization of the superficial and deep venous systems and a cursory arterial examination.

Ultrasound Technique

Vein mapping is performed with the patient supine and the arm dependent. The scan is initiated at the wrist of the nondominant arm with a tourniquet placed initially just above the wrist. In addition to using warm ultrasound gel, tapping and stroking maneuvers are used to facilitate venodilation. The veins are insonated with a 5-MHz or 7-MHz linear transducer. Veins are evaluated for any evidence of focal thrombotic, stenotic, or atretic segments. Veins are also assessed for diameter, compressibility, patency, and wall thickening. The tourniquet is sequentially moved up the arm to allow full visualization of the forearm and antecubital veins. Continuity of the venous system through the axillary and subclavian veins is also determined. Subclavian and jugular venous Doppler waveforms are analyzed for indirect evidence of central venous abnormalities. Indirect evidence of stenosis or occlusion includes diminished respiratory phasicity and diminished transmitted cardiac pulsatility. If one side is abnormal, the contralateral side is examined.

Following determination of venous anatomy acceptability, the radial, ulnar, and brachial arteries are quickly scanned with duplex ultrasonography. The scan is a cursory examination that allows for the identification of gross areas of stenosis or arterial variants such as high bifurcation of the brachial artery. Segmental arterial pressure measurements are no longer performed because of the low incidence of upper extremity inflow lesions and the prolonged time required for a complete arterial examination. Evaluation of the dominant arm is performed only when the nondominant arm evaluation is unacceptable.

Table 48-1 defines the authors' minimal anatomic requirements for construction of an autogenous fistula.

Postoperative Evaluation

According to the K/DOQI Work Group Guideline 10, "physical examination of an access graft should be performed weekly and should include, but not be limited to, inspection and palpation for pulse and thrill at the arterial, mid-, and venous sections of the graft."[4] In addition, regular access surveillance was recommended by a variety of techniques. These included, in order of decreasing preference, the following: monthly measurement of intra-access flow (measured by ultrasound dilution, conductance dilution, thermal dilution, or Doppler) or static venous dialysis pressure; monthly measurement of dynamic venous pressures; measurement of access recirculation by using urea concentrations or dilution techniques; and physical examination, evaluating

TABLE 48-1. Duplex Ultrasound Selection Criteria for Use of Upper Extremity Arteries and Veins for Dialysis Access Procedures

Venous Examination	
Venous luminal diameter	2.5 mm for AF
Venous luminal diameter	4.0 mm for BG
Absence of segmental stenoses or occluded segments	
Continuity with the deep venous system in the upper arm	
Absence of ipsilateral central venous stenosis or occlusion	

Arterial Examination	
Absence of pressure differential	20 mmHg between arms
Arterial lumen diameter	2.0 mm
Patent palmar arch	

AF, autogenous fistula; BG, bridging graft.
Reprinted with permission from Silva MB Jr, Hobson RW II, Pappas PJ, et al: A strategy for increasing use of autogenous hemodialysis access procedures: Impact of preoperative noninvasive evaluation. J Vasc Surg 27:302–308, 1998.

for persistent swelling of the arm, clotting of the graft, prolonged bleeding after needle withdrawal, or altered characteristics of pulse or thrill in a graft.

Duplex Ultrasound Surveillance

Diagnostic imaging is suggested to further evaluate any persistent abnormality. Duplex ultrasound of dialysis access is well suited to directly identify stenotic or occluded segments within the arterial inflow, conduit, and venous outflow.[22] The accuracy of DU for identification of access complications has been well established and confirmed by invasive imaging in multiple studies.[15,23-25]

Most studies have used direct measurement of diameter reduction by B-mode and color-flow imaging. Because of the turbulent, elevated flow rates through a high-volume arteriovenous fistula or graft, determination of threshold velocities corresponding to significant stenosis can be difficult to interpret. Tordoir and colleagues[15] measured frequency shifts obtained from Doppler and were able to define threshold values for angiographic diameter-reducing stenosis. Likewise, Older and colleagues[25] also developed Doppler criteria showing that 83% of greater than 50% diameter reducing lesions were detected with peak systolic velocities greater than 400 cm/sec or a peak systolic velocity ratio greater than 3.

Despite possessing an acceptable accuracy for detection of access stenosis, DU remains unproven for predicting thrombotic failure. Several investigators have reported that high-grade stenoses identified by DU in bridge grafts were associated with significantly decreased patency rates at 6 months.[16,26] However, Lumsden and colleagues questioned the efficacy of performing prophylactic angioplasty on all patients with DU-detected significant stenosis within prosthetic bridging grafts.[27] Patients with 50% stenosis or greater were randomized to elective angioplasty or clinical follow-up. Lifetable analysis showed no difference in outcomes, suggesting that the presence of an access stenosis may not necessarily predispose to conduit failure.

Conclusions

The K/DOQI Clinical Practice Guidelines have provided a standard that all those involved with dialysis access must attempt to reach. In order to reach these goals, careful preoperative evaluation and planning is required. Early referral for access placement, careful physical examination, and a meticulous preoperative duplex are important tools for meeting these guidelines. Further access management can subsequently be based on duplex ultrasound, allowing for a noninvasive, mobile, and relatively convenient method of clinical evaluation.

REFERENCES

1. Feldman HI, Kobrin S, Wasserstein A: Hemodialysis vascular access morbidity. J Am Soc Nephrol 7:523–535, 1996.
2. Fan PY, Schwab SJ: Vascular access concepts for the 1990s. J Am Soc Nephrol 3:1–11, 1992.
3. Hakim R, Himmelfarb J: Hemodialysis access failure: A call to action. Kidney Int 54:1029–1040, 1998.
4. National Kidney Foundation: K/DOQI clinical practice guidelines for vascular access (2000). Am J Kidney Dis 37(Suppl 1):S137–S181, 2001.
5. Tokars JI, Frank M, Alter MJ, et al: National surveillance of dialysis-associated disease in the United States, 2000. Semin Dial 15:162–171, 2002.
6. Matsuura JH, Rosenthal D, Clark M, et al: Transposed basilic vein versus polytetrafluoroethylene for brachial-axillary arteriovenous fistulas. Am J Surg 176:219–221, 1998.
7. Coburn MC, Carney WI Jr: Comparison of basilic vein and polytetrafluoroethylene for brachial arteriovenous fistula. J Vasc Surg 20:896–904, 1994.
8. Gibson KD, Gillen DL, Caps MT, et al: Vascular access survival and incidence of revisions: A comparison of prosthetic grafts, simple autogenous fistulas, and venous transposition fistulas from the U.S. Renal Data System Dialysis Morbidity and Mortality Study. J Vasc Surg 34:694–700, 2001.
9. Churchill DN, Taylor DW, Cook RJ, et al: Canadian hemodialysis morbidity study. Am J Kidney Dis 19:214–234, 1992.
10. Palder SB, Kirkman RL, Whittemore AD, et al: Vascular access for hemodialysis. Patency rates and results of revision. Ann Surg 202:235–239, 1985.
11. Miller PE, Tolwani A, Luscy CP, et al: Predictors of adequacy of arteriovenous fistulas in hemodialysis patients. Kidney Int 56:275–280, 1999.
12. Allon M, Lockhart ME, Lilly RZ, et al: Effect of preoperative sonographic mapping on vascular access outcomes in hemodialysis patients. Kidney Int 60:2013–2020, 2001.
13. Xue JL, MA JZ, Louis TA, et al: Forecast of the number of patients with end-stage renal disease in the United States to the year 2010. J Am Soc Nephr 12:2753–2758, 2001.
14. U.S. Renal Data System: USRDS 2002 Annual Data Report: Atlas of End-Stage Renal Disease in the United States. Bethesda, MD: National Institutes of Health, National Institute of Diabetes and Digestive and Kidney Diseases, 2002.
15. Tordoir JHM, de Bruin H, Hoeneveld H, et al: Duplex ultrasound scanning in the assessment of arteriovenous fistulas for hemodialysis access: Comparison with digital subtraction angiography. J Vasc Surg 10:122–128, 1989.
16. Strauch BS, O'Connell RS, Geoly KL: Forecasting thrombosis of vascular access with Doppler color-flow imaging. Am J Kidney Dis 19:554–557, 1992.
17. Silva MB Jr, Hobson RW II, Pappas PJ, et al: A strategy for increasing use of autogenous hemodialysis access procedures: Impact of preoperative noninvasive evaluation. J Vasc Surg 27:302–308, 1998.
18. Ascher E, Gade P, Hingorani A, et al: Changes in the practice of angioaccess surgery: Impact of dialysis outcome and quality initiative recommendations. J Vasc Surg 31:84–92, 2000.
19. Gibson KD, Caps MT, Kohler TR, et al: Assessment of a policy to reduce placement of prosthetic hemodialysis access. Kidney Int 59:2335–2345, 2001.
20. Robbin ML, Gallichio MH, Deierhoi MH, et al: US vascular mapping before hemodialysis access placement. Radiology 217:83–88, 2000.
21. Lumsden AB, MacDonald MJ, Isiklar H, et al: Central venous stenosis in the hemodialysis patient: Incidence and efficacy of endovascular treatment. Cardiovasc Surg 5:504–509, 1997.
22. Shackleton CR, Taylor DC, Buckley AR, et al: Predicting failure in polytetrafluoroethylene vascular access grafts for hemodialysis: A pilot study. Can J Surg 30:442–444, 1987.
23. Gadallah MF, Paulson WD, Vickers B, et al: Accuracy of Doppler ultrasound in diagnosing anatomic stenosis of hemodialysis arteriovenous access as compared with fistulography. Am J Kidney Dis 32:273–277, 1998.
24. Dousset V, Grenier N, Douws C, et al: Hemodialysis grafts: Color Doppler flow imaging correlated with digital subtraction angiography and functional status. Radiology 181:89–94, 1991.
25. Older RA, Gizienski TA, Wilkowski MJ, et al: Hemodialysis access stenosis: Early detection with color Doppler ultrasound. Radiology 207:161–164, 1998.
26. Sands J, Young S, Miranda C: The effect of Doppler screening studies and elective revisions on dialysis access failure. ASAIO J 38:M524–M527, 1992.
27. Lumsden A, MacDonald J, Kikeri D, et al: Prophylactic balloon angioplasty fails to prolong the patency of expanded polytetrafluoroethylene arteriovenous grafts: Results of a prospective randomized trial. J Vasc Surg 26:382–392, 1997.

Chapter 49

Thoracic Outlet Syndrome

PAUL B. KREIENBERG • DHIRAJ M. SHAH • R. CLEMENT DARLING III • BENJAMIN B. CHANG • PHILIP S.K. PATY • SEAN P. RODDY • KATHLEEN J. OZSVATH • MANISH MEHTA

- Neurogenic
- Arterial
- Venous

Thoracic outlet syndrome (TOS) encompasses a group of disorders of the upper extremity caused by compression of one of the structures in the thoracic outlet. Compression may impinge upon the brachial plexus, the subclavian artery, or the subclavian vein. Thus there are three types of thoracic outlet syndromes: neurogenic, arterial, and venous. The neurogenic type of thoracic outlet syndrome consists mainly of pain; paresthesia; and, often, weakness of the upper extremity and hand usually aggravated when the hands are used over the head. This type of thoracic outlet syndrome accounts for 90% to 95% of all patients. The arterial variant of thoracic outlet syndrome is rare and accounts for less than 5% of the cases. Bony compression of the artery results in poststenotic dilatation and aneurysm formation. These patients will generally present with thromboembolic complications related to the change in arterial structure. The venous variant also results from bony compression of the subclavian vein. Chronic repetitive trauma to the vein produces its eventual thrombosis. Each of these entities is considered briefly in this chapter.

Neurogenic Thoracic Outlet Syndrome

Mechanical compression of the brachial plexus is the principal cause of the symptoms that make up this entity. A variety of anatomic problems may produce compression of the brachial plexus. These include cervical ribs,[1] first rib, anterior scalene muscles, congenital myofascial bands and ligaments, and scar related to previous trauma (Table 49-1).

Compression of the nerve roots by these structures produces symptoms of the neurogenic thoracic outlet syndrome. These include shoulder girdle and arm pain associated with numbness and paresthesias in the ulnar distribution of the forearm and hand. If longstanding, these patients may also have wasting in thenar eminence of the hand. Thankfully, most patients do not present with extensive symptoms such as muscle wasting. The more common presentation is that of pain in the shoulder girdle and radiating down the arm. It is often worsened when patients work with their arms overhead.

Several other disorders may also have symptoms similar to these and thus should be kept in mind (Table 49-2). These include nerve compression disorders (e.g., carpal tunnel syndrome or ulnar nerve entrapment), cervical spine problems (e.g., disk herniation or spondylolysis producing radicular symptoms), and primary musculoskeletal disorders (e.g., rotator cuff tears, tendinitis, or myositis). Because these entities may produce symptoms

TABLE 49-1. Anatomic Structures That May Compress Nerves in the Thoracic Outlet

Bony	Soft Tissue
Cervical rib	Anomalous anterior scalene insertion
Long C7 transverse process	Anomalous middle scalene insertion
Abnormal first rib	Scalene muscle interdigitations
	Scalene muscle hypertrophy
	Scalenus minimus
	Abnormal ligaments or fibrous bands

very similar to the neurogenic thoracic outlet syndrome, they need to be excluded by careful physical examination and appropriate ancillary tests.

Diagnosis

The diagnosis of neurogenic thoracic outlet syndrome in patients without identifiable anatomic abnormalities is based upon the history and physical examination. The history should include whether the symptoms followed a specific trauma such as an auto accident or accident at work. Up to 70% of patients will have a history of trauma or work-related injury. Inquiry should be made as to the impact of the symptoms on the activities of daily living. Actions such as carrying objects, wearing or carrying items with shoulder straps, shampooing hair, or driving a car often cannot be done using the affected extremity. It is important to obtain information on what therapy has been tried and for what duration because often these patients are seen after their initial trial of conservative management. Often, patients are sent for strengthening exercises rather than stretching, and this may aggravate the situation. These patients are then deemed nonresponders to conservative therapy.

TABLE 49-2. Disorders Producing Symptoms Similar to Neurogenic Thoracic Outlet Syndrome

Carpal tunnel syndrome	Shoulder disorders
Ulnar nerve compression	Tendinitis
Cervical disk disease	Rotator cuff tears
Cervical spondylolysis	Myositis
Reflex sympathetic dystrophy	Biceps tendinitis
Raynaud's disease	Deltoid bursitis

A thorough physical examination is a necessity in arriving at a correct diagnosis. The patient's posture and the presence of any deformities should be noted. The neck and shoulder girdle should be examined for pain or spasm in the trapezius muscle or in the paraspinal region of the neck. The hand and fingers are examined, and grip strength is assessed. Individual tests for carpal tunnel syndrome (e.g., the Phalen test) are performed. Tenderness of the ulnar nerve at the elbow may indicate ulnar nerve entrapment.

Characteristic findings of thoracic outlet include supraclavicular tenderness. This can be elicited by palpating directly over the anterior scalene muscle or more posteriorly over the brachial plexus. A positive response reproduces the symptoms of pain and paresthesias radiating from the neck down the arm. The elevated arm stress test is a useful maneuver to try and elicit the symptoms of thoracic outlet compression. The patient is instructed to place both arms in 90 degrees of abduction and external rotation, with the shoulders braced posteriorly. The patient is then instructed to open and close the hands for three minutes. Test results are considered positive if the symptoms are reproduced. Most patients with neurogenic thoracic outlet syndrome will not be able to complete this test.

The diagnosis of thoracic outlet syndrome is usually made on clinical grounds based upon the history and physical examination. However, several ancillary tests may be useful to exclude other potential diagnoses that may produce similar symptoms.

A variety of diagnostic tests have been advocated for evaluation of the patients with presumed neurogenic thoracic outlet syndrome. Unfortunately, none of these tests is specific for thoracic outlet nerve compression. Diagnostic tests in this setting serve as ways to exclude other pathologies that may be producing the symptoms. Plain x-ray studies of the chest and cervical spine should be obtained. These will provide evidence of cervical ribs; abnormal transverse processes; and, perhaps, old bony trauma. Evidence of arthritic conditions of the spine should be noted, as should signs of degenerative disk disease of the spine. In patients with radicular symptoms wherein disk herniation may be suspected, magnetic resonance imaging (MRI) may be helpful. Newer MRI techniques employing brachial plexus coils allow determination of the site of compression and of which patients would benefit from rib resection or neurolysis.[2] Electrophysiologic studies (e.g., ulnar nerve conduction or electromyography) may be helpful in excluding other conditions, but no standard exists and there is a wide range of normal values. In practice, the authors have not found these tests to be useful in arriving at the diagnosis; many patients are referred having already had these tests performed. Sensory-evoked potentials have been proposed as a way to determine which patients may benefit from nerve decompression, but results have been disappointing.[3]

Once the diagnosis has been reached, the initial course of treatment for neurogenic thoracic outlet should be conservative and nonoperative. Initial treatment should include analgesics; anti-inflammatory medications; and muscle relaxants, if muscle spasm is present. Physical therapy should consist of heat application and ultrasound therapy. Patients should avoid postures or activities that aggravate their symptoms. Strengthening exercises should be limited to those involving the shoulder girdle to improve posture and open the thoracic outlet. Trigger point injections or scalene blocks may grant temporary relief and break the pain cycle the patients may be in while conservative measures start to provide relief. In patients with relatively new onset of symptoms, a trial of 3 to 6 months is warranted before embarking on surgical therapy.

Operative Approach

The goal of surgical therapy for neurogenic thoracic outlet is to remove the point of compression on the brachial plexus. Several treatments are purported to achieve this end, including some combination of scalenotomy, scalenectomy, first rib resection, and neurolysis. Practically speaking, the treatment depends on the operative findings, and the surgery is therefore an exploration. Treatment depends on the structure compressing the nerves. The authors elect to use the supraclavicular approach because it provides the versatility needed to perform all these procedures for thoracic outlet decompression.

To perform supraclavicular thoracic outlet decompression, the patient is placed supine on the operating room table with the neck extended and the head turned away from the operative site. A curvilinear incision is made at the base of the neck 1 cm above the clavicle. The platysma is divided, and superior and inferior flaps are created. The external jugular vein is divided and the scalene fat pad mobilized from the jugular vein and clavicle laterally. The omohyoid muscle is resected. Mobilization of these structures reveals the underlying anterior scalene muscle. The phrenic nerve should be identified and protected because it runs on the anterior scalene from lateral to medial. The scalene muscle is then divided at its attachment to the first rib, using care to protect the underlying artery. The anterior scalene muscle is then removed by continuing the dissection superiorly. The underlying brachial plexus will be observed, as will its interdigitations with muscle. Any muscle fibers that interdigitate with the middle scalene and the trunks of the plexus are also divided. The dissection proceeds superiorly until the anterior scalene is disconnected at its insertion on the transverse process. Neurolysis is then performed by removing all muscle fibers and connective tissue within the nerve trunk sheaths. Using a periosteal elevator, the anterior surface of the first rib is cleared, and using a rongeur, the rib is divided and removed anteriorly as far medial as the costochondral junction. Posteriorly, the rib is removed until the plexus is clear. In the authors' experience, rib removal is optional as long as inspection at the time of surgery reveals that it does not cause the actual compression. The wound is closed over an active drain, and a compressive bandage is placed over the wound.

Arterial Thoracic Outlet Syndrome

Arterial thoracic outlet develops because of repetitive extrinsic compression of the subclavian artery. With this compression the artery often develops poststenotic dilatation or frank aneurysms. The typical pathogenesis then is focal compression, dilation, ulceration, and thrombus formation. Therefore most of these patients will present with thromboembolic symptoms. The majority of patients will present with ischemic complications secondary to repeated episodes of embolization.[4]

Physical examination of these patients should include a thorough vascular and neurologic examination. Pulse volume recordings with digital assessment is beneficial to determine the extent of embolization. Cervical spine films and plain chest x-ray should be obtained to evaluate for the presence of a cervical rib or long C7 process. Arteriography should be undertaken to include the arch and the runoff to the hand to evaluate the digital vessels.

Most patients presenting with symptomatic arterial compromise will require first rib resection or resection of cervical rib and abnormal fibrous bands, if encountered. The abnormal segment of the artery can then be replaced with a prosthetic graft. Often, patients with digital symptoms may benefit from concomitant cervical sympathectomy.

Venous Thoracic Outlet Syndrome

Effort thrombosis of the subclavian vein is a general condition sometimes referred to as Paget-Schroetter syndrome. The syndrome is produced by repetitive trauma of the subclavian vein in the thoracic outlet. In this area the subclavian tendon and costocoracoid ligament follow the course of the clavicle, extending laterally from their origin at the claviculosternal and first chondral junction. During abduction of the arm these structures compress the vein against the first rib and scalenus anticus muscle. Patients with primary subclavian vein thrombosis are characteristically healthy, young, active individuals. Typically, they are male, usually in their 30s, with the dominant extremity involved. Most patients present with an antecedent history of unusual upper extremity positioning before the development of symptoms.[5] There is a wide range of severity and disability that can be produced by this thrombotic process. In general, the degree of disability is related to the length of the thrombosed segment and the subsequent activity level of the involved extremity. In many reports, only a small minority of patients will have little or no discomfort and swelling. This may reflect the fact that some patients undergo spontaneous recanalization or may include patients who have little continued active use of the extremity. Close to 50% of these patients are considered to have disabling symptoms that limit occupational or recreational activities.

Virchow's triad of stasis, intimal damage, and hypercoagulability readily explains the pathophysiology of this syndrome. Intimal damage can be produced by the chronic irritation of the vein by surrounding structures at the thoracic outlet. Thus treatment algorithms for this problem should include early restoration of vein patency, decompression of the thoracic outlet to correct repetitive trauma to the vein, and treatment to restore the vein to normal caliber.

Current accepted practice is to give patients identified with this syndrome thrombolytic therapy for initial dissolution of the thrombus.[6,7] When venous patency is restored and positional venography demonstrates extrinsic compression of the vein, operative decompression of the thoracic outlet should be performed as described

earlier. However, patients who undergo this decompression should also have venolysis performed to remove any chronic scarring that may be present around the vein.

Beyond thrombolysis and thoracic outlet decompression is the decision on how to mange the residual vein stenosis. Several methods for correcting intrinsic stenosis exist, including venolysis, patch angioplasty, bypass of the stenotic segment, and percutaneous transluminal angioplasty (PTA) with or without stent placement.[8] At the authors' institution the preference is for a catheter-based approach so that after lytic therapy and thoracic outlet decompression, patients with residual stenosis are treated with angioplasty and intraluminal stenting, when persistent stenosis exists.[9]

After initial diagnosis by history, physical examination, and duplex ultrasound, patients undergo venography and lytic therapy (Fig. 49-1). Venography is repeated every 6 hours until no further dissolution is seen (usually less than 24 hours). Following dissolution, patients are maintained on heparin and undergo thoracic outlet decompression. Patients who the have residual stenosis after thoracic outlet decompression undergo angioplasty (Fig. 49-2). If persistent stenosis is present after PTA, patients have stents placed and completion venography performed (Figs. 49-3 and 49-4).

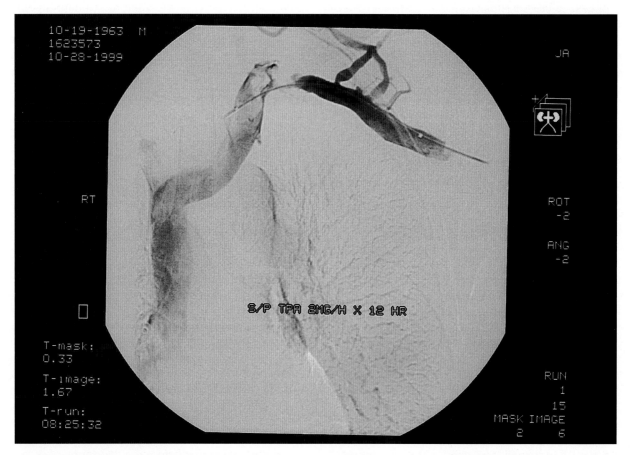

Figure 49-1. Subclavian venogram after 12 hours of thrombolytic treatment. Significant stenosis present in the patent subclavian vein. (From Kreienberg PB, Chang BB, Darling RC III, et al: Thrombolytic and surgical decompression or stent therapy for subclavian vein thrombosis. In Pearce WH, Yao JST [eds]: Advances in Surgery. New York: McGraw-Hill, 2002.)

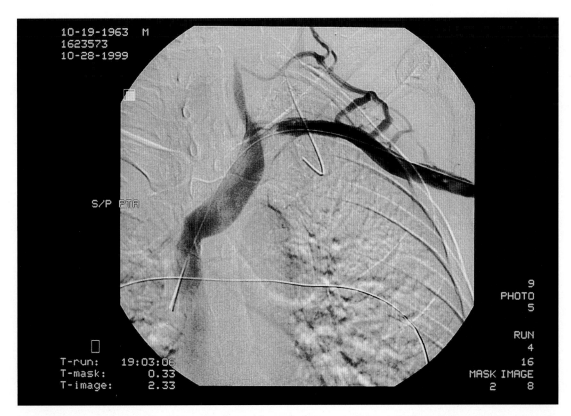

Figure 49-2. *Patient in Figure 49-1 after angioplasty of residual stenosis (10-mm balloon inflated to 10 atmospheres). Note persistent stenosis. (From Kreienberg PB, Chang BB, Darling RC III, et al: Thrombolytic and surgical decompression or stent therapy for subclavian vein thrombosis. In Pearce WH, Yao JST [eds]: Advances in Surgery. New York: McGraw-Hill, 2002.)*

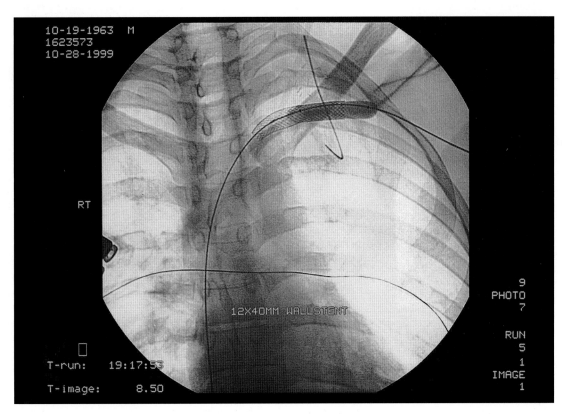

Figure 49-3. *Placement of 12 × 40 Wallstent for residual stenosis after angioplasty. (From Kreienberg PB, Chang BB, Darling RC III, et al: Thrombolytic and surgical decompression or stent therapy for subclavian vein thrombosis. In Pearce WH, Yao JST [eds]: Advances in Surgery. New York: McGraw-Hill, 2002.)*

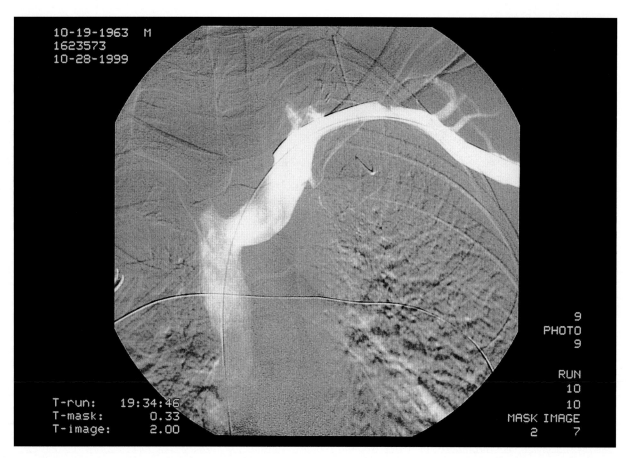

Figure 49-4. Completion venogram after angioplasty and venous stent placement. (From Kreienberg PB, Chang BB, Darling RC III, et al: Thrombolytic and surgical decompression or stent therapy for subclavian vein thrombosis. In Pearce WH, Yao JST [eds]: Advances in Surgery. New York: McGraw-Hill, 2002.)

Patients are then maintained on coumadin for 6 months. This is then discontinued unless a hypercoagulable condition exists.

REFERENCES

1. Adson AW, Coffey JR: A method of anterior approach for relief of symptoms by division of the scalenus anticus. Ann Surg 85:839, 1927.
2. Filler AG: MR neurography and brachial plexus neurolysis in the management of thoracic outlet syndromes. In Yao JT, Pearce WH (eds): Advances in Vascular Surgery. Chicago: Precept Press, 2001.
3. Komanetsky RM, Novak CB, Mackinnon SE, et al: Somatosensory evoked potentials fail to diagnose thoracic outlet syndrome. J Hand Surg 21A:662–666, 1996.
4. Cormier JM, Armane M, Ward A: Arterial complications of the thoracic outlet syndrome: 55 operative cases. J Vasc Surg 9:778–787, 1989.
5. Hurlbert SN, Rutherford RB: Primary subclavian-axillary thrombosis. Ann Vasc Surg 9, 217–223, 1995.
6. Molina JE: Need for emergency treatment in subclavian effort thrombosis. J Am Coll Surg 181:414–420, 1995.
7. Sheeran SR, Hallisey MJ, Murphy TP, et al: Local thrombolytic therapy as part of multidisciplinary approach to acute axillosubclavian vein thrombosis (Paget-Schroetter). JVIR 8:253–260, 1997.
8. Lee MC, Grassi CJ, Belkin M, et al: Early operative intervention after thrombolytic therapy for primary subclavian vein thrombosis: An effective treatment approach. J Vasc Surg 27:1101–1108, 1998.
9. Kreienberg PB, Chang BB, Darling RC, et al: Long-term results in patients treated with thrombolysis, thoracic inlet decompression, and subclavian vein stenting for Paget-Schroetter syndrome. J Vasc Surg 33:S100–S105, 2002.

Chapter 50

Clinical Applications of Intravascular Ultrasound

JASON T. LEE • GEORGE E. KOPCHOK • RODNEY WHITE

- Design and Function
- Methods and Techniques
- Clinical Utility
- Future Developments

Intravascular ultrasound (IVUS) was developed when miniaturized piezoelectric transducers were positioned at the tip of intraluminal catheters to allow for high-resolution, ultrasonic imaging of various cardiac, vascular, and hollow organ structures. Coupled with real-time computerized processing systems, IVUS catheters enable luminal and transmural cross-sectional imaging of blood vessels with high dimensional accuracy, as well as detailed information about lesion morphology (Table 50-1). The concomitant rapid expansion of minimally invasive endovascular techniques in both the coronary and peripheral vasculature has added numerous new roles for IVUS. Precise knowledge of lesion morphology and accurate visualization of vessel wall anatomy are required for endovascular procedures, and because angiography is limited by its ability to display only the outline of the vessel lumen, IVUS has emerged as a useful adjunct. In addition to providing diagnostic information, IVUS enables optimal choice of appropriate angioplasty technique, endovascular device guidance, and controlled assessment of the efficacy of interventions. Further acceptance and more widespread implementation of this modality relies on the effectiveness of IVUS to improve outcomes and minimize periprocedural complications when compared with alternative imaging modalities. This chapter reviews the design and function of available IVUS catheters, imaging techniques, and interpretation, and the present and future clinical utility in peripheral endovascular interventions.

Design and Function

The first IVUS prototypes were used to measure intracardiac dimensions and cardiac motion in the 1950s, using A-mode transducers fixed to large intraluminal catheters. Various devices (A-, B-, and M-mode) were developed for both intravascular and transesophageal imaging of vascular structures. Not until the early 1970s was intraluminal, cross-sectional imaging of vessels reported, using a multielement array transducer. To obtain a 360-degree cross-sectional image, the ultrasound beam is scanned through a full circle and the beam direction and deflection on the display is synchronized. This is achieved by one of three means: (1) a rotating transducer within the catheter connected to a motor in the ultrasound unit; (2) a rotating mirror around a fixed transducer; or (3) a phased array transducer, where multiple transducers are electronically switched.

TABLE 50-1. Lesion Morphology: Data Acquired by IVUS

Luminal diameters and cross-sectional area

Wall thickness

Lesion length, shape, and volume

Lesion position within the lumen: concentric vs. eccentric

Lesion type: fibrous (soft) vs. calcific (hard)

Presence and extent of flap, dissection, or ulceration

Presence and volume of thrombus

Current multielement IVUS catheters operate in a high-resolution B-mode and use frequencies in the range of 10 to 40 MHz, with the higher frequencies providing higher resolution but at the cost of decreased field of view and depth of penetration. The plane of imaging is perpendicular to the long axis of the catheter and provides a full 360-degree image of the blood vessel. A problem of the early phased-array devices was the electronic noise caused by the multiple wires within the catheter itself; this was because each of the elements was an independent mini-transducer needing its own connections. This problem was later overcome by incorporating a miniature integrated circuit at the tip of the catheter that provided sequenced transmission and reception without the need for numerous electrical circuits traveling the full length of the catheter. In addition to reducing the electric noise, this modification simplified the manufacturing complexity and improved the flexibility and length restrictions of the catheter.

A problem of these imaging catheters, common to all high-frequency ultrasound devices to some extent, is the inability to image structures in the immediate vicinity of the transducer (i.e., in the "near field"). Because the imaging crystals in a phased-array configuration are in almost direct contact with the structure being imaged, a bright circumferential artifact known as the "ring-down" surrounds the catheter. The ring-down artifact can be electronically removed with software adjustments, but structures within the masked region are not imaged.

Methods and Techniques

Access

The IVUS catheters can be introduced either percutaneously, through a standard vascular access sheath (5 to 10 Fr); or via an arteriotomy or venotomy during an open procedure. If large vessels proximal to the arteriotomy are to be imaged (e.g., aortoiliac imaging via a femoral cutdown), introduction through a hemostatic sheath reduces blood loss and prevents catheter damage during insertion. In most situations a retrograde common femoral artery puncture provides access to the aortoiliac segments, entire thoracic and abdominal aorta, and the coronary vasculature. Percutaneous brachial or axillary puncture provides access to upper limb vessels and may be more convenient for interrogating the thoracic aorta and aortic arch during the treatment of dissections.

IVUS catheters are available in lengths up to 125 cm, with size ranges for noncoronary catheters ranging from 6.2 to 8.0 Fr (Table 50-2). The larger 10- to 12-MHz catheters can image up to 6 cm in diameter, whereas smaller 3-Fr and wire configurations have a more limited lateral resolution. Of the various catheters currently available, the authors' institution has utilized the Volcano catheter (Jomed, Rancho Cordova, CA) and the Atlantis PV and SoniCath (Boston Scientific, Natick, MA) (Fig. 50-1).

TABLE 50-2. Specifications of Commonly Used IVUS Catheters

Size (French)	Frequency (MHz)	Length (cm)	Introducer Sheath (Fr)	Guidewire (in)
3.4	20	135	6 Fr	0.018
8.2*	10	90	9 Fr	0.038
Volcano Therapeutics Inc., Rancho Cordova, CA				
3.2	20	135	6 Fr	0.018
6*	12.5	95	8 Fr	0.035
6	20	95	8 Fr	0.035
8*	15	95	8 Fr	0.035
Boston Scientific, Natick, MA				

* Peripheral vascular use.

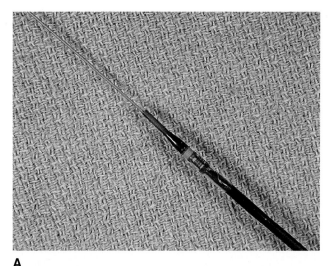

A

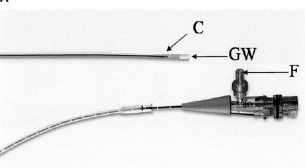

B

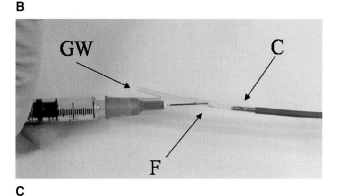

C

Figure 50-1. Commonly used peripheral vascular IVUS catheters. **A**, *Visions PV (Volcano Therapeutics Inc., Rancho Cordova, CA);* **B**, *Atlantis PV (C = catheter, GW = guidewire, F = flush port) (Boston Scientific, Natick, MA);* **C**, *Sonicath Ultra (Boston Scientific, Natick, MA, USA). Note the two types of configuration, over the wire (**A** and **B**) and the monorail system (**C**).*

Image Acquisition

IVUS catheters are advanced over a 0.025- or 0.035-inch guidewire, which allows more controlled maneuvering within the lumen of the vessel, particularly in tortuous or tightly stenotic vessels. Because of the configuration of the older mechanical rotating catheters, a central guidewire channel is not possible; these catheters have a variety of monorail and coaxial lumen options for over-

the-wire applications. Multielement array devices use a central guidewire channel, which offers advantages for catheter delivery.

Careful positioning of the catheter tip within the vessel and appropriate size matching of the device to the artery caliber are essential to optimal visualization. Image quality is best when the catheter is parallel to the vessel wall and the ultrasound beam is directed at 90 degrees to the luminal surface. Eccentric positioning of the catheter within the vessel cross-section causes the wall closer to the imaging chamber to appear more hyperechoic than the distant wall, resulting in an artifactual difference in wall thickness. Catheter centering is especially difficult in tortuous vessels, and rotational alignment may also be partly lost as the catheter meanders through the vessel. The best-quality images are generally obtained as the catheter is withdrawn through the lumen rather than during advancement.

Gray scale, real-time images are displayed on a monitor and can be recorded digitally. Measurements of vessel dimensions, luminal diameters, and cross-sectional areas can be performed by an on-line processing unit that calculates the area of the lumen outlined on still images on the monitor. A digitized pad can also be used to calculate the area from calibrated photographs of the images.

Color-Flow IVUS

One important limitation to standard IVUS catheters is its inability to clearly delineate bloodflow. A new computer software program ChromaFlo (Endosonics, Rancho Cordova, CA) is able to detect differences in the position of echogenic blood particles between images to determine flow states and to colorize the images. The software was evaluated in a study of 100 interventions, and it allowed for better recognition of the true lumen and bloodflow after angioplasty and stenting.[1] The origin of larger aortic arch branches is also more clearly outlined during interventions of the thoracic aorta. Searching for an entry site during endovascular treatment of chronic dissections or pseudoaneurysms has been aided by the color-flow IVUS (Fig. 50-2). Being able to detect flow would also be of obvious theoretical advantage during surveillance of aortic stent-grafts in looking for an endoleak, although this has yet to be well studied.

Clinical Utility

Diagnostic Applications

Two-dimensional images produced by IVUS not only outline the luminal and adventitial surfaces of vessel segments but also discriminate between normal and diseased components. In muscular arteries, the media appears as an echolucent layer sandwiched between the

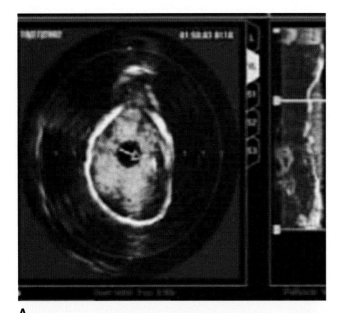

A

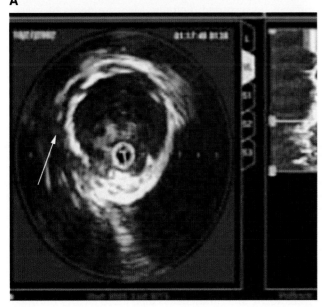

B

Figure 50-2. **A**, *Color-flow IVUS image of proximal pseudo-aneurysm of previously repaired thoracic aortic aneurysm showing breakdown of anastamosis.* **B**, *Stent-graft coverage of pseudoaneurysm. Arrow indicates previous entry site now without flow from lumen.*

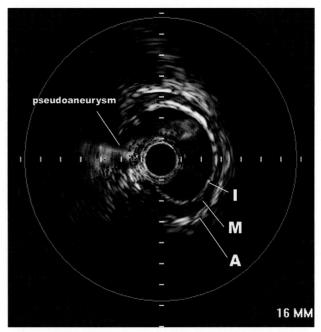

Figure 50-3. *Image of superficial femoral artery and distinct wall layers of muscular arteries (I = intima, M = media, A = adventitia). Note the large pseudoaneurysm on the color-flow image. This patient was treated with a stent to cover the neck of the pseudoaneurysm.*

more echodense intima and adventitia; it defines the outer limits of any noncalcified plaque, with the luminal circumference defining the inner limits (Fig. 50-3). This allows accurate localization and measurement of the thickness of the plaque. Small lesions (e.g., intimal flaps or tears) are well visualized because of their high fibrous tissue content and the contrasting echoic properties of surrounding blood, as well as the pulsatile bloodflow variation seen because IVUS is performed in real-time. Intraluminal thrombus can be distinguished from underlying vessel wall; it typically appears as a highly echogenic,

homogenous mass with varying image attenuation beyond its location. IVUS devices are also sensitive in differentiating calcified and noncalcified vascular lesions. Because the ultrasound energy is strongly reflected by calcified plaque, it appears as a bright image with dense acoustic shadowing behind it.

Luminal dimensions and wall thickness determined by IVUS of normal and minimally diseased arteries both in vitro and in vivo are accurate to within 0.05 mm. Determination of outer vessel diameter may be less accurate, with error margins of up to 0.5 mm. Additional studies have compared contrast angiography and IVUS for determining luminal dimensions of human arteries.[2] The luminal cross-sectional areas calculated from biplanar angiograms and measured from IVUS correlate well for normal or minimally diseased arteries, as well as for mildly elliptical lumens. In severely diseased vessels, however, angiography tends to underestimate the severity of atherosclerosis in the wall compared with IVUS.[3]

IVUS has also been used in the diagnostic assessment of several other pathologic vascular lesions. Accelerated intimal thickening in the coronary arteries of cardiac transplant recipients has been documented by IVUS when angiograms appear normal. IVUS has also been used to determine candidacy for pulmonary thromboendarterectomy as treatment for pulmonary hypertension in patients with chronic pulmonary thromboembolic disease. Intravascular tumors (e.g., vena caval extensions of renal cell carcinoma) can also be localized by IVUS to aid in planning resection. IVUS has been utilized in the trauma setting, accurately determining whether patients who have equivocal aortograms after blunt thoracic trauma have true operable lesions.[4]

Therapeutic Interventions

Long-term success of vascular procedures requires restoration of near-normal hemodynamic conditions across diseased vessel segments as a result of adequate enlargement of luminal diameters. Conventional angiography is limited in its ability to provide sensitive data regarding the effects of endovascular therapies. For meaningful critical assessment of minimally invasive catheter-based methods, both the plaque extent and consistency and the distribution of residual lesions following an intervention must be known. The advantage afforded by IVUS in evaluating lesion morphology involves accurate assessment of not only luminal dimensions but also of transmural lesion characteristics. Delineation by IVUS of the spatial distribution of the lesion in a concentric or eccentric pattern and the presence of a soft (fibrous) or hard (calcified) plaque may influence the choice of endovascular therapy as well as predict the risk of immediate or late complications (e.g., perforation, thrombosis, or restenosis). Evaluation of lesion volume before and after the procedure by IVUS provides a quantitative method to estimate the amount of lesion debulking or displacement and a reference point from which to assess the lesion recurrence/restenosis. IVUS also fulfills many of the necessary requirements of a guidance system for endovascular procedures (i.e., precise delivery and positioning of devices within target lesions). IVUS is particularly helpful in assessing the relationship of the ostia of branch vessels to the lesion that can be used as landmarks during procedures.

Percutaneous Transluminal Angioplasty

Adjunctive use of IVUS during percutaneous transluminal angioplasty (PTA) has provided a useful perspective in treating coronary and peripheral arterial occlusive disease. In a study of PTA in 16 patients with lesions of the superficial femoral artery, IVUS accurately detected the presence of dissections, plaque fractures, internal elastic lamina ruptures, and thinning of the media that occurred during PTA.[5] IVUS showed in these patients that luminal enlargement after PTA is produced by stretching of the arterial wall, whereas the volume of the lesion remains relatively constant.

The risk of restenosis after percutaneous coronary angioplasty (PTCA) has also been correlated to IVUS findings. Early restenosis following PTCA is associated with luminal thrombus, extensive dissection, and oversized balloon dilatation; whereas late restenosis correlates with residual stenosis greater than 30%, small residual lumen, undersized balloon use, concentric fibrous plaque, absence of dissection, and absence of calcification.[6] These factors are all readily identified by IVUS and illus-

trate the potential that IVUS has for enhancing PTCA procedures by allowing periprocedural decisions to be made regarding the need for additional interventions. Balloon size for PTA is often underestimated when selection is made using quantitative angiography alone, and optimal balloon size is more accurately determined by IVUS.[7] More recently, improved outcomes were documented when utilizing IVUS to delineate post-PTA dissections that were significant enough to require stents (greater than 60% residual stenosis).[8]

Intravascular Stents

Common indications for stent deployment after angioplasty are deep arterial wall dissections, elastic recoil, residual stenosis, a significant residual pressure gradient across the lesion, or plaque ulceration with local thrombus accumulation. Intravascular stents increase the patency of arterial occlusive lesions that have undergone angioplasty by reducing technical failure and restenosis rates; however, placing stents is not without risk. Inadequate stent expansion can lead to early thrombosis or stent migration, whereas overexpansion can result in excessive intimal hyperplasia or vessel perforation.

IVUS has been useful in establishing the need for stenting as well as in guiding stent deployment for both coronary and peripheral lesions. Studies have demonstrated that IVUS noted adequate stent expansion in only 13% to 20% of treated coronary lesions (satisfactory result by angiography); these required further stent expansion by balloon dilatation.[9] In peripheral vessels, angiography-guided stent deployment results in incorrect positioning or expansion in as many as 20% to 40% of cases. A recent long-term follow-up study of 52 patients who underwent balloon angioplasty and stenting of iliac stenoses documented improved long-term patency by defining the appropriate angioplasty diameter end-point and adequacy of stent deployment.[10] The residual lumen area is known to be a variable important in predicting long-term patency of endovascular procedures, and optimizing luminal dimensions by stenting is crucial.

IVUS has also been studied in carotid stenting; it was found to be complementary to angiography by more accurately visualizing stent placement and vessel wall morphology, information which is critical to deciding whether to end the procedure or proceed with further stenting.[11] IVUS can quantitatively provide accurate cross-sectional area that defines percent area stenosis at the level of the lesion. Long-term studies are still lacking as to whether IVUS will improve outcomes or decrease complication rates from carotid stenting.

Abdominal Aortic Aneurysm Endovascular Grafts

Perhaps the most important application of IVUS is in the endoluminal exclusion of abdominal and thoracic aortic aneurysms. The success of these interventions depends on appropriate patient selection, accurate preoperative and intraoperative visualization of the anatomy of the aorta, and the proper physical deployment of the devices. Experimental studies have shown that IVUS is extremely useful in choosing the site for stent-graft deployment by accurately identifying branch arteries and determining the luminal dimensions of the aorta.[12] IVUS also can detect whether full stent-graft expansion has occurred, and can provide information regarding surface topography, alignment, and movement of the graft material in the aortic lumen. In addition, several observations are commonly apparent only on IVUS; these include incomplete stent fixation (as evidenced by independent arterial wall pulsation at the stent interface), folding of unstented portions of a particular prosthesis, and motion with arterial pulsations (Fig. 50-4). Identification of such technical problems allows immediate intraoperative troubleshooting and the possibility of balloon dilatation or placement of an additional modular piece.

In the authors' own experimental series,[13] incomplete proximal balloon-expandable stent expansion was determined by IVUS in 20% of cases of endograft deployment with no apparent abnormality seen on angiography. This is an important observation, because underexpansion at the proximal or distal fixation sites can lead to endoleaks or device migration. Some 30% to 40% of abdominal aortic aneurysm (AAA) patients treated with endovascular grafts have been found to require a different diameter stent-graft on the basis of IVUS measurements over preoperative CT angiography.[14] The more accurate sizing and length measurements that IVUS provides have been suggested to lead to fewer endoleaks and secondary interventions.[15]

It is possible to place certain devices by IVUS guidance alone. Although cinefluoroscopy and IVUS are complementary in enabling expedient deployment of stent-grafts, an additional important benefit of IVUS is the potential to reduce fluoroscopy time and contrast, minimizing the radiation exposure to both personnel and the patient and minimizing the risk of renal failure. Some centers that use IVUS during aortic endovascular interventions no longer routinely perform angiography, and have not noted increased complications.[16] Longer-term studies are certainly necessary to show that routine use of IVUS during AAA repair improves outcomes and is cost-effective.

Aortic Dissections

Endovascular interventions for acute and chronic type B dissections provide an appealing alternative to open techniques that are plagued by high morbidity and mortality.[17] The deployment of an endovascular stent-graft can cover an entry site, obliterate a dissection flap, and restore bloodflow to the true lumen. IVUS confirms placement of the guidewire within the true lumen, can accurately size proximal and distal necks, and can accurately identify the anatomic landmarks of the dissection including determining the true and false lumens (Fig. 50-5). Limiting contrast in these patients is often desirable because renal compromise may be part of the pathophysiology of the dissection, and repair has been guided by IVUS alone.[18] As the spectrum of treating these devastating disorders broadens with newer endovascular techniques, the ability of IVUS to accurately delineate the anatomy will remain a necessary adjunct in the treatment of aortic dissections.

Venous Interventions

IVUS has also been studied in endovascular interventions of the venous system. Transfemoral venography for iliac vein obstruction has numerous limitations, and IVUS imaging yields findings not obvious on venography (e.g., intraluminal webs, or external compression and subsequent deformity). More importantly, IVUS provides accurate assessment of degree of iliac vein stenosis, which venography underestimates by as much as 30%.[19] This allows more appropriately sized venous stents to be placed after venoplasty.

The placement of vena caval filters for pulmonary embolus prophylaxis has also been optimized by the use of IVUS. Critically ill patients that are not candidates for transport to an angiographic suite can undergo bedside IVC filter placement with IVUS guiding the accurate deployment of the filter.[20] This obviates the need for cumbersome fluoroscopic machinery at the patient's bed-

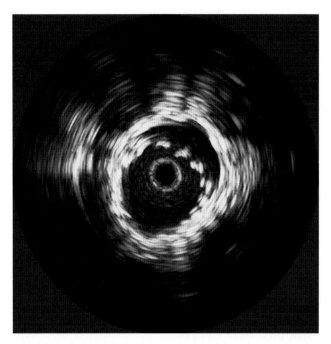

Figure 50-4. IVUS clearly demonstrates incomplete stent-graft expansion as a separation of the stent from the artery wall.

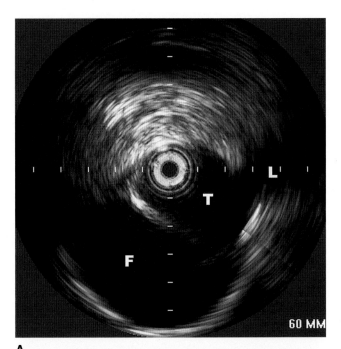

A

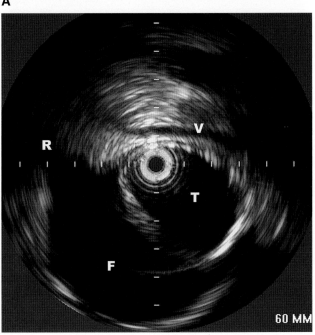

B

Figure 50-5. A, IVUS of aortic dissection delineating left renal artery (L) coming off true lumen (T). B, Right renal artery (R) noted to come from false lumen (F). Renal vein (V) also clearly visualized. Fenestration of dissection flap was performed on this patient rather than stent-graft to occlude flow to false lumen.

side, and reduces the need for contrast in critically ill patients who may have underlying renal dysfunction. Placement of IVC filters under IVUS is currently an attractive alternative to traditional methods of insertion, and the cost of the IVUS may be offset by the avoidance of angiographic suite costs.

Future Developments

Miniaturization, cost-effective manufacturing, and development of user-friendly IVUS devices are needed to enhance the utility of IVUS during vascular interventions. Development of endovascular devices with combined interventional components and IVUS transducers in the stent delivery system capable of real-time imaging during the procedure would simplify catheter exchanges, interventional techniques, and lesion assessment. Alterations in ultrasound probe placement are being developed to improve upon resolution in markedly tortuous vessels.[21] Finally, refinements in computer software and hardware will further reduce processing times and improve 2-D and 3-D image quality.

In summary, IVUS has developed rapidly from a purely diagnostic imaging modality to become an important tool capable of guiding and assessing a multitude of endovascular interventions. As interventions become increasingly complex, success will be related to the degree of accuracy of the guidance system employed during the procedure. IVUS is an integral component of current and future endovascular interventions at many centers, and although its use is currently somewhat limited by cost, its demonstrated utility may rapidly justify its clinical use.

REFERENCES

1. Irshad K, Reid DB, Miller PH, et al: Early clinical experience with color 3-D IVUS in peripheral interventions. J Endovasc Ther 8:329–338, 2001.
2. Tabbara M, White R, Cavaye D, et al: In vivo human comparison of intravascular ultrasonography and angiography. J Vasc Surg 14:496–504, 1991.
3. White RA, Donayre C, Kopchok G, et al: Intravascular ultrasound: The ultimate tool for AAA assessment and endovascular graft delivery. J Endovasc Surg 4:45–55, 1997.
4. Patel NH, Hahn D, Comess KA: Blunt chest trauma victims: Role of IVUS and TEE in cases of abnormal thoracic aortograms. J Trauma 55:330–337, 2003.
5. The SH, Gussenhoven EJ, Zhong Y, et al: Effect of balloon angioplasty on femoral artery evaluated with intravascular ultrasound imaging. Circulation 86:482–492, 1992.
6. Landau C, Lange RA, Hillis LD: Percutaneous transluminal coronary angioplasty. N Engl J Med 330:981–993, 1994.
7. Scoccianti M, Verbin CS, Kopchock GE, et al: Intravascular ultrasound guidance for peripheral vascular interventions. J Endovasc Surg 1:71–80, 1994.
8. Nishida T, Colombo A, Briguori C, et al: Outcome of nonobstructive residual dissections detected by intravascular ultrasound following percutaneous coronary intervention. Am J Cardiol 89:1257–1262, 2002.
9. Fuessl RT, Hoepp HW, Sechtem U: Intravascular ultrasonography in the evaluation of results of coronary angioplasty and stenting. Curr Opin Cardiol 14:471–479, 1999.
10. Buckley CJ, Arko FR, Lee S, et al: Intravascular ultrasound scanning improves long-term patency of iliac lesions treated with balloon angioplasty and primary stenting. J Vasc Surg 35:316–323, 2002.
11. Reid DB, Diethrich EB, Marx P, et al: Intravascular ultrasound assessment in carotid interventions. J Endovasc Surg 3:203–210, 1996.

12. Van Essen JA, van der Lugt A, Gussenhoven EJ, et al: Intravascular ultrasonography allows accurate assessment of AAA: An in vitro validation study. J Vasc Surg 27:347–353, 1998.

13. White RA, Verbin C, Kopchok G, et al: The role of cinefluoroscopy and intravascular ultrasonography in evaluating the deployment of experimental endovascular prostheses. J Vasc Surg 21:365–374, 1995.

14. Nolthenius RP, van den Berg JC, Moll FL: The value of intraoperative IVUS for determining stent graft size with a modular system. Ann Vasc Surg 14:311–317, 2000.

15. Garrett HE, Abdullah AH, Hodgkiss TD, et al: IVUS aids in the performance of endovascular repair of AAA. J Vasc Surg 37:615–618, 2003.

16. von Segesser LK, Marty B, Ruchat P, et al: Routine use of IVUS for endovascular aneurysm repair: Angiography is not necessary. Eur J Vasc Endovasc Surg 23:537–542, 2002.

17. Lee JT, White RA: Endovascular Exclusion of Descending Thoracic Aneurysms and Chronic Dissections. In Liotta D (ed): Diseases of the Aorta. Argentina: Editorial Universidad de MoRón, 2003.

18. Guidice R, Frezzotti A, Scoccianti M: IVUS-guided stenting for chronic abdominal aortic dissection. J Endovasc Ther 9:926–931, 2002.

19. Neglen P, Raju S: Intravascular ultrasound scan evaluation of the obstructed vein. J Vasc Surg 35:694–700, 2002.

20. Wellon ED, Matsuura JH, Shuler FW, et al: Bedside intravascular ultrasound-guided vena cava filter placement. J Vasc Surg 38:455–458, 2003.

21. Zanchetta M, Rigatelli G, Pedon L, et al: IVUS guidance of thoracic and complex AAA stent-graft repairs using an intracardiac echocardiography probe. J Endovasc Ther 10:218–226, 2003.

Chapter 51

Coding and Reimbursement for the Vascular Laboratory

J. DENNIS BAKER • FRANKLIN W. WEST

■ Introduction

■ Medicare Program

■ Other Programs

Introduction

Until the mid-1970s there was limited payment for vascular laboratory testing. At that point, with the rapid growth in clinical application of noninvasive techniques, insurance carriers started to provide payment for these services. There was no uniform methodology applied to determining the amount of reimbursement: Individual insurance companies developed their own payment plans using the common "usual, customary, and reasonable charges" principle. The charges billed by an individual physician were combined with the average charge for the same service by others in the area to come up with the actual amount paid. Under this system, payments to different physicians could vary widely. Linking the payment to previous charges resulted in the practice of annually increasing charges as a way of driving up the payments.

Medicare Program

General Policies

In the late 1980s, Congress reacted to the escalating costs of the Medicare program. The Omnibus Budget Reconciliation Act of 1989 called for the establishment of a national fee schedule to be used for all Medicare payments. The Health Care Financing Administration (HCFA), which was later renamed Centers for Medicare and Medical Services (CMS), adopted the methodology of the Resource-Based Relative Value Scale (RBRVS), developed by the study group under Hsiao at the Harvard School of Public Health. The new system provided a relative value for each current procedure terminology (CPT) code. For services such as diagnostic testing, relative values were provided for the technical component (payment for the cost of performing the test) and for a physician payment to cover services by the doctor providing the interpretation. Geographic adjustment factors (GAF) were developed to compensate for variations in practice costs in different parts of the country. This percentage was multiplied by the base relative value to determine the local relative value. The effect of the GAF ranged from a decrease of 18% to an increase of 24%

for the CPT codes describing noninvasive vascular procedures. The adjusted relative value was then multiplied by a dollar conversion factor to yield to actual amount of reimbursement. The "Final Rule" was published in November 1991 and became effective in January 1992. The immediate result was a substantial decrease in the payments to vascular laboratories for Medicare patients.

The creation of a national fee schedule resulted in fixing the specific dollar amount that would be paid for a given test; however, it did not determine whether or not a specific test would be paid for or not paid for. Payment policies determine the acceptable (or not acceptable) indications for a specific diagnostic test, as well as the frequency with which a given test can be repeated. HCFA passed most of the responsibility for payment policies to the local carriers. The most common system used by carriers is to publish a Local Medical Review Policy (LMRP) that specifies the conditions under which payments will be made. An important result of the delegation of these policies to the local level is that there have been wide variations in the conditions under which laboratories will be reimbursed for noninvasive testing of Medicare patients. Over the past 10 years, there have been efforts towards standardization of payment policies, but significant state-to-state variations still exist.

An important exception to the local control of payment policy is the National Correct Coding Initiative (NCCI). This initiative publishes combinations of CPT codes that are not paid when billed for simultaneous services. A private contractor for HCFA originally developed NCCI, and periodic updates continue to be carried out. Because of the private contract arrangement, it is not possible for members of national professional groups to have input before changes are made. The professional groups can only intervene after publication of an update by protesting inappropriate CPT code combinations, and some adjustments do result.

An ongoing source of frustration for many vascular laboratories is the consistent denial of some of the tests billed to Medicare. In many cases the initial denial is caused by restrictions of local payment policies. The most simple of these is repeated testing that is more frequent than allowed. Although the carriers refuse to disclose what their routine minimum repeat period is, for most practical purposes, it is 6 months. Routine follow-up examinations will be denied if done less than 6 months from the last examination. An exception that can (and should be appealed) is the situation where there is a clinical change in the patient's status requiring re-evaluation. If an appeal is to be made, one must be sure to have accurate documentation of the patient's change in status in order to back up the process. Another common problem is the rejection of a test when the patient has had the same test performed in another laboratory. At the present time, there has not been any solution to the problem of having to repeat tests because of unreliability of other facilities. One possibility to consider is to have the patient sign a waiver (Advanced Notice to Beneficiary) so that the person can be billed directly for the sum once the denial is received. This option is often not possible because the patient will either forget to mention the previous test or will refuse to sign a waiver that creates the possibility of having to pay the entire charged amount.

The other type of general problem comes with denial of claims for nonapproved indications. For a number of years, carriers have had a list of ICD9 codes that are considered approved indications for any given CPT code. In practice, a computer automatically matches the billed CPT code to the list of approved ICD9 codes. If a match is not found, the claim is automatically denied with no further review. An important point to remember is that, with few exceptions, Medicare does not pay for screening examinations. It actually takes an "act of Congress" to add a routine screening examination to the authorized list of Medicare benefits. There are beginning to be some exceptions made in the case of some screening procedures before major operations, but carriers will probably limit the screening tests to patients undergoing cardiac or major organ transplant surgery. There are specific indications that are considered appropriate by most vascular surgeons but that do not necessarily get included in local payment policies. Included in this category are vein mapping before bypass procedures, radial artery mapping for coronary operations, vein mapping for planning dialysis fistula construction, and postoperative surveillance of distal bypass grafts. Some carriers have decided to allow some or all of these indications in their local policies. Even when the test is permitted, it often may be difficult to know how to code the procedure. For example, the carrier for Southern California decided to include postcarotid endarterectomy surveillance as an allowable test but instructed that it should be coded with "carotid stenosis" as the primary diagnostic code (433.10) and "following surgery, unspecified" (V67.00) as the secondary code. Unfortunately, it is necessary to address these reimbursement problems on a carrier-by-carrier basis. This clarification is most effectively obtained by the Carrier Advisory Committee representative for vascular surgery; this person is considered the established liaison between the specialty and the carrier. This representative should specifically inquire about problem reimbursement areas and get specific instructions from the carrier as how these indications should be coded. It is important to remember that what works in one state may not work in another.

In 2002 there were two expansions of the regulations covering diagnostic testing. The first relates to ordering of tests; a treating physician or nurse practitioner must order all tests. The laboratory cannot perform a test that has not been ordered by the practitioner. The policy specifies that the order can take the form of a written document (may be sent by fax), an electronic order, or a telephone call. If a telephone call is used, both the requesting physician and the testing facility must document the telephone call in the respective copies of the patient's records. If an inappropriate test is ordered, or if the findings of the ordered test point to the need for further testing, a substitute or additional examination cannot be done without a specific order.

The other addition is a clarification of the coding for diagnosis or indication for the test. All orders for a test must include a diagnosis; the submitted claim must include a primary diagnosis. If the results of the test confirm the diagnosis of the referring physician, then this code is to be used. If the test does not confirm the diagnosis on the order, then the signs or symptoms prompting the test should be the primary code. Incidental findings can be listed, but only as secondary diagnoses. Tests ordered in the absence of signs or symptoms are screening tests, and the primary diagnosis code must reflect this fact. If a screening test yields a positive finding, this result can be coded, but only as a secondary diagnosis. (Some laboratories have misinterpreted this regulation as allowing to bill for screening tests when pathology is found. This is clearly an error.)

Medicare Part B Policies

All services provided outside of a hospital are paid under the Part B program. For noninvasive laboratories, this coverage includes all office-based and freestanding facilities. Since 1992 both the physician work and the technical components are based upon the fee schedule. Over the years there has been little change in the mechanisms and rules for Part B payments.

An important change was the definition of the Independent Diagnostic Testing Facility (IDTF) in 1997. This entity was created to replace the earlier, poorly defined Independent Physiological Laboratory, a category covering freestanding operations not associated with an office practice. Current regulations require that all units not linked to a hospital or a physician office must register with the local carrier as an IDTF. The local carrier is charged with verifying that medical supervision, technical personnel, and equipment used meet the standards for the specific tests to be performed. The carrier must perform a site visit to verify that the listed testing is indeed performed as reported. A special feature of the rules is the requirement that all nonphysician personnel performing tests must be certified. Although payment policies in some states require technologist certification, this regulation applies to all IDTFs regardless of location. The regulations were tightened in May 2001 to require that office-based laboratories that perform a substantial proportion of the workload on outside patients (i.e., patients referred just for noninvasive testing but not otherwise a part of the office practice) must register as IDTFs. (An indication from CMS officials suggests that "substantial" is more than 30% of patients examined.) Whereas Medicare claims for patients who are a part of the office practice can be billed under the group practice

number, the outside patients must be billed using the separate IDTF number.

Medicare Part A Policies

Payment for hospital-based testing services is more complex. Since the introduction of the RBRVS, the physician work component has been paid under the Part B program with the amount determined entirely by the fee schedule. The technical component (TC) for inpatient testing is not reimbursed but is considered to be included in the global hospital payment under the diagnosis-related group (DRG) system. On the other hand, the TC for outpatient tests is billed to the Part A carrier, which in a number of regions is different from the Part B carrier. To further add to the confusion, in areas where the carriers are different, the payment policies may differ, resulting in the anomaly that one hospital laboratory may be reimbursed for a procedure while a nonhospital facility across the street may be denied payment. Until recently, there was a further anomaly: The payment for TC by Part A was not controlled by the fee schedule but was a continuation of the "usual, customary, and reasonable" methodology of earlier years. As a result, many hospital-based laboratories received a TC payment that was considerably higher than that imposed by the fee schedule.

The Balanced Budget Act of 1997 mandated establishment of a prospective payment system to define payments for outpatient services, including the TC of noninvasive tests. The relevant CPT codes were assigned categories called ambulatory payment classifications (APCs). A payment rate for each APC was calculated based upon average cost data submitted by hospitals. Unlike the fee schedule, the APC payments are not linked to the conversion factor and do not have an adjustment for geographic differences. The Final Rule for the system was published in April 2000. Although the APC system finally standardizes Part A payment of TC, there are anomalies: the amount paid for complete duplex scans is lower than is reimbursed under the Part B fee schedule; on the other hand, the APC category is the same for complete and limited examinations, so that reimbursement for limited studies is substantially better for hospital facilities (Table 51-1). The authors wonder whether these anomalies will result in "gaming" of the new system by performing more limited studies. Contrary to past payment policies, the APC methodology creates a clear disincentive to performing complete studies.

Other Programs

Initially, the fee schedule was intended only for Medicare payments. During the creation of RBRVS, the American Medical Association strongly opposed application of

TABLE 51-1. Comparison of Fee Schedule and APC Technical Component Payments in 2003

Procedure	CPT	APC	TC/ Part B	TC/APC
Physiologic/ multilevel	93923	096	$110	$ 95
Physiologic/ single level	93922	096	$ 70	$ 95
Carotid scan/ complete	93880	267	$161	$134
Carotid scan/ limited	93882	267	$109	$134
Venous scan/ complete	93975	267	$208	$134
Venous scan/ limited	93976	267	$122	$134

the guidelines outside the federal program; however, by summer 1993 the organization reversed this policy. As predicted by many people, it was not long before other payers linked their reimbursements to the fee schedule, often paying some percentage of Medicare rates. These carriers have different payment policies that are often more liberal. One problem in dealing with nongovernment groups is that many do not publish their payment policies so that it is hard to deal with denied claims. The extensive growth of large scale contracting has also hurt vascular laboratories. Facilities within hospitals or large clinics may be forced to accept a discounted reimbursement negotiated as part of a large institutional contract. This type of merchandising can also hurt freestanding laboratories by the refusal of providers to negotiate contracts with individuals or small group providers.

SUGGESTED READINGS

In the past year, many of the publications covering Medicare rules and regulations have been made available on the Internet. In addition, most local carriers have established Web pages containing detailed information. These are particularly useful for finding such details as LMRPs and other information on payment policies. The following are useful Web sites:

1. The general Medicare site: www.cms.hhs.gov
2. Medicare payment systems: cms.hhs.gov/paymentsystems/
3. CMS program manuals, transmittals, and memoranda: cms.hhs.gov/manuals/
4. Medicare Policy Integrity Manual (all the details of the rules): cms.hhs.gov/manuals/108_pim/pim83toc.asp
5. Hospital Outpatient Prospective Payment System (specifics about APCs): www.cms.hhs.gov/providers/hopps/fr2000.asp
6. CMS-related laws and regulations: cms.hhs.gov/regulations/
7. CMS Medicare Learning Network (OPPS): cms.hhs.gov/medlearn/refopps.asp
8. CMS files for download: cms.hhs.gov/providers/pufdownload/default.asp#rvu
9. Quarterly provider update on Medicare issues: cms.hhs.gov/providerupdate/
10. Detailed coding guideline: www.cdc.gov/nchs/datawh/ftpserv/ftpicd9.htm#guide
11. Physicians and Health Care Practitioner's home page: cms.hhs.gov/physicians/
12. CMS Medical Review (LMRP) home page: www.cms.hhs.gov/providers/mr/lmrp.asp
13. CMS: intermediary/carrier directory: cms.hhs.gov/contacts/incardir.asp
14. LMRP home page (policies for each carrier): www.lmrp.net/
15. Current federal legislation: thomas.loc.gov/home/thomas.html
16. Federal Register: www.access.gpo.gov/su_docs/aces/aces140.html
17. Excluded parties list: www.epls.gov/

Chapter 52

Coding and Reimbursement for Interventions and Surgical Procedures

ROBERT M. ZWOLAK

The specialty of vascular surgery has evolved along with the treatment of arterial disease. Unlike some specialties where the treatment modalities defined and then limited growth, vascular surgeons have adopted to change and are therefore surviving and thriving. Because their economic survival depends on expression of complex procedures as 5-digit numbers (Current Procedural Terminology or CPT codes), this rapid growth spurt required simultaneous creation of many new codes based in the constructs of component coding.

For decades, Medicare taught surgeons that one operation should be reported with one code, regardless of the number of additional hours or incremental steps required for its successful completion. Relative values are defined for the "typical patient," and for surgeons performing complex operations, the typical patient concept ensures a huge bias for the payor. Although a skilled surgeon may shave a few minutes of time from "typical" during a straightforward operation, there is almost no limit on additional time requirements for a very complex surgical case. Thus, Medicare's argument that the hard cases and the easy cases all balance out around the typical patient is patently untrue for surgery. The curve of time and complexity is not bell-shaped, and surgeons subsidize the payor during every case that is substantially more difficult than typical.

As interventional techniques enter the world of vascular surgery, so does component coding. This system, assigned to intervention decades ago, assigns very specific codes to very specific smaller procedures, with the understanding that if a more complex procedure is performed, more than one code will be reported. To prevent duplicate payment for pre- and postservice work, multiple procedure payment reduction rules apply to the interventional procedure codes, allowing appropriate reduction. Even with this downward payment adjustment, however, providers of these services realize a refreshing link between honest work and reimbursement. In contrast to the surgical dogma of "one operation equals one code" regardless of how many extra hours the surgeon may spend, component coding provides a much more linear relationship between work and reimbursement. Although it is true that any particular intervention can require much more time than typical, the assignment of codes to smaller packets of work serves to prevent some of the huge inequities seen in traditional surgical billing. In addition, when multiple providers participate in one case, component coding offers the ability to parse the work to the correct provider. A single downside of component coding is that more cognitive knowledge is required to complete the coding itself. The information in this chapter will assist with that task.

The CPT Manual

The American Medical Association owns CPT, and all CPT codes and their descriptors are copyrighted.[1] The CPT manual is updated and revised each year in a formal process guided by the CPT Editorial Panel. The process by which new or revised CPT codes are created requires a minimum of 15 months from application to publication, and it may take much longer than that. There is no guarantee that CPT code submission will result in code creation; in fact, there is a very substantial failure rate. Vascular surgery attempted creation of a CPT code to report angioscopy for several years without success until the Society for Vascular Surgery (SVS) decided a substantial amount of intellectual capital needed to be spent on learning the process. Subsequently, SVS learned the key ingredients of successful CPT application writing, and in 1998 CPT 35400, Angioscopy during therapeutic intervention, was added. Timing was fortuitous because the subsequent 6 years saw an explosion in vascular surgery technology. With SVS CPT Advisor Anton Sidawy at the rudder, vascular surgery was able to parallel technology development with CPT code development. This meant that clinically established new procedures could flourish because there was a means to report and be reimbursed. SVS has submitted over 40 applications for new or revised Category I CPT codes in the past 7 years, and has never been turned down. This is an unparalleled record, one to be proud of. Vascular

surgeons need to thank the leaders of SVS for their insight in supporting this activity.

Selective Catheterization Codes

Vascular surgery codes are found in the Surgery/Cardiovascular System section of the CPT manual, in a subsection labeled "Arteries and Veins," starting with CPT 34001. Interventions that include transluminal angioplasty, stent placement, and injection procedures are found in the middle of this section. As counterintuitive as it may sound at first to surgeons, these catheterization and intervention codes are called "surgical" codes in the interventional world to distinguish them from radiologic supervision and interpretration codes (see following text). The rules of component coding apply to interventional "surgical" codes. With familiarity, component coding is logical and straightforward, but to the "one operation equals one code" surgeon this is a strange new world. The crux of arterial and venous coding conventions is to report the highest order artery that is catheterized intentionally in each vascular family. For arterial reporting, the aorta is considered a nonselective catheterization; first, second, and third order selective catheterization refers to the number of arterial branch points that must be negotiated, starting in the aorta, to reach the target artery. For example, catheterization of the innominate artery from the aorta is a first order selective (CPT 36215), whereas the right subclavian from the aorta is second order (CPT 36216), and advancing the catheter into the right vertebral is a third order selective catheterization (CPT 36217). Only the highest selective catheterization in each vascular family is reported. In this example, 36217 would be the only reported catheterization code. Because catheterization of multiple vascular families is reportable, one must undertake the same exercise for each successive vascular family selectively catheterized during the same procedure. There are two groups of selective arterial cath codes, one for thoracic or brachiocephalic branches (CPT 36215–36218); and the other to represent abdominal, pelvic, or lower extremity branches (CPT 36245–36248).

CPT Modifiers

Modifiers are crucially important in interventional and open surgical coding because they allow the provider to explain to the payor that multiple procedures are being reported in a rightful and honest manner. Modifiers are 2-digit alphanumerics, and they are listed on the inside cover of the CPT manual. The skilled coder has memorized most of these. Three commonly used modifiers are "-59" (distinct procedural service), "-LT" (left side), and

"-RT" (right side). Two examples in the cerebrovascular system will demonstrate the utility of modifiers. Selective catheterization of the left and right internal carotids would be reported with 36216 for the left internal (second order) and 36217 for the right internal (third order). If submitted simply as unmodified 36216 and 36217, the payor's software program will reject payment for 36216 under the assumption that the provider erroneously requested payment for a second and third order catheterization within the same vascular family. Application of modifiers 36216-LT and 36217-RT allows the payor's software to recognize that these are selective catheterizations in separate vascular families, and payment denial will be avoided. A similar situation arises with selective catheterization of the left common carotid (36215) and the left subclavian (36215). The software will reject payment for the second 36215 if no modifier is appended. Because both arteries are on the left, use of LT and RT modifiers is not appropriate. In this situation adding -59 to one of the 36215 codes (i.e., 36215 and 36215-59) is the correct approach and should result in payment for both (albeit with multiple procedure payment reduction).

S and I Codes

Radiologic supervision and interpretation codes are used to report cognitive aspects of arteriography, venography, and vascular interventions. Appropriate use of these codes implies that all required views have been obtained, images have been retained (hard copy or digital), and a thorough interpretation has been recorded. For diagnostic studies, details of selective catheterization plus enumeration of normal and abnormal findings is crucial. For therapeutic interventions, the equivalent level of detail must be included. Providers who report S and I codes without supplying substantial detail are at risk should a postpayment audit occur.

S and I codes may or may not link tightly to the catheterization codes. An example of one-to-one linkage is 75960, the intravascular stent S and I code. 75960 is reported each time a "surgical" stent deployment code is reported. CPT 37205 represents transcatheter placement of an intravascular stent, percutaneous, initial vessel. Thus 37205 and 75960 would be reported by a provider who deploys a common iliac stent and also performs the associated radiologic S and I. If a stent were also deployed in the external iliac artery of the same patient, CPT 37206 would be reported to represent stenting the second artery, and 75960 would be reported again for the associated S and I. An important caveat is that stents are reported "per vessel," not "per stent." Thus if one were to pile six stents in the left common iliac artery during a single procedure, only one stent deployment code and one S and I code would be reportable. Another important point is that multiples of the same S and I may be reported on the same day for the same patient. For instance, if stents were deployed percutaneously in both common iliacs and both external iliacs in the same patient during one procedure, the provider would report 37205 for stenting the first vessel, 37206 for stenting the additional vessel, and two 37206-59s to represent stents in two different additional vessels. CPT 75960 would be reported four times in this example, and modifiers would not be required for the S and I.

Intervention Codes

Transcatheter stent deployment codes (CPT 37205–37208) have already been introduced. Other interventional codes typically used by vascular surgeons include 35450–35476, transluminal angioplasty; 35480–35495, transluminal atherectomy; 37201, transcatheter infusion of thrombolytic therapy; 37203, transcatheter retrieval of intravascular foreign body; 37204, transcatheter occlusion or embolization; and 37250, intravascular ultrasound. Each of these has an associated S and I code. Component coding rules apply for all.

Endovascular Repair of Abdominal Aortic Aneurysm

The large family of codes used to report minimally invasive endovascular repair of infrarenal abdominal aortic aneurysm (AAA) or dissection is the product of a huge collaborative effort between SVS and Society of Interventional Radiology (SIR). The family of codes was introduced in the 2001 CPT manual, and the reporting structure follows the guidelines of component coding. Familiarity with this section of CPT is a necessity for surgeons who perform endovascular AAA repair. Particularly close attention must be given to the three introductory paragraphs in this section of the manual because they contain important reporting conventions. In brief, a typical endovascular AAA repair performed with open femoral artery exposure will be reported with four CPT codes, reflecting major activities. These are: (1) open arterial exposure, usually femoral; (2) introduction of catheter(s) into the aorta; (3) deployment of the endovascular device; and (4) radiologic S and I. Although this list was presented in temporal sequence, the actual reporting would begin with the primary code representing deployment of the main endovascular device. Thus a typical CPT report for Food and Drug Administration (FDA)-approved devices such as Medtronic AneuRx or Gore Excluder would be:

- 34802 (Endovascular repair of infrarenal AAA using modular bifurcated prosthesis, one docking limb)
- 34812-50 (Open femoral artery exposure for delivery of endovascular prosthesis, by groin incision) with the -50 modifier used to signify bilateral
- 36200-50 (Introduction of catheter, aorta) with the -50 indicating catheters introduced from both groins
- 75952 (Endovascular repair of infrarenal AAA or dissection, radiologic supervision, and interpretation)

Important reporting conventions for endovascular AAA repair include the fact that all angioplasty and stenting performed within the target zone of the endovascular prosthesis is not separately reportable. Thus, if an additional stent is required to prop open a narrow or kinked iliac limb, the surgeon cannot report that stent separately. Likewise, if a balloon angioplasty is required in a common iliac artery stenosis to allow the device carrier to pass into the aorta, that angioplasty is not separately reportable if the iliac limb of the device spans the angioplasty site. On the other hand, if angioplasty is required in the external iliac artery to allow passage of the device, and if that external iliac is not covered by the device or extensions at completion of the procedure, the angioplasty is separately reportable. In this situation, addition of the -59 modifier to the angioplasty code and the angioplasty S and I would be required for payment. Likewise, if a renal artery stent is performed simultaneous with endovascular AAA repair, both the stent and its associated S and I are reportable with -59 modifiers attached. Finally, deployment of a proximal or distal extension prosthesis (34825, 34826) is separately reportable during endovascular AAA repair, and there is a specific S and

I code for the extension (75953). Reporting extensions is done by vessel, not by stent. Thus, three proximal aortic extensions would be reported with only one 34825/75953 coding pair, whereas one extension in the aorta and one extension in the iliac would be reported as 34825 (extension in first vessel), 34826 (extension in additional vessel), and two 75953s (two extension S and Is).

Additional codes have been added to the endovascular section each year. These include 34805 to represent AAA repair using an aortouniiliac or unifemoral prosthesis; 34833 to report open iliac artery exposure with creation of a conduit; 34834 for open brachial artery exposure used to assist deployment of an infrarenal or aortic endovascular prosthesis; and 34900 for endovascular graft placement for repair of iliac artery aneurysm, pseudoaneurysm, arteriovenous (AV) malformation, or trauma. A code application submitted for 2005 will represent endovascular AAA repair using a modular bifurcated prosthesis (two docking limbs). If approved, this code will be used to report the Cook Zenith endovascular device.

Endovascular Repair of Descending Thoracic Aortic Aneurysm

As this chapter is being written, several national prospective trials of new thoracic endografts are getting under way. Because these devices are not FDA-approved, they are reported with Category III CPT codes, and the thoracic endograft code family (0033T–0040T) was introduced in 2003 (Table 52-1). The Category III designa-

TABLE 52-1. Category III Thoracic Endograft T-Code Family

Category III Code	Shortened CPT Descriptor
0033T	Endovascular repair of descending thoracic aortic aneurysm, pseudoaneurysm, or dissection; involving coverage of left subclavian artery origin, initial endoprosthesis
0034T	Endovascular repair of descending thoracic aortic aneurysm, pseudoaneurysm, or dissection; not involving coverage of left subclavian artery origin, initial endoprosthesis
0035T	Placement of proximal or distal extension prosthesis for endovascular repair of descending thoracic aortic aneurysm, pseudoaneurysm, or dissection, initial extension
0036T	Each additional extension (ZZZ add-on code)
0037T	Open subclavian to carotid artery transposition performed in conjunction with endovascular thoracic aneurysm repair, by neck incision, unilateral
0038T	S and I for endovascular thoracic repair covering left subclavian
0039T	S and I for endovascular thoracic repair not covering subclavian
0040T	S and I for extension prosthesis, each extension

tion refers to a set of temporary codes (T-codes) used to report emerging technology, services, and procedures. Cat III codes are not priced nationally, and for most there is no national coverage policy. The decision whether or not to cover Cat III procedures has been specifically delegated by Centers for Medicare and Medicaid Services (CMS) to the regional Medicare carriers.[2]

In general, it is fair to say that most regional Medicare carrier medical directors (CMDs) are predisposed to covering T-code procedures that are associated with a strong likelihood for clinical benefit, and one can hardly imagine a new procedure with greater potential benefit than endovascular thoracic aneurysm repair. Nevertheless, the default coverage policy is noncoverage. If surgeons hope to be paid for thoracic endograft procedures during these trials, they must contact their respective CMDs before the procedures are performed to explain why a positive coverage determination is appropriate. Physicians who do not contact their CMDs to discuss coverage will most assuredly not be paid. The same advice holds for hospitals in that billing department principals should contact their fiscal intermediaries in advance to discuss coverage.

Carotid Stents

Carotid angioplasty and stenting holds the distinction of having a national noncoverage decision from Medicare.[3] Under this policy, Medicare will not pay for carotid angioplasty and stenting unless the procedure is conducted under auspices of an IDE-approved trial. In the CPT realm, carotid stenting is represented by T-codes 0005T–0007T. In order for coverage and payment to evolve from its current approved trial-only status, three events must take place. First, the FDA must designate site-specific approval of a carotid stent. At the time of this writing, one stent/embolic protection device package is scheduled to undergo FDA consideration in the near future. Second, CMS must reverse its noncoverage policy. Although a coalition of eight medical and surgical specialty societies requested reconsideration for high-risk patients, CMS is unlikely to act until a final decision is reached by the FDA. Third, CPT must develop Category I CPT codes, and relative value units must be determined. During the summer and fall of 2003 the same coalition of specialty societies collaborated on a Category I CPT application for carotid stent placement with embolic protection, with a second application submitted for carotid stent without embolic protection. The status of these potential codes and the development of physician work relative value units (RVUs) will evolve throughout 2004 and, if successful, the new codes may appear in the 2005 CPT manual. As noted, however, creation of Category I codes will not result in Medicare payment unless FDA device approval and reversal of the noncoverage decision also come to pass.

Open Surgical Procedures

Many of the new CPT codes created based on SVS applications represent new and revised open surgical procedures. Lower extremity distal bypass grafts using vein conduit represent a family of codes for which Medicare reimbursement remains woefully inadequate, but to some extent, SVS has helped compensate for this by creating new add-on codes as ancillary procedures evolve. Table 52-2 provides a list of add-on codes that should be reported when a surgeon finds one or more of these additional steps necessary to create a bypass with maximal limb-salvage potential.

TABLE 52-2. Ancillary Procedures During Lower Extremity Bypass Surgery

CPT Code	Shortened CPT Descriptors (List Separately in Addition to Code for Primary Procedure
35400	Angioscopy (noncoronary vessels or grafts) during therapeutic intervention
35500	Harvest of upper extremity vein, one segment, for lower extremity or coronary artery bypass procedure
35572	Harvest of femoropopliteal vein, one segment, for vascular reconstruction procedure (e.g., aortic, vena caval, coronary, peripheral artery)
35682	Bypass graft; autogenous composite, two segments of veins from two locations
35683	Bypass graft; autogenous composite, three or more segments of veins from two or more locations
35685	Placement of vein patch or cuff at distal anastomosis of bypass graft, synthetic conduit
35686	Creation of distal arteriovenous fistula during lower extremity bypass surgery (nonhemodialysis)

New CPT Codes for 2004

Nine new Category I CPT vascular codes were created in 2004. These span applications of endovascular surgery, open upper extremity bypass surgery, an aortic reconstruction add-on code, and venous stab phlebectomy (Table 52-3).

CPT Code Applications for 2005

The SVS has submitted four Category I and four Category III CPT code applications for 2005. Already mentioned is the multispecialty collaborative effort for two CPT codes to report cervical carotid stent deployment. SVS and SIR collaborated on the aforementioned application for a three-piece modular aortic endograft repair code to be used for the FDA-approved Cook Zenith device. SVS also requested creation of a Category I code to report upper arm native hemodialysis access brachiocephalic fistula requiring two incisions and a subcutaneous tunnel.

Category III applications were submitted by SVS to report a family of T-codes to report endovascular AAA repair using a fenestrated device.

Finally, although SVS did not participate in the CPT application, new Category I codes have been requested to report radiofrequency and laser ablation of incompetent saphenous veins.

Reimbursement

Only reimbursement from CMS will be addressed here. The single most important driver of reimbursement is

accurate coding. Surgeons must learn to code traditional open surgery and intervention with equal skill. Undercoding leaves deserved money in the carrier's checking account, whereas overcoding places the surgeon at risk should a postpayment audit be undertaken. Inaccurate coding will result in inappropriate denials. Accurate coding is truly the first key.

Second, surgeons must learn about the National Correct Coding Initiative. NCCI is the formal name for what more commonly is known as "bundling." The 60,000 NCCI edit pairs block payment for a second procedure based on Medicare's impression that the work of the second procedure is embodied in the initial or main procedure. NCCI edits come in two forms, with CCI indicator "0," meaning the two procedures will never be paid simultaneously; or "1," meaning that under certain clinical circumstances the two procedures may be paid together. Providers must append the CPT modifier -59 if they believe the clinical circumstances merit simultaneous payment, and a strong justification must exist. An easy-to-use, searchable CD is available from the National Technical Information Service (NTIS) at 800-553-6847. Product number is SUB 5411, and a single issue CD costs less than $100. NCCI edits are now also available on the Internet, but these are not easily searchable. The Web site is hppt://cms.hhs.gov/physicians/cciedits/default.asp

Finally, a number of publications list Medicare RVUs and payments. One of the easiest to use is published by the American Medical Association.[4]

Conclusions

Vascular surgeons can no longer afford to code their procedures in a haphazard manner. Although the complexity of coding is increasing at least as fast as the complexity

TABLE 52-3. **New 2004 Vascular Surgery Category I CPT Codes**

CPT Code	Shortened CPT Descriptors
34805	Endovascular repair of infrarenal abdominal aortic aneurysm or dissection; using aortouniiliac or aorto-unifemoral prosthesis
35510	Bypass graft, with vein; carotid-brachial
35512	Bypass graft, with vein; subclavian-brachial
35522	Bypass graft, with vein; axillary-brachial
35525	Bypass graft, with vein; brachial-brachial
35697	Reimplantation, visceral artery to infrarenal aortic prosthesis, each artery (list separately in addition to code for primary procedure)
36838	Distal revascularization and interval ligation (DRIL), upper extremity hemodialysis access (steal syndrome)
37765	Stab phlebectomy of varicose veins, one extremity; 10–20 stab incisions
37766	Stab phlebectomy of varicose veins, one extremity; more than 20 stab incisions

of the procedures surgeons perform, it is crucial to learn the details of coding. New codes are created each year, and existing codes are revised. Vascular surgical practice is composed of Medicare beneficiaries, and Medicare payments are not keeping up with inflation. Accurate coding is the best start toward maintaining a viable practice.

REFERENCES

1. American Medical Association: Current Procedural Terminology (CPT) 2004, 30th ed. Chicago: AMA Press, 2004.
2. Department of Health and Human Services Health Care Financing Administration, Medicare Program: Revisions to payment policies under the physician fee schedule for calendar year 2002: Final rule. Federal Register 66(212):55269, 2001.
3. Tunis S: Percutaneous Transluminal Angioplasty (PTA) of the Carotid Artery Concurrent with Stenting (#CAG-00085A). Baltimore: DHHS Coverage and Analysis Group, 2001.
4. Gallagher PE, Klemp T, Smith SL: Medicare RBRVS: The Physician's Guide 2004. Chicago: AMA Press, 2004.

Chapter 53

Vascular Centers: Role of the Vascular Laboratory

M. ASHRAF MANSOUR

I n the last few years, a number of patient care issues and market forces have provided an impetus to some leading institutions of medical excellence to form vascular centers.[1-3] Several professional societies* have collaborated to hold an annual postgraduate symposium, bringing experts from the United States and Europe to discuss and promote the concept of the vascular center.[4] The idea is to have all the medical and surgical specialists, ancillary personnel, as well as testing facilities and equipment in one locale. The advantage, from the patient's point of view, is the convenience of "one-stop shopping."[5] It avoids the all too common occurrence of visiting numerous specialists in different locations, and of sometimes having the same test repeated in another physician's office. For the physician and hospital point, it provides economy of scale and avoids the need for duplication of expensive diagnostic instruments. Physicians can share offices and examination and conference rooms. Furthermore, they can potentially share the use of properly designed endovascular suites. Test results are readily available for review with patients and other specialists. Probably the most important aspect of this concept is the ability for the health care team to have direct face-to-face consultation and coordination of patient care issues. The purpose of this chapter is to give an overview of the role of an integrated vascular laboratory in the vascular center.

The Vascular Laboratory

Atherosclerosis, with its complications, is responsible for a significant number of deaths annually in the United States and developed countries.[6,7] In the United States, heart and cerebrovascular diseases are ranked first and third, respectively, among the leading causes of death. Many professional societies* have launched initiatives

---

*The American College of Cardiology, the Society of Cardiovascular and Interventional Radiology (now Society of Interventional Radiology), the Society for Vascular Medicine and Biology, the Society for Vascular Surgery, and the American Association for Vascular Surgery.

to educate the public about heart and peripheral vascular occlusive disease. The theme of early diagnosis and prevention has been underscored. The vascular laboratory plays a central role in the diagnosis and management of vascular disease.[8]

There have been many epidemiologic studies describing the intersection of disease entities in patients with systemic atherosclerosis. Dormandy and colleagues[9] reviewed several studies that show the significant overlap of medical conditions (e.g., coronary artery disease, cerebrovascular disease, and peripheral arterial occlusive disease) such that 3% to 14% of patients with any one condition have a potential of having one or more coexisting disease (Fig. 53-1).

Cerebrovascular Disease

Carotid duplex scanning is probably the most important diagnostic tool to evaluate patients with cerebrovascular disease (Fig. 53-2). Many centers of excellence depend on duplex scanning alone to select patients for endarterectomy without the need for angiography.[10] Angiography or magnetic resonance angiography (MRA) remains useful for some equivocal cases. Carotid duplex scans are also used intraoperatively as a quality assurance tool. Postoperatively, these patients are also followed in the vascular lab with scans at regular intervals. Carotid duplex scans are also useful as a screening tool for patients with other manifestations of atherosclerosis.[11] Measurement of intima-media thickness can help assess the patient's overall potential risk of cardiovascular disease. Furthermore, many patients with coronary artery disease or peripheral arterial occlusive disease have an asymptomatic carotid bruit that deserves further investigation.

Peripheral Arterial Occlusive Disease

Recording the ankle-brachial index is the first step in the diagnosis of peripheral arterial occlusive disease (PAOD).

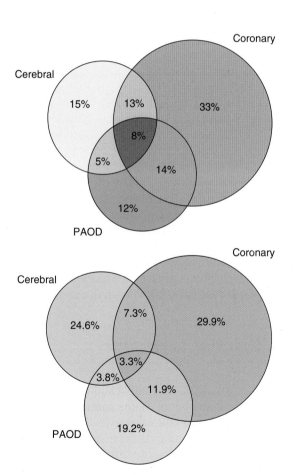

Figure 53-1. Inter-relationship of atherosclerotic disease: coronary artery disease, cerebrovascular disease, and peripheral arterial occlusive disease (From Dormandy J, Heeck L, Vig S: Lower extremity arteriosclerosis as a reflection of a systemic process: Implications for concomitant coronary and carotid disease. Semin Vasc Surg 12:118–122, 1999.)

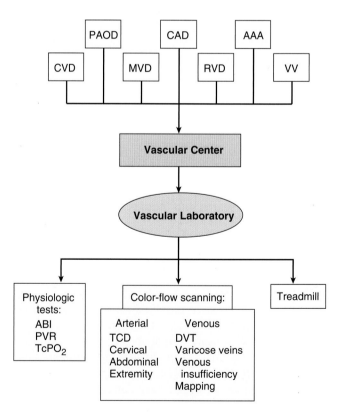

Figure 53-2. The central position of the Vascular Laboratory in the Vascular Center. CAD = coronary artery disease, CVD = cerebrovascular disease, PAOD = peripheral arterial occlusive disease, RVD = renovascular disease, MVD = mesenteric vascular disease, VV = varicose veins, AAA = abdominal aortic aneurysm.

Additional physiologic tests (e.g., pulse volume recordings) help in defining the location and cause of obstruction. The information derived from the ankle-brachial ratio helps the clinician prioritize and streamline additional testing (e.g., angiography or magnetic resonance angiography).

Many vascular laboratories are using color-flow arterial mapping as the only preoperative arterial study before recommending bypass. In the author's lab, vein mapping is often used, especially when looking for alternative donor sites such as the upper extremity. Transcutaneous oxygen measurement is often helpful to estimate the healing potential of a wound or the proper amputation level after failed bypass.

The availabilty of multiple diagnostic tools certainly enhances the ability of the vascular lab to contribute significantly to the increasing number of wound care centers.

Mesenteric and Renovascular Disease

Vascular clinicians encounter a small number of patients (less than 5% in the author's practice) with abdominal complaints that lead to investigation of the mesenteric circulation. Ideally, a color-flow scan of the celiac and superior mesenteric artery (SMA) would be the first test to determine the presence of significant obstruction in these vessels.

An increasing number of patients with poorly controlled hypertension are referred to the vascular lab for renal artery scanning. Although renal duplex scanning has proven to be one of the most challenging techniques to master, it still plays an important role in managing hypertensive patients. After intervention, whether by endovascular techniques or surgical bypass, scanning remains the ideal follow-up test.

Coronary Artery Disease

Patients presenting with a first myocardial infarction may harbor asymptomatic cerebrovascular disease or PAOD. The importance of identifying patients who could benefit from a combined coronary artery bypass and carotid endarterectomy is not lost on anyone because stroke is one of the most devastating complications after heart surgery. In patients who have decreased femoral pulses on physical examination, or absent popliteal and pedal pulses, preoperative ankle-brachial index or arterial mapping will help the surgeon select the best location to harvest the saphenous vein to avoid postoperative harvest site complications. Alternatively, if no suitable venous conduit is available, the

search for alternatives such as the radial or inferior epigastric arteries can be initiated.

Iatrogenic Pseudoaneurysms

With the increasing number of percutaneous interventions for coronary artery disease, as well as for PAOD and cerebrovascular disease, the number of iatrogenic complications at the access site seems to be increasing. The use of larger sheath sizes and the initiation of antiocoagulants or antiplatelet agents postprocedure also contribute to the problem. Most femoral or brachial pseudoaneurysms can be treated with thrombin injection, a procedure performed in the vascular lab or at bedside.

Varicose Veins and Venous Insufficiency

Since the introduction of minimally invasive techniques to treat varicose veins (e.g., radiofrequency ablation and laser-powered phlebectomy), patient acceptance appears to have grown. With these techniques, varicose vein ablation is an office-based procedure that can be safely done with proper imaging. Most of these procedures employ color-flow scanning to identify the saphenous vein in the leg for percutaneous puncture and injection of anesthetic solution. The saphenofemoral junction also needs to be clearly identified to avoid injury when the ablation catheters are passed proximally. Many physicians are now turning to portable machines for their obvious convenience and to avoid tying up the larger units that serve as the workhorses of the lab.

Clinical Research and Studies

The importance of the vascular laboratory to facilitate clinical research in atherosclerosis and vascular diseases cannot be overstated.[12] Indeed, it was pioneering labs, similar to the ones at the University of Washington and at St. Mary's Hospital in London, that tested early versions of currently available instruments. Without a properly equipped lab, it would not be possible to conduct trials of drugs for claudication or studies on the natural history of vascular disease. Through objective noninvasive studies in the lab, physicians are empowered to compare emerging treatments for vascular disease such as subendofascial perforator ligation (SEPS) or powered phlebectomy. Directors of vascular laboratories will have to embrace change and evolve with the constantly changing technologies.

Conclusions

The vascular laboratory occupies a central position in the vascular center to aid in screening, diagnosis, and management of patients presenting with vascular disease. The concept of the vascular center is to centralize patient entry into the health care system and provide efficient delivery of appropriate medical treatment.

REFERENCES

1. Becker GJ, Katzen BT: The vascular center: A model for multidisciplinary delivery of vascular care for the future. J Vasc Surg 23:907–912, 1996.
2. Hiatt WR, Creager MA, Cooke JP, et al: Building a partnership between vascular medicine and vascular surgery: A coalition for the future of vascular care. J Vasc Surg 23:918–925, 1996.
3. Whittemore A, Creager M: The vascular center at Brigham and Women's Hospital. Cardiovasc Surg 6:327–332, 1998.
4. Vascular Centers 2001: Partnering for the future of quality patient care (course syllabus). April 27–28, 2001.
5. Shah DM, Bruni K, Darling RC III: Supermarket model for vascular disease care. J Vasc Nurs 20(3):106–109, 2002.
6. Ross R: The pathogenesis of arteriosclerosis: A perspective for the 1990s. Nature 362:801–809, 1993.
7. Kadar A, Glasz T: Development of atherosclerosis and plaque biology. Cardiovasc Surg 9:109–121, 2001.
8. Jaff MR, Dorros G: The vascular laboratory: A critical component required for successful management of peripheral arterial occlusive disease. J Endovasc Surg 5:146–158, 1998.
9. Dormandy J, Heeck L, Vig S: Lower extremity arteriosclerosis as a reflection of a systemic process: Implications for concomitant coronary and carotid disease. Semin Vasc Surg 12:118–122, 1999.
10. Mattos MA, Hodgson KJ, Faught WE, et al: Carotid endarterectomy without angiography: Is color-flow duplex scanning sufficient? Surgery 116:776–783, 1994.
11. Sacco RL: Extracranial carotid stenosis. N Engl J Med 345:1113–1118, 2001.
12. Zarins CK: Unified multispecialty approach: Is it a viable response to new technology used in the care of vascular patients? J Endovasc Surg 3:364–368, 1996.

Chapter 54

How to Establish and Maintain a Database

RUSSELL H. SAMSON

As in nearly all aspects of daily life, computers can now also improve the functional efficiency of the vascular laboratory. However, not only are these benefits simply those of expediency, but rather the computer can offer many other valuable tools and opportunities. Accordingly, this chapter explores not only the computerization of the data generated by the lab, but also the additional utilities that such a vascular lab "database" offers.

What Is a Database?

The dictionary description of a database is a collection of data arranged for ease and speed of search and retrieval. In general, this requires a specific software program to be constructed to handle the requirements of the data to be studied. Once developed, this software program can be used to manipulate the data for many uses. Further, the program will also expedite the input of data. What this implies for the vascular lab is a software program that will allow the following:

1. Rapid data acquisition
2. Electronic storage of the data
3. Clinical report generation and transmittal of the report to the referring physician or test-ordering entity
4. Manipulation of the data to increase productivity of the lab and to improve patient care opportunities.

Why Does a Vascular Lab Need a Database?

In the performance of the daily routine of testing, the vascular lab generates a huge volume of data. This includes demographic data about the patient (e.g., name, address, billing information, and referring doctor particulars). It also includes test results and conclusions. For the laboratory to function efficiently, data may also be required about personnel, time and duration of tests, costs incurred, and payments received. To improve accuracy of testing, statistical data such as correlation with "gold standards" will also be necessary especially if ICAVL (Intersocietal Commission for the Accreditation of Vascular Laboratories) accreditation is to be achieved.

Although all this data can be maintained without use of a computer, the time, effort, and cost can become insurmountable, leading to lapses that can negatively impact all aspects of the laboratory's function.

How Does a Database Improve Data Acquisition and Storage?

In a paper-based lab the technologist must write down all information. This is often expedited by using preprinted forms with checkboxes, but often time is wasted in having to write out information. Further, errors can often result from handwriting problems. In a computerized database, data is entered directly (and usually, rapidly) using drop down fields, which offer choices for commonly used text or numbers (Fig. 54-1). In many cases, most of the currently available commercial vascular lab software programs also will perform some routine tasks automatically such as calculating values (e.g., ankle = brachial pressure indexes or resistance indexes). Programs will also allow commonly used phrases to be selected without having to retype them each time. This is especially helpful when generating the conclusions for the test (Fig. 54-2). Some programs will also have facilities to allow graphical representation of lesions such as carotid plaque and narrowing (see Fig. 54-2). Many will have features to allow whole tests to be copied so that only new and changed data need be entered, an enormous time saver! Increasingly, some of the most sophisticated programs will also "grab" data from the testing device directly so that the technologist does not have to enter any test data.

Busy vascular labs that are not computerized generate large amounts of paper that require significant storage space. With the cost of space now approaching $20 to $50/sq. ft in many areas, storage expenses can become prohibitive. Further, finding data, even in a well-organized system, can often be extremely time-consuming and frustrating. However, hard drives are becoming larger and cheaper, enabling years of data to be stored on a simple home computer where it can be rapidly retrieved and shared.

Clinical Report Generation

The vascular laboratory database accumulates all the information garnered about the patient. This includes demographic data, test indications, clinical manifestations, family histories, medications, test data, and conclusions. This can be manipulated by the software into a clinical report format, which can be sent to the referring entity (Fig. 54-3). Some software programs come with the reports already formatted for the various tests. Others can be customized to the preferences of the vascular lab. These reports can be printed and sent via standard mail to the referring entities. However, they can also be immediately faxed or sent via e-mail.

Data Manipulation

One of the main advantages of a computerized database registry is the ability to get immediate data not only about individual patients but also about the laboratory function as a whole. It must be realized that every field that is entered is also a data point that can be recalled for quality assurance, research, or any other intellectual pursuit. This allows the director to evaluate parameters such as timeliness of tests and report generation, patterns of referral, and test volumes. Data that may improve lab accuracy (e.g., false-negative tests and clinical correlations) can be constantly and readily reviewed on an ongoing basis. Programs may also offer scheduling modules and recall lists for patients who have missed scheduled appointments. Some will even generate form letters to the missing patients. Most commercially available programs will also provide most or all of the information required for ICAVL.

The database can also be used for research by those so inclined. Some programs will allow all data fields to be searched alone or in combination. Thus an example would be to query the database to find all diabetic patients who had an aneurysm greater than 5 cm who also had a left carotid stenosis of greater than 80%.

What You Need to Set Up a Database

The requirements of the vascular laboratory database will vary depending on the size and complexity of the

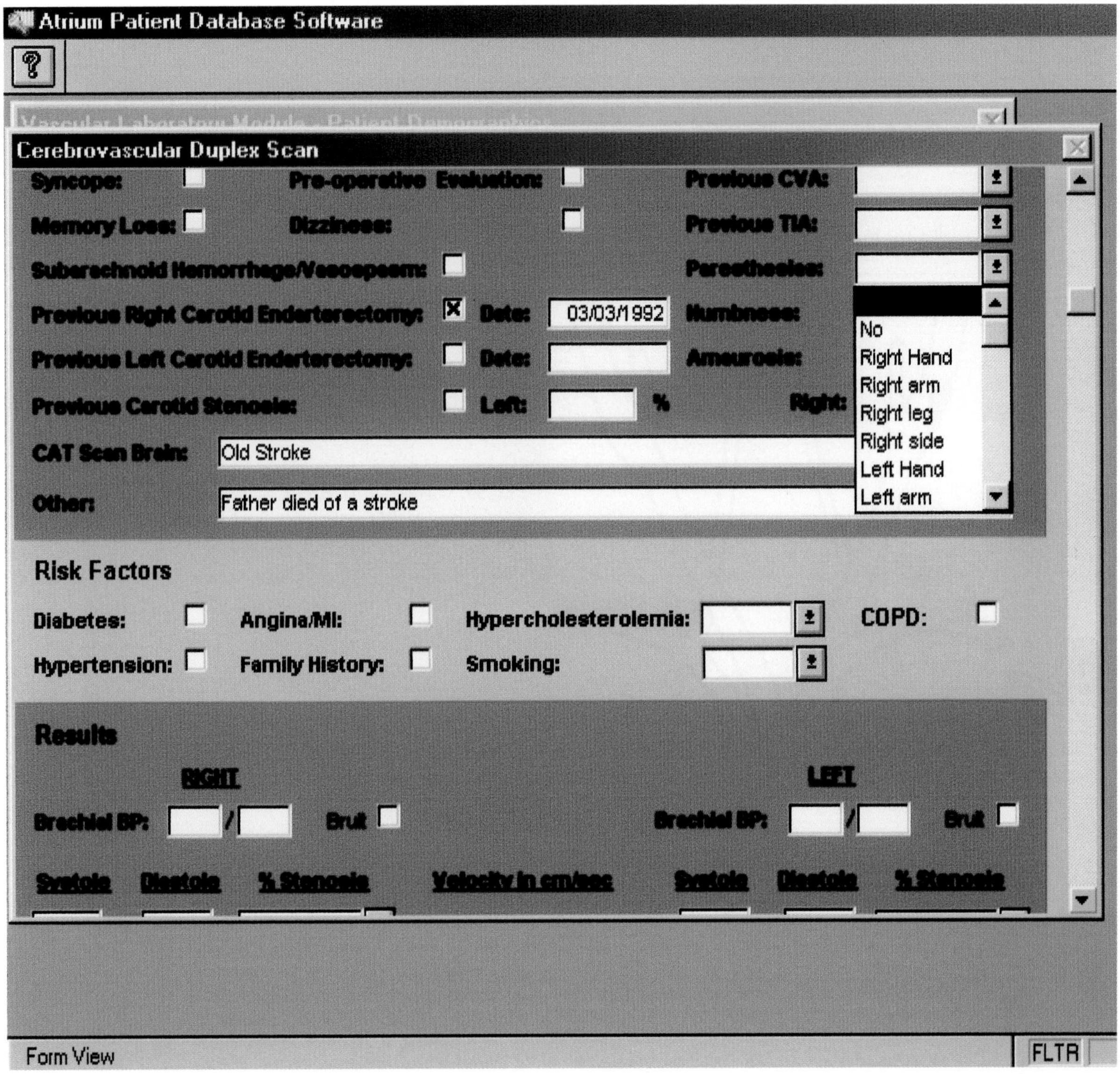

Figure 54-1. Screen capture of a database screen showing data fields. Data can be entered by clicking on a field allowing a yes/no answer, or by selecting from choices in a drop-down menu, as seen on the right of the screen where the location of numbness (e.g., no, right hand, or right arm) can be selected. Drop-down choices allow rapid entry of text in a consistent format and prevent errors in spelling and transcription. (Courtesy of AtriumNet Vaslab, Nashua, NH.)

lab. The following factors need to be considered before establishing the database:

1. The number of computer stations that will be used

2. The geographic location of these stations (e.g., same floor in the same building or different buildings across town)

3. Number of techs and interpreting physicians

4. Requirements for transmittal and sharing of data (e.g., fax, internet, phone, e-mail)

5. Patient privacy issues and HIPAA (Health Insurance Portability and Accountability Act of 1996) compliance

6. Number of tests anticipated per year

7. Compatibility with hospital data systems for in-hospital labs

It also helps to have a budget and to have at least one employee who has basic computer experience.

Once these factors have been determined, computers can be set up and networked as necessary. Although networking (i.e., joining computers together so that data can be shared) has become much easier with recent technologic advances, it generally will be advantageous to employ a network administrator. Most hospitals will have such personnel. Private labs may need to seek outside help.

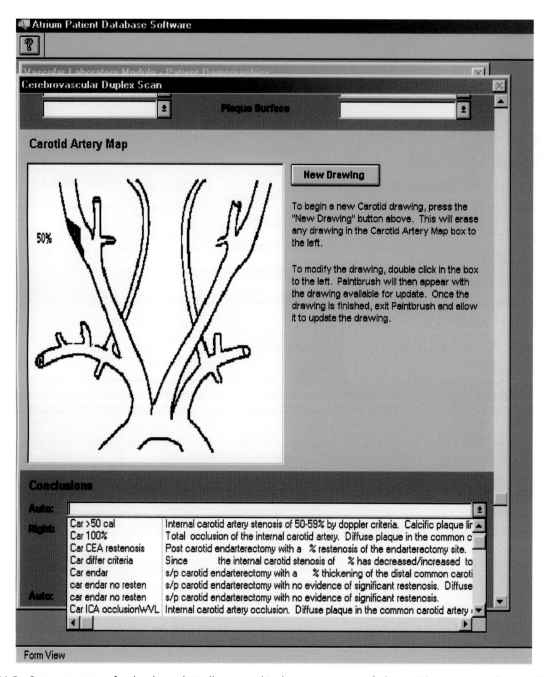

Figure 54-2. Screen capture of a database that allows graphical representation of plaque. The program also provides a drop-down field with a list of many stock conclusions that can be used to describe the blockage. (Courtesy of AtriumNet Vaslab, Nashua, NH.)

There are now many vascular lab software programs. Each has its own strengths and applicability to an individual laboratory's function. Most of these programs can be tried before purchase. Costs vary; it is important that the purchaser fully understands the pros and cons of each so that an educated purchase decision can be made. Some of the more popular programs (in alphabetical order) are AtriumNet Vaslab (Atrium Medical Corporation, Nashua, NH); Vascubase (Consensus Medical Systems, Seattle, WA); CustomLab (Reston, VA); Datacheck (DataStar Systems, Inc, Crystal Lake, IL); In Record Time (Ashland, VA); and WinVDB (Cardio-Vascular Evaluation Systems, Spring, TX).

Cerebrovascular Duplex Scan
Acuson 128XP/10v
Report Status: Final

Referral Source:	M.D.,FACS, Russell Samson	**DOB:**	09/16/1918	**Sex:**	Male
C.C.:	M.D.,Gerald John				
Primary Indication:					

Results

	RIGHT				LEFT			Drawing
Brachial BP:	151 /			**Brachial BP:**	150 /			
Bruit:	No			**Bruit:**	Yes			

Systole	Diastole	% Stenosis	Velocity in cm/sec	Systole	Diastole	% Stenosis
			Origin ICA			
72	14	1-49%	Proximal ICA	134	33	50-59%
			Mid ICA			
			Distal ICA			
			Proximal CCA			
			Mid CCA			
123	14		Distal CCA	86	13	
			Bulb			
84	0		Subclavian	115	0	
183	13		Ext. Carotid Artery	158	0	
45	11		Vertebral Artery	38	10	
	0.6		ICA/CCA Ratio		1.6	
	0.8		Resistance Index		0.75	
Prograde			Vertebral Flow			Prograde
heterogeneous			Plaque Composition			heterogeneous
irregular			Plaque Surface			irregular

(Drawing shows labels: 45%, 50-59%, 25%, 35%)

Conclusions

Right:

Internal carotid artery stenosis of 1-49% by spectral analysis and approximately 45% by gray scale. The common and external carotid arteries have less than 50% stenosis by gray scale. Normal subclavian and vertebral arteries. No significant change since 03/07/02.

Left:

Internal carotid artery stenosis of 50-59% by doppler criteria. The common and external carotid arteries have less than 50% stenosis by gray scale. Normal subclavian and vertebral arteries. No significant change since 03/07/02.

[signature]	1/30/2003 2:06:23 PM	**Technologist:** Kathie Merigliano, RVT
M.D.,FACS, Russell Samson	**Date Signed**	

Your Company Name Goes Here
Your Company Address Goes Here
Your Company 2nd Address Line Goes Here

Figure 54-3. Representative cerebrovascular duplex scan clinical report sent to referring physicians.

What to Do if You Don't Want to Purchase an Established, Commercially Available Database

Some vascular labs may prefer to start from scratch and custom design their own programs. There are programs that are generic database compilers, such as Microsoft Access and Microsoft Excel (Bellevue, WA). Even novices can sometimes develop simple databases using these programs. However, in general, these will not be adequate for anything more than basic data collection. Software programmers can use these to develop complex databases; this can be very costly, but may be more suitable for some institutions. Under these circumstances, the lab personnel must be sure in advance of what information they want to collect and process, and in what format it needs to be collected. It is advisable to lay out a diagram of all the features that will be required. Like building a house, it is more costly to make changes or additions after the framework has been completed. Further, if data has been collected and then must be modified, serious errors may result.

The Ten Commandments of Databases: Do's and Don'ts

1. Learn the software before entering patient information. It is advisable to be aware of all the features of the software before entering definitive patient data. Accordingly, it is mandatory that one read the instruction manual that comes with the package. Many users jump right in without doing this, only to find that their valuable data is not functional. Before starting, most programs will require some basic information to be entered. This will usually include information such as names of technologists and reading physicians and demographics about the lab. In order to become well versed in the program, try entering some test patient data using easily identifiable imaginary patient names. Then use the "delete-patient" feature before entering actual patient data.

2. Always back up the program. Data should be backed up daily. Most programs will have a back-up facility included with the software. Ideally, a copy of the data should be maintained away from the laboratory as well. This can be done by copying the data to a storage medium such as a CD that can be kept off-site. There are also data storage areas that can be accessed for a fee through the Internet.

3. Try to live with the software that you buy and avoid customization if possible. When the software company updates their product or brings out a new version, customized features may not be supported. On the other hand, some programs will allow the user to add fields to collect data or information that the programmers may not have thought of. For example, the laboratory may want to collect information about their patients' cholesterol levels. These are called user-defined fields and will be supported by future upgrades. The ability to add such fields without assistance from programmers is a very valuable benefit offered by such software. However, before adding such a field, always think about what your goal is in seeking this added information and make sure you define in advance the choices that can be entered into the field. If only free-form text can be entered, always doublecheck spelling, because just one misspelled letter will prevent that data from being retrieved at a later date.

4. Keep up with the latest versions. Changes in Medicare rules, new research advances, and ICAVL requirements are constantly changing the laboratory environment. Out-of-date software can result in unusable information.

5. Get in the habit of entering the data directly into the computer rather than writing information down and then entering data. This will prevent transcription errors from occurring.

6. Use the shortcuts that the program may offer. For example, some programs will allow an old test to be copied to a new data sheet when a patient comes back for a repeat study. Then only new data or changes need be entered.

7. For users who are not "mouse" proficient, learn to use the keyboard shortcut keys.

8. Remember the adage that "garbage in is garbage out." Proof your entries!

9. Use all the features that the program provides you. Many programs are very sophisticated and can produce organizational aids such as logbooks and activity reports. Maintaining paper trails in addition to the electronic data is an unnecessary waste of time.

10. Don't despair when you first start using these programs; they will become second nature with time.

Glossary

AAA: abdominal aortic aneurysm
ABI: ankle brachial index
ACA: anterior cerebral artery
ACC: American College of Cardiolgy
ACR: American College of Radiology
ACS: American College of Surgeons
AHA: American Heart Association
APG: air plethysmography
ASHD: atherosclerotic heart disease
AT: acceleration time
AVF: arteriovenous fistula
AVP: ambulatory venous pressure
AXBIFEM: axillobifemoral bypass

B-mode: brightness mode in ultrasound

CA: celiac artery
CAD: coronary artery disease
CBT: carotid body tumor
CC: cubic centimeter, equal to a milliliter
CCA: common carotid artery
CEA: carotid endarterectomy
CEAP: classification of venous
    insufficiency (clinical, etiologic,
    anatomic, pathophysiologic)
CFA: common femoral artery
CFS: color-flow scanning
CFV: common femoral vein
CHA: common hepatic artery
CHF: chronic heart failure
CIA: common iliac artery (CIV for the vein)
CM: centimeter
CPT: current procedural terminology
CRF: chronic renal failure
CT: computerized tomography
CTA: computerized tomography
    angiography
CVA: cerebrovascular accident
CVI: chronic venous insufficiency
CW Doppler: continuous-wave Doppler

DFA: deep femoral artery
    (DFV for the vein)
DP: pressure difference (gradient)
DSA: digital subtraction angiography

DU: duplex ultrasound
DVT: deep vein thrombosis

ECA: external carotid artery
EDV: end-diastolic velocity
EF: ejection fraction
EIA: external iliac artery (EIV for the vein)
ESRD: end-stage renal disease

FA: false aneurysm (or pseudoaneurysm)
FEM-FEM: femorofemoral (e.g., fem-fem
    bypass)
FEM-POP: femoropopliteal (e.g., fem-pop
    bypass)
FMD: fibromuscular dysplasia
    (also flow-mediated dilatation)
FV: femoral vein

GSV: great saphenous vein

ICA: internal carotid artery
ICAVL: Intersocietal Commission for the
    Accreditation of Vascular
    Laboratories
ICD-9: International Classification of
    Diseases, 9th edition
ICU: intensive care unit
IIA: internal iliac artery (IIV for the vein)
IJV: internal jugular vein
IMA: inferior mesenteric artery
IMT: intimamedia thickness
ISCVS: International Society for
    Cardiovascular Surgery
IVC: inferior vena cava

LR: likelihood ratio

MCA: middle cerebral artery
ML: milliliter (equal to one cubic
    centimeter)
MM: millimeter
MRA: magnetic resonance angiography
MRI: magnetic resonance imaging

NPV: negative predictive value

OR: odds ratio

PAOD: peripheral arterial occlusive disease
PE: pulmonary embolism
PI: pulsatility index
PPG: photoplethysmography
PPV: positive predictive value
PRF: pulse repetition frequency
PSV: peak systolic velocity
PV: portal vein
PVD: peripheral vascular disease
PVR: pulse volume recording
PTA: percutaneous transluminal angioplasty
PTFE: polytetrafluoroethylene (generic
    structure for graft material such as
    Goretex and Impra)

RAR: renal aortic ratio
RI: restistivity index
RR: relative risk
RT: refilling time
RVF: residual volume fraction

SFA: superficial femoral artery
SIR: Society for Interventional Radiology
SMA: superior mesenteric artery
SMV: superior mesenteric vein
SSV: small saphenous vein (formerly
    lesser saphenous vein)
SVC: superior vena cava
SVS: Society for Vascular Surgery
SVT: superficial vein thrombosis

TAV: time average velocity
TCD: transcranial Doppler
TIA: transient ischemic attack
TOS: thoracic outlet syndrome

VA: vertebral artery
VA: Veterans Administration
VF or Q: volume flow
VFI: venous filling index
Vr: velocity ratio
VTE: venous thromboembolism
VV: venous volume

Index

Note: Page numbers followed by f indicate figures; those followed by t indicate tables.